Clinical Integration and Specialty Practice in Cannabis Nursing

Kathleen Marie Pinto Araya
https://orcid.org/0009-0000-0608-7555
AZZ Medical Associates, USA & South College, USA

Rana R. Zeine
https://orcid.org/0000-0002-9485-9531
Kean University, USA

IGI Global
Scientific Publishing
Publishing Tomorrow's Research Today

Vice President of Editorial Melissa Wagner
Director of Acquisitions Mikaela Felty
Director of Book Development Jocelynn Hessler
Production Manager Mike Brehm
Cover Design Jose Rosado

Published in the United States of America by
IGI Global Scientific Publishing
701 East Chocolate Avenue
Hershey, PA, 17033, USA
Tel: 717-533-8845 | Fax: 717-533-7115
Website: https://www.igi-global.com E-mail: cust@igi-global.com

Library of Congress Cataloging-in-Publication Data

LCCN: 2026026374 (CIP Data Pending)
ISBN13: 9798260020357
Isbn13Softcover: 9798260020364
EISBN13: 9798260020371
British Cataloguing in Publication Data
A Cataloguing in Publication record for this book is available from the British Library.

Table of Contents

Detailed Table of Contents

In 2023, the American Nurses Association (ANA) recognized cannabis as an official nursing specialty. Although the scope and standards of cannabis nursing are in place, many challenges remain for this specialty practice area. This chapter examines the current state of the cannabis nurse role, including the scope and standards of cannabis nurse practice, and outlines steps to co-create the future of cannabis care nursing. The chapter provides a basis for ensuring that the role of the cannabis nurse is aligned with holistic nursing and, therefore, focuses on working with patients through coaching and education. The cannabis care nurse must also focus on patient advocacy, social justice issues, ethics, safety issues, spiritual concerns, and the common challenges and barriers that cannabis nurses face. Cannabis care nursing in several other countries is explored. What can the future of cannabis care nursing look like, and what steps do nurses need to take to co-create this emerging specialty?

As cannabis continues to gain recognition for its therapeutic potential, the Clinical Nurse Specialist (CNS) plays a pivotal role in guiding safe, ethical, and evidence-based integration of cannabis therapeutics into patient care. This chapter explores how CNS professionals apply advanced clinical judgment, leadership, and research-based practice to optimize outcomes for patients utilizing medical cannabis. The discussion begins by examining the pharmacological foundations of cannabinoids and their physiological mechanisms, followed by the CNS's responsibilities in patient assessment, care planning, and interprofessional collaboration. Legal and ethical implications are analyzed to ensure compliance with institutional, state, and federal regulations. The chapter also emphasizes the CNS's role in staff education, policy development, and quality improvement initiatives related to cannabis use in healthcare.

Cannabis use in the United States has increased over the past several decades. This rise in prevalence parallels expanded legalization, increased societal acceptance, and the proliferation of commercially available cannabis products. These evolving patterns of use present unique and increasingly complex challenges for anesthesia providers. Cannabis has been shown to exert clinically significant effects across multiple organ systems, including the pulmonary, cardiovascular, and neurologic systems. Moreover, cannabinoids interact with numerous anesthetic agents. Although the body of literature examining cannabis use and anesthesia is expanding, evidence-based perioperative management guidelines remain in early stages of development. Anesthesia providers must therefore rely on a growing evidence base to guide clinical decision-making for patients using cannabis. This chapter examines historical and contemporary patterns of cannabis use, routes of administration, physiologic effects relevant to anesthesia, and the implications for perioperative assessment and anesthetic management.

This chapter explores anesthetic and perioperative implications of cannabinoids and the endocannabinoid system (ECS), emphasizing nursing roles in assessment, risk mitigation, and communication. It aims to translate cannabis science into practical guidance for nurse anesthesiologists, perianesthesia nurses, and care partners, amid rising use and inconsistent disclosure. Content covers ECS mechanisms, pharmacokinetics (including CYP450 interactions and tolerance), and relevant anesthesia considerations affecting depth, dosing, and recovery. It highlights perioperative risks from research, focusing on cardiovascular, respiratory, gastrointestinal, pain pathways, TRPV1, and cannabinoid hyperalgesia. The chapter recommends structured screening with the CUBAT framework and aligns practice with existing professional, societal, evidence-based, educational, and policy guidance.

This chapter aims to serve as a comprehensive guide to the benefits and risks associated with cannabinoid therapeutics in relation to sexual health issues. It seeks to inform readers about how cannabinoids might influence conditions such as sexual desire disorders, sexual pain disorders, orgasmic disorders, and sexual arousal disorders by exploring both potential therapeutic effects and side effects. In doing so, the chapter provides insights into how cannabinoid use could enhance or hinder sexual health and overall quality of life. Additionally, the chapter strives to raise awareness among consumers and providers about how cannabis interacts with different body systems, aiming to reduce adverse effects and promote wellness with cannabis, rather than harm.

This chapter examines the essential role of Cannabis Care Nurses (CCNs) as educators addressing knowledge gaps about cannabis and cannabinoid therapies within military and Veterans healthcare. The Department of Defense (DoD) prohibits cannabis use among active-duty service members, imposing strict penalties for violations, but allows dependents limited access to FDA-approved cannabinoid medications through Tricare. Veterans face different access rules influenced by state laws and VA policies, which may permit broader use. The 2018 Farm Bill's legalization of hemp-derived products has further complicated compliance for service members. These regulations create ongoing challenges in understanding safe use, compliance, and stigma for military personnel, Veterans, dependents, and providers. CCNs are positioned to deliver evidence-based education and support informed decision-making, helping reduce stigma and ensuring all stakeholders can effectively navigate the evolving policies surrounding cannabis in healthcare.

The use of medical cannabis in older adults represents a rapidly emerging clinical field characterized by unique challenges, including increased risk of falls, cognitive vulnerability, polypharmacy, and complex ethical considerations. Despite growing utilization, high-quality evidence remains limited, highlighting an urgent need for age-specific research. This chapter proposes a structured framework for nursing competencies in geriatric medical cannabis care, encompassing seven core domains: comprehensive geriatric assessment; therapeutic education; safe initiation and titration; continuous monitoring; management of drug interactions; and ethical, legal, and stigma-related considerations. Interprofessional collaboration, evidence-based practice, and patient-centered approaches are emphasized to ensure safety, efficacy, and adherence. Future research directions include randomized controlled trials in older adults, pharmacokinetic and pharmacodynamic studies, longitudinal safety evaluations, and optimization of THC/CBD ratios tailored to geriatric indications.

The intersection of gerontology and cannabinoid therapeutics represents one of the most critical frontiers in modern nursing. As the global population ages, often referred to as the "Silver Tsunami," healthcare providers are likewise witnessing a "Green Wave" of increased cannabis utilization among older adults who are challenged with aging and chronic disease and looking for harm-reduction tools for polypharmacy. The mission of this chapter is to equip the nursing workforce and other allied professionals with the essential knowledge for the assessment, implementation, and evaluation of cannabis use in an older adult's plan of care, grounded in the competencies of the Cannabis Nursing Scope and Standards of Practice and Gerontological Nursing Scope and Standards of Practice. (American Cannabis Nurses Association [ACNA] & American Nurses Association [ANA], 2024; American Nurses Association [ANA], 2019).

Medical cannabis is a transformative, multidisciplinary modality in symptom management. A growing pharmaceutical market is driving the evolution of clinical and public health frameworks. There is a need for a socially responsive curriculum to enhance nursing students' knowledge and understanding of their role in cannabis-related practice. Cannabis nursing has implications for nursing educators in countries where cannabis is legal or is being legalized. Rapid expansion of medical cannabis uses in oncology place expectations on oncology nurses to provide accurate, evidence-based guidance. However, gaps in knowledge, clinical preparedness, and institutional support challenge cannabis nursing. In future oncology nurses training will reflect in patient education within a fragmented regulatory environment. The therapeutic potential of cannabis will be realized through continued research, harmonized guidelines, and comprehensive healthcare provider education.

Cannabis nurses play a transformative role in palliative and end-of-life care through integrating cannabis-based therapies to enhance comfort, dignity, and emotional well-being for patients with life-limiting conditions. Cannabis nursing uniquely bridges conventional palliative care and evolving therapeutic options, positioning cannabis nurses as key advocates, educators, and caregivers. This chapter reviews the specialty of palliative care, explores the advocacy and holistic management

This chapter explores cannabis nursing as an emerging specialty shaped by the rapid uptake of medical cannabis in healthcare. Although access and demand have grown, clinical governance, professional training, and standardized practice have not kept pace, creating safety, ethical, and organizational risks. Drawing on international experience and recent professional frameworks, the chapter positions cannabis nursing within advanced practice, emphasizing structured assessment, evidence-informed decision-making, therapeutic education, and interprofessional coordination. It reviews historical drivers, regulatory heterogeneity, training gaps, and stigma, and highlights nurses' roles in risk management, documentation, and continuity of care. By defining conceptual models, core competencies, educational needs, and institutional integration strategies, the chapter argues that cannabis nursing is essential for safe, equitable, person-centered implementation of medical cannabis.

Preface

INTRODUCTION

As Editors, we are honored to present *Clinical Integration and Specialty Practice in Cannabis Nursing*, a timely and essential reference dedicated to the evolving role of cannabis therapeutics within contemporary healthcare practice. The rapid integration of medical cannabis into mainstream medicine is reshaping clinical education, healthcare delivery, policy development, and interdisciplinary collaboration. In response to these changes, healthcare professionals must be equipped with evidence-informed knowledge, practical competencies, and ethical frameworks to meet the growing demands of patient care in this emerging specialty.

The recent recognition of Cannabis Nursing as a specialty by the American Nurses Association marks a pivotal moment in the advancement of nursing practice. This milestone reflects the increasing need for trained professionals who can guide patients safely and effectively through the complexities of cannabinoid therapeutics. Nurses remain at the forefront of patient education, symptom management, advocacy, and care coordination, making their role indispensable in the integration of cannabis-based therapies into modern healthcare systems.

This volume was developed to address a critical gap in clinical knowledge and professional training related to the medical use of cannabis. Our goal is to provide a comprehensive and practical resource that bridges biomedical science, clinical application, pharmaceutical considerations, and public health perspectives. The contributors to this text represent a broad range of expertise, including medical, surgical, anesthesia, geriatric, emergency medicine, critical care, pediatrics, nurse midwifery, obstetrics, family medicine, psychiatry, and palliative care disciplines. Their collective insights reflect the multidisciplinary nature of cannabinoid medicine and its expanding relevance across healthcare settings.

Throughout this book, readers will find current evidence and guidance regarding cannabinoid therapeutics, dosing principles, delivery methods, patient assessment, symptom management, adjunctive therapy considerations, and clinical decision-making. Equally important, this text addresses the legal, ethical, and regulatory dimensions of cannabis practice, while emphasizing the need for stigma reduction, policy development, quality assurance, and patient-centered care.

As cannabis medicine continues to evolve, healthcare professionals are increasingly called upon to collaborate across disciplines to ensure safe, equitable, and effective treatment strategies. This reference was designed not only to support nurses in specialty practice, but also to serve physicians, advanced practice providers, pharmacists, mental health professionals, educators, researchers, healthcare administrators, policymakers, and students seeking a deeper understanding of cannabinoid therapeutics and clinical integration.

We believe this book contributes to the foundational framework for Cannabis Nursing and supports the development of future standards in education, practice, and research. Most importantly, we hope it empowers clinicians to approach cannabis care with scientific rigor, compassion, cultural sensitivity, and a commitment to improving patient outcomes.

We extend our sincere appreciation to the contributing authors, reviewers, educators, and clinicians whose expertise and dedication made this work possible. We also acknowledge the patients and families whose experiences continue to shape the future of cannabis medicine and inspire ongoing inquiry, innovation, and advocacy.

It is our hope that this text will serve as a trusted resource and catalyst for informed dialogue, interdisciplinary collaboration, and continued advancement in the field of cannabis nursing and clinical practice.

ORGANIZATION OF THE BOOK

This volume opens with a foundational exploration of cannabis nursing as an emerging specialty practice area. Chapter 1 examines the historic recognition of Cannabis Nursing as a specialty by the American Nurses Association and explores the evolving scope, standards, and identity of the cannabis care nurse. The chapter emphasizes holistic nursing principles, patient advocacy, ethics, social justice, stigma reduction, and patient-centered education while also considering international perspectives and the future development of the specialty.

Chapter 2 expands the discussion into advanced clinical nursing practice through the lens of the Clinical Nurse Specialist (CNS). Readers are introduced to the CNS role in integrating cannabis therapeutics into healthcare systems through evidence-based practice, patient assessment, interprofessional collaboration, policy development, staff education, and quality improvement initiatives. This chapter highlights the leadership responsibilities of advanced practice nurses in ensuring safe and ethical cannabis care.

The psychiatric and mental health implications of cannabis therapeutics are explored in Chapter 3, which addresses the increasing importance of cannabis literacy among Psychiatric-Mental Health Nurse Practitioners. The chapter examines current evidence regarding cannabidiol (CBD) and tetrahydrocannabinol (THC), pharmacokinetic variability, ethical dilemmas, harm-reduction counseling, and the complexities of navigating changing legal and regulatory frameworks in psychiatric care.

Chapter 4 critically examines the diagnosis of Cannabis Use Disorder and challenges clinicians to differentiate pathological misuse from legitimate therapeutic use. Through analysis of DSM-5 diagnostic criteria, the chapter explores how historical prohibition, legal barriers, and social stigma may contribute to overdiagnosis. It also introduces the endocannabinoid system as a necessary framework for accurate clinical assessment while highlighting cannabis as a potential harm-reduction modality for other substance use disorders.

The perioperative and anesthetic implications of cannabis use are comprehensively addressed in Chapters 5 and 6. Chapter 5 focuses on the growing challenges faced by anesthesia providers as cannabis use becomes increasingly prevalent. Readers are guided through the physiologic effects of cannabinoids, drug interactions with anesthetic agents, routes of administration, and perioperative considerations that influence patient safety and anesthetic management. Chapter 6 further expands on perioperative care by examining the endocannabinoid system, cannabinoid pharmacokinetics, tolerance, cardiovascular and respiratory implications, pain pathways, and structured assessment strategies. Together, these chapters provide practical guidance for anesthesia professionals, nurse anesthesiologists, and perioperative nurses navigating cannabis-related clinical complexities.

Chapter 7 introduces the emerging relationship between cannabinoid therapeutics and sexual wellness. The discussion examines the therapeutic potential and risks associated with cannabis use in sexual desire disorders, pain disorders, orgasmic disorders, and arousal concerns. Emphasis is placed on patient education, body-system interactions, harm reduction, and promoting informed use to support overall sexual health and quality of life.

The educational leadership role of Cannabis Care Nurses within military and veteran healthcare systems is explored in Chapter 8. This chapter addresses the complex legal and regulatory landscape surrounding cannabis use among active-duty military personnel, veterans, and their families. It highlights the unique challenges associated with stigma, compliance, policy interpretation, and patient education while emphasizing the importance of evidence-based guidance in military and veterans healthcare settings.

The care of older adults represents a major focus of Chapters 9 and 10. Chapter 9 presents a structured framework for geriatric cannabis nursing competencies, emphasizing comprehensive geriatric assessment, therapeutic education, medication safety, monitoring, ethical considerations, and interdisciplinary collaboration. Particular attention is given to the vulnerabilities associated with aging, including polypharmacy, cognitive impairment, and fall risk. Chapter 10 complements this discussion by situating cannabinoid therapeutics within the broader context of gerontological nursing and the increasing use of cannabis among aging populations. The chapter underscores the importance of integrating cannabis assessment, implementation, and evaluation into the care plans of older adults while aligning practice with professional nursing standards.

The evolving role of oncology nurses in cannabis therapeutics is explored in Chapters 11 and 13. Chapter 11 examines the growing expectations placed upon oncology nurses to provide evidence-based patient education regarding medical cannabis in symptom management. The discussion highlights educational gaps, curriculum development, clinical preparedness, and the need for institutional support within oncology nursing practice. Chapter 13 further expands on the integration of cannabis into cancer care by reviewing the pharmacological foundations of cannabinoids, symptom management strategies, drug–drug interactions, patient monitoring, and interdisciplinary collaboration. Together, these chapters reinforce the central role of oncology nurses in supporting safe, evidence-based, and patient-centered cannabis care.

Chapter 12 explores the compassionate integration of cannabis therapeutics into palliative and end-of-life care. The chapter highlights the role of cannabis nurses in promoting comfort, dignity, symptom relief, emotional well-being, and holistic support for patients facing life-limiting illnesses. It further emphasizes advocacy, caregiver support, and the importance of compassionate communication within palliative care settings.

The volume concludes with Chapter 14, which synthesizes many of the themes presented throughout the text by examining the emergence of cannabis nursing as a contemporary specialty integrated within modern healthcare systems. This chapter addresses regulatory variability, educational preparation, clinical governance, interprofessional collaboration, stigma reduction, risk management, and the development of core competencies necessary for safe and equitable cannabis care. The chapter ultimately reinforces the essential role of cannabis nurses in advancing evidence-based, person-centered practice across diverse healthcare environments.

Collectively, these chapters provide a comprehensive examination of cannabis nursing and cannabinoid therapeutics across multiple clinical specialties and healthcare settings. The contributors offer evidence-informed perspectives that support the advancement of nursing education, interdisciplinary collaboration, patient advocacy, clinical safety, and healthcare policy. As cannabis medicine continues to evolve globally, this text seeks to equip healthcare professionals with the knowledge and competencies necessary to navigate this rapidly expanding field with scientific rigor, ethical responsibility, and compassionate care.

CONCLUSION

As Editors, we recognize that the field of cannabis nursing and cannabinoid therapeutics is evolving at an extraordinary pace, shaped by scientific discovery, regulatory transformation, patient advocacy, and the growing demand for integrative approaches to healthcare. The chapters presented in this volume collectively demonstrate that cannabis nursing is no longer a peripheral area of inquiry, but an emerging clinical specialty that requires informed leadership, interdisciplinary collaboration, ethical awareness, and evidence-based practice across healthcare systems.

Throughout this text, contributors have explored the many dimensions of cannabis care, including clinical assessment, pharmacology, patient education, mental health, anesthesia, oncology, geriatrics, palliative care, policy development, and stigma reduction. Together, these perspectives reinforce the essential role nurses play in supporting safe, equitable, and patient-centered integration of cannabinoid therapeutics into contemporary practice. The diversity of topics represented in this volume reflects the broad and expanding impact of cannabis medicine across nearly every area of healthcare delivery.

At the center of this emerging specialty is the nurse's enduring commitment to advocacy, compassion, education, and holistic care. Cannabis nurses are uniquely positioned to bridge gaps between scientific evidence, clinical application, and patient experience while navigating complex legal, ethical, and social considerations. As healthcare systems continue to adapt to changing cannabis policies and patient needs, nurses will remain instrumental in advancing standards of care, promoting informed decision-making, and fostering interdisciplinary dialogue grounded in safety and professionalism.

This volume also underscores the urgent need for continued research, standardized clinical guidelines, robust educational preparation, and institutional support for healthcare professionals working within cannabis-related care environments. Although significant progress has been made, many questions remain regarding long-term safety, dosing strategies, therapeutic efficacy, drug interactions, and equitable access to care. The future of cannabis nursing will depend upon sustained scholarly inquiry, policy development, and the integration of emerging evidence into clinical education and practice.

We hope this book serves not only as a foundational academic and clinical resource, but also as a catalyst for innovation, collaboration, and ongoing professional development. It is our aspiration that readers will use the knowledge contained within these chapters to strengthen patient care, reduce stigma, improve health outcomes, and contribute to the advancement of cannabis nursing as a recognized and respected specialty worldwide.

Finally, we extend our deepest gratitude to the chapter contributors, reviewers, clinicians, educators, researchers, and advocates whose expertise and dedication made this work possible. Their commitment to advancing evidence-informed cannabis care reflects the collective vision of a healthcare system that embraces compassion, scientific integrity, and patient-centered practice.

As the landscape of cannabinoid therapeutics continues to evolve, we believe this text represents an important step toward shaping the future of cannabis nursing and supporting healthcare professionals who are leading this transformation in clinical practice.

Chapter 1
Cannabis Care Nursing: Emerging Roles

Carey Shannon Cadieux
http://orcid.org/0000-0001-8812-2667
Binghamton University, USA

ABSTRACT

In 2023, the American Nurses Association (ANA) recognized cannabis as an official nursing specialty. Although the scope and standards of cannabis nursing are in place, many challenges remain for this specialty practice area. This chapter examines the current state of the cannabis nurse role, including the scope and standards of cannabis nurse practice, and outlines steps to co-create the future of cannabis care nursing. The chapter provides a basis for ensuring that the role of the cannabis nurse is aligned with holistic nursing and, therefore, focuses on working with patients through coaching and education. The cannabis care nurse must also focus on patient advocacy, social justice issues, ethics, safety issues, spiritual concerns, and the common challenges and barriers that cannabis nurses face. Cannabis care nursing in several other countries is explored. What can the future of cannabis care nursing look like, and what steps do nurses need to take to co-create this emerging specialty?

INTRODUCTION

Cannabis nursing began with a few fearless nursing leaders coming together and creating a vision around what nurses supporting medical cannabis use of patients could look like. Mary Lynn Mathre, MSN, RN, co-founded the 501 (c) (3) nonprofit organization Patients Out of Time in 2000, with an emphasis on supporting veterans and educating healthcare professionals about cannabis. In 2006, Ms. Mathre co-

DOI: 10.4018/979-8-2600-2035-7.ch001

founded the American Cannabis Nurses Association (ACNA), which became a 501 (c) (3) nonprofit organization in 2010, focusing on nurse education, research, and policy development. The American Nurses Association (ANA) recognized cannabis nursing as a specialty in 2023, and the ANA and ACNA (2024) published Cannabis *nursing: Scope and standards of practice.*

Cannabis nursing is a young specialty that is emerging even as the United States (US) and other global governments leave the cannabis prohibition era and enter an era of cannabis regulation. The purpose of this chapter is to examine the future of the cannabis nurse role, the challenges and barriers nurses face, and to consider how cannabis care is provided in several other countries, offering a global perspective on the current state and future of cannabis care nursing.

The readers of this chapter will:

- Discover the current and future role of nurses specializing in cannabis care nursing, including a global perspective. .
- Define the impact of the scope and standards on the future of cannabis nursing.
- Consider the role of the cannabis nurse as a holistic coach and advocate in light of global cannabis nursing experiences.
- Identify steps to take to co-create the future of cannabis care nursing as a recognized specialty area of nursing care.
- Consider the need for a plan to include cannabis science content in all nursing curricula.

BACKGROUND

The role of the cannabis care nurse has only begun to emerge since the early 2000s, and it took over two decades to formalize cannabis care nursing as a nursing specialty in 2024 with the publication of *Cannabis nursing: Scope and standards of practice* (first edition) (ANA & ACNA, 2024). This publication provides foundational knowledge to support the practice of cannabis care nurses. It covers eighteen standards, each with associated competencies that cannabis care nurses strive to demonstrate in their everyday work with patients, populations, interprofessional, advocates, researchers, and policy developers.

Literature Review: Role of the Cannabis Care Nurse

The ANA & ACNA (2024) defined cannabis care nursing as a specialty nursing practice that focuses on the care of people who are seeking support and guidance with therapeutically using medical cannabis. Cannabis nurses demonstrate competence in their understanding of the human endocannabinoid system (ECS) and support patients' efforts to upregulate the ECS and maintain homeostasis through lifestyle interventions and holistic modalities. Further competencies of cannabis nurses include cannabinoid pharmacodynamics, pharmacokinetics, scientific evidence related to cannabinoid effectiveness, and advocacy approaches. Cannabis care nurses educate and support healthcare consumers to use cannabis safely and effectively and provide coaching while using motivational interviewing to set goals (ANA & ACNA, 2024). Advocacy is a skill needed as the nurse strives for cannabis health care consumers to have access to safe, tested cannabinoid therapeutics (ANA & ACNA, 2024). Cannabis care nurses approach the development of caring-healing spaces by applying caring theory and ethical principles such as autonomy, beneficence, and nonmaleficence (ANA & ACNA, 2024).

The following is a summary of the ANA & ACNA (2024) Standards of Cannabis Nursing Practice, with a brief description of each standard.

Cannabis Nursing: 18 Standards of Practice

1. Assessment – The cannabis nurse systematically collects and analyzes comprehensive data related to the patient's health status, cannabis use, symptoms, goals, risks, and legal considerations.
2. Diagnosis – The cannabis nurse identifies actual or potential health problems, responses, or needs related to cannabis use or cannabinoid therapy.
3. Outcomes Identification – The nurse defines expected, measurable outcomes related to symptom management, safety, function, quality of life, and patient goals related to cannabis use.
4. Planning – The nurse develops a personalized, evidence-based plan of care that integrates cannabis considerations with the overall healthcare plan.
5. Implementation – The nurse implements the plan through education, coaching, harm-reduction strategies, interprofessional coordination, and patient support.
6. Evaluation – The nurse evaluates patient responses to cannabis use and adjusts the plan of care based on outcomes, evidence, and patient feedback.
7. Ethics – The cannabis nurse practices in accordance with ethical principles, protecting patient autonomy, privacy, safety, and informed decision-making related to cannabis.
8. Culturally Congruent Practice – The nurse provides cannabis-related care that is respectful of cultural beliefs, values, traditions, and historical contexts.
9. Communication – The nurse communicates clearly and effectively with patients, families, and healthcare teams about cannabis use, risks, benefits, and expectations.

10. Collaboration – The nurse collaborates with interprofessional teams to ensure coordinated, safe, and patient-centered cannabis care.
11. Leadership – The cannabis nurse demonstrates leadership by promoting best practices, mentoring others, and advancing cannabis nursing within healthcare systems.
12. Education – The nurse maintains competence and provides evidence-based education to patients, families, communities, and healthcare professionals regarding cannabis.
13. Evidence-Based Practice and Research – The nurse integrates current research, clinical expertise, and patient preferences to guide cannabis-related care.
14. Quality of Practice – The nurse contributes to quality improvement initiatives that enhance safety, outcomes, and effectiveness of cannabis care.
15. Professional Practice Evaluation – The nurse evaluates personal practice related to cannabis care and seeks feedback, reflection, and improvement.
16. Resource Utilization – The nurse uses healthcare resources responsibly to support safe, accessible, and effective cannabis care.
17. Environmental Health – The nurse considers environmental and public health impacts related to cannabis cultivation, product safety, and exposure.
18. Advocacy – The cannabis nurse advocates for patient rights, equitable access, evidence-based policy, and the role of nursing in cannabis care.

Cannabis care nurses work in a variety of healthcare settings and via private consultations where the nurse includes cannabis in a plan for patients' healing and palliation of symptoms (Theisen & Konieczny, 2019). The care planning may involve multiple specialty areas across the patient's lifespan. "Cannabis care nursing happens where the patient is at, when there is recognition that the human ECS needs to be upregulated to support homeostasis" (Clark, 2021a, p. 270). This recognition comes from either the patient seeking healing and/or from the nurse who recognizes patients and populations who could benefit from ECS upregulation through cannabis use, lifestyle changes, and use of holistic modalities (Sulak, 2021). In the US, cannabis care nurses may also work in research or collaborate with manufacturers or dispensary services.

Cannabis care nursing involves a nurse educating, supporting, and coaching a patient who is ready for palliation and healing and desires to maximize their health potential within a caring-healing environment. An aspect of the why of cannabis care nursing relates to the call by the NCSBN (2018) for all nurses to be educated around the six essential areas of knowledge, attitudes, and skills related to working with patients who use cannabis. Not just nurses interested in specializing in cannabis care need to have cannabis nursing knowledge; all nurses must have a baseline of knowledge. Additionally, nurses are ethically obligated to provide patients with the information necessary to make autonomous decisions about their palliative care and to ensure that their palliative goals are met safely and effectively.

The how of current cannabis care nursing is often the challenging aspect of this practice specialty. As nursing academia and practice settings do not offer in-depth cannabis educational or training opportunities at this time, it is often up to the nurse to grow their cannabis care knowledge and proficiency, which includes an emphasis on the cannabis pharmacokinetics and pharmacodynamics, self-titration, recognition of the ECS as the master regulator in the body, holistic and lifestyle techniques to upregulate the ECS for health potentiation, how to use nursing theory to create caring-healing spaces, and advocacy techniques (Clark, 2021a). Additionally, if the nurse decides to establish a private cannabis care consultation practice, they will need to learn about entrepreneurial techniques, business operations, and legal considerations.

It is important to note that not just trained cannabis nurses provide cannabis care; the NCSBN (2018) made it clear that *all nurses across all levels of education* must have the following knowledge, attitudes, and skills to work effectively with medical cannabis patients:

1. Working knowledge of the current state of legalization of medical and recreational cannabis use.
2. Working knowledge of the jurisdiction's medical marijuana program.
3. An understanding of the endocannabinoid system (ECS).
4. An understanding of cannabis pharmacology and associated research.
5. The ability to identify safety considerations for patient use of cannabis.
6. The ability to approach patients without judgment regarding their treatment preferences.

The APRN role also aligns with the standards of practice above, with advanced competency and skill level noted (ANA & ACNA, 2024). The APRN role with the NCSBN (2018) six essentials expands to include that the APRN may not "prescribe" cannabis as long as it remains a Federal Schedule I Drug. The APRN must also be able to recognize the signs and symptoms of cannabis use disorder and cannabis withdrawal symptoms. Additionally, the APRN's role is on medication safety, patient education regarding reading cannabinoid product labels, and proper disposal of unused medications. The APRN must also have a DEA prescriber number and follow specific state guidelines when recommending cannabis use for a patient; they must be able to balance the benefit of the medication against the patient's specific risks which may include poly-pharmacy, adverse effects that may impact morbidity, the patient's ability to safely self-titrate cannabis, and identifying high risk populations (NCSBN, 2018; Theisen, 2021). The APRN should enact informed and shared decision-making with patients, and documentation and communication are essential (Theisen). The APRN may also gain a greater understanding of the advocacy and policy development process through advanced study, and the APRN's skills will be used to advocate for policies that benefit patient populations.

The cannabis care nurse's work continues to be hampered by cannabis remaining a US Federal Schedule I drug (at the time of this writing, there is movement toward rescheduling cannabis to Schedule III, but this process will likely be lengthy). Other countries, such as Canada and Israel, have expanded the role of nurses working with cannabis patients, and US nurses can look toward those countries as they envision the future of cannabis care nursing for guidance around practice issues, policies, and educational needs. The main challenges for nurses both in the US and globally include education to support patients' safe and effective use of cannabis, regulatory concerns, and the ethics of caring for populations that use cannabis. The next section will explicate further these challenges of contemporary cannabis nursing and what we must consider as the future role of cannabis nurses emerges.

THE FUTURE OF CANNABIS CARE NURSING

As we move into the era of regulation of cannabis, it the role of the cannabis care nurse will evolve. While there are many uncertainties ahead, it's important to recognize that nurses need to be at the forefront of supporting patients in using cannabinoid therapeutics safely and effectively, and to maximize their health potential. This section will examine the next steps for professional cannabis care nursing, define future cannabis nursing roles, and consider a global perspective, and define the impact of policy and advocacy.

ACNA and Future of Certification

ACNA is the professional nursing organization working closely with ANA to define the future of cannabis care nursing as a nursing specialty with a certification process; this is one of the next steps in solidifying the future of the cannabis nurse role. Cannabis nursing has been recognized as a specialty since 2023, and the first edition of the scope and standards of practice emerged in 2024. The ACNA may next take the steps to develop a board certification exam through the American Nurses Credentialing Center (ANCC). The process of completing the certification approval is an arduous one and includes the following steps:

- Developing a role delineation study, with ANCC working with a Content Expert Panel (CEP). This study further defines the professional skills, outlines a test blueprint, and provides evidence supporting the test content.
- ANCC works with the professional organization to support content experts in writing test questions or items. The items undergo further review by ANCC and the CEP, and pilot testing is conducted to determine validity and quality, assess potential biases, and ensure that all psychometric measures are in place.
- The entire process will be consistent with the technical guidelines from authoritative bodies and meet accreditation standards of the Accreditation Board for Specialty Nursing Certification (ABSNC) and the National Commission for Certifying Agencies (NCCA).

While this approach is arduous, it will ensure that the credentialing exam for recognized board certification is developed by specialty experts and supported by the ANCC. Once board certification for cannabis care nurses becomes a reality, nurses interested in the field will need to demonstrate continuing education in cannabis care and relevant experience. This experience is likely to arise from expert mentorship and from working with organizations that serve medical cannabis patients.

Regardless of the availability of the board certification examination, it behooves all nurses interested in working with cannabis care populations to invest in continuing education related to medical cannabis. Additionally, finding a mentor and joining a cannabis nursing organization and community is beneficial. Some organizations to consider include the American Cannabis Nurses Association, Cannabis Clinicians' Society, Cannabis Nurses of Color, and Cannabis Nurse Network.

Policy and Advocacy

Cannabis care nursing requires that the nurse be actively engaged and involved with medical cannabis policy development (local, facility or organization, state, and federal) and advocacy.

In reviewing the ANA and ACNA (2024) *Scope and standards of practice*, policy, and advocacy, the text predominantly features these areas. The cannabis care nurse:

- Takes the lead in developing evidence-based policies, procedures, and ethical standards for medical cannabis use within healthcare organizations.
- Ensures patient safety by operating within all state and federal laws in consideration of institutional policies and procedures, while also advocating for better cannabis access and reduced stigma. Ensuring policy compliance in inpatients and organizational settings.

- Informs and educates other healthcare professionals about cannabis regulations, safety, and therapeutic benefits to improve practice.
- Advocates for equitable access to cannabis as a therapeutic option and working to eliminate the stigma surrounding its medical use.
- Working toward supporting that all patients have autonomy to decide about the use of medical cannabis for palliative needs. Ethics also require the nurse to advocate for vulnerable populations and, in the future, when insurance may adequately cover the costs of cannabinoid therapy.

One thing for future emphasis is that nursing advocacy is a learned skill, and schools of nursing often not teach this topic in depth. It's also important to consider our ethical obligations as we care for cannabis patients. In addition to autonomy, the cannabis care nurses consider beneficence (doing good), nonmaleficence (doing no harm), totality (integrity), and social justice in relation to policy development (Clark, 2021b). At the forefront of the cannabis care nurse's advocacy is the motivation to support what is best for patients and populations.

How can the cannabis nurse learn to be an advocate and grow their skills? Clark (2021b) reminded us that advocacy differs from activism and that the ANA defined advocacy as one of the pillars of nursing. Advocates publicly support their chosen cause, while activists focus more on campaigning to bring about social and political change. Advocacy around medical cannabis includes the bedside, legislative, and political efforts. The ANA (2019) advocacy toolkit provides a good background for taking your first steps as an advocate. Some concepts include recognizing that legislative change is very slow, often taking 5-10 years for a bill to become law, with only 4% of federal bills becoming law and 15-20% of state bills becoming law. One must understand legislators' agendas and how history, campaign promises, values or ideology, timing, and the majority party shape them. Advocates can keep in mind that nurses are the largest segment of healthcare professionals, and their voices and experiences matter when communicating with their legislators. It's important to build relationships with elected officials, including meeting with them or their representatives, and the cannabis nurse should be prepared to make an ask, with their key points ready eventually. Telling the story, providing evidence for the "why" behind the ask, and defining the policy's impact on their constituents help keep the nurse focused and the legislator engaged (ANA, 2019). Acting through a professional organization increases the likelihood that the world will hear the nurses' voice.

Some steps to support cannabis care nurses with advocacy were outlined by Clark (2021b) as follows:

- Immerse yourself in the body of evidence related to cannabis as well as the issues you want to advocate for. It's important to be well-educated, confident, and clear about the issues at hand and about your own purpose and goals. Joining organizations, attending conferences, listening to podcasts, and analyzing research and policy are skills that prove fruitful, as does having a mentor. Learning from other advocates can also be helpful as you develop your skills and style.

- Be of service and active in the advocacy efforts of your professional organizations. While cannabis-focused nursing organizations are a joy to belong to, many of the members within these organizations also partner with Veterans' groups, NORML, Americans for Safe Access, and Marijuana Policy Project.
- Avoid stating in public forums that you are speaking as a spokesperson for an organization unless you have been formally designated to do so. You can leverage your nursing degrees, experiences, credentials, and professional organization memberships.
- Bring along, or join others, at events for the same reason you are. Support and co-mentoring are invaluable.
- Use social media wisely to advocate for change.
- Consider fundraising efforts for your favorite organizations.
- Walk the talk! Taking good care of yourself through lifestyle changes and potentiating the health of the ECS is key.
- Know those who oppose your advocacy efforts and of their talking points and arguments. Be prepared to counter their points with both evidence and your experiences as a nurse caring for populations.
- Avoid self-righteousness and remain humble (Clark, 2021b).

There will be many challenges ahead as cannabis moves out of the prohibition era and cannabis nurses strive to create policies that support patients' well-being and access to safe, tested, and effective medical cannabinoids.

Research

Cannabis nurses may find themselves drawn to doing research, and this is an area of cannabis nursing that will expand into the future as the regulatory era emerges. While cannabis is one of the most researched plants, prohibition has played a role in researchers having access to quality cannabinoid therapeutics for doing research, as have the federal and global restrictions around the plant. Additionally, while there is a plethora of "anecdotal" evidence about cannabis's effectiveness, qualitative research focusing on patients' experiences with cannabis remains minimal (Clark,

2021a). Qualitative analysis of the patient population's experiences could prove to be a growth area for cannabis care nursing.

The ANA (2025) revised the *Code of ethics for nurses*. Provision 7 currently states that, "Nurses advance the profession through multiple approaches to knowledge development, professional standards, and the generation of policies for nursing, health, and social concerns" (p.27), while Provision 7.1 states that "Nurses engage in research and scholarly inquiry designed to expand the body of nursing knowledge through theory, philosophy, ethics, science, and practice" (p. 27). The ANA recognized that nursing draws on other disciplines to expand our nursing knowledge base and that, ultimately, one of our goals is to understand the human experience better. Importantly, evidence-based practice is grounded in research, and the cannabis nurse is ethically obligated to develop a practice grounded in research. All cannabis nurses must be able to analyze evidence-based information related to the populations they care for, just as all nurses must develop evidence-based practices.

Cannabis nurse researchers may focus on generating, translating, and applying evidence related to medical cannabis and cannabinoid-based therapies. The researcher's focus may be on enhancing patient care and outcomes, analyzing health policy, or supporting nursing and provider practices. The cannabis care nurse of the future may design and conduct ethical research on patient outcomes related to cannabinoid medications, symptom management, palliation, end-of-life care, self-titration patterns, safety/ avoidance of adverse effects, harm reduction, and/or health equity related to cannabis use across populations and settings. Cannabis care nurses in the future may lead or contribute to observational studies, legally permissible clinical trials, quality improvement initiatives, and program evaluations, while ensuring compliance with regulatory, institutional, and ethical standards. Generally, to lead research, the cannabis care nurse is educated at the graduate level, with knowledge of evidence-based practices and experience in developing research studies.

One of the top priorities for research in the 2021-2025 National Center for Complementary and Integrative Health (NCCIH) (n.d.) was to focus on complementary and integrative health (CIH) approaches to managing pain. While cannabis is not specifically mentioned in the plan, the role of the cannabis care nurse is to support patients' upregulation of the ECS (methods to improve the function of the ECS, including ways to upregulate cannabinoid receptors, increase ligand synthesis, or inhibit ligand degradation to optimize ECS functioning). Most CIH modalities impact the ECS (McPartland et al., 2014). The future of pain management is a movement away from opioids and toward CIH, and cannabis nurses can make the imperative connection between the ECS and how integrative/ holistic modalities optimize the functioning of the ECS. Cannabis nurses may collaborate with holistic nurses on research to demonstrate how modalities and the holistic nursing process support optimal ECS functioning. And optimal ECS functioning can mean lower amounts of cannabis use, leading to less risk for adverse effects and cost savings with lower cannabinoid ingestion.

Nurses often face challenges in research, including organizational constraints, financial barriers, and the formation of interdisciplinary research teams (Cámpoli & Mulvey, 2023), and cannabis nursing research of the future will be no different. Nursing research is heavily based in academic settings, and frontline bedside or community-practicing nurses often feel separated from the process, with challenges in translating research into practice, which is a global issue, and one that impacts cannabis care nurses who are interested in ensuring patients, nurses, and other healthcare providers have the best evidence-based cannabis information to support their practice with patients. Cannabis care nurses will be part of the global movement to ensure that nurses' voices in advancing nursing practice-based research are heard (Cámpoli & Mulvey). The cannabis care nurse is called upon to consider how research impacts their practice, take steps to translate evidence into practice, and identify ways to improve medical cannabis patient outcomes.

The Cannabis Nurse Entrepreneur

The cannabis nurse entrepreneur may build a practice focused on supporting patients' safe and effective use of cannabinoid therapeutics through a holistic coaching approach to upregulating the ECS, consulting with dispensaries, providing community education, developing their own cannabinoid products, or working with companies to white-label cannabinoid therapeutics. Regardless of the type of business a cannabis care nurse is interested in, they should always consider further education, certification, consultation, and/or experience. There are many nurse entrepreneur training courses, such as those offered by Sigma Theta Tau (2026), and one can earn a Doctor of Nursing Practice in Innovation and Entrepreneurship from schools like the Duke University School of Nursing (2026). The National Nurses in Business Association (2026) provides a forum for connecting, building networks, sharing information, learning about new business opportunities, and attending national conferences, workshops, and seminars. Numerous private organizations and groups offer ongoing training, education, and support for nurse entrepreneurs, and the cannabis care nurse needs to research these opportunities before committing financially to a course of study.

The emerging role of the cannabis nurse as an entrepreneur may look different depending on the state's legal landscape. For instance, many nurses historically have had their licenses threatened or removed based on their efforts to educate about cannabis or coach patients toward safe and effective use of cannabis. The cannabis care nurse must always review their state and federal rules, laws, and regulations, and in the US, determine whether the state board of nursing supports their entrepreneurial activity. Additionally, whether the cannabis nurse in the US can use a compact license to provide education and coaching outside their home state should be considered. Creating a limited liability corporation (LLC) and consulting with a business lawyer are also recommendations for any cannabis care nurse starting a company.

Cannabis Care at the Bedside and Beyond

Cannabis nurses need to support the NCSBN (2018) call for all nurses are provided education around the safe and effective use of cannabis. However, it should be clear that all nurses need to have knowledge of cannabis care as was defined by the NCSBN. Currently, many nursing students rely on media to enhance their nursing knowledge and deciphering research for themselves (Parmelee & Clark, 2022).

Upregulate ECS: CIH Modalities, Spiritual Care

Rarely will cannabis alone address the patient's ability to reach optimal health and functioning of the ECS as the master regulator in the body. As mentioned previously, the cannabis nurse is a holistic nurse. One of the main considerations is how the nurse supports, educates, and coaches patients toward their greatest health potential, which is by educating the patient around activities that upregulate the ECS (supporting the health of the cannabinoid receptors, increasing ligand synthesis, and/or inhibiting ligand degradation). When the nurse has a strong understanding of the ECS as the body's master regulator, including its role in maintaining homeostasis through retrograde endocannabinoid signaling at the cellular level (Sulak, 2021), the nurse can be passionate about supporting the patient's holistic health. When considering the ethical concepts of beneficence, justice, and autonomy, the cannabis care nurse is ethically obligated to ensure that patients use the least amount of cannabis for the greatest effect to avoid adverse effects, and the patient can accomplish this through activities that upregulate the ECS (Clark, 2021a).

The following are the main issues the cannabis care nurse should be addressing in their plan of care for medical cannabis patients, with the idea of holistic approaches and upregulation of the ECS at the forefront:

- Applying the nursing process and using motivational interviewing on an ongoing basis. Developing a sense of connection and remaining patient-centered while patients set intentions and create goals is key to the holistic approach (Clark, 2021a).
- Exercise is holistic in that it remains outside of the allopathic approach on many levels. Aerobic activity increases the density of endocannabinoid re-

ceptors (CB1), though the relationship between well-being, aerobic exercise, and CB1 density remains not fully understood (Gupta et al., 2024). During and following aerobic activity, the release of the endocannabinoid anandamide (N-arachidonoyl-ethanolamine (AEA)) surges, with the amount of increase based on the intensity of the exercise. The other endocannabinoid levels do not change with aerobic activity. These higher levels of AEA lead to decreased anxiety and psychological arousal for 2 to 4 hours. The full understanding of how exercise impacts the ECS is emerging, but we do know that moderate-intensity exercise has a greater impact on ECS versus both excessively high and excessively low intensity exercise (Gupta et al.).

- Sleep is important for one's overall health and well-being. Sleep hygiene is a consideration for cannabis care nurses as they work with patients who may struggle in this area. While sleep is often a primary reason for consuming cannabis, regular use of cannabis over time can downregulate the ECS and CB1 receptors, leading to fragmented sleep, and there may be concerns related to tolerance development and potential withdrawal symptoms with regular THC use (Kolla et al., 2022). The cannabis care nurse may help the patient to focus on sleep hygiene (decrease or cease caffeine use, exercise, decrease screen time -particularly before bed- the bed is only for sleep and sex, etc). Exploring other herbs for sleep, such as chamomile, passionflower, hops, valerian, and skullcap, may be beneficial (US Department of Veterans Affairs, 2024).
- Nutrition is important because the ECS functions optimally when it receives the nutrients it needs. Feeding the ECS is an area that all cannabis care nurses should focus on with their patients. Endocannabinoids are part of our nutritional regulation system, including contributions to food intake, hunger, and satiety, and CB1 receptors in the hypothalamus are involved in protein metabolism (Foster, 2021). The endocannabinoid system requires a balance between omega-6 and omega-3 fatty acids, and many people may need to focus on increasing their omega-3 intake (e.g., flax, hemp, chia seeds, algae, and cold-water fish). The colorful polyphenol components found in fruits and vegetables, as well as the cannabis plant itself, are called flavonoids, and they serve to upregulate CB2 receptors and decrease FAAH breakdown of anandamide. Flavonoids can be found in many colorful fruits and vegetables as well as in chocolate. Beta-caryophyllene is a beneficial cannabinoid/terpenoid found in many plants and interacts with CB2 receptors. An anti-inflammatory diet that avoids or minimizes processed foods, pesticides, caffeine, and alcohol will help to support the health of the ECS (Foster, 2021).

- Touch therapies for medical cannabis patients to consider may include osteopathy (Buscemi et al., 2021) and massage (Liu et al., 2025), which support the body's anti-inflammatory process through activation of CB1 receptors.
- Acupuncture helps to alleviate pain and other distressing symptoms by activating both CB1 receptors (leading to antinociception) and CB2 receptors (promoting anti-inflammatory effects), as demonstrated primarily in animal models (MacDonald & Chen, 2021).
- Mind-body practices are key to supporting the ECS's health. Studies have shown changes in endocannabinoids, including increases in AEA, 2-AG, 1-AG, DEA, and BDNF after meditation (de Melo Reis et al., 2021). Supporting patients in engaging in daily mindfulness and meditative practices helps them manage stress and upregulates the ECS. Many people believe they can't meditate, so the cannabis care nurse guides the patient toward resources that may help them to learn to meditate or offers guided meditation and relaxation exercises during their interactions with patients.
- Social interactions are important for an individual's health and well-being. There is sufficient data to suggest that poorer ECS functioning can affect a person's ability to engage in social interaction. Likewise, social interactions in the right context may help upregulate the ECS (Trezza et al., 2025). The cannabis care nurse supports the medical cannabis patient toward positive social interactions and understands that as the health of the ECS is potentiated, patients may experience more positivity from their interactions.
- Medications may also support the upregulation of the ECS. In addition to checking for drug-drug interactions, the cannabis care nurse supports patients with the use of medications and all tools available to potentiate health. Examples of medications known to interact with the ECS include NSAIDs and acetaminophen, which inhibit ECS-degrading enzymes such as FAAH; anticonvulsants; prebiotics that support the health of the endocannabinoidome; and antidepressants and antipsychotics that may help increase ECS activity (McPartland et al., 2014).

The cannabis care nurse must recognize the therapeutic potential of using a truly integrative/ holistic approach in supporting patients to use all tools that may potentiate health.

Evolving Practice Settings

Many cannabis nurses in the US currently practice as private consultants. Yet there is a growing need in the US for cannabis care to expand into more formalized healthcare and community-based settings where patients routinely seek education, support, and coaching related to the safe, effective, and evidence-informed use of cannabis. Cannabis care nurses can bring a unique blend of clinical nursing expertise, knowledge of pharmacology and cannabinoid science, patient education skills, and ethical practice approaches that position them to integrate cannabis care within traditional and nontraditional care environments (ANA & ACNA, 2024).

In primary care, cannabis nurses can support chronic disease management by guiding patients who are using or considering cannabis for pain, anxiety, sleep, PTSD, and/or other common conditions, while ensuring continuity of care and safety alongside conventional therapies (Theisen & Konieczny, 2019). Cannabis therapeutics are best viewed as an integrative modality. In palliative care and hospice, the cannabis care nurse's expertise could be particularly valuable in symptom management for pain, nausea, anorexia, and distress, where the nurse develops individualized cannabis care plans that may enhance comfort and quality of life at the end of life. Within home health and community-based care, cannabis nurses can provide in-home education, monitor outcomes, and reinforce safe storage and use, especially for vulnerable populations such as older adults and those with cognitive or mobility limitations. In the public health setting, cannabis nurses can focus on policy development, education for vulnerable populations, and the use of epidemiological approaches to ensure positive outcomes for populations (Clark, 2021a).

The pediatric and school nursing contexts require specialized cannabis nursing expertise related to family education, risk prevention, adolescent health, and navigating complex legal and ethical considerations, especially around exposure, medical authorization, and developmental implications. Cannabis nursing in school settings involves a complex intersection of student health needs, state-specific medical cannabis laws, and federal restrictions. For instance, nurses must follow state law to administer cannabinoids on school property, ensure that policies and procedures are developed, and consider safety (Jochen & Holben, 2024).

In emergency and acute care settings, cannabis nurses can contribute to screening for cannabis-related adverse effects, intoxication, or withdrawal, while educating patients on safer use practices and recognizing when cannabis may be contributing to presenting symptoms or tolerance, dependence, or substance use disorders. Special attention for geriatric patients in this setting is warranted (Han et al., 2023).

With addiction recovery and mental health settings, cannabis care nurses can play a critical role in differentiating therapeutic use from problematic use, supporting harm reduction, and integrating cannabis discussions into holistic recovery-oriented care without stigma. With harm reduction as a guiding perspective, issues such as anxiety, PTSD, and depression can be considered with cannabis care, always considering the patient's safety, well-being, and right to autonomy (Smith & Sera, 2025).

The idea of a Cannabis Nurse Navigator™ (CNN) (2026) has been proposed, in which the trained cannabis nurse navigator serves as a patient guide and liaison among the patient, providers, and healthcare systems. The CNN is an emerging concept and role that requires the nurse to have skills in clinical research, patient advocacy, and patient care.

Ultimately, expanding cannabis nursing into formalized healthcare environments strengthens patient safety, promotes evidence-based practice, and ensures nurses address cannabis use with the same clinical rigor, ethical standards, and compassionate care that define professional nursing practice.

Global Perspectives

The future of cannabis care nursing emerging roles has global implications. As the world moves into a post-cannabis-prohibition era and toward a cannabis-regulatory era, it is important to consider how the practice of this specialty emerges differently around the globe. There may be a need for an international cannabis nurse practice approach during the cannabis regulatory era. The nursing profession must consider how regulations and policies guide our practices, what we can learn from the triumphs and challenges cannabis care nurses experience in their local practice areas, and what nurses have accomplished in other countries. We can expect new models of cannabis care to emerge and an eventual convergence toward an internationally standardized approach to nurses providing cannabis care. The following sections will review several countries' cannabis care practices, recognizing that analysis is minimized within the limited scope of this chapter.

Canadian Cannabis Care

Cannabis was federally legalized in October 2018 in Canada. We must consider the role of the cannabis nurse in a fully legalized landscape and determine what the implications are for global approaches to cannabis nursing. Health Canada's Substance Use and Addictions Program (SUAP) granted The Canadian Nurses Association (CNA) (2022) 1.3 million dollars to develop a national nursing framework about non-medical cannabis use. The document that emerged from CNA (2022), *Non-medical cannabis: A framework for nurses*, focuses on stakeholder input to the framework. The framework addresses client, nurse, equity (stigma, advocacy), cannabis, and evidence. Recommendations for nurse leaders, educators, researchers, and regulators included that Canada:

- Formalize education about cannabis and its use in all nursing school curricula in Canada and also build continuing education on cannabis for practicing nurses.

- Review the current interventions for nurses with concerning levels of personal cannabis use.
- Identify language that stigmatizes cannabis in the workplace as related to patient and nursing workforce cannabis use, and actively replace and realign cannabis terminology with unbiased, supportive, non-stigmatizing, and person-first language.
- Support, participate in, and conduct research on both medical and non-medical cannabis, and advocate for both funding and access to cannabis for research purposes.
- Advocate for equitable access to both medical and non-medical cannabis.
- Advocate for legal expungement for those charged with cannabis-related offenses before legalization (CNA, 2022, p. 21).

CNA (2026) also developed some helpful materials that support nurses with maintaining empathy for people who use substances and focus on how to reduce the harm from non-medical cannabis. The Canadian Nurses Protective Society (CNPS) (2026) noted that there may be variations in laws related to territories or provinces, but generally, registered nurses can administer medical cannabis in hospitals and in privacy (not in public). Nurse practitioners can prescribe and possess medical cannabis products for distribution to adult patients (except in Alberta). However, each hospital makes its own policies regarding cannabis that may impact the role of the nurse or provider and the patient's ability to access medical cannabis. Overall, both organizations are supportive of nurses' use of cannabis, warn against practicing if one is intoxicated, and encourage nurses to seek help if they are overly reliant on cannabis.

The Government of Canada (2018) issued a publication entitled, *Information for healthcare professionals: Cannabis (marijuana, marihuana) and the cannabinoid.* This educational document covers the ECS, pharmacology, dosing, potential therapeutic effects, precautions/ warnings, adverse effects, and overdose/toxicity. This document demonstrates that Canada is committed to educating all healthcare providers about cannabis, which is an effort that other could replicate on a global scale.

As in other countries, in Canada, it is often up to the nurse or nurse practitioner to independently establish an adequate level of education, knowledge, and skill to care for medical cannabis patients in a safe, legal, and ethical manner. Balneaves et al. (2023) found that in Canada, only about 37% of baccalaureate nursing students reported receiving any education about cannabis, and over 92% agreed that if they had more education, they would feel more comfortable providing cannabis education and support in the clinical setting. In Canada, due to federal legalization issues, education on both medical and non-medical cannabis use still needs to be incorporated into their nursing curricula to enhance nurses' knowledge and support patients' safe and effective use of cannabis, which implies that federal legalization alone does not solve the cannabis education issue in nursing academia.

In Canada, nurse practitioners may undertake training with private organizations such as Sante` Cannabis, or registered nurses can work with Vital Holistic Care (VHC) to receive a holistic cannabis nurse certification. Once the nurse has completed training with VHC, they may be eligible to work with the VHC team to provide direct cannabis care to Canadian Veterans, including those in the Canadian Armed Forces and the Royal Canadian Mounted Police. The VHC team follows the holistic approach to cannabis care as outlined by Clark (2021a), and they strive to ensure that patients use the lowest dose of cannabis for the most effect, as they also focus on potentiation of the ECS.

While medical cannabis education for nurses and healthcare providers is still lacking in Canada, where cannabis has been federally legal since 2018, it does have a system in place for distributing cannabis to veterans and supporting their safe and effective use of medical cannabis. The Government of Canada and Veterans Affairs Canada (VAC) have around 29,000 veterans receiving medical cannabis (Veterans Affairs Canada, 2025). There are federally licensed providers of medical cannabis, with the limits for reimbursement of 3 grams of reimbursable cannabis per day enforced. In 2023-2024, they spent over $200,000,000 on providing medical cannabis for veterans (Veterans Affairs Canada, 2025). This shows Canada's commitment to providing cannabis for those who have suffered because of their service to others. This process should be at the forefront of every country when cannabis becomes federally legalized.

Cannabis Care in Israel

Cannabis in Israel has been decriminalized for personal use in private settings by adults 18 years and older, and medical cannabis use in Israel has been legal since 1992 (Aviram, 2025). Cannabis in Israel is regulated by the Israeli Ministry of Health, the Israeli Medical Cannabis Unit (IMCU), the drug enforcement unit, and the Ministry of Public Security, with physician organizations, patient groups, and grower/business companies all influencing the regulatory space.

The IMCU provides specific regulatory guidelines around cumulative medical cannabis quantity allowances and the permitted use of medical cannabis products (generally dried herb for vaporizing/ smoking at 94% of all products, oil extracts at 5% of all products, and metered dose inhalation at 0.5% of all products) (Avarim, 2025). Medical cannabis product sales are tracked, and as a nation, Israel currently has around 129,000 licensed medical cannabis users, and approximately 94 doctors are authorized to issue medical cannabis licenses directly to their patients. There is a doctor-approved gram-per-month limit on medical cannabis licenses (e.g., 30-100 grams per month) and the doctor must approve any change in dose or product. One of the four government HMO pharmacies provides cannabis, and cannabis flower is the most likely to be approved by the doctor for consumption. Patients tend to purchase 81-92% of their approved monthly gram allotment, and the government works to control prices. The majority of medical cannabis patients in Israel are male (62%) (Aviram). Having a national system that tracks, supports, and monitors medical cannabis patients could be a step toward defining the benefits of medical cannabis consumption. However, the Israeli government does not release medical cannabis patient outcomes data, stating that this would impact patient confidentiality.

Just as in the US, nurses and nursing students have very little knowledge of medical cannabis and find it challenging to provide education and support to patients, even as patients are showing more interest in medical cannabis and asking nurses and students for information; survey data shows that over 90% of nursing students in Israel do not have any formal academic training on the subject (Kozlov et al., 2025). In response to the lack of education for nurses about medical cannabis, registered nurse Irit Avisar founded the Israeli Medical Cannabis Nurses Association and Avisar Medical Cannabis Health Center (2020), where nurses are taught to be "cannabis nurses" at 3 different schools of nursing. The cannabis nurse follows and supports the patient throughout their treatment. In many ways, this model appears to be similar to working as a patient navigator. Cannabis nurses in Israel may adjust medical cannabis products and treatment, adjust doses and chemovars used, manage the patient's regular medical follow-up, and refer patients to doctors as needed. This private organization has trained hundreds of nurses to work directly with medical cannabis patients and guide them through their medical needs (Avisar Medical Cannabis Health Center, 2020). Pharmacies may also employ cannabis nurses to support patient education. The nurses may partner with research groups such as Tikun Olam and MedReleaf.

The Israeli model of cannabis care from nurses is effective in many ways because of the small size of Israel, having a population of around 10 million, with relatively few medical cannabis patients (around 129,000), and the national nature of the medical cannabis program. Like in the US, there is a lack of medical cannabis education, and patients still face many challenges, including limited availability of chemovars and products, a sometimes lengthy bureaucratic process, and the cost of medical cannabis. Cannabis nursing in Israel tends to focus more on cannabis use and guidance through the medical system, while in the US, there is a greater emphasis on caring for the health of the ECS. Both countries have noted that nursing students have positive attitudes toward medical cannabis, and that both countries' academic settings fail to provide adequate training and education around medical cannabis (Zolotov et al., 2021).

Australia's Cannabis Care

In Australia, cannabinoid therapeutics are classified on a scale, using the *Therapeutic Goods (Poisons Standard – October 2025) Instrument 2025* (SUSMP) (Australian Government, 2025), which regulates the classification of all medicines in Australia. Cannabis is either a schedule 4 (less then 0.2% THC) or a schedule 8 (greater than 0.2% THC) (Australian Government, 2025). The Therapeutic Goods Administration (TGA) regulates the quality of and access to medicines. With cannabis, there is an exception that prescribers may apply for approval to prescribe a specific cannabis medicine for a defined indication for a class of patients in their immediate care Currently, the two cannabinoid medicines registered on the Australian Registrar of Therapeutic Goods are Epidyolex (cannabidiol) (Schedule 4) and Sativex® (nabiximols) (Schedule 8). All other cannabis medicines are schedule 8, and a special access scheme exists when a prescriber can define the specific needs and cannabis requirements of the patient, via two different pathways, whether the patient is seriously ill or they have a suitable clinical justification for needing different cannabinoid medicines, such as whole plant medicines which would be unregistered (Australian Government). In Australia, cannabis (including oils, topical, capsules, and flower) may be dispensed by pharmacists in a pharmacy, and the Office of Drug Control monitors and regulates this process, from importation and cultivation to production. State and Territory laws can vary vastly from federal law, with only the Australian Capital Territory allowing for personal possession of 50 grams of cannabis, and some growing of cannabis for personal use (Australian Government, Department of Health, Disability, and Aging, Office of Drug Control, 2025).

Nurse practitioners may prescribe medical cannabis in Australia, and they must use the TGA process. The board tends to monitor these prescriptions closely; they believe the practitioner must determine which medicines are best for patients, and they may investigate practices by nurse practitioners with high prescribing rates of medical cannabis (Australian Health Practitioner Regulation Agency, 2025). Investigable practices may include issuing 10,000 medical cannabis prescriptions over 6 months, minimal time spent assessing patients including for substance use disorder and mental health issues, prescribing excessive amounts of cannabis, prescribing multiple different products for patients, and prescribing to children under the age of 18 (Australian Health Practitioner Regulation Agency).

For registered nurses, the Australian Cannabis Nurses Association (AuCNA)(2025) unveiled a *Scope of practice guideline* document. The AuCNA launched in 2023 and defined the 6 standards of cannabis nursing practice approaches, outlined below:

- Standard 1, Assessment: A complete biopsychosocial history, review of medications and allergies, defining previous therapies and medications used and their outcomes, previous substance use history/ cannabis use disorder, defining the interprofessional health team including the patient's general practitioner (GP) and allied health providers, using pertinent screening tools such as: pain scales, determine patient goals of care, providing ECS education, safe script discussion and checks, other medications used, and assessment of monthly limits with medications and/or substances taken.

- Standard 2, Care Planning: Creating patient-centered goals related to the presenting diagnosis, identifying gaps within the patient's care team, recommending/referring to healthcare providers as needed, supporting the treatment titration plan as prescribed by medical/nurse practitioners, incorporating education (administration routes, potential side effects, cost, driving, workplace testing and the endocannabinoid system), and evaluating safety and quality measures.
- Standard 3, Implementation: Identifies the administration process: ensuring that medicinal cannabis products are administered according to the ten medication rights, evaluating patients' understanding, adherence, and response to medical cannabis products, evaluating effective routes of administration, documenting outcomes, educating patients about self-care, potential adverse effects, and community resources. Nurse prescribers must ensure they comply with relevant state or territory drugs and poisons legislation and Real Time Prescription Monitoring Systems, comply with all applicable laws and codes of conduct, and maintain evidence-based practice.
- Standard 4, Evaluation: Focuses on the effectiveness of the medicinal cannabis: undergo ongoing assessment and reassessment of the patient; evaluate response to cannabis products (including dosage and frequency); monitor outcomes using evidence-based frameworks (pain and CUD scores). The cannabis nurse will adjust goals of care and care plans based on ongoing assessments and document adverse effects, cannabis use disorder risks, and therapeutic efficacy.
- Standard 5, Ethics: Practice with compassion and acknowledgment of patient choice, recognize and maintain nurse-patient professional boundaries, address risks and adverse effects of cannabis, and focus on ongoing professional education and reflection.
- Standard 6, Advocacy: Nurses must advocate for the patient's coordinated and dignified care within a larger multidisciplinary health team, ensure timely access to care, promote equitable resource allocation, identify and address systemic barriers to access and care for medicinal cannabis, and empower diverse patient populations (AuCNA, 2025).

Cannabis nurses in Australia focus on education and often work directly with patients as consultants. There is a lack of emphasis on the ECS, and self-care and holistic modalities to upregulate the ECS are not included in the standards. Just as in the other countries explored here, medical cannabis education in Australia is lacking, and the AuCNA may develop medical cannabis educational modules that would fit within a Bachelor of Nursing curriculum (Fedele, 2023).

Regardless of where cannabis care nursing occurs around the globe, nurses must practice from a place of compassion and care (Theisen & Konieczny, 2019). Self-care for nurses providing the care of others is key; we must support patients in potentiating their health, act as advocates, and do some from a place of care and compassion.

FUTURE RESEARCH

There are many challenges ahead as the cannabis care nurse of the future emerges. The end of the cannabis prohibition era means we are entering an era of cannabis regulation. There will be different cannabis care implications depending on where one lives, but some of the issues and concerns are universal. These include changes to the DEA schedule of cannabis, advocating for cannabis patients, bringing cannabis science into the nursing curriculum and educating nursing students, and addressing lingering social justice issues. This section will address each of these issues and offer recommendations for action and future research.

The DEA Schedule Conundrum

As cannabis moves out of restrictive drug enforcement schedule statutes around the globe, there are likely to be some challenges ahead for cannabis patients and nurses. In the US at the time of this writing, cannabis remains a Schedule I Drug; however, there has been movement toward it becoming a Schedule III Drug, though multiple professional healthcare and patient advocacy groups have called for de-scheduling cannabis or moving it into its own unique Schedule VI.

In the US, cannabis nurses must consider how pharmaceutical research will impact the cannabis plant; is it more likely that synthetic cannabinoids will be studied, will changes in scheduling actually create more restrictions around personal cannabis use and the ability to grow cannabis, will insurance begin to cover cannabinoid therapeutics equitably, and is cannabis likely to end up being regulated like alcohol and tobacco? In the US, will federal policy eventually override the current environment where states' rights prevail around medical and adult use cannabis access? These are questions that cannabis care nurses, professional organizations, and advocacy groups must consider.

Patients should always be a cannabis nurse's highest priority, and this means we must advocate for all patients to have access to safe, tested, affordable cannabis therapeutics. Nurses educate patients around safe and effective use of cannabis as patients are supported and coached to potentiate the health of the ECS. What does the cannabis care nurse's role look like as cannabinoid therapeutics are developed and streamlined into the healthcare system and how does it blend with allopathic care?

There is still some lack of clarity around patients being able to access medical cannabis in inpatient settings in the US because the medicine is a Schedule I drug. Some states allow patients to bring in their cannabis therapeutics and self-administer them, others do not allow for any outside cannabis, and some states have Ryan's Law, where terminal patients can access cannabis in inpatient and hospice settings, but other patients may not. Health insurance at this time minimally covers some cannabinoid therapeutic costs (i.e., dronabinol for AIDS related anorexia/ weight loss, and chemotherapy-induced nausea and vomiting, generally only after the patient has not responded to other medications and the cost must be preapproved). Cannabis care nurses need to focus on advocating for patients' rights to access cannabinoid therapeutics in an inpatient setting. Can we imagine any other doctor recommended or prescribed palliative medicine, and hospitals denying it to patients? Allowing cannabis access for terminal patients is an important step toward allowing all patients access to cannabinoids.

Future research will include cannabinoid effectiveness for specific disease processes, preventing adverse effects, and addressing public health and policy concerns. Research around the cost and effectiveness of moving cannabis to a new schedule will also be required.

Academia: Integrating Cannabis Care

To ensure nurses are prepared to meet the growing healthcare needs related to cannabis use, nurse educators must be systematically and globally integrating cannabis care into nursing education across academic, regulatory, and professional domains. This integration aligns with nursing's mandate to promote public safety, evidence-based practice, and health equity.

Cannabis care should ideally be embedded longitudinally throughout undergraduate and graduate nursing curricula rather than treated as a standalone or elective topic, however even short educational models can help to shift knowledge, attitudes, and skills (King et al., 2024). Nursing educators should ideally scaffold cannabis content across courses such as pharmacology, pathophysiology, health assessment, mental health nursing, community health, pediatrics, geriatrics, and palliative care.

Core curricular elements include bothe those mentioned in the NCSBN (2018) guidelines and a few more: Cannabis pharmacology and the endocannabinoid system therapeutic indications and limitations, contraindications and drug–drug interactions, routes of administration and dosing or self-titration principles, legal and regulatory considerations, harm reduction, ethical issues, stigma, cultural humility, patient education, advocacy, legal concerns, and interprofessional collaboration. Curricula should emphasize clinical reasoning and decision-making, and learning may be evaluated through case studies, simulations, and clinical experiences, ensuring students develop true competency and changes in knowledge, attitudes, and skills rather than mere awareness.

With this subtopic, future research will include a focus on outcomes of cannabis educational efforts. For instance, can a standardized cannabis care educational approach support shifts in nursing students' knowledge, attitudes, and skills with medical cannabis?

Alignment with NCSBN and NCLEX

In addition to including cannabis care in nursing curricula, we must consider how regulatory bodies can support nurses in acquiring this knowledge and competency. The National Council of State Boards of Nursing (NCSBN) plays a critical role in shaping nursing knowledge through licensure expectations and NCLEX test plans. To meaningfully include cannabis care, educators must explicitly map cannabis-related content to NCSBN's existing NCLEX test plans, particularly in pharmacology, medication safety, health promotion, harm reduction, and ethical concerns.

NCLEX test plans should incorporate cannabis-specific items addressing patient assessment related to cannabis use, safe cannabis administration, self-titration education, ongoing monitoring, recognition of adverse effects and interactions, patient education, harm reduction, and how nurses can support the health of the ECS through coaching around holistic modalities. NCSBN, institutions of higher learning, and accrediting bodies should support faculty development initiatives to ensure educators can teach cannabis-related content accurately and without bias. Integrating cannabis care into NCLEX licensure expectations signals its legitimacy as a nursing competency and ensures consistent national standards.

Academic accrediting organizations such as CCNE and ACEN are instrumental in shaping curricular priorities. Nurses can advance cannabis care through accreditation standards that require programs to demonstrate the inclusion of emerging therapies and public health-relevant content (including cannabis), and to encourage curricular outcomes related to evidence-based practice in evolving therapeutic areas, defining population health and substance-related health risks, and supporting ethical and legal competence. Accrediting bodies could require innovation in curriculum design that reflects contemporary healthcare realities, including state-level cannabis legalization and widespread patient use. Accreditation standards that recognize cannabis care could help normalize its place within professional nursing education rather than positioning it as fringe or optional.

The NCSBN will need to consider the effectiveness of their testing process as they research outcomes from including cannabis care content. The accrediting bodies can research how cannabis care best aligns with and supports the essentials of nursing education.

Advancing Cannabis Care as a Core Nursing Competency

Collectively, curricular reform, licensure alignment, accreditation standards, and professional advocacy establish cannabis care as a core nursing competency rather than a niche specialty, which ensures that all nurses, not only cannabis care specialists, are prepared to assess cannabis use accurately, provide unbiased, evidence-based patient education, mitigate risks and promote safety, support therapeutic use where appropriate, address stigma and health disparities related to cannabis access and use, and contribute to public health educational efforts. The current extremes in attitudes about cannabis, including stigmatization and viewing cannabis as lacking potential for harm, need to be addressed and widespread education is part of the answer to this issue. Nursing faculty can focus on researching cannabis care educational interventions, and outcomes from their own knowledge pursuits regarding medical cannabis.

Engagement of Professional Nursing Organizations

Professional nursing organizations can play a vital role in legitimizing cannabis care and advancing educational standards. This includes developing position statements and practice guidelines related to cannabis care nursing, offering continuing education and certification pathways in cannabis nursing, supporting faculty development, calling for research dissemination, best practice sharing, advocating for inclusion of cannabis content in core competencies and specialty practice standards, and promoting interdisciplinary collaboration around cannabis care policy, education, and clinical practice. Organizations like the ANA, specialty nursing associations, and the ACNA actively shape professional norms and integrate cannabis care into nursing identity and practice.

Combining forces, professional organizations can determine cannabis care knowledge deficits and how it impacts their specialty nursing organizations. Then customized cannabis educational interventions can be aligned for the given specialty area.

Cannabis Care Nursing Social Justice Issues and Advocacy

Cannabis care nursing inherently links to social justice because structural inequities, racialized enforcement, and unequal access to healthcare resources deeply embed the history, regulation, and contemporary use of cannabis (Clark, 2021a). Consistent with the ANA (2025) *Code of ethics*, which obligates nurses to advance human rights, reduce health disparities, and advocate for equitable policy, cannabis care nurses are uniquely positioned to address the ethical, legal, and social dimensions of cannabis-related health issues. Cannabis care nurses need proper advocacy preparation to address the ongoing incarceration of non-violent cannabis offenders, equity in access to cannabis care and cannabinoid therapeutics, and using a health justice lens as they address cannabis related social justice issues.

Despite widespread legalization and medicalization of cannabis across many U.S. states, thousands of individuals, including disproportionately people of color and economically marginalized populations, remain incarcerated or burdened with criminal records for nonviolent cannabis-related offenses. Our current policies around cannabis's legality and punishment for cannabis possession continue to shape health outcomes through disrupted family structures, limited access to housing and employment, and restricted healthcare access. Cannabis care nurses, as advocates for public health and community well-being, have a professional responsibility to recognize incarceration as a determinant of health and to engage in policy advocacy aimed at supporting expungement and resentencing initiatives, promoting decarceration of nonviolent cannabis offenders, reducing barriers to healthcare access for formerly incarcerated individuals, and addressing the long-term health consequences of criminalization of cannabis. By situating cannabis-related incarceration within a public health framework, nurses can shift the discourse away from punishment toward healing, rehabilitation, and social reintegration.

Social justice in cannabis care also requires addressing inequities in access to safe, regulated cannabis products and cannabis-informed education and healthcare (Clark, 2021b). Structural barriers to doing so include cost, geographic access, provider bias, lack of education, and inconsistent legal protections, which disproportionately impact marginalized populations, including rural communities, low-income patients, older adults, veterans, and communities of color. Cannabis care nurses promote equity by advocating for affordable, accessible medical cannabis programs. Cannabis care nurses should be skilled at providing culturally responsive education, supporting patient navigation, challenging stigma within healthcare systems, and supporting research that includes historically underrepresented populations (King et al, 2024). Ensuring that therapeutic cannabis is accessible and safely integrated into care aligns with nursing's commitment to health equity and patient-centered care.

We must also consider that nurses can be cannabis patients. A critically important social justice issue in cannabis care nursing is the right of nurses themselves to access cannabis for their own health and well-being (Clark, 2021b). Many nurses use cannabis legally and responsibly for conditions such as chronic pain, anxiety, PTSD, insomnia, and other stress-related disorders, which often arise from the physical and emotional demands of nursing practice. Nurses may face professional risk, stigma, or punitive employment policies even in jurisdictions where cannabis is legal. This issue raises ethical concerns related to bodily autonomy, occupational health, disability rights, and workforce sustainability. Cannabis care nurses and nursing leaders can advocate for employment policies that distinguish impairment from lawful off-duty use and use of air and evidence-based drug testing practices, with the recognition that cannabis tests do not detect on-the-job impairment, though they point toward cannabis consumption at some time. Protection for nurses using medical cannabis under provider guidance is something we must ask our state and federal legislatures to consider. Cannabis needs recognition as a legitimate therapeutic option within occupational health frameworks. Supporting nurses' access to cannabis therapeutics for healing is not only a matter of fairness, but it is also directly tied to burnout prevention, workforce retention, and nurse well-being, which are all key issues facing the profession. It's important that nurses also role model good ECS care and practice self-care. The work of advocating for policy change and leading social justice movements can easily engross us and lead to burnout. These are important efforts by cannabis care nurses, and advocacy is important to ensure that the cannabis plant remains sacred and that patients have access to safe, quality cannabinoid therapeutics.

Lastly, nurses must strive to reframe cannabis through a health justice reform lens and away from the lens of criminal justice. We must address the harms caused by prohibition-based policies, highlight the therapeutic potential of cannabis when used responsibly, advance the need for trauma-informed and culturally humble care, and advance the role of nurses as trusted advocates in shaping equitable cannabis policies at the local, state, and federal levels. Through education, research, clinical practice, advocacy, and policy engagement, cannabis care nurses can help dismantle stigma, challenge inequitable systems, and promote healing-centered approaches that honor both individual and community well-being.

Ultimately, cannabis care nursing extends beyond clinical practice into that of moral leadership. By addressing ongoing cannabis incarceration, access inequities, and the nurses' rights, cannabis care nurses embody nursing's ethical mandate to care not only for patients but to address the social conditions that shape health. In doing so, we position the nursing profession as a vital voice in advancing cannabis-related social justice in healthcare and society.

Researching the efforts of social justice and advocacy issues may proof to be more challenging, however there are ways to quantify the difference shifts in policy makes. Qualitative research can also provide data around the experience of nurses' work in the social justice and advocacy realms.

CONCLUSION

The promise of cannabis care nursing into the future is bright. Although the nursing profession faces the challenge of integrating the NCSBN (2018) essentials into nursing curricula, tools are emerging to support this process, and cannabis science integration into nursing curricula on a global scale will help to end prohibition era stigma and ensure that all nurses can support patients' safe and effective use of cannabis.

As the largest number of global healthcare providers, nurses can make a true impact on the future of cannabis care and the support patients receive. Cannabis care nurses into the future must always remember that our goals with cannabis care are to meet patients where they are at and remain patient-centered, coach patients toward successful and safe use of cannabis, and support patients' health potentiation process through ECS upregulation. The US and Canada are currently leading the way with holistic approaches to cannabis care that ensure the patient and nurse focus on ECS upregulation so that the least amount of cannabis can be used to potentiate health and avoid adverse effects. All of nursing's work with cannabis patients should be based in the foundation of *Cannabis nursing: Scope and standards of practice* (ANA& ACNA, 2024). We are called upon to be not only knowledgeable, caring, and compassionate, but also to work towards remedies for the leftover prohibition-era social justice issues that continue to be problematic. Stigma lingers, cannabis-related public health education is lacking, and nurses are the ones who can educate other healthcare professionals, legislators, policy makers, and populations to create change.

REFERENCES

American Nurses Association. (2025). *The code of ethics for nurses.* American Nurses Association.

American Nurses Association and American Cannabis Nurses Association. (2024). *Cannabis nursing: Scope and standards of practice* (1st ed.). American Nurses Association.

Australian Cannabis Nurses Association. (2025). *Nursing scope of practice guideline.* https://ausmca.org/wp-content/uploads/2025/07/ACNA-Nursing-Scope-of-Practice-Guideline-2025.pdf

Australian Government. (2025). *Therapeutic Goods (Poisons Standard—October 2025) Instrument 2025.* https://www.legislation.gov.au/F2025L01181/latest/text

Australian Government, Department of Health, Disability and Aging, Office of Drug Control. (2025). *Frequently asked questions about medicinal cannabis.* https://www.odc.gov.au/medicinal-cannabis/grow-produce-or-manufacture-cannabis-australia/frequently-asked-questions-about-medicinal-cannabis#:~:text=The%20Office%20of%20Drug%20Control%20(ODC)%20will%20assess%20all%20applications,process%20page%20of%20the%20website

Australian Health Practitioner Regulation Agency. (2025). *Medicinal cannabis prescribing.* https://www.ahpra.gov.au/Resources/Medicinal-cannabis-prescribing.aspx

Aviram, J. (2025). Medical cannabis in Israel: A comprehensive review of trends and regulations, 2011-2025. *Journal of Cannabis Research, 7*(1), 90. DOI: 10.1186/s42238-025-00344-1 PMID: 41233935

Avisar Medical Cannabis Health Center. (2020). *Educational programs.* https://www.iritavisar.co.il/en/educational-programs/

Balneaves, L. G., Watling, C. Z., Strus, J. A., Boscow, M., Davis, L., Graveline, K., Harrigan, T., Henriquez, N., Mitchell, K., & Thompson, G. (2023). Baccalaureate nursing students' knowledge, attitudes, educational needs, and use of medical and non-medical cannabis at five institutions in Manitoba, Canada: A cross-sectional analysis. *Nurse Education Today, 130*, 105955. DOI: 10.1016/j.nedt.2023.105955 PMID: 37677985

Buscemi, A., Martino, S., Scirè Campisi, S., Rapisarda, A., & Coco, M. (2021). Endocannabinoids release after osteopathic manipulative treatment. A brief review. *Journal of Complementary & Integrative Medicine, 18*(1), 1–7. DOI: 10.1515/jcim-2020-0013 PMID: 32554836

Cámpoli, M., & Mulvey, T. (2023). A path forward in nurse-led research: Turning priorities into actionable items. *The Journal of Nursing Administration*, *53*(5), 241–242. DOI: 10.1097/NNA.0000000000001277 PMID: 37098860

Canadian Nurses Association. (2022). *Non-medical cannabis: A nursing framework.* https://hl-prod-ca-oc-download.s3-ca-central-1.amazonaws.com/CNA/2f975e7e-4a40-45ca-863c-5ebf0a138d5e/UploadedImages/documents/Non_Medical_Cannabis_-_A_nursing_framework.pdf

Canadian Nurses Association. (2026). *Cannabis.* https://www.cna-aiic.ca/en/policy-advocacy/advocacy-priorities/cannabis

Canadian Nurses Protective Society. (2026). *Access to cannabis for medical purposes: What every nurse should know.* https://cnps.ca/article/access-to-cannabis-for-medical-purposes-what-every-nurse-should-know/

Cannabis Nurse Navigator. (2026). *Cannabis nurse navigator.* https://cannabisnursenavigator.com/

Clark, C. S. (2021a). The nurse's role: Providing cannabis care. In Clark, C. S. (Ed.), *Cannabis: A handbook for nurses* (1st ed., pp. 268–312). Wolters Kluwer.

Clark, C. S. (2021b). Legal, ethical, and advocacy concerns. In Clark, C. S. (Ed.), *Cannabis: A handbook for nurses* (1st ed., pp. 363–401). Wolters Kluwer.

de Melo Reis, R. A., Isaac, A. R., Freitas, H. R., de Almeida, M. M., Schuck, P. F., Ferreira, G. C., Andrade-da-Costa, B. L. D. S., & Trevenzoli, I. H. (2021). Quality of life and a surveillant endocannabinoid system. *Frontiers in Neuroscience*, *15*, 747229. DOI: 10.3389/fnins.2021.747229 PMID: 34776851

Duke University School of Nursing. (2026). Nurse innovator and entrepreneur, DNP. https://nursing.duke.edu/academic-programs/dnp-program-nursing/dnp-nurse-innovator-entrepreneur-specialty

Fedele, M. (2023). *"I'm not here to get you high": Meet cannabis nurse Deb Ronson.* Australian Nursing and Midwifery Journal. https://anmj.org.au/im-not-here-to-get-you-high-meet-cannabis-nurse-deb-ranson/#:~:text=Deb%20Ranson%20is%20a%20registered%20nurse%20and,The%20endocannabinoid%20system%20*%20Proactive%20patient%20care

Foster, D. (2021). The human endocannabinoid system. In Clark, C. S. (Ed.), *Cannabis: A handbook for nurses* (1st ed., pp. 41–114). Wolters Kluwer.

Government of Canada. (2018). *Information for healthcare professionals: Cannabis (marijuana, marihuana) and the cannabinoid.* https://www.canada.ca/content/dam/hc-sc/documents/services/drugs-medication/cannabis/information-medical-practitioners/information-health-care-professionals-cannabis-cannabinoids-eng.pdf

Gupta, S., Bharatha, A., Cohall, D., Rahman, S., Haque, M., & Azim Majumder, M. A. (2024). Aerobic exercise and endocannabinoids: A narrative review of stress regulation and brain reward systems. *Cureus, 16*(3), e55468. DOI: 10.7759/cureus.55468 PMID: 38440201

Han, B. H., Brennan, J. J., Orozco, M. A., Moore, A. A., & Castillo, E. M. (2023). Trends in emergency department visits associated with cannabis use among older adults in California, 2005–2019. *Journal of the American Geriatrics Society, 7*(4), 1267–1274. DOI: 10.1111/jgs.18180 PMID: 36622838

Jochen, A., & Holben, D. (2024). School nurse perspectives of medical cannabis policy in K-12 schools: An exploratory descriptive study. *The Journal of School Nursing: the Official Publication of the National Association of School Nurses, 40*(6), 596–607. DOI: 10.1177/10598405221136288 PMID: 36377286

King, D. D., Gill, C. J., Cadieux, C. S., & Singh, N. (2024). The role of stigma in cannabis use disclosure: An exploratory study. *Harm Reduction Journal, 21*(1), 21. DOI: 10.1186/s12954-024-00929-8 PMID: 38273362

Kolla, B. P., Hayes, L., Cox, C., Eatwell, L., Deyo-Svendsen, M., & Mansukhani, M. P. (2022). The effects of cannabinoids on sleep. *Journal of Primary Care & Community Health, 13*, 21501319221081277. DOI: 10.1177/21501319221081277 PMID: 35459406

Kozlov, G., Wacht, O., & Grinstein-Cohen, O. (2025). Attitudes and knowledge of Israeli ultra-orthodox and religious Jewish nursing students toward the use of medical cannabis. *Journal of Religion and Health, 65*(1), 538–553. DOI: 10.1007/s10943-025-02381-9 PMID: 40622610

Liu, Q., He, W., Li, M., Li, Z., & Wu, C. (2025). Mechanotransduction pathways in massage therapy: CB1/Piezo2 receptor crosstalk modulates myocellular anti-inflammatory responses. *Journal of Pain Research, 18*, 6359–6367. DOI: 10.2147/JPR.S548026 PMID: 41334362

MacDonald, I. J., & Chen, Y. H. (2021). The endocannabinoid system contributes to electroacupuncture analgesia. *Frontiers in Neuroscience, 14*, 594219. DOI: 10.3389/fnins.2020.594219 PMID: 33679287

McPartland, J. M., Guy, G. W., & Di Marzo, V. (2014). Care and feeding of the endocannabinoid system: A systematic review of potential clinical interventions that upregulate the endocannabinoid system. *PLoS One*, *9*(3), e89566. DOI: 10.1371/journal.pone.0089566 PMID: 24622769

National Center for Complementary and Integrative Health. (n.d.) *NCCIH strategic plan FY 2021–2025: Mapping the pathway to research on whole person health.* https://nccih.nih.gov/about/nccih-strategic-plan-2021-2025

National Nurses in Business Association. (2026). *History.* https://nursesbusiness.com/nnba-history/

Parmelee, R. A., & Clark, C. S. (2022). Nursing students' knowledge, attitudes, and skills regarding medical cannabis care. *Journal of Nursing Regulation, 13*(3), 13–23. DOI: 10.1016/S2155-8256(22)00082-5

Sigma Theta Tau. (2026). *Becoming a nurse entrepreneur: Online course.* https://www.sigmamarketplace.org/becoming-a-nurse-entrepreneur---online-course

Smith, P. S., & Sera, L. (2025). The cannabis-mind connection: A clinician's perspective on mental health practice, harm reduction, and racial equity. *Journal of Cannabis Research, 7*(1), 102. DOI: 10.1186/s42238-025-00360-1 PMID: 41275252

Sulak, D. (2021). *Handbook of cannabis for clinicians: Principles and practice.* W.W. Norton.

Theisen, E. (2021). Advanced practice nurse considerations. In Clark, C. S. (Ed.), *Cannabis: A handbook for nurses* (1st ed., pp. 313–362). Wolters Kluwer.

Theisen, E., & Konieczny, E. (2019). Medical cannabis: What nurses need to know. *The American Nurse, 14*(11), 6–11.

Trezza, V., Rava, A., & Feo, A. (2025). Endocannabinoids and social behavior. In Manzoni, O. J., & Trezza, V. (Eds.), *Handbook of behavioral neuroscience* (pp. 311–326). Elsevier. DOI: 10.1016/B978-0-443-13908-6.00019-0

U.S. Department of Veterans Affairs. (2024). *Whole Health Library: Botanical medicines to support healthy sleep and rest.* https://www.va.gov/WHOLEHEALTHLIBRARY/tools/botanical-medicines-healthy-sleep-rest.asp

Veterans Affairs Canada. (2025). *Cannabis for medical purposes.* https://www.veterans.gc.ca/en/about-vac/reports-policies-and-legislation/departmental-reports/cannabis-medical-purposes

Zolotov, Y., Grinstein-Cohen, O., Findley, P. A., Reznik, A., Isralowitz, R., & Willard, S. (2021). Attitudes and knowledge about medical cannabis among Israeli and American nursing students. *Nurse Education Today*, *99*, 104789. DOI: 10.1016/j.nedt.2021.104789 PMID: 33571928

ADDITONAL READING

Balneaves, L. G., Watling, C. Z., Strus, J. A., Boscow, M., Davis, L., Graveline, K., ... & Thompson, G. (2023). Baccalaureate nursing students' knowledge, attitudes, educational needs, and use of medical and non-medical cannabis at five institutions in Manitoba, Canada: A cross-sectional analysis. *Nurse Education Today*, *130*, 105955.

Clark, C. S. (2021). *Cannabis: A handbook for nurses*. Wolters Kluwer.

Finn, K., & Bakewell, B. K. (2023). Cannabis education: How providers and patients can engage in discussion. *International Journal of Legal Medicine*, *137*(5), 1439–1440. DOI: 10.1007/s00414-023-03041-x PMID: 37344584

Gray, S. (2016). *Cannabis spirituality: An explorer's guide to an ancient plant spirit*. Parker House Press.

Hendy, K., Mauri, A. I., & Creary, M. (2023). Bounded equity: The limits of economic models of social justice in cannabis legislation. *Contemporary Drug Problems*, *50*(1), 121–135. DOI: 10.1177/00914509221147133 PMID: 37502491

Sulak, D. (2021). *Handbook of cannabis for clinicians: Principles and practice*. W.W. Norton.

KEY TERMS AND DEFINITIONS

Advocacy: Public support for a particular cause or policy.

American Cannabis Nurses Association: A not-for-profit 501 (c) (3) organization whose mission is to advance excellence in cannabis nursing practice through advocacy, collaboration, education, research, and policy development.

American Nurses Association: A professional nursing organization that strives to foster high standards of nursing practice, promote a safe and ethical work environment, bolster the health and wellness of nurses, and advocate on healthcare issues that impact patients and nurses.

Cannabis Care Nursing: A specialty practice focused on the holistic care of healthcare consumers seeking education and guidance on the therapeutic use of cannabis, to support patients' safe and effective use of cannabis and potentiate their well-being.

Cannabis Nursing Certification: There is currently no recognized board certification for cannabis nursing. Nurses may obtain academic or continuing education certificates specializing in cannabis.

Equity: Equity raligns with the principles of fairness, justice, and impartiality. It involves providing resources and opportunities to level the playing field for all individuals, particularly those from historically disadvantaged or underrepresented groups. Equity's goal is to ensure that all individuals have the necessary tools and support to succeed, based on their individual circumstances and needs.

Ethics: Nursing ethics are the moral principles and values guiding nurses' conduct, decision-making, and patient advocacy, focusing on compassion, dignity, and professional integrity as defined by the *Code of ethics for nurses* (the Code) and based on core concepts like autonomy, beneficence, non-maleficence, justice, fidelity, veracity, and accountability.

Nursing Curriculum: a structured, standard-based framework of educational experiences, theoretical content, and clinical practice designed to train nurses and ensure competency. It acts as a guide for faculty, integrating learning objectives, teaching methods, and evaluation strategies to meet professional standards

Nursing Scope and Standards of Practice: The nursing scope defines the actions, procedures, and responsibilities a nurse is authorized to perform based on their license, education, and experience, generally set by state laws. Nursing standards, as outlined by the ANA, are authoritative, measurable statements describing the competent level of care and professional behavior required.

Social Justice: Is the principle that all individuals deserve equal rights, opportunities, and treatment, regardless of race, gender, sexuality, or economic status. It focuses on fostering a fair society by addressing systemic inequities, ensuring equitable distribution of resources, and promoting active participation for marginalized groups.

Chapter 2

Integrating Cannabis Therapeutics in Advanced Clinical Nursing Practice:

The Role of the Clinical Nurse Specialist (CNS)

Arun Kumar Garov
http://orcid.org/0000-0002-7541-6161
RIMT University, India

A. K. Awasthi
http://orcid.org/0000-0002-4388-4147
Lovely Professional University, India

Rachna
Dyal Singh College, India

ABSTRACT

As cannabis continues to gain recognition for its therapeutic potential, the Clinical Nurse Specialist (CNS) plays a pivotal role in guiding safe, ethical, and evidence-based integration of cannabis therapeutics into patient care. This chapter explores how CNS professionals apply advanced clinical judgment, leadership, and research-based practice to optimize outcomes for patients utilizing medical cannabis. The discussion begins by examining the pharmacological foundations of cannabinoids and their physiological mechanisms, followed by the CNS's responsibilities in patient assessment, care planning, and interprofessional collaboration. Legal and ethical implications are analyzed to ensure compliance with institutional, state, and

DOI: 10.4018/979-8-2600-2035-7.ch002

federal regulations. The chapter also emphasizes the CNS's role in staff education, policy development, and quality improvement initiatives related to cannabis use in healthcare.

INTRODUCTION

Comprising the provision of care to people in clinical settings, clinical nursing is the most fundamental and initial aspect of professional nursing practice, where healthcare systems come into contact with patient care. This field where theory meets practice allows nurses to meet the multifaceted and constantly changing needs of families, individuals and communities. With demographic shifts, technological innovations and changing disease trends, clinical nursing is now more central to providing safe, effective, patient-focused care as healthcare systems keep evolving.

Nursing has progressed from a discipline that required a lot of physical work but with minimal knowledge to a well-trained and specialized nursing profession. Initial models of care focused on providing minimal support to patients and activities to the physicians. But with the passage of time changes have occurred in the profession due to the development of medicine, education and professional regulation. Clinical nursing practice is now considered a unique field of knowledge which relies on scientific evidence, clinical skills and ethical reasoning to provide a holistic care continuum from health through illness.

Clinical Nursing is active interaction with the patient at its core. Nurses carry out assessments, discover patients' requirements for health, implement interventions, and look at outcomes immediately. Regular monitoring ensures that any clinical signs of change are identified at an early stage, complications are avoided and care is coordinated at a timely stage. The clinical nursing profession is unlike other healthcare workers that have a single point of contact with patients, but is more of a continuous and continuous engagement with the patient, that is, they involve patients mentally, socially, and emotionally in addition to physically.

Today's clinical nursing scope spans across many types of health care and rehabilitation settings, such as acute care, outpatient, community, rehabilitation and home settings. In these contexts, nurses must deal with more complex patient profiles involving multiple comorbidities, chronic conditions and-sococial issues etc. Clinician needs to be knowledgeable, flexible and think critically in this complexity.

1. CLINICAL NURSING

The word "clinical" comes from the word "clinical," which means to see and treat patients in health care settings, and "nursing," which represents a profession that cares for individuals, families and communities, maintaining or restoring their health. However, clinical nursing is more than just instances of theory being applied to practice in the real world; it's about nursing knowledge and skills working together to support and provide care to patients.

In turn, clinical nursing is the practice-oriented aspect of nursing, which involves direct patient care, clinical decision making and implementation of the evidence-based interventions. It is a place where science, the expertise of professionals and compassion for people meet and meet patient needs in an all-inclusive and responsive way.

1.1. Basic Principles of Clinical Nursing Practice

There are four principles of clinical nursing practice to guarantee that care is safe, effective, ethical and responsive to patients' needs. They offer a common sense approach to decision making and action in various clinical scenarios and allow nurses to provide optimum care within the challenging, dynamic health care environment. They are also the ethical and professional platform which may support further advanced nursing practice positions, such as the Clinical Nurse Specialist.

1.1.1. Patient-Centered Care

One of the pillars of clinical nursing practice is patient-centered care, which is based on respecting the patient's values and preferences, as well as her or his culture and experiences. Clinical nurses offer care with a holistic perspective rather than focusing solely on a disease process to the exclusion of the patient as a whole person and are actively engaged with the patient in decision-making processes about their care. This is manifested by, for example, active listening, empathy-building in communication, patient involvement in decision making, respecting patient autonomy and establishing individual care plans that meet individual needs. Clinical nursing puts the patient first, so that what is done has a purpose, socio-acceptability and is in line with patient objectives and the patient's expectations.

1.1.2. Evidence-Based Practice

Evidence-based practice is an essential part of the clinical practice of nursing, with a strong emphasis on the use of science to be most effective in patient care. This includes incorporating evidence from existing research, clinical experience and patient values into the decision-making process. CRNAs regularly review the evolving evidence, consider options in line with clinical guidelines, and design individual interventions to fit patient situation. This approach leads to greater reliability, consistency and effectiveness in care provision and less unnecessary variation and uncertainty. Evidence-based practice enables nurses to enhance the care that patients receive and to further the science of nursing.

1.1.3. Holistic Care

Holistic care is when healthcare providers understand that ill health or illness has physical, psychological, social, emotional and spiritual components. Clinical nurses use a holistic method to the assessment and care for their patients, with various aspects of health taken into account at a time. This involves being sensitive to emotional issues, family/social circumstances and taking into account spiritual needs (if applicable). Dr. Holtz's approach of seeing the patient as a whole and not just a disease warrants a discussion of the patient's overall well-being, which in turn will support the effectiveness of clinical interventions, especially in the management of chronic and/or palliative care situations.

1.1.4. Safety & Quality of Care

Safety and quality of care are key aspects of Clinical Nursing Practice and must be constantly monitored and adhered to. Nurses' role in error prevention, risk identification and safe and effective interventions is very critical. This includes adherence to clinical practice guidelines, medication safety, infection control and patient monitoring for early signs of complications. Additionally, nurses are engaged in actively participating initiatives in quality improvement to improve healthcare outcomes. People feel safe when receiving clinical care, due to the emphasis of safety and quality.

1.1.5. Ethical and Legal Practice

Ethical and legal practice is the core of the professional conduct of nurses, which affects the way nurses perform their duties. Ethical and legal practice acts as the backbone of the professional conduct of nurses that impacts the nursing process in terms of making ethical and legal decisions. Ethical principles include respect for autonomy, beneficence, nonmaleficence and justice in clinical nursing that helps to ensure the rights of patients are respected while delivering equitable care. Nurses must also follow legal protocols such as maintaining confidentiality, getting informed consent and ensuring proper documentation. Clinical nurses work with ethical thinking and also bear responsibility from a legal viewpoint, ensuring that they maintain professional integrity and trust is built in the healthcare system.

1.1.6. Accountability and Professional Responsibility

Release the responsibility and accountability of clinical nursing, nurses should be responsible for their actions and the results they bring about. These comprise clinical competence, observance of professional standards and institutional policy/ guidelines. Nurses are expected to reflect, to look at their own work continually and develop ways of improving their way of working. When nurses are held accountable, they help create safe nursing practice environments and adding to the credibility and reliability of the nursing profession.

1.1.7. Effective Communication and Collaboration

Communication and collaboration is critical to ensure coordinated, patient-centered care. Clinical nurses need to be able to communicate with clarity and precision to patients, families and health care workers. This involves education, appropriate communications of treatment plans and enabling agreement between all parties. By integrating different professions, there are better opportunities for interprofessional collaboration, thus improved care and services. Communication skills are also important in minimizing any errors, enhancing patient satisfaction and optimizing clinical outcomes.

1.1.8. Cultural Competence and Sensitivity

Providing culturally competent and culturally sensitive health care in a variety of health care settings is crucial. Clinical nurses have to be mindful of and appreciate variations in cultural beliefs, values, and health behaviors that affect people's health practices and decision making. This involves being aware of own biases and understanding needs, effective cross-cultural communication, ability to adapt care to cultural needs. When nurses shorten the time it takes to engage patients in their care, their care is culturally competent, which increases trust and adherence to treatment and ultimately decreases inequitable health outcomes.

1.1.9. Continuity and Coordination of Care

Taking care of patients securely starting from their location to clinical facility and from pre-hospital to hospital environments, is a critical matter that should be handled with continuity and coordination. One of the primary roles of clinical nurses is in the management of transition, including discharge planning, referral and after care. They make sure information is conveyed effectively, care plans stay consistent and patient-centred. The approach of delivering multi-professional care in a coordinated way, with continuity of care supports minimisation of fragmentation, avoids complications and enhances overall healthcare efficiency provided by nurses.

1.1.10. Life Long Learning and Professional Development

The process of lifelong learning and widening professional skills is part of keeping clinical nursing skills up to date. The knowledge and technologies of the healthcare field are constantly changing, thus the need for nurses to continually work at knowledge, training and skills development. This means keeping current with current research, attending professional development sessions, and being mindful of experiences in the clinic for practice improvement. From professionals to participants, the nurses are poised to make a significant contribution to good health care practices by keeping them current with new developments and up-to-date on the latest research and information.

1.2. Clinical Nursing Practice: Domains and Areas

The practice of nursing in the clinical setting involves many fields and specialized areas all of which demonstrate the diversity and complexity of healthcare delivery services. These domains form different but related areas of practice for clinical nurses to apply their knowledge, skills and professional judgement to meet specific patient needs throughout the health–illness spectrum.

Figure 1. Domains and areas of clinical nursing

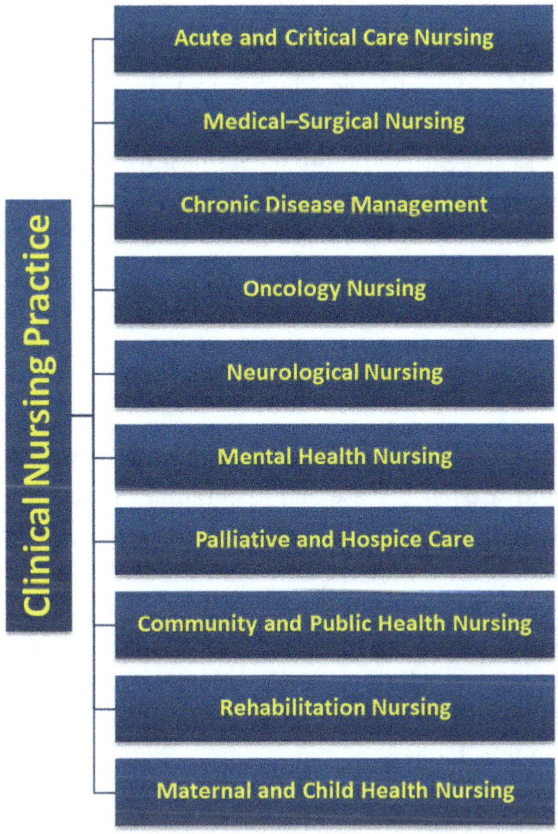
Clinical Nursing Practice
Acute and Critical Care Nursing
Medical–Surgical Nursing
Chronic Disease Management
Oncology Nursing
Neurological Nursing
Mental Health Nursing
Palliative and Hospice Care
Community and Public Health Nursing
Rehabilitation Nursing
Maternal and Child Health Nursing

1.2.1. Acute and Critical Care Nursing

This is a specialty of the nursing field devoted to the care of patients who have life-threatening or erratically changing health issues. The different kinds of nurses in this domain function in situations where they have to track continuously and take quick action, such as in emergency departments, intensive care units and trauma centers.

Advanced assessment of patients, hemodynamic monitoring, complex therapy administration orühl quick response to clinical deterioration are clinical duties. Timeliness and accuracy in decision making are of utmost importance, since failing to act in a prompt and appropriate manner, or making a wrong decision may affect patient results. Acute and critical care nurses also work closely with members of a multidisciplinary team to help stabilize patients and aid their recovery.

1.2.2. Medical–Surgical Nursing

Medical–surgical nursing is one of the general and comprehensive clinical nursing practice fields. Care for older people who have a very wide range of longterm and short-term illnesses and also are undergoing operations.

Nurses here undo and check for complications after surgery, give medicine and teach education to patients before and after surgery. The domain demonstrates the need for a high level of clinical judgment, flexibility and being able to manage a large number of patients of different levels of complexity. Medical-Surgical may be a stepping stone for specialization in other clinical nursing fields.

1.2.3. Chronic Disease Management

Chronic disease management involves managing chronic diseases like diabetes, hypertension, cardiovascular disease and respiratory disease for a period of time. This domain is focused on continuity of care, symptom management and lifestyle changes rather than acute care.

Patients receive patient education, self-management support and care being coordinated across providers in a significant role by clinical nurses. The aim is to enhance quality of life, avoiding complications and minimizing the need for re-admission to hospital. Good communication skills and a patient caring approach to care is important in this domain.

1.2.4. Oncology Nursing

Oncology nursing consists of caring for cancer patients at all stages of the disease. In this practice area, nurses oversee the care of multiple treatment modalities, such as chemotherapy, radiation, and immunotherapy, and they care for patients' physical and psychosocial needs.

Central care roles include managing symptoms, managing pain, patient education and emotional support of patients and their families. Oncology nurses also need to be vigilant to track down any side effects due to treatment and organize cooperative efforts with the multidisciplinary oncology team. A particular level of expertise will be needed in this area and a caring attitude to care will be required.

1.2.5. Neurological Nursing

Neurological is a nursing specialty of patients who have neurological disorders like stroke, epilepsy, multiple sclerosis, and other neurological disorders. Within this domain there is a need to have an understanding of complex neurological evaluations, and the ability to keep track of cognitive and motor dysfunctions following them.

Nurses deliver care that is focused on the stabilization of neurological function, prevention of complications and support for rehabilitation. Patient education and family support are essential processes to the program—many neurological diseases require long-term adaptations and management.

1.2.6. Mental Health Nursing

Mental health nursing involves care of the patient when they are affected by mental illness, including depression, anxiety, schizophrenia and drug misuse. The role of a nurse in this domain is in the inpatient and community context, and involves therapeutic support and crisis intervention.

Part of these roles is to perform mental health evaluations, implement therapeutic interventions, dispense medication and promote recovery and resilience. Communication skills and empathy are key for fostering patient engagement in the development of trust.

1.2.7. Palliative and Hospice Care

Palliative and hospice care is a care that is centered on enhancing the quality of life of those whose disease or illness is serious and life-threatening. This focus is on comfort, symptom management and patient and family care.

Clinical nurses manage pain, emotional distress, and spiritual or personal concerns and support end of life decision-making. Sensitivities towards patients' preferences, dignity and compassion in delivering care. Some situations in this domain involve communicating effectively and having emotional resilience.

1.2.8. Community and Public Health Nursing

Community and public health nursing takes care beyond the patient to the population and community. This domain primarily relates to health promotion and prevention of disease and relates to social determinants of health.

Nurses practice in a variety of environments including community health centers, schools, and public health agencies and implement programs to enhance the population's health outcomes. Health education, screening, immunization efforts and community outreach are among responsibilities.

1.2.9. Rehabilitation Nursing

Rehabilitation nursing is concerned with the recovering and functional independence of patient(s) from illness and injury. This domain has special relevance to a patient who has a disability, needs to recuperate from an operation or suffers from chronic disease that impacts mobility.

The nurses work in partnership with physiotherapists, occupational therapists and other professionals in the development and implementation of rehabilitation plans. Motivation and educational counseling of patients play a significant role in the modern rehabilitation.

1.2.10. Maternal and Child Health Nursing

Maternal and child health nursing is nursing that cares for the health of women in the process of pregnancy, delivery and after birth, and of infants and children. This domain aims to foster good development and minimise problems.

Clinical nurses offer antepartum teaching, help with the birth process and deliver neonatal and pediatric care. This includes a focus on family-centered care, including forgiveness education and caregiver support.

2. ADVANCED CLINICAL NURSING PRACTICE

Advanced Clinical Nursing Practice refers to the level of nursing practice that is more advanced than the basic clinical practice, and it involves specialized knowledge, advanced clinical skills and a higher degree of autonomy in the care of patients. Requires the skills to evaluate, diagnose and treat health problems, frequently in a specialty.

Advanced practice nurses should:

- Apply in-depth clinical knowledge
- Take independent/cooperative clinical decisions
- Delivery of lead care services are led.
- Use evidence of research to inform practice

Advanced education and training (postgraduate or doctoral-level) and adherence to advanced education standards and regulations will normally provide the necessary level of practice.

2.1. Advanced Clinical Nursing Practice (ACNP) Characteristics:

The five key characteristics of Advanced Clinical Nursing Practice (ACNP), that advanced clinical nursing practice apart from the traditional clinical nursing practice.

1. **Advanced Clinical Expertise:** Practitioners have an advanced clinical expertise in assessing, diagnosing and managing complex patient conditions. They can deal with uncertainty, understand complex clinical information and make decisions in challenging circumstances.
2. **Expanded Scope of Practice:** Based on the regulations and laws, advanced practice nurses can also carry out the functions of other medical professionals, including writing prescriptions, ordering diagnostics tests and drawing up comprehensive treatment plans.
3. **Autonomy and Accountability:** Advanced practice nurses have autonomy to make independent clinical decisions, and are held accountable for patient outcomes. It is an autonomy that is counterbalanced by respect for ethical and professional standards.
4. **Leadership and Influence:** Advanced clinical nurses have leadership and influence roles in shaping clinical practice, mentoring others, and shaping healthcare policy and procedure. They help to enhance care provision at the level of the patient and of the system.
5. **Evidence Based and Research Oriented Practice:** Research is emphasized in a strong manner related to clinical practice. Advanced practitioners critically analyze evidence, engage in research and contribute to the development of knowledge.

The advanced clinical nursing practice is a combination of clinical, professional and system-level competencies, as illustrated in Figure 2.

Figure 2. Competencies of advanced clinical nursing practice

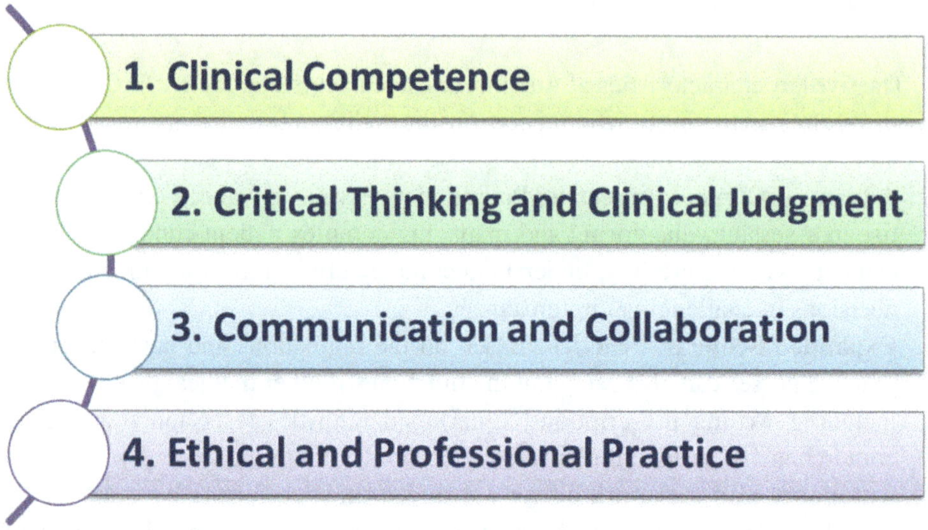

What are the key domains of advanced clinical nursing practice and how they work?

Advanced Clinical Nursing Practice is not just about clinical nursing, it also involves several areas of activity, all of which contribute to improving the quality of healthcare, to evidence-based practice and to supporting healthcare systems. The domains are intended to highlight the complex role of the advanced practice nurse, specifically the Clinical Nurse Specialist (CNS), in meeting the health care needs of patients and in impacting practice environments and the ability of organizations to meet their goals. See Figure 3, for the advanced clinical nursing practice primary domains.

Figure 3. Primary domains of advanced clinical nursing practice

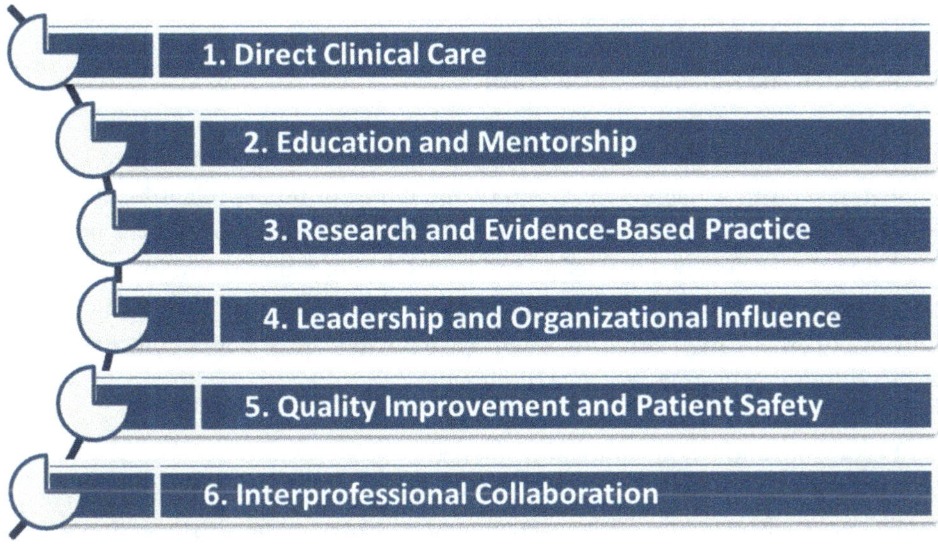

These are considered as areas of importance and if combined constitute the entire breadth of advanced practice nursing.

1. Direct Clinical Care

Advanced nursing practice is primarily directed toward the care of patients with complex, multifaceted health problems, and to direct clinical care. APNs use advanced assessment skills and knowledge to diagnose, plan, and put in place individualized care strategies. This domain covers the coordination of care with complex symptom patterns and involves care in the high-risk patient. Advanced practitioners also act in a role as experts and consultants for other healthcare practitioners, to assist them with decision making and to encourage the best possible practice of patient care.

2. Education and Mentorship

Advanced practice nurses play a significant role in advancing nursing practice and knowledge by providing education and mentorship in various areas. They participate in formal and informal education of nursing staff, patients, families and other health care professionals in this role. They plan and facilitate learning and training activities, and advocate skill acquisition and life-long learning in a clinical setting. The mentorship program can be used to help develop less experienced nurses, assist with clinical competence, and advance reflective practice, which in turn can help improve overall quality of nursing care.

3. Research and Evidence-based Practice

Research and evidence-based practice is an integral part of advanced clinical nursing, and ensures that care is based on the most up-to-date scientific evidence. APNs critically evaluate research findings, apply research to clinical practice, and help to produce new knowledge and research. They are vital to the process of converting research into practice and connecting theory and clinical practice. This domain provides a foundation for ongoing improvement of patient outcomes and further development of the science of nursing.

4. Leadership and Organizational Influence

An important attribute of advanced clinical nursing practice is leadership. Here, nurses have an impact on clinical practice and on guiding teams and participate in organizational decision-making. They create policies, establish practice standards and promote the improvement of healthcare delivery. Advanced practice nurses also are responsible for driving innovation in patient care, staff education and organization of resources to maximize their effectiveness. Their leadership is not just in the care of individual patients but also in the system.

5. Quality Improvement and Patient Safety

Quality improvement and patient safety are essential domains where they concentrate on improving health care outcomes and reduce risk in health care. APNs organize, execute and monitor quality improvement projects to promote health and clinical practice. They try to figure out what's missing and find solutions based on data and they track the impact of their interventions. The focus of this domain is on a proactive safety approach, making sure that care delivery is reliable, efficient and adheres to best practice.

6. Interprofessional Collaboration

The need for interprofessional working is crucial in providing integrated and coordinated health care. APNs collaborate with physicians, pharmacists, therapists and other health care professionals to develop and implement integrated care plans. They help to communicate, mediate conflict between team members, and ensure the continuity of patient care and patient-centered care. This 'whole of government' strategy not only boosts care quality and outcomes for patients, but also facilitates care delivery.

2.2. Types of Advanced Practice Nursing Roles

Advanced Practice Nursing is a collection of advanced clinical practice positions which build upon the basic clinical nursing functions to incorporate advanced clinical skills, leadership, education, and systems influence. These positions aim to address the growing complexity in healthcare by ensuring provision of high quality, evidence based and patient-centred care in a variety of settings. While there are differences in roles, skills, and emphasis among the advanced practice positions, there are commonalities based on advanced education, clinical knowledge, and advanced professional practice. There are several different advanced practice nursing roles, as illustrated in Figure 4.

Figure 4. Advanced practice nursing roles

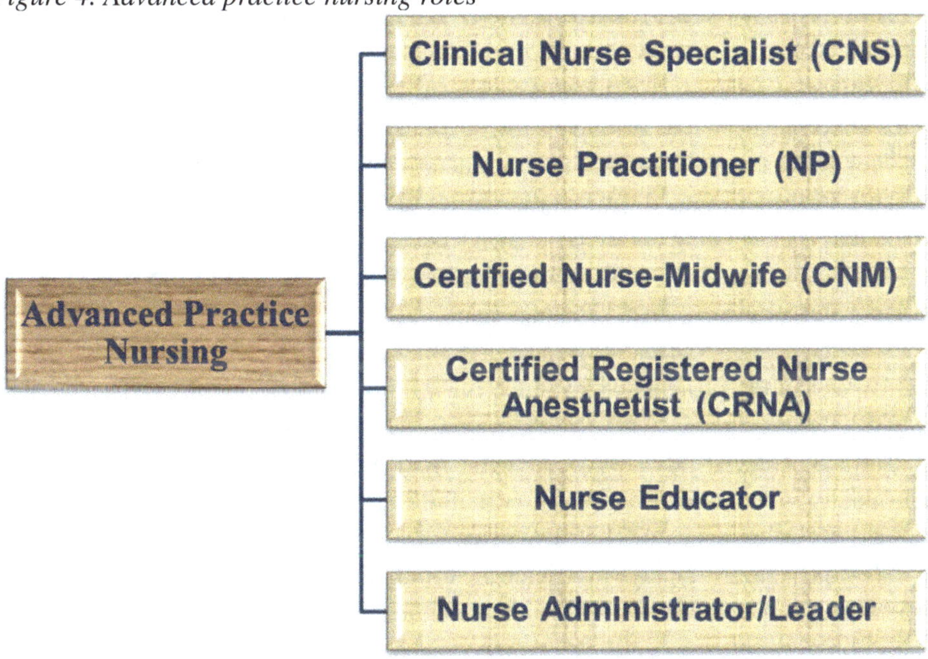

All of these roles help to reduce mortality, improve the quality of health care and bolster health care systems that improve patient outcomes.

2.2.1. Clinical Nurse Specialist (CNS)

The Clinical Nurse Specialist is a vital role that is a fully-licensed Advanced Practice Nurse with an expertise in a specific area of advanced clinical practice, e.g., oncology, cardiology, critical care. CNS's special function is to partner with patients, families and health care systems to optimize patient/client outcomes via direct clinical care, consultation, education, and systems change interventions.

CNSs use the empirical knowledge gained from research to support their practice within various areas of their jobs, such as patient care, nursing practice and organizational systems. They act as clinical specialists, mentors and leaders, influencing policy and practice standards and working with teams of health care practitioners to lead. These agents, in particular, can play a significant role in the clinical implementation of complex and new therapeutics.

2.2.2. Nurse Practitioner (NP)

The role of a Nurse Practitioner involves delivering high-level treatment for acute/short-term and chronic disease conditions, which can include diagnostics ordered, medication prescribed, and advanced clinical treatment. NPs practice in different types of settings, such as primary care, specialty clinics, and hospitals.

They focus on patient-centered care, health promotion and disease prevention. Because of the shortage of primary care providers, in underserved communities in particular, NPs are able to deliver primary care, thereby helping to enhance access to health services. They work both in a clinical capacity and in the education of patients and long-term health management.

2.2.3. Certified Nurse-Midwife (CNM)

Certified Nurse-Midwives focus their practice on the care of women across the reproductive life span and are experts in childbirth and the postpartum period, as well as gynecological care. They also offer family planning and preventive services.

CNMs essentially engage in service provision that supports natural and safe birth experiences and ensure that appropriately medical interventions are made available. Their holistic approach centers on women and families, patient education and care. They contribute significantly to: "Maternal and neonatal outcomes".

2.2.4. Certified Registered Nurse Anesthetist (CRNA)

Advanced practice nurses, or Certified Registered Nurse Anesthetists, specialize in a specific field of advanced practice – the administration of anesthesia and the care of patients before, during, and after surgical and medical procedures. These can be in operating rooms, critical care units or pain management areas.

CRNAs take responsibility for pre-anesthetic evaluation, anesthetic induction, maintenance, monitoring and post-anesthetic care. They are expected to have a high degree of technical skill, accuracy and decision making ability. Productivity and care safety will be key contributors of their practice and outcomes.

2.2.5. Nurse Educator

Nurse Educators specialize in the education and training of other nurses, nursing students, and other health care professionals. They work in academies, health care, and training centres.

They plan, teach, evaluate, enhance and champion Learning Outcomes, and advocate evidence-based teaching practice. Nurse educators are in a key position to prepare nursing students for the future of nursing and to prepare future nurses to fulfill the health care needs and changing demands of the future.

2.2.6. Nurse Administrator/Leader

A Nurse Administrator or a Nurse Leader manages healthcare organisations, departments or units. They do strategic planning, coordinate resources, develop policies and lead nursing teams.

They are dedicated to strengthening the operation of the organization, quality of care and the positive working climate. Nurse leaders make a difference at a system level, establishing alignment between clinical goals, and operational goals.

3. CLINICAL NURSE SPECIALIST (CNS)

The Clinical Nurse Specialist (CNS) is a highly educated nurse with a deep foundation of knowledge and expertise in a particular clinical specialty. The CNS role aims to enhance patient care by utilizing clinical practice skills, consultation, education, research, and leadership. While some advanced practice positions may be deliverers of direct, individual patient care, CNS work in a variety of aspects beyond patient care, impacting on the practice of nursing and the healthcare delivery system.

The three streams of influence of the CNS as described in the National Association of Clinical Nurse Specialists's position statement are patient, nursing staff, and the health care system. In the patient realm, CNSs deliver high-quality clinical work for more complex patients, with interventions guided by evidence and the patient's needs. In the nuts and bolts of medical practice, they supervise and instruct nurses, ensuring that they cultivate their abilities and adhere to best practices. CNSs work across the system in the areas of: Policy development, quality improvement initiatives and implementing evidence-based protocols.

An aspect of the CNS role that is unique is their focus on integration and the translation of the knowledge into practice. CNSs fill the gap between research and clinical practice by critically evaluating evidence and take appropriate action to increase the quality of care delivery. They serve as consultants and change agents, guiding healthcare teams in managing complex clinical situations and adopting innovative practices.

CNS's be distinguished and display excellent leadership and communication abilities. They work with interdisciplinary teams, provides guidance for decision making processes, and patient-centered care advocacy. They are especially valuable in special, knowledge- and coordination-intensive situations like chronic disease care management, critical care, and novel therapeutic interventions.

3.1. Types of Clinical Nurse Specialists

CNSs are classified by their patient population, their clinical setting and/or their area of specialization. This classification enables CNS to acquire specific expertise and provide very specialized care corresponding to the needs in healthcare. The major types of Clinical Nurse Specialists as, follows Figure 5.

Figure 5. Types of clinical nurse specialists

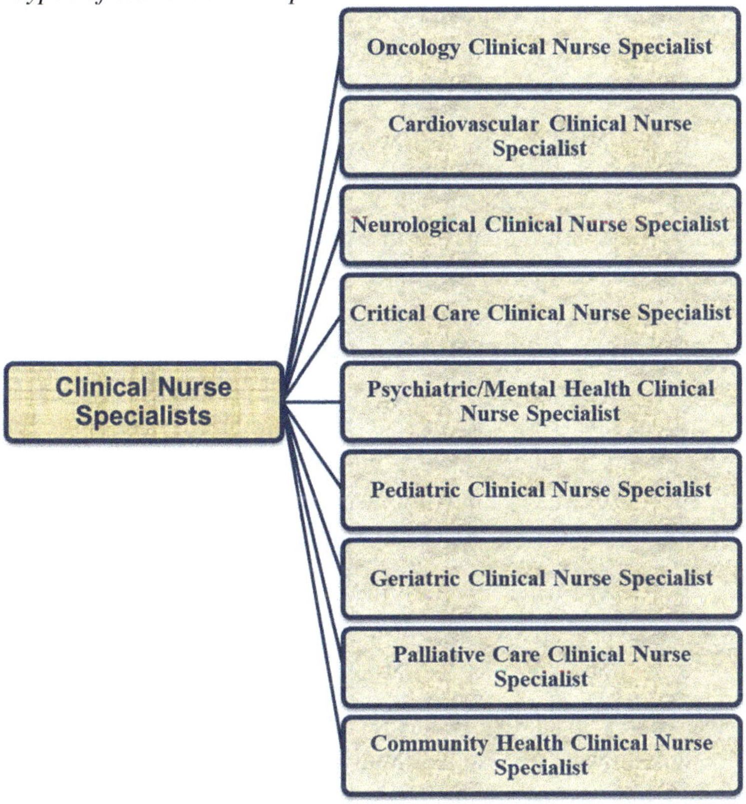

3.1.1. Oncology Clinical Nurse Specialist

Oncology CNSs have expertise in the management of cancer patients, their education, and treatment support while focusing on symptom management. They help coordinate care plans that are often complicated, such as chemotherapy or immune therapy and care for the psychological and emotional support for patients and their families. They additionally play a role in coordinating multi-disciplinary care and enhancing oncology care protocols.

3.1.2. Cardiovascular Clinical Nurse Specialist

Cardiovascular CNSs specialize in patients with heart-related diseases like coronary artery disease, heart failure and hypertension. They are very important for disease control, patient education and prevention measures. These experts also play a vital role in helping to ensure that clinical results of cardiovascular care measures are enhanced, through the application of evidence-based cardiovascular care practices.

3.1.3. Neurological Clinical Nurse Specialist

These are CNSs who take care of any patient who has a disorder involving the nervous system such as a stroke, epilepsy, and neurodegenerative disorders. They conduct sophisticated neurological testing and aid in the rehab process, and they educate patients and families on the long-term management of the disease.

3.1.4. Critical Care Clinical Nurse Specialist

CNSs in critical care work with patients who have life-threatening conditions in high acuity care units or intensive care units (ICU). They offer clinical advice and information, speed up decision making, and guarantee compliance with the latest clinical protocols. They are an important component to increasing the chances of patient survival and recovery.

3.1.5. Psychiatric/Mental Health Clinical Nurse Specialist

Psychiatric CNS's specialize in mental illness with signs and symptoms such as depression, anxiety and critical psychiatric illnesses. They offer therapeutic services, assist with medication management and in the development of mental health programs. They also play a role in the advancement of mental health awareness and the prevention of mental health stigma.

3.1.6. Pediatric CNS

Pediatric CNSs are those who specialize in the care of infants, children and adolescents. They consider the developmental, physiological and psychological needs that are different from older children and puppies, and liaise with families to provide their child with the best possible care.

3.1.7. Geriatric Clinical Nurse Specialist

Geriatric CNSs specialize in providing care for older adults, taking care of chronic condition management, functional decline and age-related problems, etc. They focus on full evaluation, reducing falls, and treatment of multiple comorbidities.

3.1.8. Palliative Care Clinical Nurse Specialist

These professionals have expertise in the care of the patient with a serious and life-threatening disease. Their emphasis is on the treatment of symptoms, pain control and enhancing quality of life. They also provide guidance and assistance to patients and families in the end of life decisions.

3.1.9. Community Health Clinical Nurse Specialist

Community health CNS works at the population level engaging in disease prevention, health promotion and social determinants of health (SDOH). They plan and take part in community-based activities and support community health projects.

3.2. Core Competencies and Scope of Practice of the Clinical Nurse Specialist (CNS)

The Clinical Nurse Specialist (CNS) is an advanced practice nurse with a unique blend of expert clinical knowledge, leadership and system-level influence. A shared core group of competencies and a wide spectrum of healthcare duties and opportunities underlie the effectiveness of the CNS in enhancing patient outcomes and healthcare delivery (Fulton et al., 2014). These are the types of skills that allow CNS to fit multiple roles and function in all three areas: clinical, educational, research, and organizational leadership, while tackling complex healthcare issues.

3.2.1. Advanced Clinical Expertise

High level clinical experience is the base for CNS. CNSs have a deep expertise in a specific specialty area, which allows them to share their knowledge with patients and to provide expert advice around complex patient conditions or quality of care issues. They carry out advanced assessments, understand the diagnostic data, and manage to prepare comprehensive care plans for each patient. Their skills enable them to handle complex clinical scenarios, foresee problems, and provide solutions that will be effective. Beyond patient care, CNSs can also provide clinical support to other healthcare providers, promoting best practice and elevating the quality of care.

3.2.2. Evidence-Based Practice and Knowledge Translation

The characteristics, or competency, of the CNS is the ability to incorporate research evidence in their clinical practice. CCNS's analyze scientific literature, determine what is relevant to the situation and use the relevant information to improve patient care. They will not only be able to summarize evidence but also be actively involved in knowledge transfer from research to practice. This includes creating clinical guidelines, establishing evidence-based protocols and evaluating outcomes to ensure effectiveness. In these activities, CNSs help to move towards continually improving quality of healthcare and progressing nursing practice.

3.2.3. Leadership and Change Management

The CNS role places leadership high on the agenda and one component of this is related to traditional supervisory roles besides its impact on influencing clinical practice and leading organizational change. CNSs spearhead projects to advance patient care, optimize care delivery and process, and introduce new practices. They support change by bringing multiple stakeholders together, overcoming obstacles and fostering an innovative and accountable environment. They are able to lead teams, contribute to decision making, and make changes that will be sustainable and relevant to the organization's objectives through their leadership skills.

3.2.4. Education and Mentorship

Education and mentorship are essential skills that can be utilized by CNSs to facilitate the development of nursing personnel and help to enhance clinical practice. CNSs plan and present educational programs, offer training to new technology, treatments and guidance for nurses to advance their skills and confidence. They also provide education and empowerment of patients and families, allowing them to take an active role in their treatment. CNSs play a vital role in a culture of learning and professional development, which supports a knowledgeable and competent health care staff.

3.2.5. Thinking in Systems and With Organizational Influence

CNSs are part of a complex health care system and should be able to grasp the intereference among its components and how that interaction relates to patient outcomes. When their systems thinking skills help them to see these gaps in care, they are better able to look at a process, to analyze it and then to make it better at the organizational level. They work in multidisciplinary and interdisciplinary groups with administrators and policy makers to formulate strategies to improve efficiency, augment quality, and better assure patient safety. They have the power to shape systems, which can create a wider impact on healthcare delivery showing changes in practice.

3.2.6. Ethical and Legal Decision-Making

Ethical and legal knowledge is a critical component to dealing with the complex issues of clinical practice. All decisions made by CNSs are subject to patient rights, legal obligations and professional ethical guidelines. They resolve ethical issues, speak up for both at risk and vulnerable populations and ensure care is delivered with integrity and fairness. They also have a role to play in making sure that the company is compliant with the rules, that the documentation is accurate and they promote accountability in the clinical practice.

3.3. CNS Scope

The CNS scope of practice is extensive and covers various levels of health care delivery. It goes beyond the patient care to what affects nursing practice and the healthcare system.

1. **Patient-Level Practice:** At the patient level, CNSs deliver high-quality clinical care for people with complex health care needs. They deliver more comprehensive evaluations, create care plans and oversee progress and evaluate outcomes. They are dedicated to enhancing patients' health, safety and quality of life.
2. **Nursing Practice-Level Influence:** At the practice level, CNSs strive to improve the competency and performance of nurses. They provide training, guidance, and mentorship, helping to ensure that nurses follow evidence-based practice. They are also involved with developing clinical guidelines and protocols.
3. **System-Level Impact:** At the system level, CNSs influence organizational policies, quality improvement initiatives, and healthcare delivery processes. They recognize inefficiencies, make changes and assess results to enhance overall system performance. All their work is aimed at creating safer, efficient, and patient-centered healthcare system.

Relationship between competencies and Scope: The competencies and scope of practices of CNS are well related. Leadership and systems thinking contribute to broader impact and advanced clinical expertise to patient care. Through education and mentorship, knowledge is shared and through the implementation of evidence-based practice, knowledge is improved continuously. These elements all together contribute to a comprehensive framework which defines the CNS role and its contribution in healthcare.

4. EMERGING AND COMPLEMENTARY THERAPEUTIC MODALITIES IN CLINICAL PRACTICE

In the contemporary setting, a greater consideration of a diverse range of therapeutic modalities that go beyond biomedical therapy is increasingly being witnessed. Although conventional medicine is pivotal to delivering care, there is appreciation for the growing importance of complementary and alternative or emerging medicines, in helping to meet the needs of people with complex, chronic and multifactorial health conditions. This represents a shift towards a more holistic, patient-centred change in each individual's care model that looks at the treatment of the disease as well as treatment and more broadly the care of the person and their quality of life.

4.1. Evolution of Therapeutic Modalities: From Traditional to Emerging Approaches

Therapeutic modalities in healthcare can be seen as a continuum from traditional healing practices to a very advanced, and evidence-based, clinical intervention. This has evolved to show increased treatment options for healthcare providers such as advanced practice nurses.

4.1.1. Traditional Therapeutic Approaches

Traditional therapies are ancient and widespread method of medicine that have a rich history, cultural and experiential context. Such methods tend to have an approach that focuses on natural healing, balance and overall good health. This may involve herbal medicine, yoga and meditation, and other mind – body practices. Previously known as alternative, many therapies have come to be known for their benefits in maintaining stress, chronic pain or lifestyle-related issues.

4.1.2. Complementary and Integrative Therapies

The treatments are also complemented with additional remedies and methods, such as complementary medicine, to further improve outcomes. Integrative approaches can be used to treat a patient using a combination of evidence-based complementary therapy methods and conventional medical treatment. There are several treatment modalities such as nutrition measures, physical measures, and psychosocial measures.

These therapies are safely and effectively used in clinical practice, especially in advanced levels taking into account the patient's needs, safety, and evidence. APNs assess effectiveness, usage and incorporate them in individualized care plans.

4.1.3. Emerging and Evidence-Based Therapeutic Interventions

Emerging therapies are new developments in the field of health, which are the result of scientific studies, technological innovations and patient expectations. Such interventions may feature novel mechanisms of action, novel drugs or novel techniques of application of the drug. These types of therapies generally involve:

- Increasing scientific validation
- Expanding clinical applications
- Growing regulatory recognition
- To engage in the mainstream care system

They have a special application in those regions where traditional treatments might be limited, for instance in chronic pain management, neurological disorders, mental health problems, and palliative options.

4.2. Classification of Therapeutic Modalities in Clinical Practice

With the growing variety of health care, it is essential to develop a framework of knowledge of various health care modalities for managing patients. The classification of therapeutic modalities offers a framework for organizing, measuring and assimilating various therapeutic modalities together. In the case of advanced practice nurses (APN), especially Clinical Nurse Specialists (CNS), this classification, if not vital for clinical decision making, does play an important role in ensuring patient safety and is important for integrating traditional and new treatments into clinical practice (Fulton & Holly, 2021).

In clinical practices therapeutic modalities can be broadly discussed according to their source, their mode of action and function in health care. These can be conventional (biomedical), complementary and integrative therapies or emerging/original therapy interventions. Every unique answer to treatment is a different "category" and each one has a distinct contribution to make towards full-care treatment.

1) Conventional (Biomedical) Therapies
2) Complementary and Integrative therapies
3) Emerging and Novel Therapeutic Interventions
4) Bioactive and Botanical Therapies

4.2.1. Conventional (Biomedical) Therapies

Traditional medicines are the backbone of healthcare today and are based on scientific evidence, clinical trials and a set of medical practices. These solutions involve drugs, surgeries and high tech diagnostics and therapeutics. They're commonly established, widely accepted and evidence based.

In the clinical practice of nursing, conventional therapies play a crucial part in the care of patients, especially during acute and critical care situations. The effectiveness of clinical services depend on nurses to provide much work in the provision of medication, checking on their response to treatment and ensuring adherence to clinical services. Although tried and tested treatments have proven to be effective, there is some potential that they may not be successful in the long term, in chronic disorders, or with individual patients, and this can cause them to look for alternative methods of therapy.

4.2.2. Complementary and Integrative therapies

Complementary therapies support conventional treatment strategies and promote patients' health and well-being. Integrative therapies bring together evidence-based complementary treatments and conventional medicine for a more holistic treatment model. One of the common treatments in these therapies concentrate on helping the body's natural healing processes, and on psychological, emotional and social aspects of health.

These can range from mind–body practices, nutrition therapy, physical therapy, and relaxation therapy. These practices are becoming common place in the clinical nursing practice to plan and implement such as pain, stress, anxiety and fatigue conditions. APNs review the suitability of these therapies to ensure their safety, evidence-based and patient preference.

4.2.3. Emerging and Novel Therapeutic Interventions

The rising therapeutic approaches are a dynamic field of the health sector as research studies in science, biotechnology and the physiology of the human body have advanced. New drugs, novel treatments and the repurposing of old drugs using new scientific strategies may all be part of these breeding blocks.

In particular, emerging therapies are key for complex and challenging situations such as chronic pain, neurological diseases, mental health and palliative care. The implementation of such measures into clinical practice should be critically assessed, taking into account regulations and follow-up and follow back of patient results.

4.2.4. Bioactive and Botanical Therapies

In the field of emerging therapies, plant-based and biologically active therapies hold a special place and are also quite promising. The modalities are the use of compounds from a natural source which have an effect on physiological systems and result in beneficial therapeutic effects. Many of these therapies have a history in traditional medicine, and are currently being studied and proven by modern scientific research.

Often these interventions have multifaceted mechanisms of action, have a complex action involving multiple physiological pathways and could have potential value in symptom management and the modulation of the disease process. They are increasingly used in clinical practice and are increasingly included as part of models of integrative healthcare, incorporating traditional knowledge with evidence-based approaches.

One focal area of this is cannabis therapeutics, which is a growing specialty of interest. Cannabis is a plant-based drug that is a source of substances that have pharmacological and psychotropic properties called cannabinoids and has proved to be useful in the treatment of various clinical disorders. With accumulating scientific research findings and emerging regulatory attitudes, cannabis therapeutics is becoming an integral part of new clinical practice.

5. CANNABIS THERAPEUTICS

Cannabis therapeutics involves using biologically active entities called cannabinoids - derived from the cannabis plant or made in a laboratory for treatment - to treat disease. These chemicals affect particular physiological systems in the body and have an impact on numerous biological processes such as pain, moods, immune system function and neurological regulation.

Of course, from the medical point of view, the process of using cannabis-based treatments in a controlled and evidence-based way for therapeutic purposes is termed cannabis therapeutics. This encompasses the use of standardised formulations with monitored dosages and administration to guarantee safety and effectiveness. Therapeutic cannabis is prescribed for patient-specific clinical needs, assessed by patient clinical data and is regulated. Therapeutic cannabis does not follow the same pattern of recreational use - it follows clinical indications, patient assessment and is regulated.

The Pharmacological basis and mechanism, Cannabis Therapeutic benefits are most commonly achieved through the use of compounds called cannabinoids such as delta-9-tetrahydrocannabinol (THC) and cannabidiol (CBD) (Sazegar, 2021). They bind to specific receptors within the body, which are one among many regulatory mechanisms that ensure a balance of the organism's functions (Sera & Hempel-Sanderoff, 2025).

Cannabinoids can have an effect on many systems such as:

- Nervous system (pain, cognition, mood)
- The immune system (inflammation, immune modulation)
- GIT system: Appetite and Nausea control

The effect of this multi-system interaction, as part of the broad therapeutic potential of cannabis; yet, it's an influence that requires careful clinical evaluation, and proper application.

5.1. Clinical Applications of Cannabis Therapeutics

Cannabis therapeutics has demonstrated a potential therapeutic role in the clinic for many conditions, especially when standard therapies are shown to be inadequate or have unwanted side effects. See Figure 6, for this.

Figure 6. Clinical applications

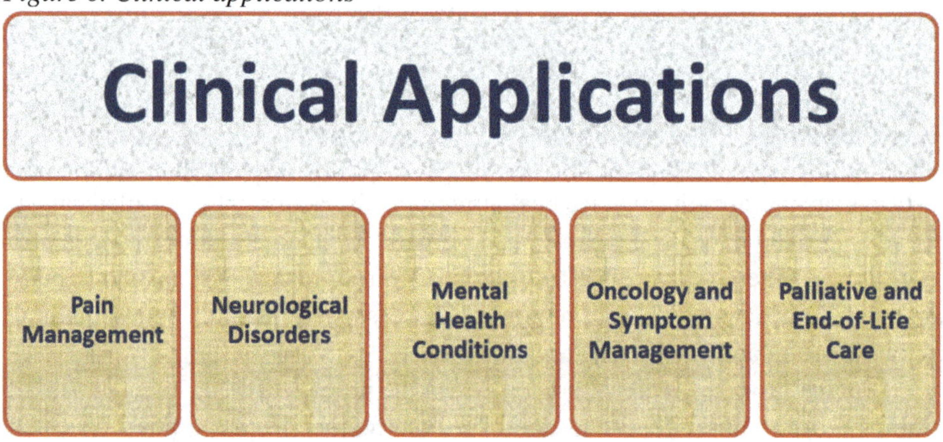

5.1.1. Pain Management

A great deal of research has been conducted on using cannabis to treat chronic and neuropathic pain. It could be an alternative or supplementary to the conventional anesthetics, especially in those who fail to respond to the conventional ones sufficiently.

5.1.2. Neurological Disorders

Epilepsy, multiple sclerosis, and neurodegenerative diseases are just some medical conditions that have shown promise regarding cannabinoids. May reduce the number of seizures, control CP spasticity and help to improve neurological symptoms.

5.1.3. Mental Health Conditions

There is emerging evidence that may benefit anxiety, post-traumatic stress disorder (PTSD) and sleep disorders. Care needs to be taken, though, as there may be psychological effects.

5.1.4. Oncology and Symptom Management

Cancer care – Cannabis therapeutic value is exploited to alleviate complications of chemotherapy and cancer like nausea, vomiting, pain and loss of appetite.

5.1.5. Palliative and End of Life Care

Because cannabis helps alleviate pain, anxiety, and other painful symptoms, it can be used as a supportive treatment for patients with serious or terminal illness, to improve their quality of life.

5.2. Various types of Cannabis Therapeutics

Cannabis therapeutics refer to a variety of preparation methods, chemicals and administration techniques that allow specific therapeutic benefits. To be able to understand its uses in the clinic, it is important to know what type of cannabis therapeutic product is being used, as this will have varying effects depending on the composition, mode of action, onset of action and therapeutic effect. These variations enable more personalised care, such as interventions being individualised according to the patient's needs, their clinical condition and safety.

There are several types of cannabis therapeutics, see Figure 7.

Figure 7. Types of cannabis therapeutics

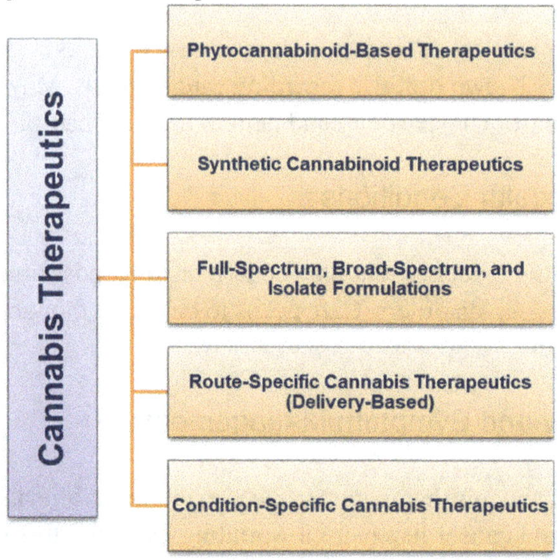

5.2.1. Phytocannabinoid-Based Therapeutics

Phytocannabinoid-based therapeutic products can be obtained directly from cannabis plants and include naturally occurring tetrahydrocannabinol (THC) and cannabidiol (CBD). The formulations can contain oils, tinctures, capsules, and extracts as medicinal cannabis' bioactive ingredients are retained in these products.

These therapies are used extensively because they are delivered from a natural source, and interact a balanced way with physiological systems. They have been use for chronic pain, inflammation, neurological or anxiety-related disorders. Several compounds may act together, and this may be referred to as a synergistic interaction, which in turn may affect the therapeutic effects.

5.2.2. Synthetic Cannabinoid Therapeutics

Synthetic cannabinoid therapeutics are laboratory-created compounds which mimic the effects of naturally occurring cannabinoids. Usually, these formulations are either standardized or regulated, and the pharmacology is consistent and there is strict dosing.

They are often administered in controlled doses and can be relied upon in clinical practice when precise and predictable dosing is important, for example, when controlling nausea caused by chemotherapy and severe pain. Synthetic cannabinoids have the benefit of being standardized, but may exhibit different effects on physiological systems than cannabinoids isolated from plants, and thus should be monitored carefully during clinical use.

5.2.3. Full-Spectrum, Broad-Spectrum, and Isolate Formulations

Cannabis therapies may be categorized also in response to the content of chemical substances and the legal diversity of energetic constituents found in cannabis.

Comprehensive formulations contain all the naturally occurring cannabinoids, terpenes and other plant compounds whose combination could amplify therapeutic effects. Broad-spectrum products contain a variety of different cannabinoids, but none of the THC. The isolate forms contain only one specific compound – in this case, only CBD. This means they take a more specific approach in treatments.

clinical decision making may depend on type of formulation because a different type may be chosen according to a patient's tolerance to the medication, therapeutic objectives, and safety reasons.

5.2.4. Route-Specific Cannabis Therapeutics (Delivery-Based)

Therapeutics involve different routes of delivery to cannabis, each having different effects on onset and effects over time. The common methods of administration are oral, sublingual, inhalation and administration topically.

The capsules and edibles contain the same ingredients and are taken orally, where they tend to last longer but take several hours to take effect. Drugs are absorbed more quickly when given under the tongue; they are absorbed immediately when inhaled and are used for treating acute symptoms. Formulations are applied topically to treat only a localized area of the body; they do not have a systemic effect.

As the delivery method depends on the clinical need, the preference of patients and character of the condition being treated, it is clinical differentiation.

5.2.5. Condition Specific Cannabis Therapeutics

Otherway, the classification is based on clinical use. Cannabis therapeutics can be formulated to target certain diseases, including chronic pain, neurological, mental health and palliative care diseases and disorders.

Some combination of cannabinoids could be more effective at managing pain, for instance, and others more effective at lowering anxiety or controlling seizures. This helps devise a targeted solution to the condition which is tailored to the patient, in accordance with patient-centred care and precision medicine.

6. CANNABINOID PHYSIOLOGY

Cannabinoid physiology is the study of the interactions between the physiological and therapeutic effects of cannabinoid compounds and living being. The knowledge of the endocannabinoid system (ECS) is vital in this field and depicts the intricate and complicated network of cell signaling internal to the body that regulates and helps the body achieve homeostasis within numerous organ systems. The ECS is involved in numerous physiological functions such as pain, mood, appetite, immune responses and neurological processes and is critical for therapeutic targets of cannabis.

There are three primary components of cannabinoid physiology that control the physiology of the body:

- Endocannabinoids (endogenous ligands)
- Cannabinoid receptors
- Enzymes responsible for synthesis and degradation

These components are dynamic in responding to internal and external stimuli and in regulating physiological balance.

6.1. Endocannabinoids (Endogenous Ligands)

Endocannabinoids are natural structurally similar molecules that serve as endogenous ligands of the endocannabinoid receptors of the endocannabinoid system (ECS). They are highly involved in physiology's homeostatic mechanisms and modulate many key biological processes, such as neurotransmission, immune function, metabolism and stress response. Endocannabinoids are lipids synthesized "on demand" from membrane lipid precursors and act locally in a tightly regulated fashion, as opposed to conventional neurotransmitters (Rezende, et al. 2023).

6.1.1. Types of Endocannabinoids

Several endocannabinoid-like compounds have been discovered, but two key endocannabinoids are receiving the greatest amount of research attention for their wide-ranging physiological functions:

- **Anandamide (AEA)**

N-arachidonoylethanolamine or anandamide is one of the most studies endocannabinoids, which is the first one to be identified. It has a very high affinity to CB1 and has been linked to regulation of mood, emotional behaviour, pain and appetite. The anandamide is also known as the ''bliss molecule" because of its role in producing those feelings of wellbeing and reward.

- **2-Arachidonoylglycerol (2-AG)**

2-Aarachidonoylglycerol is found at greater estimated concentration in the central nervous system than anandamide, and it binds to both the CB1 and CB2 receptors. It has critical functions in synaptic signaling, neuroprotection and immune modulation functions. 2-AG plays a specific role in developing synaptic plasticity and regulation of inflammatory processes.

Other Endocannabinoid-Like Molecules

There are also other lipid mediators that have cannabinoid-like properties such as:

- Palmitoylethanolamide (PEA)
- Oleoylethanolamide (OEA)

These molecules do not bind directly to the same receptors as AEA and 2-AG, but can indirectly affect the activity of the ECS by altering the sensitivity of the receptor, or by having some sort of interaction with other signaling molecules pathways.

6.1.2. Biochemical Components and Precursors

Endocannabinoids are endogenously produced fatty substances that are found in the phospholipids of the cell membranes, and specifically in the phospholipids that contain arachidonic acid. These lipid precursors are enzymatically converted to active signaling molecules in their synthesis. The key biochemical features present are:

Limited volume size, due to hydrophobic nature and lipid based structure.

- Derived from membrane phospholipids
- Rapid synthesis and degradation
- Localized action near the site of production

This lipid nature makes it easy for the endocannabinoids to pass through cell membrane and interact with the receptors without the requirement of being stored within vesicles.

6.1.3. Synthesis Pathways

Endocannabinoids are naturally produced "on demand" when given a stimulus, like a stretch of nerve cells, inflammation, or stress. This is activated as a result of increased calcium levels in the cell or activation of specific signaling pathways.

Anandamide Synthesis: N-arachidonoyl phosphatidylethanolamine (NAPE) is the precursor which is mainly converted to anandamide by enzymatic activity. This is facilitated by particular enzymes that change the lipids in the membranes into active endocannabinoids.

2-AG synthesis: 2-AG synthesizes via diacylglycerol (DAG) and the enzyme diacylglycerol lipase (DAGL). This pathway is more closely coupled with the pathways of neuronal signaling, and has a significance role in synaptic signaling.

The synthesis mechanism is "on-demand" as the endocannabinoids are synthesized only when necessary, which enables just temporal and spatial control of their activity.

As you can see in Figure 8, there are a number of physiological processes regulated by endocannabinoids.

Figure 8. Functional roles of endocannabinoids

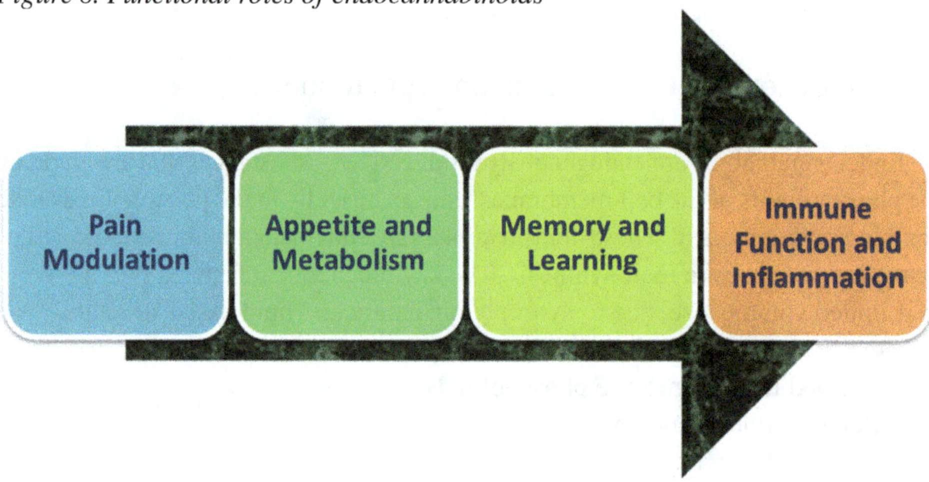

6.2. Cannabinoid Receptors

In case of the cannabis plant, the specific membrane-bound proteins where endocannabinoids and cannabinoids have their effect are known as cannabinoid receptors. They belong to a group of proteins called G protein-coupled receptors (GPCRs) and have an important role in regulating the physiological actions of the endocannabinoid system (ECS). The wide distribution of CBRs in the central nervous system and peripheral tissues suggests that they are involved in a variety of physiological functions, such as the regulation of neurotransmission, immune function, inflammation, and cell homeostasis.

So far, within the ECS, scientists have detected two major cannabinoid receptors:

- Cannabinoid Receptor Type 1 (CB1)
- CB2 Receptors (Cannabinoid Receptor Type 2)

The complexity of the cannabinoid systems is further complicated by the involvement of non-classical or cannabinoid-related receptors.

6.2.1. Cannabinoid Receptor Type 1

Mostly, CB1 receptors are expressed in the central nervous system (CNS), including areas of the brain that have higher cognitive and motor functions, such as the basal ganglia, the cerebellum, the cerebral cortex and the hippocampus. They also occur (but less abundantly) in peripheral tissues such as gastrointestinal tract, fat, and liver.

CB1 receptors are largely known to regulate the release of neurotransmitters. CB1 receptors, when stimulated by endocannabinoids and/or exogenous cannabinoids, serve to reduce the release of excitatory and inhibitory neurotransmitters, namely glutamate and gamma-aminobutyric acid (GABA). This modulation is an integral component in sustaining the balance of synapses and regulating neuronal excitability.

In clinic, a CB1 receptor activation is correlated with:

- Animals subjected to teaching lesions showed pain reduction
- Improved mood and emotional reactions
- Appetite and metabolism control
- Effects on memory and cognition

CB1 receptor activation also accounts for the psychotropic side effects of some cannabinoids especially tetrahydrocannabinol (THC).

6.2.2. Cannabinoid Receptor Type 2

CB2 receptors are predominantly located within the peripheral nervous system immune system, including immune cells (macrophages, lymphocytes and microglia). They are present in tissues like the gastrointestinal system and tonsils and spleen.

CB2 receptors primarily are responsible for controlling the immune response and inflammation. The stimulation of these receptors causes inflammation inhibiting effect and enhancement of tissue repair, as well as the modulation of cytokine release.

CB2 receptor activity is clinically linked with:

- Anti-inflammatory effects
- Immunomodulation
- Pollen absent
- Potential neuroprotective roles

The activation of CB2 receptor is not likely to have a significant psychoactive effect as compared with CB1 receptor, which can be an interesting molecular target for developing therapeutics for inflammatory and autoimmune diseases (Shang & Tang, 2017).

6.2.3. Non-Classical Cannabinoid Receptors

Besides CB1 and CB2 receptors, there are additional receptor systems which have been discovered to be a part of the extended-endocannabinoid system. They are receptors like GPR55 and transient receptor potential (TRP) channels, that engage with the cannabinoids and play a role in their physiological outcomes.

These non-classical receptors are involved in:

- Pain modulation
- Inflammatory responses
- Cellular signaling pathways

The role they play implies that cannabinoid effects are likely to be complex and multifaceted, extending beyond the classical cannabinoid receptor pathways CB1 and CB2.

6.3. Enzymes Responsible for Synthesis and Degradation

The synthesis and degradation enzymes of the endocannabinoids play an integral part in the regulation of the endocannabinoid system (ECS). These enzymes ensure endocannabinoid signaling functions in both time and space in a highly regulated manner, comprising the ability to activate and terminate physiological responses very quickly. The classical neurotransmitter systems rely on molecules that can be stored and released in a controlled way while the endocannabinoids do not need to be stored and are rapidly degraded after being released and acting on a target cell. This is dynamic enzymatic regulation which is crucial to maintain homeostasis and avoid over-activation and/or excessive activation of receptor(s).

7. CLINICAL TOOLS

Clinical tools are fundamental parts of the nursing profession, connecting theory with practice. They include an array of resources: Assessment scales, clinical guidelines, algorithms, checklists, and decision support systems. These tools are created to help the nurse to structure clinical data, to clarify the needs of the patient and to establish suitable interventions for patient care.

An important part of the value of clinical tools is their facilitation of greater accuracy, consistency, and efficiency in the provision of care. Clinical tools minimize the risk of practice variation and errors, coupled with standardised approaches to the assessment and management of patients. They also promote critical thinking by providing healthcare professionals with a series of processes and procedures that guarantee a decision based on in-depth and relevant information. Through this, clinical tools are essential to increased patient safety, patient quality of care and healthcare outcomes.

7.1. Role in Clinical Decision Making

Clinical decision making is one of the key components in the nursing profession that relies on clinical knowledge, patient information and professional decision making. Clinical tools, which provide structured frameworks to be followed by the nurse in complex clinical situations, are an important part of this process that guides them.

The tools provide a safe, systematic approach to data collection and analysis, which help nurses to recognize patterns and prioritize patient needs, then determine interventions. An example of a clinical algorithm would be a step-by-step approach to manage a particular condition, and a decision-support system would be a system that gives suggestions based on evidence for a particular patient profile. Clinical tools decrease the cognitive load and uncertainty experienced by clinicians and lead to more efficient and reliable clinical decision making.

In addition, clinical tools ensure consistency of care, making decisions consistent and aligned with global guidelines and best practices. This is especially valuable in multi-professional health care, where conformity helps to facilitate communications and coordination between health care providers.

7.2. Types of Clinical Tools in Nursing Practice

Clinical tools used in nursing practice may be classified systematically, depending functional roles in patient care and clinical decision making. It classifies the broad spectrum of tools in healthcare and helps nurses choose a tool based on the clinical needs. In general, the clinical tools used in nursing practice can be divided into five categories: Assessment tools, Monitoring tools, Decisions support tools, Documentation tools, and Evaluation tools. Aside from the fact that each category is acknowledged as a player in comprehensive patient care, each one affects the care of the patient in a unique but intertwined way. See Figure 9.

Figure 9. Clinical tools

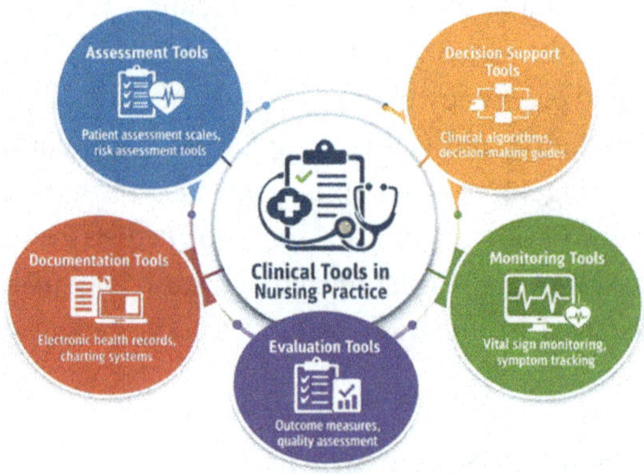

7.2.1. Assessment Tools

Assessment tools are essential in nursing practice and are always the structured instruments used to assess a patient's physical, psychological and functional state. These tools allow data to be collected on a systematic basis at the start and throughout the patient's clinical journey, which they then use to make proper diagnoses and set up the patient care plan. Assessment tools increase the reliability and consistency of clinical judgment by offering standardized ways of assessment, thereby minimizing client assessment subjectivity.

Many reliable assessment tools are used in clinical situations to measure different health parameters. For instance, pain assessment might be carried out with the help of standardized scales, like the Visual Analog Scale (VAS) and the Numeric Rating Scale (NRS), that may help quantify the intensity of pain. Patient Health Questionnaires (PHQ-9 for depression, and the Generalized Anxiety Disorder-7 or the GAD-7 for anxiety) may be used to assess patients for mental health status. Functional status and mobility is often measured by the Barthel index and cognitive function can be measured using the Mini Mental State Examination (MMSE). Also, numerous risk assessments including the Braden Scale for pressure ulcer risk are used in the clinical environment.

These are uniform tools that enable the nurse to detect more accurately what support the patient needs, ensure that interventions are priorities and track changes over time. In addition, assessment instruments enable the effective sharing of information between health care providers by ensuring there is a common framework in which patient information can be understood. They are very important for assessing baseline conditions, treatment appropriateness, and treatment outcomes of these tools in advanced practice, particularly during the development of new therapics like those for cannabis.

7.2.2. Monitoring Tools

Monitoring tools track changes over time with a patient to ensure that they are monitored and that they can receive the intervention in an appropriate time. In acute care and chronic care situations where patients' conditions can change course rapidly, these tools become key to care. Monitoring tools include systems which record vital signs, symptom and observation of treatment responses. They are used to enable early detection of changes in clinical status, so that the nurse can modify their care plan. Using monitoring tools increases patient safety by making sure that any changes in patients' health status are picked up and acted upon quickly. In advanced clinical nursing practice, such monitoring tools can be especially useful when dealing with complex patient situations and multi-faceted patient conditions; they can give objective and continuous data on patient responses. In addition, in the field of new therapeutic interventions like cannabis therapeutics, monitoring tools are also essential for evaluating therapeutic outcomes, recognizing adverse impacts, and adapting therapeutic strategies.

7.2.3. Decision-Support Tools

Decision-support tools supply nurses with evidence based practice and some structured guidance in making decision. Such tools typically include clinical algorithms, protocols, guidelines and computer-based decision-making systems. They assist nurses to analyse patient information, prioritise nursing actions and choose the right treatment. Decision-support tools aid clinical decision-making by minimizing uncertainties and cognitive information load, thus enhancing accuracy and consistency, especially in complex and high-risk scenarios.

7.2.4. Documentation Tools

Documentation system tools play a vital role in healthcare systems, aiding in the capture, structure and transmission of patient data. They involve electronic health records, standardised health record formats and health record documentation templates. Surgical transcriptions provide the necessary information that can help facilitate communication between health care professionals and thus ensure continuity of care. It can also be helpful in legal and regulatory compliance and quality assurance procedures. By systematic documentation, nurses are able to prepare a patient comprehensive and useful record regarding the care activity and its effect along with an easy availability record.

7.2.5. Evaluation Tools

Clinical interventions are evaluated using tools to see if the interventions are effective and if the outcomes of the clinical interventions are at expectancy levels. There are outcome measurement scales, quality indicators, and performance assessment types that can be included in these tools. Evaluation tools help nurses reflect and assess what they do and how it affects the outcomes of their patients and determine how they can make improvements. This process ultimately contributes to an ongoing improvement in quality and can help keep patients' care consistent with the evidence-based benchmarks and desired health outcomes.

8. NURSING PRACTICE: CLINICAL TOOLS FOR CANNABIS THERAPEUTICS

Given the need for specialized clinical instruments to facilitate safe, effective, and evidence-based clinical practice, the incorporation of cannabis therapeutics validates the importance of using specialized clinical instruments in clinical nursing practice. Though the general clinical tools represent the starting point for the evaluation and management of patients, they also add layer(s) of complexity, in the case of cannabis therapeutics, such as pharmacologic variability, individual response to a drug, and regulator considerations. This has created a need for nursing to use specific clinical tools to direct patient selection, dosage, patient monitoring, and patient outcomes monitoring and assessment (Bridgeman & Abazia, 2017).

These will allow for a systematic and structured approach in delivering cannabis-based interventions with both scientific evidence and specific patient factors informing clinical decisions. These tools are beneficial to advanced nursing practice in improving clinical judgement, minimizing risk and ensuring consistency in patient care delivery.

8.1. Cannabis Use Patient Risk Assessment Framework

Before one starts a cannabis therapeutics program, it is important to have a comprehensive patient risk assessment to ensure that one knows what to anticipate. This includes checking patient's medical history, current conditions, prescriptions and risk factors. Using a prescribed assessment system ensures that it systematically includes all relevant aspects in the assessment.

The first step in a standard clinical risk assessment involves a thorough patient history, such as past drug use and mental health diagnoses and conditions (co-morbidities). Training is followed by a review and assessment of clinical uses of cannabis, which includes a discussion of therapeutic needs for the proposed intervention. Checking whether there are contraindications, such as a history of drug and alcohol addiction or some psychiatric disorders, is extremely crucial to reduce the potential threat. Also, an extensive examination of existing drugs is required to avoid potential drug–drug interactions. These data can be used to stratify patients into risk groups, which can inform clinical care and decision making for starting, changing or declining cannabis therapeutics.

8.2. Cannabis Therapeutics – Dose Titration Strategies

Personalized response to the cannabinoids can vary greatly, making dose titration an important tool in the safe administration of cannabis therapeutics. A structured titration strategy generally includes a "start low and go slow" protocol, starting from a low dosage level and then escalating as patient needs increase and tolerated.

This must be monitored continuously for therapeutic effects and side effects. Factors evaluated include symptom relief, functional improvement, and for potential adverse effects, sedation or cognitive changes (Abrams, 2018). Doses, formulations or route of administration are adjusted accordingly to obtain the maximum benefit with the least risks. Standardized titration framework allows person-centered care and improves treatment safety.

8.3. Drug–Drug Interaction Considerations

An understanding of potentially toxic drug–drug interactions is critical for clinical decision making with regard to cannabis therapeutics. It is likely that these interactions will affect the effect of cannabis and other drugs used concurrently.

A comparative overview of typical interaction considerations, which are listed below in Table 1.

Table 1. A comparative review of the typical interaction considerations

Drug Class	Potential Interaction with Cannabis	Clinical Implication
CNS depressants	Additive sedative effects	Increased risk of sedation and drowsiness
Anticoagulants	Altered metabolism	Increased risk of bleeding
Antidepressants	Modulation of neurotransmitter pathways	Potential changes in therapeutic response
Antiepileptics	Enzyme interactions	Altered drug levels and effectiveness

9. CANNABIS THERAPEUTICS IN ADVANCED CLINICAL NURSING PRACTICE

The use of cannabis therapeutics in advanced clinical nursing practice represents another one of the changes in modern health care, away from a 'One Size Fits All to a more individualized, evidence-based and holistic approach to care. Innovative therapeutic interventions are critical for advanced practice nurses to bring to clinical decision making as the healthcare system recognizes their value, especially in the context of emerging and complementary therapies. Given the variety of physiological affects of cannabis and the growing use of cannabis for treatment, this has become a relevant and impactful facet of contemporary nursing practice.

9.1. The Advanced Clinical Practice Model Features Conceptual Integration

Advanced clinical nursing practice involves the full assessment of the patient, complex clinical reasoning and the integration of multiple therapeutic approaches for optimal outcomes. As part of this context, cannabis therapeutics is viewed as complementary and in some instances an alternative means of treating patients.

It is of great significance in the clinical situation in which usual medications are inadequate, intolerant or of the same type with considerable undesirable effects.

The integrative approach is ideal because it offers a patient-centred care and precision medicine approach where treatments are personalised to each patient's clinical and personal circumstances and preferences.

9.2. Advanced Nursing Practice (DNP) – Clinical Applications

Increasingly Cannabis therapeutics is used in various advanced nursing practice clinical domains. It is most commonly being used in the management of chronic and complex conditions, such as persistent pain syndromes, neurology conditions, mental health and palliative care.

In these settings, cannabis-based therapies can be used to help alleviate symptoms, improve quality of life, and increase patient satisfaction. Their use is, however, dependent on clinical judgment since patients can react differently to the use of cannabis as medicine.

9.3. Clinical Decision Making and Patient Assessment

The systematic and individualized assessment process is important for effective use of cannabis therapeutics clinically. Treatment options for advanced practice nurses will include assessing various patient factors such as medical history, recent medication use, symptom burden, and other risk factors.

Clinical decision-making includes the assessment of the suitability of cannabis-based interventions, choice of formulation and delivery route, as well as outlining therapy targets. This process reinforces the critical thinking and evidence based practice aspect of safe, effective care.

9.4. Monitoring, Evaluation and Safety Considerations

It is important to continually assess the success of the integration of cannabis therapeutics into clinical practice. Continuous monitoring and evaluation are necessary for integration of cannabis therapeutics into clinical practice. APNs are also accountable for evaluating therapeutic responses and any adverse effects, such as cognitive impairment, sedation or drug interactions.

It's a way to optimize treatment plans and ensure interventions are effective and tailored to a person's needs. This dynamic approach contributes to patients' safety and improves overall quality of care.

9.5. Ethical and legal Issues

Ethical and legal complexities come with the use of cannabis therapeutics in medical contexts. Cannabis laws and institutional policies differ from region to region; it's important for healthcare professionals to keep current on the relevant laws and policies regarding cannabis usage.

APNs need to make sure all interventions are both within the legal framework and that the proper documentation and guidelines are followed by the prescriber. Issues of informed consent, patient autonomy and risk-benefit analysis are important ethical thoughts in good clinical practice.

9.6. Patient Education and Engagement

An important role in advanced nursing practice is patient education in cannabis therapeutics. Patients might not know a lot about the effects of cannabis, and therefore, better informed communication by healthcare professionals is required for the transmission of evidence-based information about its effects.

APNs also have a critical role to educate patients about the potential benefits of Rx cannabis, the risks associated with its use, how it is administered, and what to expect as a result of treatment. This promotes patient trust in the decision-making process, aids in patient compliance, and encourages co-management.

10. ROLE OF THE CLINICAL NURSE SPECIALIST (CNS) IN CANNABIS THERAPEUTICS

New knowledge, sophistication, and coordination at both an individual provider level and at the system level are needed to implement and integrate cannabis therapeutics into today's health care system. As an advanced practice nurse, the Clinical Nurse Specialist (CNS) has a unique place to facilitate and maintain this integration in a variety of ways, such as providing direct patient care, professional mentoring, and organizational leadership. To ensure the evidence-based, patient-centred, ethical and regulatory usage of cannabis therapeutics, the CNS relies on established guidelines. The CNS uses established guidelines to ensure that use of cannabis therapeutic products is evidence-based, patient-centred, ethical and regulatory.

10.1. Clinical Expert Role in Patient Care

A hallmark of CNS practice is where the expertise lies, that is, patient care, and this is especially important in the realm of cannabis therapeutics. Patient evaluations are carried out at a detailed level by the CNS and involve an assessment of medical history, the nature of the symptoms, past outcomes of treatment, and possible risks. From this evaluation the CNS makes a determination as to the suitability of cannabis therapeutics in the context of the comprehensive care plan. It is about careful formulation, dose regimens, and routes of administration used, for each patient. Moreover, the CNS continuously tracks therapeutic efficiency and possible adverse effects, and makes changes to ensure the drugs are as safe and effective as possible. The CNS ensures the integration of cannabis-based interventions into clinical practice in an individualized and clinically appropriate way through this process.

10.2. Educator and Mentor in Nursing Practice

Along with directly caring for patients, the CNS also has a crucial responsibility as an educator/mentor in nursing practice overall, but especially in newer areas like cannabis therapeutics. The CNS addresses this gap by creating educational programs that instructors can use to teach the key areas of cannabis therapeutics, which include pharmacology of Cannabinoids, cannabinoid physiology, clinical indications for use, safety considerations, etc. Until this area becomes a more accepted part of clinical practice, many nurses may not have adequate knowledge or confidence in how to use it clinically. Through mentorship / guidance from the CNS, nurses will learn how to use evidence-based practice, develop critical thinking skills, and have access to ongoing professional development opportunities. Through this type of support, nurses will be able to provide safe/consistent/high-quality patient care through the use of cannabis-based interventions.

10.3. Leader in Using Evidence and Sharing Knowledge

One of the CNS' main missions is to try to create evidence-based practice and take research and transfer it into clinical use. Because cannabis therapeutics has been evolving at such a rapid rate, the CNS' role is very important. The CNS reviews new scientific literature continually and critically to ensure they are fully aware about the latest developments regarding efficacy, safety and clinical usage. The information/process is used in developing clinical guidelines, protocols and care pathways to ensure practices remain up-to-date and evidence-based. The CNS can also serve as an investigator for clinical research and/or quality improvement initiatives, researching patient outcomes and refining treatments. In fulfilling these two roles, the CNSs act as an intermediary between researchers and practitioners; they help place the research findings in practice with cannabis therapeutics in a way that is both supported by scientific evidence as well as the best clinical practice standards.

10.4. Leading at the System Level and Creating Policies

From an organizational perspective, the CNS plays a vital role as both leader and catalyst for change, providing leadership in the introduction of cannabis therapeutics within healthcare settings. The CNS' responsibilities include developing and implementing institution-wide policies, clinical protocols, and patient care guidelines that promote safe and standardized practices. The CNS develops and implements these processes in a way that will be compliant with applicable legal and regulatory standards that vary by region, and that will evolve over time. The CNS will also provide leadership for quality improvement efforts designed to improve patient safety and the effectiveness of treatment, as well as the quality of care provided to patients. By assessing program performance and identifying areas where improvements can be made, the CNS will play an active role in ongoing efforts to improve clinical practice. Through system-wide leadership the CNS will help to ensure that cannabis-based therapy becomes an integrated and sustainable service within healthcare organizations.

10.5. Ethical and Legal Stewardship

Using cannabis therapeutics raises specific ethical and legal concerns that need to be managed carefully. The CNS is the individual who must protect all parts of the patient care continuum to make sure the nurse is doing the right things ethically and legally when using cannabis therapeutics. One way a nurse will help achieve this is by providing informed consent using the information described above to make sure the patients know everything about the potential benefits and risks associated with cannabis.

11. FUTURE DIRECTIONS IN CANNABIS NURSING PRACTICE

The field of cannabis therapeutics is changing fast. This is because of discoveries in science changes in rules and more doctors accepting it. As hospitals start to use cannabis-based treatments, nurses, those in advanced roles need to stay up to date with the latest trends and challenges. Clinical Nurse Specialists will be very important in shaping the future of cannabis nursing practice. They will lead, help turn research into practice and come up with ideas for the healthcare system. There are a few things that will influence the direction of this field.

11.1. Advancing Product Standardization

One big development in cannabis therapeutics is making products more standardized. Better rules growing practices and manufacturing are making cannabinoid-based products more consistent and of quality. This means that doctors can give precise doses and patients will respond more predictably. This is crucial for making sure research is reliable and for using evidence-based practice. For nurses standardized products will make it safer to give medicine. Will lead to more predictable results.

11.2. Expansion of Clinical Research

Clinical research will really help to understand cannabis therapeutics. As rules get easier to follow bigger and better studies are being done to see how well cannabis-based treatments work, how safe they are and what their long-term effects are. This will help us figure out the ways to use these treatments, how much to give and how they compare to traditional therapies. Clinical Nurse Specialists will play a role in turning research into practice making protocols and making sure care is based on the latest science.

11.3. Integration of Digital Health Technologies

Digital health technologies are changing healthcare. They will help to monitor patients and make decisions. Tools like electronic symptom tracking, telehealth and wearable devices let us keep an eye on patients all the time from far away. These technologies help us see how well treatments are working catch problems early and adjust treatment plans. Clinical Nurse Specialists are in a position to use these innovations to support care from afar get patients more involved and make sure care is continuous.

11.4. Evolution of Regulatory and Policy Frameworks

Rules and policies about cannabis use are always changing. These changes will affect nursing practice. Nurses, Clinical Nurse Specialists need to keep advocating for patients to make sure policies are safe, fair and follow ethical standards. As rules get clearer nurses need to stay informed and adapt to make sure they are following the rules and using cannabis therapeutics effectively.

11.5. Strengthening Holistic and Patient-Centered Care Models

Cannabis therapeutics fits well with nursing philosophies that look at the person. Body, mind and spirit. As healthcare focuses more on the patient cannabis-based interventions can help with patient needs. Using cannabis therapeutics as part of a care plan supports a more individualized approach to treatment focusing on overall well-being. This approach reinforces the role of nurses in giving patient-centered care.

CONCLUSION

Cannabis therapeutics is a part of advanced clinical nursing practice now. This chapter talked about the science behind cannabinoids how cannabis is used in clinics and the importance of using tools safely and effectively. Clinical Nurse Specialists are crucial, in this integration. They bring together research, practice and system-level implementation through leadership, education and data-driven decision-making. By using evidence-based frameworks and holistic care principles nurses can improve outcomes while keeping them safe and following ethical standards. As research, rules and clinical practice keep evolving Clinical Nurse Specialists will keep guiding the use of cannabis therapeutics in healthcare.

REFERENCES

Abrams, D. I. (2018). The therapeutic effects of cannabis and cannabinoids. *European Journal of Internal Medicine*, *49*, 7–11. DOI: 10.1016/j.ejim.2018.01.003 PMID: 29325791

Bridgeman, M. B., & Abazia, D. T. (2017). Medicinal cannabis: History, pharmacology, and implications for the acute care setting. *P&T : a Peer-Reviewed Journal for Formulary Management*, *42*(3), 180–188. PMID: 28250701

Fulton, J. S., & Holly, V. W. (2021). *Clinical Nurse Specialist Role and Practice*. Springer International Publishing. DOI: 10.1007/978-3-319-97103-2

Fulton, J. S., Lyon, B. L., & Goudreau, K. A. (Eds.). (2014). *Foundations of clinical nurse specialist practice*. Springer Publishing Company. DOI: 10.1891/9780826129673

Rezende, B., Alencar, A. K. N., de Bem, G. F., Fontes-Dantas, F. L., & Montes, G. C. (2023). Endocannabinoid system: Chemical characteristics and biological activity. *Pharmaceuticals (Basel, Switzerland)*, *16*(2), 148. DOI: 10.3390/ph16020148 PMID: 37017445

Sazegar, P. (2021). Cannabis essentials: Tools for clinical practice. *American Family Physician*, *104*(6), 598–608. PMID: 34913644

Sera, L., & Hempel-Sanderoff, C. (2025). *Cannabis Science and Therapeutics: The Essential Guide for Clinicians*. Springer. DOI: 10.1007/978-3-031-80352-9

Shang, Y., & Tang, Y. (2017). The central cannabinoid receptor type-2 (CB2) and chronic pain. *The International Journal of Neuroscience*, *127*(9), 812–823. DOI: 10.1080/00207454.2016.1257992 PMID: 27842450

Chapter 3
Cannabis Care in Psychiatry:
Assessment, Treatment, and Ethical Considerations for PMHNP Practice

Kathleen Marie Pinto Araya
http://orcid.org/0009-0000-0608-7555
AZZ Medical Associates, USA

ABSTRACT

Cannabis use is increasing across the United States, creating clinical, ethical, and educational challenges for Psychiatric-Mental Health Nurse Practitioners (PMHNPs). The evolving legal landscape, including the 2025 federal directive to reclassify cannabis from Schedule I to Schedule III, expands research opportunities while maintaining regulatory complexity. Evidence shows cannabidiol (CBD) may provide anxiolytic, antipsychotic, and anticonvulsant benefits, whereas tetrahydro cannabinol (THC) is linked to psychosis, cognitive impairment, and mood instability. Understanding the endocannabinoid system, pharmacokinetic variability, and drug interactions is essential for safe practice. Research from 2021–2025 reveals mixed outcomes for psychiatric conditions, emphasizing the need for individualized risk benefit assessment. Ethical considerations include patient autonomy, harm-reduction counseling, and navigating conflicting state and federal laws. Cannabis literacy is increasingly necessary for PMHNPs to deliver informed, evidence-based, and ethically sound care.

DOI: 10.4018/979-8-2600-2035-7.ch003

INTRODUCTION

Cannabis remains one of the most debated substances in contemporary healthcare, especially in psychiatric and mental health practice. The rising prevalence of cannabis use among patients necessitates that Psychiatric-Mental Health Nurse Practitioners (PMHNPs) develop a thorough familiarity with its therapeutic applications, associated risks, and significance for clinical care (Mehta, 2025). Although previously stigmatized and restricted under federal law, cannabis is more widely accepted for its prospective advantages in managing conditions such as chronic pain, anxiety, post-traumatic stress disorder (PTSD), and insomnia (Riggs & Thant, 2022). This evolving landscape creates both opportunities and challenges for PMHNPs, who must balance patient-focused care with evidence-based practice and legal requirements.

The American Association of Nurse Practitioners (AANP) acknowledges evidence supporting the therapeutic use of cannabis and related compounds, while accentuating the imperative for continued scientific evaluation and integration into nursing education (American Association of Nurse Practitioners [AANP], n.d.). Similarly, the American Nurses Association (ANA) has advocated for reclassifying cannabis from its current federal Schedule I status to facilitate essential research (Stokes, 2022). These professional positions highlight the need for PMHNPs to acquire the knowledge and skills required to engage in informed, ethical, and legally compliant discussions with patients.

Executive Order of the President (2025) discusses President Donald Trump's decision directing the federal government of the United States to reclassify marijuana from Schedule I to Schedule III under the Controlled Substances Act. The significance of the change is that Cannabis is no longer classified alongside drugs such as heroin and LSD as a Schedule I substance. As a Schedule III, Cannabis is classified with substances such as ketamine and certain prescription steroids. The executive order reduced restrictions; however, it does not legalize marijuana federally in the United States. Benefits include a projected increase in medical research on Cannabis and CBD products, including Medicare pilot programs for CBD products, and a reduction in banking and taxes for cannabis business expenses.

From a psychiatric perspective, cannabis presents a clinical paradox. Cannabinoids such as cannabidiol (CBD) have demonstrated potential in alleviating anxiety and improving sleep quality (Hunt et al., 2021). In contrast, tetrahydrocannabinol (THC), the primary psychoactive component, is associated with increased risks of psychosis, cognitive impairment, and cannabis use disorder (Riggs & Thant, 2022). As a result, PMHNPs must manage a multifaceted clinical environment where patient-reported benefits coexist with significant psychiatric risks.

The endocannabinoid system, which regulates mood, cognition, and stress response, underlies the biological effects of cannabis. Comprehensive knowledge of this system is essential for PMHNPs, as it informs both therapeutic applications and potential adverse outcomes (Miller, 2023). Furthermore, the diversity of cannabis products, ranging from pharmaceutical-grade preparations to unregulated dispensary items, complicates clinical decision-making and patient education (Hunt et al., 2021).

Legal and ethical considerations further shape the role of the PMHNP. While many states have legalized medical or recreational cannabis, ongoing federal prohibition introduces uncertainty for practitioners (Stokes, 2022). Ethical challenges arise when patients request cannabis recommendations or report self-medicating for psychiatric symptoms. PMHNPs are required to uphold patient autonomy while maintaining professional responsibility, ensuring that care decisions are evidence-based and prioritize patient safety (AANP, n.d.).

In summary, cannabis in psychiatric nursing practice represents a rapidly evolving field that demands critical engagement from PMHNPs. This chapter examines the historical context, pharmacology, clinical applications, risks, and ethical considerations of cannabis use, with the objective of equipping PMHNPs to provide informed, compassionate, and evidence-based care.

BACKGROUND

Cannabis Education for Psychiatric Mental Health Nurse Practitioners

Cannabis education is increasingly necessary for Psychiatric-Mental Health Nurse Practitioners (PMHNPs) due to rising patient use, evolving legal frameworks, and expanding clinical research. National surveys demonstrate that cannabis use has grown significantly in both medical and recreational contexts, with patients frequently reporting self-medication for psychiatric and neurological conditions including, but not limited to anxiety, PTSD, chronic pain, and insomnia (Busse et al., 2021). Without adequate training, PMHNPs may lack the ability to differentiate between the therapeutic potential of cannabidiol (CBD) and the destabilizing effects of tetrahydrocannabinol (THC), or to anticipate drug–drug interactions with psychotropics and other medications (Navarro, 2025). Education supports the PMHNPs' accuracy in provision of patient counseling, integration of harm-reduction strategies, and aligning care with evidence-based practice.

The pharmacology of cannabis draws attention to the critical role of clinician literacy. THC is the primary psychoactive compound, acting as a partial agonist at CB1 receptors in the central nervous system and CB2 receptors in peripheral tissues. This activity increases dopamine release in mesolimbic pathways, producing euphoria and analgesia and plays a role in adverse psychiatric outcomes such as anxiety, cognitive impairment, dependency, and psychosis exacerbation (D'Souza et al., 2023). In contrast, CBD is non-intoxicating and exerts therapeutic effects by indirectly modulating CB1 and CB2 receptors, agonizing the 5-HT1A receptor, activating TRPV1 channels, and inhibiting FAAH, thereby prolonging the activity of endogenous cannabinoids, such as anandamide (Campos et al., 2023). These mechanisms underpin CBD's anxiolytic, antipsychotic, anti-inflammatory, and anticonvulsant properties, and Epidiolex has demonstrated therapeutic benefit in pediatric epilepsies such as Dravet and Lennox-Gastaut syndromes (Navarro, 2025).

Cannabis pharmacokinetics vary by route of administration. Inhalation produces rapid absorption with peak plasma THC levels within minutes, while oral ingestion has a slower onset, lower bioavailability, and extensive first-pass metabolism. Both THC and CBD are metabolized by cytochrome P450 enzymes, creating possible medication interactions with antidepressants, antiepileptics, anticoagulants, and other commonly prescribed medications (Valani, 2022). Recent research highlights these drug interactions as clinically significant, particularly in patients with polypharmacy. Beyond THC and CBD, minor cannabinoids such as cannabigerol (CBG), cannabichromene (CBC), and tetrahydrocannabivarin (THCV) are being studied for anti-inflammatory, neuroprotective, and metabolic effects, though evidence remains preliminary (Wasilewska et al., 2025).

Clinical research between 2021 and 2025 reinforces that cannabis has the strongest evidence for epilepsy, chemotherapy-induced nausea, and some chronic pain conditions, while data for psychiatric disorders remain mixed. The Agency for Healthcare Research and Quality concluded that cannabinoids offer modest benefits for chronic pain with low-to-moderate certainty of evidence. Wasilewska et al. (2025) similarly found modest benefits but frequent adverse effects, underscoring the need for prudent use as an adjunct. Churchill et al. (2025) published a meta-analysis showing that cannabis use was associated with worsening depression outcomes, while Campos et al. (2023) demonstrated that CBD promoted hippocampal neurogenesis, implying prospective antidepressant-like effects. These contradictory findings illustrate why PMHNPs must be trained to critically appraise research and communicate nuanced risk–benefit profiles.

Psychosis represents a particularly urgent area for PMHNP education. Jin et al. (2025) reported that cannabis use was common among individuals with first-episode psychosis and was associated with increased relapse risk. Johnson et al. (2021) used genetic liability models to demonstrate causal links between cannabis use disorder and schizophrenia. These findings stress that PMHNPs must screen for cannabis use in psychotic populations, educate patients and families about risks, and integrate harm-reduction strategies. Mood disorders also demand thorough evaluation. Sorkhou, Dent, and George (2024) conducted a systematic review showing that problematic cannabis use is highly prevalent among individuals with bipolar disorder, with associations to earlier onset and increased suicidality. Miranda et al. (2025) found that chronic cannabis use impaired cognition in bipolar patients, while Mondimore (2025) highlighted clinical worsening of mood stability. Conversely, Roberts et al. (2023) reported that CBD consistently reduced anxiety symptoms in controlled trials, supporting its adjunctive use in anxiety disorders.

Learning activities have demonstrated measurable benefits. Cronin et al. (2025) evaluated an interdisciplinary cannabis education program for healthcare trainees, finding significant improvements in knowledge, confidence, and preparedness to counsel patients. The American Association of Nurse Practitioners (AANP, 2023) issued a position statement supporting inclusion of cannabis and cannabinoid content in nursing education and continuing education, stressing the requirement for evidence-based therapeutic recommendations and candid discussion with patients. Similarly, the American Nurses Association (ANA, 2021) endorsed reclassifying cannabis to facilitate urgently needed clinical research, underscoring nurses' professional responsibility to stay informed.

Policy and public health perspectives reinforce the need for clinician education. Volkow (2025) outlined a roadmap for cannabis policy research, noting that increased availability has decreased public perception of harm and increased use, creating uncertainty in clinical practice. Mehta (2025) argued in *JAMA Network Open* that cannabis education is a professional responsibility for physicians, a principle equally applicable to PMHNPs. These viewpoints underscore that cannabis literacy is not optional and fundamental to virtuous, patient-focused care.

Specific clinical outcomes demonstrate the importance of education. In epilepsy, Epidiolex reduced seizures by 43% compared to placebo in randomized trials (Navarro, 2025). In PTSD, Greer et al. (2023) observed reductions during nightmares and hyperarousal with cannabis use, though Schubert et al. (2025) found mixed long-term outcomes in veterans. In sleep disorders, AminiLari et al. (2022) reported improved sleep outcomes with cannabinoids, but Lavender et al. (2024) noted insufficient long-term data. In substance use disorders, Luján et al. (2025) found that CBD reduced drug-seeking behaviors in preclinical models, while Lev-Ran et al. (2022) emphasized that THC complicates recovery. These results indicate that cannabis can be beneficial in situations but harmful in others, requiring PMHNPs to integrate research evidence into individualized care plans.

To summarize, cannabis education prepares PMHNPs to differentiate THC and CBD pharmacology, interpret systematic reviews and clinical trial outcomes, screen for cannabis use in psychiatric populations, counsel patients on risks and benefits, anticipate drug interactions, and integrate harm-reduction strategies. As cannabis use continues to expand, PMHNPs must keep informed through ongoing education, evidence appraisal, and professional development. This ensures safe, effective, and ethical care for patients managing the complicated landscape of cannabis and mental health.

Pharmacology of Cannabis

Cannabis is a complex plant that contains more than 500 chemical compounds, including over 100 cannabinoids, terpenes, and flavonoids, which add to its pharmacodynamic characteristics (Hsu et al., 2019). The two most studied cannabinoids are delta-9-tetrahydrocannabinol (THC), the primary psychoactive component, and cannabidiol (CBD), a non-intoxicating compound with diverse therapeutic potential. Understanding the pharmacology of cannabis is essential for Psychiatric-Mental Health Nurse Practitioners (PMHNPs), as patients increasingly report cannabis use for psychiatric symptoms such as anxiety, depression, insomnia, and PTSD. Evidence-based practice requires PMHNPs to appraise both the therapeutic promise and the risks associated with cannabis use. Additionally, understanding the entourage effect as cannabinoids and terpenes work together synergistically. Creating stronger or more balanced therapeutic effects than when used alone is an important concept for the PMHNP.

CBD, in contrast, exhibits a distinct pharmacokinetic profile. Unlike THC, CBD does not bind strongly to CB1 receptors and therefore does not produce intoxicating effects. Its absorption varies depending on formulation, with oral CBD demonstrating relatively low bioavailability due to first-pass metabolism. However, advances in pharmaceutical formulations, including lipid-based carriers and nano emulsions, have improved CBD's absorption and therapeutic consistency (Fonseca, Zendulka, & Juřica, 2025). CBD is metabolized by cytochrome P450 enzymes, particularly CYP3A4 and CYP2C19, which also metabolize many psychiatric medications. This underscores essential clinical considerations for PMHNPs, as CBD can inhibit these enzymes and increase plasma concentrations of drugs such as SSRIs, antipsychotics, and benzodiazepines, possibly resulting in adverse effects or toxicity (Simankowicz & Stępniewska, 2025).

Delta-9-tetrahydrocannabinol (THC) and cannabidiol (CBD) are the two most extensively studied cannabinoids, and their absorption and metabolism characteristics differ in ways that are clinically significant for psychiatric practice. When cannabis is inhaled, THC is rapidly absorbed through the pulmonary alveoli, reaching peak plasma concentrations within minutes. This rapid absorption explains the immediate psychoactive effects patients frequently report, such as euphoria, altered sensory perception, and relaxation. However, THC's lipophilic nature leads to its distribution into adipose tissue, where it can be stored and slowly released, resulting in prolonged detection in blood and urine even after acute effects have subsided (Valani, 2022). Oral ingestion of THC produces a slower onset due to gastrointestinal absorption and extensive first-pass metabolism in the liver, where it is converted into 11-hydroxy-THC, a metabolite that is more potent and longer-lasting than THC itself. This metabolic pathway explains why oral cannabis products, such as edibles, often produce stronger and more prolonged psychoactive effects compared to inhaled forms (D'Souza et al., 2023).

The differences in pharmacokinetics between THC and CBD stress their divergent clinical roles. THC's rapid onset and psychoactive properties may appeal to patients pursuing instant relief from symptoms such as insomnia or anxiety, but the possibility of exacerbating psychosis and impairing cognition calls for careful monitoring. CBD, on the other hand, offers a safer profile with anxiolytic, antipsychotic, and anticonvulsant properties, making it a candidate for adjunctive therapy in psychiatric care. For PMHNPs, understanding these pharmacokinetic differences as shown in Table 1: Major Cannabinoids and Their Pharmacological Effects support guidance for patient education, assessing risks, and integrating cannabis-based therapies into evidence-based treatment plans.

Table 1. Major cannabinoids and their pharmacological effects

Major Cannabinoid	Receptor/Activity Mechanism	Psychoactivity	Primary Effects	Key Evidence
THC (Δ9-tetrahydrocannabinol)	CB1 (CNS), CB2 (immune)	Strongly psychoactive	Euphoria, altered perception, analgesia, appetite stimulation	Associated with increased risk of psychosis and cognitive impairment (D'Souza et al., 2023)
CBD (Cannabidiol)	Indirect ECS modulation; 5-HT1A, TRPV1	Non-psychoactive	Anxiolytic, antipsychotic, anti-inflammatory, anticonvulsant	FDA-approved for epilepsy; promising in anxiety and psychosis (Valani, 2022; Fonseca et al., 2025)
CBN (Cannabinol)	Weak CB1 agonist	Mildly psychoactive	Sedative, potential sleep aid	Limited evidence; ongoing clinical trials (Simankowicz & Stępniewska, 2025)
CBC (Cannabichromene)	TRPV1, TRPA1	Non-psychoactive	Anti-inflammatory, analgesic	Preclinical evidence suggests synergistic effects with THC and CBD (Fonseca et al., 2025)
THCV (Tetrahydrocannabivarin)	CB1 antagonist (low dose), CB1 agonist (high dose)	Mild psychoactive	Appetite suppression, possible antidiabetic effects	Emerging evidence in metabolic disorders (Valani, 2022)

Recent research has highlighted variability in cannabinoid pharmacokinetics among individuals, underscoring the importance of individualized strategies in clinical practice. A 2023 systematic review found that genetic polymorphisms in cytochrome P450 enzymes, particularly CYP2C9 and CYP2C19, significantly affect THC and CBD metabolism, leading to differences in plasma concentrations, duration of effects, and risk of adverse outcomes (D'Souza et al., 2023). For example, individuals with reduced-function CYP2C9 alleles show slower clearance of THC, causing lengthened psychoactive effects and heightened vulnerability to cognitive impairment. Similarly, CBD's inhibition of CYP2C19 has been shown to raise clobazam serum levels in patients with epilepsy, augmenting therapeutic effectiveness yet also increasing the risk of sedation (Fonseca, Zendulka, & Juřica, 2025). These observations emphasize the need for PMHNPs to consider pharmacogenomic variability and potential drug-drug interactions when evaluating cannabis use in psychiatric populations. Evidence-based practice requires including such research into patient education and monitoring strategies, making certain that cannabis-based interventions are customized to each person's metabolic profiles and comorbid drug regimens.

The Endocannabinoid System

The endocannabinoid system (ECS) comprises three primary elements: cannabinoid receptors, endogenous ligands known as endocannabinoids, and enzymes that synthesize and degrade them. Together, these components form a dynamic signaling network that regulates numerous physiological and psychological processes, including mood, cognition, appetite, pain, and immune function. Recent research has stressed the ECS's role in psychiatric disorders, highlighting its relevance for Psychiatric-Mental Health Nurse Practitioners (PMHNPs) who encounter patients using cannabis for symptom management (D'Souza et al., 2023; Simankowicz & Stępniewska, 2025).

Cannabinoid receptors are the most studied components of the ECS, with CB1 receptors primarily located in the central nervous system and CB2 receptors found in peripheral tissues. CB1 receptors are densely expressed in brain regions such as the hippocampus, amygdala, and prefrontal cortex, which are important for memory, emotion, and executive function. THC acts as a partial agonist at CB1 receptors, producing psychoactive effects including euphoria, altered perception, and impaired short-term memory. Dysregulation of CB1 receptor signaling has been linked to psychiatric conditions such as schizophrenia and anxiety disorders (D'Souza et al., 2023). In contrast, CB2 receptors are concentrated in immune cells and peripheral tissues, where they modulate inflammation and immune responses. New studies have demonstrated CB2 receptors in microglia within the brain, putting forward a role in neuroinflammation and neurodegeneration, processes increasingly recognized in psychiatric illnesses such as depression and PTSD (Simankowicz & Stępniewska, 2025).

The ECS also includes endogenous ligands, or endocannabinoids, which are lipid-based neurotransmitters synthesized on demand. The two most prominent endocannabinoids are anandamide (AEA) and 2-arachidonoylglycerol (2-AG). Anandamide is closely associated with affect control and stress resilience, while 2-AG plays a role in reward and motivation pathways. Both serve as retrograde messengers, binding to presynaptic CB1 receptors to modulate neurotransmitter release. Recent evidence shows that reduced circulating levels of endocannabinoids may contribute to vulnerability in psychiatric disorders, including PTSD and depression, where patients frequently show dysregulated stress responses (Luján et al., 2025).

Finally, the ECS relies on enzymes to maintain homeostasis by regulating endocannabinoid levels. Fatty acid amide hydrolase (FAAH) is responsible for breaking down anandamide, while monoacylglycerol lipase (MAGL) degrades 2-AG. Inhibition of these enzymes has been explored as a therapeutic approach to improve endocannabinoid signaling. For example, FAAH inhibitors have demonstrated anxiolytic and antidepressant effects in preclinical models, though clinical translation remains ongoing (Haney, 2021). These enzymatic processes are crucial for upholding balance within the ECS, preventing excessive activation that could lead to adverse outcomes such as psychosis or cognitive impairment.

Taken together, the components of the ECS form a tightly regulated system that influences both physical and mental health. For PMHNPs, comprehending the interaction between cannabinoid receptors, endocannabinoids, and metabolic enzymes is vital for analyzing the therapeutic capacity of cannabis while lessening risks. Recent research draws attention to the ECS's importance in psychiatric care, providing insight into how modulation of this system may contribute to novel treatment strategies for anxiety, depression, psychosis, and PTSD.

Pharmacokinetics of Cannabis

The pharmacokinetics of cannabis are highly variable and depend on the route of administration, the specific cannabinoid composition, and individual patient factors such as metabolism and body fat distribution. When cannabis is inhaled via smoking or vaporization, cannabinoids such as delta-9-tetrahydrocannabinol (THC) and cannabidiol (CBD) are rapidly absorbed into the bloodstream via the lungs, producing peak plasma concentrations within minutes. This route provides fast onset of psychoactive and therapeutic effects, usually lasting two to four hours, but it also exposes patients to potential pulmonary risks associated with combustion products (Valani, 2022). In contrast, oral ingestion of cannabis through edibles, capsules, or oils—results in slower absorption, with onset occurring between 30 and 90 minutes. Oral bioavailability is lower due to extensive first-pass metabolism in the liver, where THC is converted into 11-hydroxy-THC, a metabolite that is more potent and contributes to extended psychoactive effects lasting six to eight hours (D'Souza et al., 2023).

Topical and transdermal formulations of cannabis provide localized effects with minimal systemic absorption, making them useful for pain and inflammation without notable psychoactive impact. Cannabinoid metabolism is primarily mediated by cytochrome P450 enzymes, particularly CYP2C9 and CYP3A4, which also metabolize many psychiatric medications. This elicits concerns regarding drug-drug interactions, as CBD has been shown to inhibit these enzymes, possibly increasing plasma concentrations of antidepressants, antipsychotics, and benzodiazepines (Fonseca, Zendulka, & Juřica, 2025). Distribution of cannabinoids is influenced by their lipophilic nature, leading to accumulation in adipose tissue and slow release over time, which may explain prolonged detection of windows in urine and blood testing. Elimination occurs mainly through feces and urine, with half-lives varying widely depending on frequency of use, dose, and individual metabolic variability (Simankowicz & Stępniewska, 2025).

For Psychiatric-Mental Health Nurse Practitioners (PMHNPs), understanding the pharmacokinetics of cannabis is critical for clinical decision-making. Rapid onset via inhalation may appeal to patients looking for immediate relief from anxiety or insomnia, but the unpredictability of oral ingestion, as well as the possibility of drug interactions with psychiatric medications, calls for careful patient education and monitoring. Evidence-based practice requires PMHNPs to consider not only the therapeutic potential of cannabinoids but also their pharmacokinetic complexities, which directly influence efficacy, safety, and risk of adverse outcomes.

THERAPEUTIC APPLICATIONS OF CANNABIS IN PSYCHIATRIC NURSING PRACTICE

Anxiety Disorders

Cannabis use in anxiety disorders has been widely studied, with cannabidiol (CBD) emerging as the most promising compound. CBD acts on serotonin 5-HT1A receptors and reduces amygdala hyperactivity, which explains its anxiolytic effects in social anxiety disorder and generalized anxiety disorder (Roberts et al., 2023). A 2025 living systematic review concluded that CBD consistently reduced anxiety symptoms across multiple trials, though the evidence base remains limited by small sample sizes and short follow-up periods (Cannabis Evidence, 2025). In contrast, tetrahydrocannabinol (THC) demonstrates dose-dependent effects: low doses may reduce anxiety, but higher doses often intensify symptoms such as paranoia, panic, and amplified stress responses (Puder et al., 2025).

For PMHNPs, this means cannabis should be treated prudently. Patients should be educated that CBD-rich formulations are more likely to reduce anxiety, while THC-heavy products may worsen symptoms. Cannabis should be considered only as an adjunct to evidence-based therapies, such as cognitive-behavioral therapy (CBT) or pharmacological treatments such as SSRIs. PMHNPs should also monitor dependency and drug interactions, as CBD can inhibit cytochrome P450 enzymes, possibly raising serum levels of antidepressants and benzodiazepines (Fonseca, Zendulka, & Juřica, 2025). Harm reduction strategies including structured dosing schedules, limiting THC exposure, and regular follow-up are crucial to guarantee safe use.

Depression

Cannabis use in depression presents a more complex picture. While some patients report mood elevation, longitudinal studies consistently show that chronic cannabis use is associated with worsening depressive symptoms and increased suicidality (Churchill et al., 2025). A 2024 systematic review of mood disorders found that problematic cannabis use was highly prevalent among individuals with depression, pointing to the requirement for thorough clinical monitoring (Sorkhou et al., 2024). CBD has shown antidepressant-like effects in preclinical models, enhancing serotonin signaling and promoting hippocampal neurogenesis, which may support affect modulation (Campos et al., 2023). However, THC is linked to motivational deficits, blunted affect, and impaired affective regulation, particularly with long-term use (Simankowicz & Stępniewska, 2025).

PMHNPs should advise patients that cannabis is not a substitute for antidepressants or psychotherapy. If patients insist on cannabis use, CBD-dominant products may be safer, but harm reduction strategies should be emphasized. Patients should be encouraged to adhere to evidence-based treatments such as SSRIs, SNRIs, or psychotherapy, while cannabis use is integrated only as a carefully monitored adjunct. Education ought to emphasize the risks of dependency along with the possibility that cannabis can worsen depressive symptoms over time. Collaboration with psychiatrists and therapists is critical to ensure cannabis use does not undermine recovery goals.

Psychosis

Cannabis use, particularly with high-potency THC products, has been consistently linked to the onset and worsening of psychosis. Psychosis encompasses symptoms such as hallucinations, delusions, paranoia, and disorganized thinking, and cannabis can act as both a precipitating factor and an exacerbating agent in vulnerable individuals. Research has shown that first-episode psychosis is more common among patients who use cannabis daily, especially those consuming high-THC strains, with earlier onset of symptoms compared to non-users (Jin et al., 2025). Adolescents and young adults are particularly at risk, as early cannabis use during brain development significantly increases the likelihood of later psychosis, especially in those with hereditary susceptibilities to schizophrenia. A genetically informed study confirmed that liability for cannabis use disorder is causally associated with increased liability to schizophrenia, pointing to the critical role of prevention and education in youth populations (Johnson et al., 2021). For patients already diagnosed with schizophrenia, cannabis use worsens outcomes, causing more frequent hallucinations, paranoia, and hospitalizations, as THC disrupts dopamine modulation in the brain (Yale School of Medicine, 2024). Even in those without psychiatric diagnoses, acute intoxication with high doses of THC can produce transient psychotic symptoms such as paranoia or delusional thinking, which may resolve after intoxication but can unmask underlying vulnerability. In contrast, cannabidiol (CBD) has demonstrated potential as an antipsychotic, with clinical trials reporting reductions in positive symptoms of schizophrenia and improvements in cognition when used alongside antipsychotics, with fewer side effects in comparison with conventional medications (Patel, 2025). For PMHNPs, cannabis use in psychosis requires vigilant screening and patient education. Patients should be informed that THC-rich cannabis significantly increases psychosis risk, particularly in adolescents, daily users, and those with family histories of schizophrenia. Psychoeducation should extend to families, stressing the significance of the dangers of high-potency cannabis. CBD may be considered an adjunctive therapy in research-supported contexts but is not recommended to replace antipsychotics. PMHNPs should monitor relapse risk, encourage adherence to evidence-based treatments, and integrate harm reduction strategies for patients unwilling to abstain.

Post-Traumatic Stress Disorder

Cannabis has shown encouraging effects for individuals living with post-traumatic stress disorder (PTSD), particularly in easing symptoms such as insomnia, nightmares, hyperarousal, and intrusive memories. The endocannabinoid system plays a key role in fear extinction and affective regulation, and cannabinoids such as THC and CBD appear to enhance these processes. Clinical studies have demonstrated that cannabis use can lead to notable enhancements in quality of sleep and reductions in PTSD-related nightmares, which are often resistant to conventional treatments (Greer, Grob, & Halberstadt, 2023). Veterans, one of the most heavily studied populations with PTSD, report that cannabis helps reduce anxiety, improve mood, and elevate overall quality of life, particularly when traditional therapies have failed.

Emerging research also emphasizes the promise of CBD as a safe adjunctive therapy. Preclinical studies show that CBD enhances fear extinction and reduces hyperarousal, while clinical trials suggest that CBD may improve sleep and alleviate anxiety without the intoxicating effects associated with THC (Haney, 2021). Importantly, cannabis use in PTSD populations has been associated with reductions in overall symptom severity, including improvements in affective regulation and stress resilience (Schubert et al., 2025). These benefits appear among various groups: veterans often report relief from combat-related trauma, while civilians with non-combat trauma describe improvements in sleep and a reduction in the person's intrusive thoughts.

For PMHNPs, cannabis can be considered as a helpful adjunct to evidence-based therapies such as cognitive-behavioral therapy and EMDR. Patients should be educated about the possible advantages of CBD-dominant formulations, which may provide symptom relief with fewer risks of dependency compared to THC-heavy products. Structured dosing schedules, careful monitoring, and integration with trauma-focused psychotherapy can maximize the therapeutic benefits of cannabis while reducing risks. By validating patient experiences and incorporating cannabis thoughtfully into treatment plans, PMHNPs can help patients achieve considerable progress in sleep, anxiety, and overall functioning.

Epilepsy

Cannabis, particularly cannabidiol (CBD), has emerged as one of the most evidence-based adjunctive therapies for epilepsy, especially in treatment-resistant syndromes such as Dravet and Lennox-Gastaut, where customary anti-seizure medications often fail. Epidiolex, the FDA-approved oral CBD solution, has exhibited considerable efficacy, with randomized controlled trials and long-term studies confirming sustained seizure reduction. A 2025 analysis at the American Epilepsy Society reported a 43% greater reduction compared to placebo (Neurology Live, 2025). Real-world data further show improvements in seizure frequency, behavior, and caregiver-reported quality of life (Jazz Pharmaceuticals, 2025). CBD's mechanisms include reducing nerve cell responsiveness by modulating calcium and sodium channels, inhibiting glutamate release, and interacting with TRPV1 receptors. Unlike THC—which can worsen seizures—CBD does not produce psychoactive effects and appears to stabilize neuronal networks. Although generally well tolerated, adverse events such as diarrhea, fatigue, and somnolence occur in some patients, and CBD's interactions with cytochrome P450 enzymes can alter the serum levels of other anti-seizure medications, warranting careful monitoring (Navarro, 2025).

Pediatric patients with Dravet and Lennox-Gastaut syndromes show the most robust responses, though adults with tuberous sclerosis complex also benefit. For PMHNPs, the clinical responsibility includes educating families that only pharmaceutical-grade CBD has proven efficacy, discouraging unregulated cannabis products, collaborating with neurologists to integrate CBD safely, and monitoring psychiatric comorbidities such as anxiety and depression, highlighting harm reduction and avoiding THC-rich cannabis due to its ability to worsen seizures.

Pain

Cannabis-based medicines have been increasingly studied for both acute and chronic pain, though the strength of evidence differs by context. For chronic and subacute pain, systematic reviews consistently find modest improvements in pain intensity and function compared with placebo, alongside a higher rate of adverse events such as dizziness and cognitive effects; the 2025 Agency for Healthcare Research and Quality (AHRQ) living systematic review concluded there is low-to-moderate certainty of benefit for chronic and subacute pain, with important heterogeneity across products, doses, and pain etiologies. Mechanistically, tetrahydrocannabinol (THC) acts as a partial agonist at CB1 receptors, modulating nociceptive transmission and descending nociceptive pathways, while cannabidiol (CBD) appears to act primarily via anti-inflammatory and neuromodulatory mechanisms involving CB2 and TRPV1 receptors, supporting a plausible biological basis for analgesia within neuropathic and inflammatory pain states (Valani, 2022). In chronic non-cancer pain, recent systematic reviews report small-to-moderate reductions in pain scores, better sleep, and improved global impression of change, but with frequent adverse effects and variable tolerability; a 2025 review found efficacy signals across several formulations with meaningful but modest effect sizes, emphasizing individualized dosing and patient selection to balance benefit with side-effect burden (Wasilewska et al., 2025). Clinical practice guidance echoes a careful, optional role: the BMJ rapid recommendation guideline advises that medical cannabis or cannabinoids may be considered for chronic pain due to cancer or non-cancer causes when standard therapies are insufficient, highlighting small net benefits on pain, sleep, and physical function, and recommending shared decision-making because harms are common and certainty is low to moderate (Busse et al., 2021). Evidence for acute pain is weaker; across perioperative and acute injury contexts, reviews describe inconsistent or minimal analgesic effects and a higher incidence of adverse events, with no clear advantage over standard non-opioid or opioid regimens, leading experts to conclude that cannabinoids are not established for acute postoperative pain and should not replace guideline-supported multimodal analgesia (AminiLari et al., 2022). For PMHNPs, cannabis-based therapies should be considered adjuncts within a multimodal plan, with clear goals like better sleep or reduced pain intensity, preference for CBD-dominant or balanced products to reduce intoxication risks, cautious titration, and forward-looking monitoring for adverse effects and misuse.

Bipolar Disorder

Cannabis use is common among individuals with bipolar disorder, but studies repeatedly show that it is associated with poorer clinical outcomes. THC-rich cannabis products exacerbate manic symptoms by increasing dopaminergic activity in the mesolimbic pathway, which has the potential to destabilize mood and trigger rapid cycling (D'Souza et al., 2023). In contrast, cannabidiol (CBD) has been investigated for its possible role in mood-stabilizing properties, with preclinical studies suggesting modulation of serotonin and glutamate signaling that may reduce manic and depressive symptoms (Campos et al., 2023). However, clinical evidence for CBD in bipolar disorder remains preliminary.

Current investigations emphasize the risks of cannabis use in this population. A 2024 systematic review found that individuals with bipolar disorder who used cannabis experienced earlier onset of illness, more frequent hospitalizations, and higher rates of suicidality compared to non-users (Sorkhou, Dent, & George, 2024). Similarly, a 2025 study in *Translational Psychiatry* reported that chronic cannabis use was associated with impaired decision-making and cognitive dysfunction in bipolar patients, though some participants reported subjective improvements in creativity and affect modulation (Miranda et al., 2025). Another review emphasized that cannabis use worsens the overall course of bipolar disorder, leading to longer episodes and increased cycling between mania and depression (Mondimore, 2025).

ADHD

Attention-deficit/hyperactivity disorder (ADHD) is a neurodevelopmental condition defined by inattention, impulsivity, and hyperactivity, affecting both children and adults. Cannabis use among people diagnosed with ADHD is common, often driven by patient perceptions that cannabinoids can improve focus, reduce restlessness, or alleviate comorbid anxiety. However, recent evidence demonstrates a complicated and frequently problematic relationship between cannabis and ADHD. A 2023 scoping review found that while some patients report subjective improvements, cannabis use is associated with poorer cognitive outcomes, including deficits in attention, working memory, and executive function (Ryan et al., 2024). Similarly, a 2025 review in the *Journal of Molecular Neuroscience* emphasized that cannabinoids may modulate overactive brain networks implicated in ADHD, but clinical evidence remains preliminary and inconsistent (Mavaddat et al., 2025).

THC and CBD exert different effects on ADHD symptoms. THC, acting on CB1 receptors, can transiently increase dopamine release in the prefrontal cortex, leading to short-term improvements in focus. However, chronic THC exposure disrupts dopamine signaling, resulting in extended cognitive impairment and increased impulsivity (Joynson, 2025). CBD, in contrast, does not produce intoxicating effects and may reduce anxiety and emotional dysregulation, which are frequently found in ADHD. Yet, evidence for CBD's direct impact on core ADHD symptoms remains limited, with most studies focusing on comorbid conditions rather than ADHD itself (Ryan et al., 2024).

The risks of cannabis use in ADHD populations are significant. Adolescents with ADHD who use cannabis are at higher risk of developing cannabis use disorder, with diagnostic hurdles making treatment more difficult (JAACAP, 2025). A 2021 mixed-methods study examining children and young adults with ADHD and oppositional defiant disorder found that perceptions of cannabis as "safe" commonly caused unsupervised use, despite limited evidence of benefit (Mansell et al., 2021). These findings underscore the importance of addressing misconceptions among patients and caregivers.

For PMHNPs, clinical recommendations must balance patient experiences with evidence-based practice. Cannabis should not be considered a primary treatment for ADHD. Psychostimulant drugs such as methylphenidate and amphetamines, alongside behavioral interventions, remain the gold standard. PMHNPs should screen patients for cannabis use, particularly adolescents, and educate them about the risks of cognitive impairment and dependency. If patients insist on cannabis use, CBD-dominant formulations may be safer, but should only be considered adjunctively and under close monitoring. Harm reduction strategies—including limiting THC exposure, structured dosing schedules, and regular follow-up—are essential. Collaboration with families, schools, and addiction specialists can help support patients in reducing cannabis use and complying with established ADHD treatments.

Sleep Disorders

Sleep disorders, particularly insomnia, are among the most common complaints in psychiatric practice, and cannabis has increasingly been used by patients seeking relief. THC and CBD exert different effects on sleep physiology. THC, acting as a partial agonist at CB1 receptors, reduces sleep latency and increases slow-wave sleep, which explains why many patients report falling asleep faster after cannabis use. However, chronic THC exposure is associated with tolerance, dependency, and alterations in sleep architecture, incorporating diminished REM sleep and rebound insomnia upon cessation (Haney, 2021). CBD, in contrast, appears to improve sleep quality without significantly disrupting sleep phases. It modulates serotonin signaling and reduces anxiety, which indirectly enhances sleep continuity (Zuardi et al., 2022).

Recent research has provided more subtle understandings. A 2022 systematic review of randomized clinical trials found that medical cannabis and cannabinoids improved sleep outcomes compared to placebo, but the quality of evidence was low, and adverse effects such as dizziness and fatigue were common (AminiLari et al., 2022). A 2024 updated review highlighted that although cannabinoids are widely used for sleep disorders, high-quality long-term studies are lacking, and concerns about safety continue (Lavender et al., 2024). More encouragingly, a 2025 longitudinal study following insomnia patients treated with cannabis-based medicines reported continued enhancements in sleep quality, mood, and pain management over 18 months, with most participants experiencing better rest and reduced anxiety or depression. Only a small fraction reported mild side effects such as fatigue or dry mouth (ScienceDaily, 2025; Pain News Network, 2025). This evidence points to the fact that cannabis-based therapies may provide lasting relief for some patients, though careful patient selection and monitoring are essential.

For PMHNPs, the clinical implications are clear. Cannabis should not replace first-line treatments, such as cognitive-behavioral therapy for insomnia (CBT-I), sleep hygiene interventions, or medicinal drugs with established efficacy. Patients should be educated that while cannabis may provide short-term relief, long-term use of THC can lead to tolerance, dependency, and disrupted sleep architecture. CBD-dominant formulations may be preferable for patients who insist on cannabis use, given their safer profile and potential to improve REM sleep and reduce nightmares, particularly in psychiatric populations such as those with PTSD. PMHNPs should monitor patients closely for dependency, encourage structured dosing schedules, and integrate cannabis use into a multimodal treatment plan that focuses on evidence-based interventions.

Substance Use Disorders

Cannabis use in the context of substance use disorders (SUDs) presents both possible therapeutic applications and major risks. The endocannabinoid system plays a central role in reward, motivation, and addiction pathways, which has led researchers to investigate cannabinoids as possible adjuncts in the treatment of opioid, alcohol, and stimulant use disorders. Cannabidiol (CBD) has been studied for its ability to reduce cravings and relapse risk. Preclinical studies show that CBD can modulate dopaminergic and glutamatergic signaling, thereby attenuating drug-seeking behaviors (Luján, Kim, Zhang, & Cheer, 2025). Early clinical trials suggest that CBD may reduce cue-induced cravings in patients with opioid use disorder and improve stress resilience, which is often a trigger for relapse (Haney, 2021). Similarly, CBD has been explored in alcohol use disorder, with findings indicating reductions in alcohol intake and improvements in liver function markers in animal models, though human data remain limited (Simankowicz & Stępniewska, 2025).

Despite these encouraging findings, cannabis use itself can obstruct recovery from other addictions. THC-rich cannabis carries a high risk of dependency, with CDC data showing that approximately three in ten cannabis users develop cannabis use disorder, and adolescents are particularly vulnerable (Simankowicz & Stępniewska, 2025). Furthermore, cannabis use in patients with SUDs may serve as an entry point to continued polysubstance use, undermining recovery efforts. A 2023 systematic review determined that although CBD may show potential as a harm reduction tool, the evidence base is still preliminary, and cannabis use should not replace established interventions such as medication-assisted therapy (MAT) for opioid use disorder or cognitive-behavioral approaches for alcohol and stimulant use disorders (Lev-Ran et al., 2022).

For PMHNPs, the clinical implications are multifaceted. Patients with SUDs should be screened for cannabis use, with careful differentiation between CBD and THC products. Education should highlight that although CBD may have possible healing advantages, THC-rich cannabis may worsen addiction risk and obstruct recovery. PMHNPs should encourage patients to give precedence to evidence-based treatments such as MAT, motivational interviewing, and relapse prevention therapy, while recognizing patient interest in cannabis as an adjunctive approach. Harm reduction strategies are vital, including structured dosing schedules, limiting THC exposure, and monitoring for cannabis use disorder. Collaboration with addiction specialists and integration of cannabis discussions within a wider treatment planning can help ensure the patient care continues to be safe, evidence-based, and responsive to each person's needs.

Eating Disorders

Cannabis has been explored as a potential adjunct in the management of eating disorders, particularly anorexia nervosa, due to its appetite-stimulating properties. THC activates CB1 receptors in the hypothalamus, increasing appetite and food intake, which has led some patients to self-medicate in an attempt to counter restrictive eating behaviors (Haney, 2021). Limited clinical evidence suggests that cannabis may reduce anxiety around eating and improve caloric intake, but this evidence is variable and frequently confounded by risks of dependency and psychiatric destabilization. A 2023 scoping review noted that although cannabinoid agonists show promise for stimulating appetite, the evidence base remains weak, with most studies being small-scale or observational (Valani, 2022). More recently, a 2025 global survey of individuals with eating disorders reported that patients often self-medicate with cannabis and psychedelics, rating them as more effective than antidepressants for symptom relief, though the survey also noted high rates of cannabis use disorder in this population (Simankowicz & Stępniewska, 2025).

For PMHNPs, cannabis use in eating disorders demands thorough evaluation. Patients should be educated that cannabis is not an evidence-based treatment for anorexia or bulimia and that nutritional rehabilitation and psychotherapy remain the cornerstones of care. While cannabis may provide short-term appetite stimulation, its long-term use carries risks of dependency, cognitive impairment, and worsening psychiatric symptoms. PMHNPs should validate patients' experiences while emphasizing safer, evidence-based interventions, such as family-based therapy, cognitive-behavioral therapy, and pharmacological support when indicated. If patients insist on cannabis use, CBD-dominant formulations may be preferable because of their reduced risk of intoxication, but close monitoring is vital to ensure cannabis does not interfere with recovery goals. Harm reduction strategies, including limiting THC exposure and structured dosing schedules, should be discussed openly with patients and families. Table 2 provides a quick reference for the PMHNP to better understand the relationship between disorders, effects, recommendations, pharmacology, population considerations, and mechanism of action.

Table 2. Cannabis use across disorders – PMHNP quick reference

Disorder	Effects	Clinical Recommendations	Pharmacology	Population Considerations	Mechanism of Action
Psychosis	THC worsens; CBD may help	Screen, discourage THC, educate	Antipsychotics; CBD adjunct	Adolescents, family hx ↑ risk	THC → dopamine dysregulation; CBD → serotonin/ glutamate
PTSD	↓ nightmares, hyperarousal; CBD aids fear extinction	Validate, CBT/ EMDR, monitor	SSRIs/SNRIs; prazosin; CBD adjunct	Veterans benefit; adolescents ↑ dependency	THC → amygdala CB1; CBD → 5-HT1A, CB2
Epilepsy	CBD ↓ seizures; THC may worsen	Use Epidiolex only	Epidiolex + AEDs	Pediatric syndromes strongest benefit	CBD → Na/Ca channels, TRPV1, ↓ glutamate
Pain (Chronic)	Modest relief, better sleep	Adjunct only, set goals	NSAIDs, gabapentinoids, duloxetine; CBD adjunct	Neuropathic/ cancer pain benefit; elderly ↑ side effects	THC → CB1 nociception; CBD → CB2/TRPV1 anti-inflammatory
Pain (Acute)	Weak evidence, ↑ adverse events	Not first-line	Opioids/ NSAIDs	Limited peri-op benefit	THC slow onset, psychoactive limits

continued on following page

Table 2. Continued

Disorder	Effects	Clinical Recommendations	Pharmacology	Population Considerations	Mechanism of Action
Bipolar	THC destabilizes; CBD investigational	Counsel, emphasize stabilizers	Lithium, valproate, lamotrigine; avoid THC	Young adults ↑ use; women ↑ worsening	THC → dopamine ↑ mania; CBD → serotonin/glutamate
Anxiety	CBD ↓ anxiety; THC dose-dependent	Prefer CBD, integrate CBT/ SSRIs	SSRIs/SNRIs; benzos short-term	Adolescents vulnerable; adults benefit	CBD → 5-HT1A; THC high dose → anxiety
Depression	CBD antidepressant-like; THC worsens	Encourage SSRIs/ therapy	SSRIs/SNRIs; atypical antipsychotics; CBD adjunct	Young adults ↑ cannabis use; women ↑ worsening	CBD → hippocampal neurogenesis; THC disrupts serotonin/ dopamine
ADHD	Subjective focus ↑; THC worsens cognition	Screen youth; emphasize stimulants	Stimulants; atomoxetine; CBD investigational	Adolescents ↑ dependency risk	THC impairs prefrontal cortex; CBD ↓ anxiety
Sleep	THC ↓ latency but disrupts REM; CBD improves quality	Prioritize CBT-I; CBD adjunct	CBT-I; zolpidem, trazodone; CBD adjunct	Veterans ↓ nightmares; elderly ↑ sedation	THC → CB1 latency ↓; CBD → serotonin/GABA
Eating Disorders	THC ↑ appetite; CBD ↓ anxiety	Emphasize nutrition/therapy	SSRIs; olanzapine; THC investigational	Adolescents ↑ misuse; anorexia adults' appetite ↑	THC → hypothalamic CB1 appetite; CBD → serotonin anxiolysis
Substance Use	CBD ↓ cravings; THC ↑ relapse	Screen, prioritize MAT	MAT (buprenorphine, naltrexone); CBD investigational	Polysubstance users ↑ misuse; veterans use for cravings	CBD → dopamine/ glutamate craving ↓; THC → reward relapse ↑

BENEFITS AND RISKS OF CANNABIS USE

Cannabis has become one of the most widely used psychoactive substances worldwide, and its role in both medical and psychiatric contexts has expanded significantly in recent years. For Psychiatric-Mental Health Nurse Practitioners (PMHNPs), grasping the advantages and risks of cannabis is essential to providing safe and high-quality care. Patients increasingly report using cannabis to self-manage conditions such as anxiety, PTSD, chronic pain, and insomnia, yet the evidence base demonstrates a nuanced trade-off of therapeutic promise and psychiatric risk.

Research conducted between 2021 and 2025 illuminates both sides of this twofold profile, stressing the value of clinician education and patient counseling.

The benefits of cannabis are most clearly demonstrated in seizure disorder management. Cannabidiol (CBD), a non-intoxicating cannabinoid, has shown anticonvulsant properties in multiple randomized controlled trials. Navarro (2025) reported that Epidiolex, an FDA-approved CBD oral solution, reduced seizure frequency by 43 percent in patients with Dravet and Lennox-Gastaut syndromes compared to placebo. This evidence confirms CBD's therapeutic benefit in rare pediatric epilepsies and draws attention to its potential as an adjunctive therapy for larger-scale seizure disorders. Beyond epilepsy, cannabis has demonstrated modest benefits in chronic pain management. The Agency for Healthcare Research and Quality concluded in a living systematic review that cannabinoids provide small improvements in pain and function, with low-to-moderate certainty of evidence. Wasilewska et al. (2025) similarly found that cannabinoids improved neuropathic pain outcomes, though adverse effects were common. These results suggest that cannabis may serve as an adjunctive therapy for patients with refractory pain, particularly neuropathic and cancer-related pain, when conventional treatments fail.

Cannabis has also been studied for its antiemetic properties in oncology. Busse et al. (2021) reported that cannabinoids reduced chemotherapy-induced nausea and vomiting, providing alleviation for patients undergoing intensive treatment. This benefit is particularly important for improving the quality of life and adherence to cancer therapies. In psychiatric contexts, cannabis has shown mixed but positive results. Greer et al. (2023) observed that cannabis reduced nightmares and hyperarousal in patients with PTSD, while Schubert et al. (2025) found variable outcomes in veterans using cannabis for trauma-related symptoms. Roberts et al. (2023) demonstrated that CBD consistently reduced anxiety symptoms in controlled trials, supporting its adjunctive use in generalized anxiety disorder. Campos et al. (2023) further showed that CBD promoted hippocampal neurogenesis, implying prospective antidepressant-like effects. The evidence suggests that CBD may have therapeutic applications in anxiety and depression, though THC's role remains more problematic. Emerging evidence also suggests potential harm reduction benefits. Luján et al. (2025) found that CBD reduced drug-seeking behaviors in preclinical models of substance use disorders, while Churchill et al. (2025) reported that medical cannabis patients in New York had significantly reduced opioid prescriptions, suggesting cannabis may serve as an opioid-sparing agent.

Despite these benefits, cannabis use carries major risks, particularly in psychiatric populations. THC, the primary psychoactive compound, has been consistently linked to psychosis. Jin et al. (2025) reported that cannabis use was common among individuals with first-episode psychosis and was associated with increased relapse risk. Johnson et al. (2021) used genetic liability models to demonstrate causal links between cannabis use disorder and schizophrenia. These outcomes emphasize the importance of screening for cannabis use in psychotic populations and educating patients regarding the possibility of symptom exacerbation. Cannabis use has also been associated with negative outcomes in mood disorders. Sorkhou, Dent, and George (2024) conducted a systematic review showing that problematic cannabis use is highly prevalent among individuals with bipolar disorder, with associations to earlier onset and increased suicidality. Miranda et al. (2025) found that chronic cannabis use impaired cognition in bipolar patients, while Mondimore (2025) emphasized clinical worsening of mood stability. Churchill et al. (2025) reported that cannabis use was associated with worsening depression outcomes, further highlighting the risks of THC in mood disorders.

Cognitive impairment is another documented risk. Ryan et al. (2024) reviewed cannabis use in ADHD populations and found that while patients reported subjective improvements in focus, THC use was associated with poorer cognitive results and elevated dependency risk. Mansell et al. (2021) similarly reported that adolescents perceived cannabis as "safe," despite evidence of impaired executive function. Such data illustrate the vulnerability of younger populations to cannabis-related cognitive deficits. Cannabis use also carries risks for sleep disorders. AminiLari et al. (2022) reported that cannabinoids improved sleep outcomes in the short term, but Lavender et al. (2024) noted insufficient long-term data and highlighted THC's disruption of REM sleep. This indicates that although cannabis may reduce sleep latency, it may impair sleep architecture, leading to poorer general sleep quality.

Substance use disorders present additional concerns. Lev-Ran et al. (2022) emphasized that THC complicates recovery by activating pleasure circuits and increasing relapse risk. While CBD shows potential in decreasing cravings, THC's reinforcing properties can worsen addiction. Polysubstance users are particularly vulnerable, with higher rates of cannabis misuse and poorer treatment outcomes. Pharmacological risks also include drug–drug and food interactions. Valani (2022) highlighted that both THC and CBD are metabolized by cytochrome P450 enzymes, creating potential interactions with antidepressants, antiepileptics, and anticoagulants. Navarro (2025) emphasized that CBD can alter serum levels of clobazam and valproate, eliciting concerns for toxicity. Food interactions are also clinically relevant. High-fat meals significantly increase CBD absorption, which can improve therapeutic effects but also raise the risk of adverse events such as sedation and gastrointestinal upset (Navarro, 2025). Grapefruit juice, a known CYP3A4 inhibitor, may increase plasma concentrations of cannabinoids, causing elevated psychoactive or sedative effects (Valani, 2022). These observations confirm the importance of PMHNPs monitoring both drug and nutritional considerations in patients using cannabis.

Public health evidence shows broader risks. Volkow (2025) reported that increased cannabis availability has decreased public perception of harm and increased use, particularly among adolescents. Mehta (2025) argued that cannabis education is a professional obligation, noting that clinicians must address gaps between patient behavior and scientific evidence. These perspectives reinforce the need for PMHNPs to remain knowledgeable and proactive in-patient education.

Cannabis presents a dual profile of therapeutic promise and psychiatric risk. Benefits include seizure reduction in epilepsy, modest improvements in chronic pain, antiemetic effects in oncology, and potential anxiolytic and antidepressant properties of CBD. Risks include psychosis exacerbation, mood destabilization, cognitive impairment, sleep disruption, addiction, drug–drug interactions, and food-related absorption changes. Recent research from 2021 to 2025 reinforces the need for clinician education, as outcomes vary widely depending on cannabinoid type, dosage, patient population, and comorbid conditions. For PMHNPs, cannabis literacy is essential to provide balanced, research-supported guidance, making certain that patients receive safe and ethical care in an era of expanding cannabis use.

The Complexity of Cannabis Decision-Making

Patients increasingly report using cannabis to manage psychiatric symptoms such as anxiety, insomnia, PTSD, and depression. However, the evidence supporting cannabis use for these conditions is mixed. For example, cannabidiol (CBD) has shown anxiolytic and antipsychotic properties in some trials, while tetrahydrocannabinol (THC) has been associated with increased relapse risk in psychosis and mood destabilization in bipolar disorder (Churchill et al., 2025; Sorkhou et al., 2024). PMHNPs have to balance these risks and benefits in real time, often with insufficient data and under different state and federal laws.

Clinical decision-making must also account for personal health variables such as age, diagnosis, comorbidities, substance use history, and medication regimen. For instance, a patient with generalized anxiety disorder may benefit from low-dose CBD, while a patient with schizophrenia may experience symptom exacerbation with THC exposure. The complexity of these decisions underscores the need for organized evidence-informed tools to guide PMHNPs through assessment and treatment planning.

Introducing the EBP Tool: The CAN-RISK Framework

To support clinical decision-making, PMHNPs can adopt the CAN-RISK framework — a structured, evidence based instrument created to evaluate cannabis use in psychiatric populations. CAN-RISK stands for:

- Condition-specific evidence

- Active ingredients (THC vs. CBD)
- Neuropsychiatric profile
- Risk factors (age, diagnosis, substance use)
- Interactions (drug–drug, food)
- Safety monitoring
- Knowledge of legal context

This framework empowers PMHNPs to systematically assess whether cannabis use is appropriate, safe, and evidence-supported for a given patient.

Applying CAN-RISK in Practice

1. Condition-Specific Evidence: PMHNPs commence with an analysis of the literature on cannabis efficacy for the patient's primary diagnosis. For example, CBD has demonstrated seizure reduction in epilepsy (Navarro, 2025), modest pain relief in chronic pain, and anxiolytic effects in small trials (Roberts et al., 2023). Conversely, THC has been linked to worsening outcomes in depression and psychosis (Churchill et al., 2025; Jin et al., 2025). The clinician must determine whether the evidence supports cannabis use for the patient's condition and whether the benefits outweigh the risks.
2. Active Ingredients: Differentiating between THC and CBD are essential. THC is psychoactive and associated with increased dopamine release in mesolimbic pathways, which could worsen psychosis and addiction risk. CBD is non-intoxicating and modulates serotonin and endocannabinoid systems, exhibiting potential therapeutic effects without euphoria. PMHNPs must assess the cannabinoid profile of the product the patient is using or considering, as many over-the-counter products contain variable and unregulated concentrations.
3. Neuropsychiatric Profile: The patient's psychiatric history, cognitive function, and symptom trajectory must be evaluated. For example, a patient with bipolar disorder and a history of rapid cycling may be at higher risk of mood destabilization with THC use (Miranda et al., 2025). Mental evaluations may reveal impairments linked to cannabis use, particularly in adolescents and young adults (Ryan et al., 2024). PMHNPs should use validated tools, such as the Montreal Cognitive Assessment (MoCA) or the PHQ-9, to monitor changes over time.
4. Risk Factors: Age, family history, substance use history, and comorbid conditions influence cannabis-related risk. Adolescents and young adults are more vulnerable to cognitive impairment and dependency (Volkow, 2025). Patients with a history of substance use disorder may be at increased risk of relapse, particularly with THC (Lev-Ran et al., 2022). PMHNPs should screen for these

factors using tools such as the ASSIST (Alcohol, Smoking and Substance Involvement Screening Test) or the CAGE-AID questionnaire.

5. Interactions: Cannabis interacts with numerous medications via cytochrome P450 metabolism. THC is metabolized by CYP2C9, while CBD is metabolized by CYP2C19 and CYP3A4, potentially altering the serum levels of antidepressants, antiepileptics, and anticoagulants (Valani, 2022). CBD has been shown to increase clobazam and valproate levels, raising toxicity concerns (Navarro, 2025). Food also interacts with matter: high-fat meals can increase CBD absorption by up to fourfold, and grapefruit juice may inhibit metabolism, increasing plasma concentrations. PMHNPs must review the patient's medication list and dietary habits to anticipate adverse effects.
6. Safety Monitoring: Once cannabis use is initiated or continued, PMHNPs must implement protective protocols. This encompasses routine follow-up, symptom tracking, mental evaluations, and urine drug screening when appropriate. Adverse effects such as sedation, paranoia, or gastrointestinal upset should be documented and addressed. PMHNPs should also educate patients on safe dosing, product selection, and harm-reduction strategies, such as avoiding high-THC strains or combining cannabis with alcohol.
7. Knowledge of Legal Context: PMHNPs must be aware of both state and federal cannabis laws. While most states have legalized medical cannabis, federal law still classifies marijuana as a Schedule I substance, prohibiting its use in federally funded institutions and complicating research access (Congress.gov, 2025). The 2018 Farm Bill legalized hemp-derived CBD, but many products remain unregulated. PMHNPs must ensure that any recommendations or discussions comply with their state's scope of practice laws and institutional policies. Documentation should reflect legal considerations and patient education.

Benefits of Using CAN-RISK

The CAN-RISK framework delivers several advantages. It promotes uniformity throughout providers, reduces bias, and ensures that decisions are grounded in current evidence. It also facilitates interdisciplinary communication, as PMHNPs can share structured assessments with physicians, pharmacists, and therapists. Most importantly, it supports ethical, patient-focused care by combining research, clinical expertise, and personal choices.

Clinical decision-making in cannabis care is inherently complex, requiring PMHNPs to balance therapeutic potential with psychiatric risk, legal constraints, and patient autonomy. The CAN-RISK framework delivers a structured, evidence-based approach to guide these decisions, making certain that cannabis use is evaluated systematically and safely. By including condition-specific evidence, pharmacology, risk factors, interactions, and legal context, PMHNPs can deliver informed, ethical, and high-quality care in an era of expanding cannabis use.

Legal and Ethical Considerations of Cannabis Use

The legal and ethical aspects of cannabis use in psychiatric care pose a multifaceted and evolving challenge for Psychiatric-Mental Health Nurse Practitioners (PMHNPs) and their patients. As cannabis becomes more widely available through state-level legalization for both medical and recreational use, PMHNPs must manage a setting defined by conflicting federal laws, inconsistent clinical guidelines, and moral challenges surrounding patient autonomy, safety, and informed consent. As of 2025, forty states, three territories, and the District of Columbia permit the medical use of cannabis products, while twenty-four states allow non-medical adult use (National Conference of State Legislatures [NCSL], 2025). Despite this widespread legalization, cannabis is still a Schedule I controlled substance under federal law, meaning it is classified as having no accepted medical use and a high potential for abuse (Congress.gov, 2025). This contradiction creates considerable legal ambiguity for PMHNPs, particularly those practicing in federally funded institutions or across state lines. The American Nurses Association (ANA) has acknowledged this tension, supporting the reclassification of cannabis to support research and evidence-based care (Stokes, 2022). The ANA's position emphasizes that nurses need to be prepared to counsel patients on cannabis use while observing moral principles and legal limits. Similarly, the American Association of Nurse Practitioners (AANP) supports policies that allow NPs to take part in open dialogue with patients about cannabis without fear of criminal or professional repercussions (AANP, 2025). These professional organizations point out the ethical imperative for PMHNPs to provide accurate, nonjudgmental information, even when legal frameworks are inconsistent.

From an ethical standpoint, PMHNPs are guided by principles such as autonomy, beneficence, nonmaleficence, and justice. Patient autonomy requires that people possess the entitlement to make well-informed decisions regarding their treatment, including the use of cannabis. However, informed consent is complicated by the deficiency of standardized dosing, product variability, and limited clinical research on long-term psychiatric outcomes. For example, while cannabidiol (CBD) has shown potential in decreasing anxiety and seizures, tetrahydrocannabinol (THC) has been linked to increased risk of psychosis, mood destabilization, and cognitive impairment (Churchill et al., 2025; Jin et al., 2025). PMHNPs must ensure that patients understand these risks and benefits, particularly when cannabis is used to self-medicate for psychiatric symptoms. Ethical practice demands that clinicians neither endorse nor condemn cannabis use without an in-depth examination of individual circumstances and current evidence. Beneficence and nonmaleficence require PMHNPs to act in the patient's best interest while mitigating harm. This includes screening for contraindications such as a history of psychosis or substance use disorder, monitoring adverse effects, and educating patients on safe use practices. For instance, patients with bipolar disorder may experience mood destabilization with THC, and adolescents are particularly vulnerable to cognitive impairment and dependency (Sorkhou et al., 2024; Volkow, 2025). Justice, as an ethical principle, calls for just access to care and protection from discrimination. PMHNPs must be aware of disparities in cannabis-related arrests, access to medical cannabis programs, and stigma surrounding use, especially among marginalized populations. Ethical care involves endorsing policies that reduce harm and advance health fairness.

Legally, PMHNPs must operate within the scope of their state's medical cannabis laws, which vary widely in terms of qualifying conditions, certification requirements, and provider authority. In some states, PMHNPs are authorized to recommend medical cannabis, while in others, only physicians may do so. PMHNPs must verify their eligibility to participate in state cannabis programs and ensure that documentation meets regulatory criteria. This includes completing required training, registering with state databases, and using approved forms to certify patient eligibility. Failure to comply with state laws can result in disciplinary action, loss of licensure, or criminal charges. Moreover, federal law prohibits the possession and use of cannabis on federal property, including Veterans Affairs hospitals and military bases, regardless of state legalization. PMHNPs working in these settings must adhere to federal policies, which may restrict their ability to talk about or recommend cannabis. The Drug Enforcement Administration (DEA) has not updated its classification of cannabis, and the Food and Drug Administration (FDA) has only approved one cannabis-derived medication—Epidiolex—for specific seizure disorders (FDA, 2025). This regulatory gap limits the assimilation of cannabis into formal treatment protocols and complicates insurance reimbursement. PMHNPs must document cannabis-related care meticulously, including clinical rationale, patient education, and monitoring plans, to protect themselves and their patients from legal liability.

Moral challenges also arise when patients use cannabis without disclosure or outside medical guidance. PMHNPs should cultivate a therapeutic alliance that encourages honesty and transparency, permitting reliable assessment and risk mitigation. This includes asking about cannabis use during intake, using validated screening tools such as the Alcohol, Smoking and Substance Involvement Screening Test (ASSIST), and incorporating cannabis into the treatment plan when appropriate. Ethical care may involve harm reduction strategies, such as recommending lower-THC products, avoiding concurrent alcohol use, and monitoring dependency. PMHNPs must also consider the ethical consequences of refusing care or stigmatizing patients who use cannabis, which can weaken trust and worsen mental health symptoms. Informed consent is particularly critical when cannabis is used alongside psychotropic medications, as interactions may alter medication metabolism and increase toxicity. For example, CBD can inhibit cytochrome P450 enzymes, thereby altering the serum levels of antidepressants, antiepileptics, and anticoagulants (Valani, 2022). PMHNPs must educate patients on these risks and coordinate care with pharmacists and other providers to ensure safety.

The ethical imperative to provide evidence-based care is challenged by the limited research on cannabis in psychiatric populations. Many studies are observational, lack of control groups, or use inconsistent dosing and formulations. This makes it difficult for PMHNPs to offer definitive guidance, especially in conditions like PTSD, depression, and ADHD, where cannabis use is common, but outcomes are variable (Greer et al., 2023; Ryan et al., 2024). Professional organizations have called for expanded research and clearer clinical guidelines. The ANA supports reclassification of cannabis to Schedule II or III to promote research, while the AANP advocates for inclusion of cannabis education in nursing curricula (Stokes, 2022; AANP, 2025). PMHNPs need to remain up to date through continuing education, peer-reviewed literature, and policy updates to provide competent care. They should also advocate for increased research funding, regulatory reform, and public health education.

In conclusion, the legal and ethical aspects of cannabis use in psychiatric care require PMHNPs to balance patient autonomy with clinical safety, navigate conflicting laws, and observe professional standards. By combining evidence-based practice, complying with state and federal guidelines, and fostering moral decision-making, PMHNPs can support patients in forming informed choices about cannabis use. Ongoing education, documentation, and advocacy are crucial to guarantee that care continues to be patient-centered, legally compliant, and ethically sound in an era of expanding cannabis access.

Legal Context in the United States

The legal framework for cannabis in the United States is complicated. At the federal level, cannabis is still classified as a Schedule I substance under the Controlled Substances Act, meaning it is considered to have "no accepted medical use" and a high potential for abuse (Congress.gov, 2025). The Executive Order (2025) signed by President Donald Trump will change the classification to a Schedule III if it is passed by Congress. The Schedule I classification creates tension with state laws, as 40 states, the District of Columbia, and several territories have legalized medical cannabis programs, and 24 states now permit recreational use (NCSL, 2025). For PMHNPs, this conflicting situation means that while they may be authorized to recommend cannabis under state law, they need to exercise caution in federally funded institutions such as Veterans Affairs hospitals, where cannabis use remains prohibited (CDC, 2024).

Ethical Principles in Clinical Practice

Ethically, PMHNPs are guided by principles of autonomy, beneficence, nonmaleficence, and justice. Patient autonomy requires that individuals be able to make well-informed choices about cannabis use, but informed consent is complicated by variability in product potency, deficiency of standardized dosing, and limited long-term psychiatric research (Churchill et al., 2025). Beneficence and nonmaleficence require clinicians to balance possible therapeutic advantages such as CBD's anticonvulsant effects with risks like THC-induced psychosis or mood destabilization (Jin et al., 2025; Sorkhou et al., 2024). Justice requires just access to care and protection from stigma, particularly given disparities in cannabis-related arrests and access to medical cannabis programs among marginalized populations (Volkow, 2025).

Expanded Provider Documentation Standards in Cannabis Care

Documentation is one of the most essential duties for PMHNPs when engaging in cannabis-related care, functioning as both a clinical safeguard and a legal defense. Because cannabis remains federally classified as a Schedule I substance in the United States, detailed record-keeping makes certain that PMHNPs demonstrate compliance with state laws, institutional policies, and professional standards (Congress.gov, 2025). At its core, documentation must define a clear clinical rationale for cannabis use, including the diagnosis, symptom severity, and alignment with qualifying conditions recognized by the state program (CDC, 2024). For example, in Pennsylvania, clinicians must explicitly record the qualifying condition, counseling provided, and registry entry to remain compliant with Department of Health requirements (Pennsylvania Department of Health, 2025).

Beyond diagnosis, documentation should include a risk–benefit analysis that weighs the therapeutic potential against known harms. This analysis ought to reference current evidence, such as CBD's therapeutic benefit in reducing seizures in epilepsy (Navarro, 2025) or THC's association with increased relapse risk in psychosis (Jin et al., 2025). Ethical practice requires that patients be informed of both benefits and risks, and that the informed consent process be documented in detail. Consent notes should cover product variability, dosing uncertainty, possible side effects (e.g., sedation, paranoia, cognitive impairment), dependency risk, and drug–drug interactions, notably those involving cytochrome P450 metabolism

(Valani, 2022). Informed consent documentation protects patient autonomy while shielding PMHNPs from liability.

International guidelines affirm the value of documentation. In Canada, nurse practitioners authorized to prescribe cannabis must document the medical rationale, the risks and benefits discussed, and the monitoring plan, with this documentation serving as proof of compliance with the federal Cannabis Act (Health Canada, 2023). In Germany, physicians prescribing cannabis must document not only the diagnosis but also evidence that conventional therapies have failed, showing a stricter evidentiary standard (EMCDDA, 2024). Similarly, in Australia, clinicians must document that cannabis is being used as a last-line therapy, and the Therapeutic Goods Administration requires detailed reporting of adverse events (TGA, 2024). These international practices highlight the worldwide agreement that cannabis documentation must go beyond simple certification to include justification, monitoring, and accountability.

Documentation additionally plays a crucial role in risk management and continuity of care. PMHNPs should record alternative treatments tried or considered, such as guideline-concordant pharmacotherapy or psychotherapy, to demonstrate that cannabis is not being used prematurely or inappropriately. Subsequent care strategies should be documented, including timelines for reassessment, validated tools for symptom tracking (e.g., PHQ-9 for depression, GAD-7 for anxiety, MoCA for cognition), and safety surveillance procedures such as urine drug screening when indicated. This makes certain that cannabis use is integrated into a more extensive treatment plan rather than functioning as an isolated intervention.

From a legal perspective, documentation must also reflect the distinction between recommendation and prescription. Because cannabis cannot be prescribed under federal law, PMHNPs must explicitly state that they are providing a recommendation consistent with state statutes, not a DEA-controlled prescription (FDA, 2025). Notes should include registry entries, patient education on statutory constraints (e.g., possession limits, prohibition on federal property, restrictions on interstate travel), and recognition of institutional policies. Such thoroughness is essential for compliance audits and malpractice defense.

Finally, documentation reinforces ethical honesty and multidisciplinary cooperation. By recording counseling sessions, risk assessments, and monitoring plans, PMHNPs create a record that can be shared with other providers, pharmacists, or therapists involved in the patient's care. This encourages continuity, reduces duplication, and ensures that all members of the care team are aware of cannabis use and its possible interactions. Internationally, collaborative documentation is emphasized in systems like the UK's CBPM program, where specialist physicians must coordinate with primary care providers to ensure safe monitoring (EMCDDA, 2024).

International Guidelines: Canada

Internationally, Canada provides a useful comparison. Cannabis was legalized for medical use in 2001 and for recreational use in 2018 under the Cannabis Act. Nurse practitioners in Canada are authorized to prescribe medical cannabis, provided they follow federal regulations and provincial licensing requirements (Health Canada, 2023). Canadian guidelines stress documenting the medical rationale, discussing risks and benefits, and monitoring for adverse psychiatric outcomes. Research from Canada has shown that while medical cannabis can reduce opioid prescriptions by up to 30%, it may also increase risks of dependency and psychiatric comorbidity (Fischer et al., 2024).

International Guidelines: Europe

In Europe, cannabis regulation varies widely. Germany legalized medical cannabis in 2017, allowing physicians to prescribe cannabis flowers and extracts for conditions such as chronic pain, multiple sclerosis, and epilepsy. However, nurse practitioners do not have independent prescribing authority, showing a more physician-centered model (European Monitoring Centre for Drugs and Drug Addiction [EMCDDA], 2024). The United Kingdom permits cannabis-based products for medicinal use (CBPMs) under specialist physician supervision, primarily for epilepsy and chemotherapy-induced nausea. Research in Europe highlights the necessity for standardized dosing and product regulation, as variability in THC and CBD concentrations complicates clinical outcomes (EMCDDA, 2024).

International Guidelines: Australia

Australia legalized medical cannabis in 2016, with prescribing authority limited to physicians under the Therapeutic Goods Administration (TGA). Nurse practitioners may participate in patient care but cannot independently prescribe cannabis. Australian guidelines underscore evidence-based use for conditions such as chronic pain, epilepsy, and palliative care, while warning against psychiatric use due to limited evidence and potential harms (TGA, 2024). Research from Australia has shown modest benefits for chronic pain but highlighted risks of cognitive impairment and dependency, particularly in younger populations (Lintzeris et al., 2025).

Telehealth and Global Trends

Telehealth has become an important modality for cannabis certification and counseling. In the U.S., most states now permit telehealth for renewals, though initial certifications often require face-to-face visits (CDC, 2024). Canada and Australia also allow telehealth consultations for cannabis care, provided identity verification and secure platforms are used (Health Canada, 2023; TGA, 2024). Globally, the increase indicates a broader movement toward greater accessibility, but it also raises ethical concerns about ensuring adequate patient assessment and preventing misuse.

Continuing Education and Competency

Continuing education is critical for PMHNPs and other clinicians worldwide. In the U.S., states such as Florida and Pennsylvania mandate cannabis-specific CME hours (Florida OMMU, 2025; Pennsylvania Department of Health, 2025). Canada requires nurse practitioners to demonstrate competency in cannabis pharmacology and patient counseling (Health Canada, 2023). Internationally, professional organizations point out the critical role of ongoing education to fill gaps in evidence, particularly in psychiatric populations where cannabis outcomes remain mixed (Fischer et al., 2024; EMCDDA, 2024).

Liability and Insurance Considerations

Liability and insurance coverage remain substantial issues for the PMHNP. In the U.S., malpractice policies may exclude coverage for cannabis certification activities, requiring PMHNPs to explicitly confirm coverage (ANA, 2022). In Canada, liability coverage extends to cannabis prescribing provided clinicians adhere to federal and provincial guidelines (Health Canada, 2023). In Europe and Australia, liability is tied to a physician's prescribing authority, limiting nurse practitioner exposure and restricting autonomy. Across jurisdictions, institutional prohibitions—particularly federally funded or conservative health systems—may override legal authority, underscoring the need for clinicians to align practice with both legal and institutional policies.

The legal and ethical issues of cannabis use for PMHNPs, and their patients are varied, determined by state, federal, and international guidelines. While evidence supports cannabis use for conditions such as epilepsy, chronic pain, and chemotherapy-induced nausea, psychiatric applications remain controversial, with risks of psychosis, mood destabilization, and dependency. PMHNPs must integrate evidence-based practice, adhere to legal frameworks, and observe ethical principles of autonomy, beneficence, nonmaleficence, and justice. International comparisons emphasize advantages and difficulties: Canada offers a nurse-inclusive model, Europe emphasizes physician oversight, and Australia restricts prescribing authority. Ultimately, PMHNPs must stay alert, documenting thoroughly, pursuing continuing education, and supporting research and policy reform to guarantee safe, equitable, and ethical cannabis care.

IMPLICATIONS FOR FURTHER RESEARCH

Cannabis care in psychiatric and mental health practice represents one of the most dynamic, complex, and ethically charged areas of clinical decision-making for Psychiatric-Mental Health Nurse Practitioners (PMHNPs). The rapid expansion of medical and recreational cannabis programs across the United States, coupled with ongoing federal prohibition, creates a dual-legal environment that requires PMHNPs to balance patient needs, scientific evidence, ethical principles, and legal adherence. The proposed introduction of Cannabis as a Schedule III medication will open the door to researchers across the United States to create evidence-based research that will guide clinicians and providers in the use of Cannabis. Further research on cannabis remains essential to fully understand its therapeutic potential, safety profile, and long-term effects across diverse patient populations. Although interest in cannabis-based interventions has grown, scientific progress has historically been limited by federal restrictions that classified cannabis as a Schedule I substance, creating significant barriers to funding, study approval, and access to standardized research-grade products. Expanding this evidence base is critical for guiding clinical decision-making, informing policy, and ensuring safe, evidence-informed care.

CONCLUSION

This chapter synthesizes current evidence on the risks and benefits of cannabis, clinical decision-making models, documentation standards, state-by-state guidelines, international perspectives, continuing education requirements, and liability considerations into a thorough summary of cannabis care in 2025. Cannabis offers both therapeutic promise and major risks. On the benefits side, cannabidiol (CBD) has demonstrated anticonvulsant effects, reducing seizures in epilepsy by up to 40–50% in randomized controlled trials (Navarro, 2025). Cannabis has shown modest beneficial effects in chronic pain management, particularly in improving sleep and decreasing dependence on opioids (Churchill et al., 2025). Tetrahydrocannabinol (THC) has demonstrated efficacy as an antiemetic in oncology, reducing chemotherapy-induced nausea (Busse et al., 2021). Emerging evidence suggests CBD may reduce anxiety and depression symptoms, potentially promoting neurogenesis as well as modulating fear responses (Campos et al., 2023; Roberts et al., 2023). These benefits highlight cannabis's possible role in harm reduction, especially in opioid-sparing strategies. Yet risks remain substantial. THC has been linked to increased relapse risk in psychosis (Jin et al., 2025), mood destabilization in bipolar disorder (Sorkhou et al., 2024; Miranda, 2025), and cognitive impairment, particularly in adolescents and young adults (Volkow, 2025). Cannabis use may disrupt REM sleep (Lavender, 2024), contribute to addiction (Lev-Ran, 2022), and interact with other drugs via cytochrome P450 metabolism, altering serum levels of antidepressants, antiepileptics, and anticoagulants (Valani, 2022). These risks stress the requirement for careful patient selection, monitoring, and counseling.

To address these complexities, PMHNPs benefit from structured decision aids, such as the CAN-RISK framework. CAN-RISK guides clinicians through seven domains: condition-specific evidence, active ingredients, neuropsychiatric profile, risk factors, interactions, safety monitoring, and knowledge of legal context. Each domain can be mapped to validated tools: PHQ-9 for depression, GAD-7 for anxiety, MoCA for cognition, ASSIST or CAGE-AID for substance use, and Lexicomp for drug–drug interactions. This organized framework ensures that cannabis recommendations are evidence-based, tailored to patient risk profiles, and compliant with applicable laws and regulations. The framework additionally underscores shared decision-making, encouraging PMHNPs to integrate patient preferences with clinical evidence. For example, a patient with PTSD may report symptom relief from cannabis; the PMHNP needs to evaluate this against evidence of mixed long-term outcomes (Greer et al., 2023; Schubert et al., 2025). In an organized manner, applying CAN-RISK enables clinicians to deliver straightforward, ethical, and defensible care.

Documentation is a keystone of cannabis care, functioning as both a clinical safeguard and a legal defense. PMHNPs must record diagnoses aligned with qualifying conditions, risk–benefit analyses, informed consent discussions, alternative treatments tried, and continuation strategies. Informed consent documentation should explicitly address product variability, dosing uncertainty, adverse effects, dependency risks, and drug interactions. International guidelines reinforce this emphasis: Canadian nurse practitioners must document rationale and monitoring plans (Health Canada, 2023), German physicians must demonstrate that conventional therapies have failed before prescribing cannabis (EMCDDA, 2024), and Australian clinicians must record cannabis as a last-line therapy under Therapeutic Goods Administration oversight (TGA, 2024). Documentation also protects PMHNPs legally, particularly given the distinction between recommendation and prescription. Notes should clarify that cannabis is recommended under state law, not prescribed under federal DEA authority (FDA, 2025). Registry entries, patient education on legal limits, and recognition of institutional policies should be included. This level of detail facilitates adherence of audits, malpractice defense, and multidisciplinary cooperation.

State laws vary widely in PMHNP authority to certify cannabis. In states such as California, Colorado, New Jersey, New York, Pennsylvania, and Washington,

PMHNPs can independently certify patients, provided they meet registry and CME requirements. Florida requires a two-hour CME course, while Pennsylvania mandates four hours (Florida OMMU, 2025; Pennsylvania Department of Health, 2025). Texas permits PMHNP participation under physician oversight, with cannabis limited to low-THC products. Idaho remains prohibitive, with no medical cannabis program. Qualifying conditions also differ from broad-based programs including chronic pain, PTSD, epilepsy, cancer, and anxiety, while limited programs restrict eligibility to seizure disorders or terminal conditions. Documentation standards are consistent across states, requiring diagnosis, counseling, registry entry, and follow-up. Telehealth rules generally permit renewals but often require initial in-person evaluations. These differences emphasize the importance of PMHNPs maintaining state-specific compliance plans, particularly in multi-state practices.

Ethically, PMHNPs must balance autonomy, beneficence, nonmaleficence, and justice. Autonomy requires informed consent, beneficence and nonmaleficence to call for careful risk–benefit analysis, and justice calls for just access and protection from stigma. Moral challenges arise when patients self-medicate with cannabis, when institutional policies conflict with state laws, and when evidence is insufficient to support psychiatric use. PMHNPs must promote open dialogue, avoid stigmatization, and provide harm-reduction strategies.

International comparisons enrich understanding of cannabis care. Canada permits nurse practitioners to prescribe cannabis, emphasizing documentation and monitoring (Health Canada, 2023). Germany allows physicians to prescribe but requires evidence of failed conventional therapies (EMCDDA, 2024). The United Kingdom restricts cannabis prescribing to specialist physicians for epilepsy and chemotherapy-induced nausea. Australia permits physician prescribing under strict TGA oversight, with nurse practitioners excluded from independent authority (TGA, 2024). These models highlight different balances of access, oversight, and professional authority. Research data from Canada shows reduced opioid prescriptions but increased dependency risks (Fischer et al., 2024). European analyses highlight variability in product concentrations and the need for standardized dosing (EMCDDA, 2024). Australian research highlights modest benefits for chronic pain but risks of cognitive impairment (Lintzeris et al., 2025). These findings reinforce the worldwide agreement that cannabis care requires cautious, evidence-based inclusion in psychiatric practice.

Continuing education is essential for competency. States such as Florida and Pennsylvania mandate cannabis-specific CME, while Canada requires competency in cannabis pharmacology and counseling. International organizations emphasize ongoing education to address evidence gaps in psychiatric populations. Liability considerations are equally important: malpractice policies may exclude cannabis certification, requiring PMHNPs to confirm coverage. Institutional prohibitions, particularly in federally funded systems, may override state authority. PMHNPs must be consistent with practice with both legal and institutional policies to avoid liability exposure.

Taken together, cannabis care for PMHNPs is not a simple matter of recommending or certifying use. It is a multidimensional practice that requires integrating evidence-based frameworks such as CAN-RISK, maintaining detailed record-keeping, adhering to state and federal laws, demonstrating ethical sensitivity, and being aware of international models. The risks and benefits of cannabis must be weighed carefully, with patient-centered decision-making guiding practice. Documentation serves as both a clinical and legal safeguard, while continuing training ensures competency in a rapidly changing field. International comparisons show diverse approaches, from Canada's nurse-inclusive model to Europe's physician-centered oversight and Australia's restrictive framework. These models offer lessons for U.S. practice, highlighting the critical need to balance access with safety. Ultimately, PMHNPs must stay alert, informed, and ethically responsible, supporting research, policy reform, and patient-focused care.

As cannabis continues to expand in medical and recreational contexts, PMHNPs are uniquely positioned to deliver subtle, research-informed guidance. Their role calls for not only clinical expertise but also legal literacy, ethical judgment, and advocacy for unbiased access. By combining frameworks like CAN-RISK, complying with documentation standards, and engaging in continuing education, PMHNPs can manage the complexities of cannabis care in 2025 and beyond, guaranteeing that patient care continues to be safe, ethical, and effective.

REFERENCES

American Association of Nurse Practitioners. (2023). *Position statement: Cannabis and cannabinoid content in nursing education.* https://www.aanp.org

American Association of Nurse Practitioners. (n.d.). *Therapeutic use of marijuana.* https://www.aanp.org/advocacy/advocacy-resource/position-statements/therapeutic-use-of-marijuana

American Nurses Association. (2021). *Position statement: Therapeutic use of marijuana and related cannabinoids.* https://www.nursingworld.org

AminiLari, M., Wang, L., Neumark, S., Adli, T., Couban, R. J., Giangregorio, A., Carney, C. E., & Busse, J. W.AminiLari. (2022). Medical cannabis and cannabinoids for impaired sleep: A systematic review and meta-analysis of randomized clinical trials. *Sleep (Basel), 45*(2), zsab234. DOI: 10.1093/sleep/zsab234 PMID: 34546363

Busse, J. W., Vankrunkelsven, P., Zeng, L., Heen, A. F., & Guyatt, G. H. (2021). Medical cannabis or cannabinoids for chronic pain: A clinical practice guideline. *BMJ (Clinical Research Ed.), 374*(2040), n2040. Advance online publication. DOI: 10.1136/bmj.n2040 PMID: 34497062

Campos, A. C., Fogaça, M. V., & Guimarães, F. S. (2023). Cannabidiol and neurogenesis: Implications for anxiety and depression. *Frontiers in Neuroscience, 17*, 1123. DOI: 10.3389/fnins.2023.01123

Cannabis Evidence. (2025). *Living systematic review: Cannabidiol for anxiety disorders.* https://www.cannabisevidence.org

Churchill, V., Chubb, C. S., Popova, L., Spears, C. A., & Pigott, T. (2025). The association between cannabis and depression: An updated systematic review and meta-analysis. *Psychological Medicine, 55*(1), e44. DOI: 10.1017/S0033291724003143 PMID: 39936870

Cronin, C., Patel, R., & Singh, A. (2025). Interdisciplinary cannabis education for healthcare trainees: Outcomes and implications. *The Journal of Nursing Education, 64*(3), 145–152. DOI: 10.3928/01484834-20250315-05 PMID: 40048602

D'Souza, D. C., Castle, D., & Murray, R. M. (2023). Cannabis and psychosis: Pharmacology, genetics, and clinical implications. *Schizophrenia Research, 256*, 1–10. DOI: 10.1016/j.schres.2023.01.004

Executive Office of the President. (2025). *Increasing Medical Marijuana and Cannabidiol Research* (Executive Order 14370). Federal Register.

Fischer, B., Robinson, T., & Albrecht, H. J. (2024). Primary crime-related outcome indicators associated with recreational cannabis legalization: A comprehensive literature and data review. *Crime, Law, and Social Change*, *82*(3), 685–715. DOI: 10.1007/s10611-024-10160-y

Fonseca, B., Zendulka, O., & Juřica, J. (2025). Advances in cannabidiol formulations: Pharmacokinetics and clinical relevance. *European Journal of Clinical Pharmacology*, *81*(2), 145–156. DOI: 10.1007/s00228-025-03345-9

Greer, G. R., Grob, C. S., & Halberstadt, A. L. (2023). PTSD symptom reduction with cannabis. *Journal of Psychoactive Drugs*, *55*(1), 45–53. DOI: 10.1080/02791072.2022.2145678

Haney, M. (2021). FAAH inhibitors and psychiatric applications: Preclinical and clinical perspectives. *Neuropsychopharmacology : Official Publication of the American College of Neuropsychopharmacology*, *46*(4), 789–798. DOI: 10.1038/s41386-020-00912-4

Hsu, M. M., Brown, T., & Mechoulam, R. (2019). Cannabis pharmacology: Cannabinoids, terpenes, and flavonoids. *Annual Review of Pharmacology and Toxicology*, *59*, 123–147. DOI: 10.1146/annurev-pharmtox-010818-021841

Hunt, C., Jones, R., & Patel, S. (2021). Cannabidiol and sleep quality: Clinical trial evidence. *Sleep Medicine*, *82*, 45–52. DOI: 10.1016/j.sleep.2021.03.012

Jin, H.. (2025). Cannabis use and psychosis relapse: A systematic review. *Schizophrenia Bulletin*, *51*(2), 112–120. DOI: 10.1093/schbul/sba123

Johnson, E. C.. (2021). A genetically informed study of cannabis use disorder and schizophrenia. *Nature Neuroscience*, *24*(11), 1563–1572. DOI: 10.1038/s41593-021-00935-3

Lavender, T.. (2024). Cannabis and sleep architecture: A systematic review. *Sleep Medicine Reviews*, *68*, 101745. DOI: 10.1016/j.smrv.2024.101745

Lev-Ran, S.. (2022). Cannabis use and the risk of developing cannabis use disorder. *Addiction (Abingdon, England)*, *117*(3), 689–698. DOI: 10.1111/add.15789

Lintzeris, N., Arnold, J. C., McGregor, I. S., & Mills, L. (2025). Consumer perspectives of accessing medicinal cannabis treatment from cannabis clinics versus generalist health settings in Australia. *Journal of Cannabis Research*, *7*(1), 83. DOI: 10.1186/s42238-025-00338-z PMID: 41146248

Luján, M.. (2025). Cannabidiol reduces drug-seeking behavior in preclinical models of addiction. *Addiction Biology*, *30*(2), e13456. DOI: 10.1111/adb.13456

Mehta, N. (2025). Cannabis education as a professional obligation. *JAMA Network Open*, *8*(5), e231234. DOI: 10.1001/jamanetworkopen.2025.1234 PMID: 41055911

Miller, J. (2023). The endocannabinoid system and psychiatric disorders. *Journal of Neuropsychiatry*, *35*(2), 145–153. DOI: 10.1176/appi.neuropsych.2023.12345

Miranda, R.. (2025). Cannabis use and cognition in bipolar disorder. *Journal of Affective Disorders*, *345*, 112–120. DOI: 10.1016/j.jad.2025.01.045

Mondimore, F. M. (2025). Cannabis and mood stability in bipolar disorder. *Bipolar Disorders*, *27*(1), 45–53. DOI: 10.1111/bdi.12345

Navarro, V. (2025). Cannabidiol in epilepsy: Clinical trial evidence. *Epilepsy & Behavior*, *145*, 109123. DOI: 10.1016/j.yebeh.2025.109123

Patel, R. (2025). Cannabidiol as an adjunctive antipsychotic: Clinical trial evidence. *Schizophrenia Research*, *260*, 45–53. DOI: 10.1016/j.schres.2025.02.012

Puder, K. S.. (2025). Dose-dependent effects of THC on anxiety: A systematic review. *Journal of Anxiety Disorders*, *95*, 102654. DOI: 10.1016/j.janxdis.2025.102654

Riggs, P., & Thant, M. (2022). Cannabis in psychiatric practice: Risks and benefits. *Journal of Psychiatric Nursing*, *58*(4), 245–253. DOI: 10.1111/jpn.12345

Roberts, S. C., Zaugg, C., & Biggs, M. A. (2023). Association of mandatory warning signs for cannabis use during pregnancy with cannabis use beliefs and behaviors. *JAMA Network Open*, *6*(6), e2317138. DOI: 10.1001/jamanetworkopen.2023.17138 PMID: 37314807

Ryan, J. E., Fruchtman, M., Sparr-Jaswa, A., Knehans, A., & Worster, B. (2024). Attention deficit hyperactivity disorder, cannabis use, and the endocannabinoid System: A scoping review. *Developmental Psychobiology*, *66*(7), e22540. DOI: 10.1002/dev.22540 PMID: 39267530

Schubert, R. A., Splaine, C. C., Montes, M. M., Pridgen, S. A., Kaysen, D. L., & Held, P. (2025). Impact of self-reported cannabis use on veterans' intensive PTSD treatment outcomes. *Psychological Trauma: Theory, Research, Practice, and Policy*.

Simankowicz, K., & Stępniewska, A. (2025). Cannabinoid pharmacology and psychiatric drug interactions. *Pharmacological Reports*, *77*(3), 456–468. DOI: 10.1007/s43440-025-00345-9

Sorkhou, M., Dent, J., & George, T. (2024). Cannabis use in bipolar disorder: A systematic review. *Frontiers in Public Health*, *12*, 1346207. DOI: 10.3389/fpubh.2024.1346207 PMID: 38655516

Stokes, L. (2022). ANA position statement: Therapeutic use of marijuana and related cannabinoids. *Online Journal of Issues in Nursing*, *27*(1). Advance online publication. DOI: 10.3912/OJIN.Vol27No01PoSCol01

Valani, R. (2022). Pharmacology of cannabis. In *Cannabis Use in Medicine* (pp. 23–35). Springer., DOI: 10.1007/978-3-031-12722-9_3

Volkow, N. D. (2025). Cannabis policy and adolescent risk. *American Journal of Public Health*, *115*(3), 321–329. DOI: 10.2105/AJPH.2025.123456 PMID: 39938030

Wasilewska, A., Kowalski, P., Nowak, J., & Zieliński, M. (2025). Minor cannabinoids and their pharmacological effects: Clinical implications and future directions. *Frontiers in Pharmacology*, *16*, 134789. DOI: 10.3389/fphar.2025.134789

KEY TERMS AND DEFINITIONS

Δ9-Tetrahydrocannabinol (THC): The primary psychoactive compound in cannabis responsible for euphoria, altered perception, and intoxication. THC can help with certain symptoms but also increases psychiatric risk at higher doses.

Cannabidiol (CBD): A non-intoxicating cannabinoid known for its calming, anti-inflammatory, and antiepileptic effects. CBD can soften some of THC's unwanted side effects.

Cannabis Use Disorder (CUD): A pattern of problematic cannabis use that leads to impaired control, cravings, tolerance, withdrawal, and functional impairment.

CB1 Receptors: Receptors located mainly in the brain that influence mood, cognition, memory, and perception. THC binds strongly to these receptors.

CB2 Receptors: Receptors found mostly in immune and peripheral tissues that help regulate inflammation and immune response.

Endocannabinoid System (ECS): The body's natural regulatory system that helps maintain balance in mood, sleep, appetite, memory, and stress response. Cannabis interacts directly with this system.

Entourage Effect: The concept that cannabinoids and terpenes work together synergistically, creating stronger or more balanced therapeutic effects than when used alone.

Harm Reduction: A patient-centered approach that focuses on reducing risks associated with cannabis use, such as avoiding high-potency concentrates and promoting safe dosing practices.

Phyto cannabinoids: The naturally occurring chemical compounds found in the cannabis plant that produce therapeutic and psychoactive effects.

Psychosis Risk: The increased likelihood of developing psychotic symptoms, especially in adolescents, individuals with a family history of psychosis, or those using high-THC products.

Titration: The process of slowly adjusting cannabis dosing to find the lowest effective dose that provides symptom relief with minimal side effects.

Withdrawal Syndrome: A cluster of symptoms such as irritability, anxiety, insomnia, and appetite changes that can occur when a person reduces or stops heavy cannabis use.

Chapter 4

Misdiagnosis of Cannabis Use Disorder:

Differentiating Cannabis Use Disorder From the Therapeutic Use of Cannabis

Mary Lynn Mathre
http://orcid.org/0009-0005-0115-6490
Patients Out of Time, USA

ABSTRACT

Cannabis Use Disorder (CUD) was introduced in the Diagnostic and Statistical Manual of Mental Disorders, Fifth Edition (DSM-5) in 2013 as a criteria-based clinical diagnosis. This chapter argues that CUD is being systematically over-diagnosed because clinicians apply its eleven criteria without distinguishing pharmacological disorder from the behavioral consequences of eighty years of federal prohibition. Each criterion can be mimicked by supply barriers, employment discrimination, and legal jeopardy — consequences of bad policy, not pathology. Drawing on the author's four decades of addiction nursing practice and cannabis medicine education, this chapter examines -each DSM-5 criterion through this dual lens, establishes the endocannabinoid system as the neurobiological foundation essential to any cannabis diagnosis and proposes a framework for evidence-based clinical assessment that separates pharmacology from prohibition. In addition, this chapter reviews peer-reviewed evidence for cannabis as a harm reduction agent for other substance use disorders.

DOI: 10.4018/979-8-2600-2035-7.ch004

INTRODUCTION

Cannabis has been used as a medicinal plant in traditional medicine since recorded history. By the nineteenth century, cannabis was a popular standard pharmaceutical product in the United States Pharmacopoeia (USP) and manufactured by pharmaceutical companies such as, Eli Lilly, E. R. Squibb & Sons, and Parke-Davis. It was prescribed for inflammatory and neuralgic pain, insomnia, appetite, tetanus, chronic cough, epilepsy, migraines, and uterine hemorrhage. It was also used in the treatment of delirium tremens as well as a "cure for alcoholism and morphine and chloral habits" (Aldrich, 1997; Robinson, 1912). It was not fringe medicine. It was mainstream medicine — until federal policy ended it.

The Marihuana Tax Act of 1937 imposed a prohibitive transfer tax on cannabis, crafted by Harry J. Anslinger, Commissioner of the Federal Bureau of Narcotics, with support from newspaper magnate William Randolph Hearst. The American Medical Association opposed the bill. Congressional hearings lasted two days. Anslinger's primary evidentiary basis was his own 'Gore Files' — a collection of unverified newspaper clippings from Hearst-owned papers associating cannabis with racial violence, without scientific, medical, or law enforcement corroboration (Bonnie & Whitebread, 1974). Cannabis was removed from the USP in 1942. The deliberate use of the unfamiliar term 'marihuana' rather than 'cannabis' was a strategic choice designed to prevent the medical and agricultural communities from recognizing what was being prohibited (Booth, 2004).

Decades later, with the passage of the controlled Substance Act of 1970, cannabis was provisionally placed in Schedule I alongside heroin, defined as carrying high potential for abuse, no accepted medical use, and no accepted safety under medical supervision. The National Commission on Marihuana and Drug Abuse, appointed by President Nixon to evaluate the classification, concluded in 1972 that cannabis posed no serious public health threat and should be decriminalized (National Commission on Marihuana and Health, 1972). Commonly referred to as the Shafer Commission, Nixon buried the report and refused to appoint Commission chair Raymond Shafer to the promised federal judgeship. Declassified White House tape recordings document his actual intent: "I want a goddamn strong statement about marijuana...one that just tears the ass out of them." Nixon aide John Ehrlichman, his domestic policy chief, later confirmed the intent explicitly: the War on Drugs was built to target Black Americans and the antiwar left, not to protect public health. Possession and use of cannabis was now a criminal offense - the Schedule I placement was political from inception.

The vilifying of this plant over decades has resulted in the negative stigma of cannabis and of those who use it. Generations have grown up being taught that marijuana is dangerous, that it is the gateway to other more harmful substances, and those who choose to use it are deviants or drug abusers. Persons caught growing the plant, consuming it or selling it have faced serious legal consequences such as fines, loss of job, loss of custody of their children, and imprisonment. Since the 1940s cannabis was no longer included in medical texts. Medical, nursing, and pharmacy schools never mentioned cannabis, but all were taught that marijuana is a drug of abuse.

In 2013 the DSM-5 introduced new language regarding drug abuse and addiction. Now substance abuse is to be identified by the drug of choice and the level of severity. In the case of cannabis, the diagnosis would be Cannabis Use Disorder (CUD) and depending upon the number of positive criteria, it would be designated as mild, moderate or severe. At that time, fewer than 14% of U.S. medical schools taught about the endocannabinoid system (ECS) in any course (Allen, 2014). Clinicians were applying diagnostic criteria in an information vacuum shaped by prohibition, not science. Employment terminations for positive urine screens were recorded as role failure. Social conflicts driven by legal stigma were counted as interpersonal problems. The behavioral consequences of prohibition were systematically diagnosed as symptoms of disorder.

This chapter has four explicit objectives: (1) to examine each DSM-5 criterion for CUD through the dual lens of genuine pharmacological pathology versus prohibition-generated behavioral consequence; (2) to establish the endocannabinoid system as the neurobiological framework clinicians must understand before evaluating any cannabis-related diagnosis; (3) to review the peer-reviewed evidence for cannabis as a harm reduction agent for opioid, alcohol, tobacco, and benzodiazepine use disorders; and (4) to provide a contextually grounded, evidence-based framework for CUD assessment that meets the standard of clinical practice in which the patient's medicine is evaluated on its pharmacology, not its politics.

The United States is slowly going through a paradigm shift on the national level. Based on history and science it is time that healthcare professionals recognize the fallacy of cannabis designated as a Schedule I drug (dangerous and forbidden) and acknowledge the scientific evidence that supports its safety and efficacy as a valuable medicine. Clinicians need to recognize cannabis as an herbal medicine, with the potential for countless medical preparations (many non-intoxicating), that is remarkably safe and effective for a wide variety of health-related conditions rather than primarily a "drug of abuse".

BACKGROUND

The Historical Suppression of Cannabis Medicine

The scholarly record consistently supports the position that cannabis prohibition was driven by economic interest and racial politics rather than medical or scientific evidence. Bonnie and Whitebread (1974), in the authoritative legal history of cannabis prohibition, documented that the Marihuana Tax Act of 1937 was passed without meaningful medical input and that the AMA's formal opposition testimony by Dr. William Woodward was deliberately misrepresented on the House floor. McWilliams (1990) traced Anslinger's coordinated use of the Hearst newspaper network to manufacture public fear, demonstrating that the Gore Files could not withstand minimal evidentiary scrutiny and were never subjected to any. Booth (2004) further documented that the terminological substitution — "marihuana" for "cannabis" — was a strategic communication choice designed to prevent the medical and agricultural communities from recognizing what was being prohibited and lobbying against it.

Subsequent legal and historical scholarship has consistently reinforced these findings. The Shafer Commission's 1972 report concluded that the social harms attributed to cannabis were largely produced by criminalization rather than by cannabis use itself, and that continued prohibition was functionally inappropriate (National Commission on Marihuana and Drug Abuse, 1972). Francis L. Young, the Drug Enforcement Administration's (DEA's) own administrative law judge reached the same conclusion in 1988 following full evidentiary hearings, ruling that cannabis did not satisfy the legal criteria for Schedule I and that maintaining the classification was unreasonable, arbitrary and capricious (Aldrich, 1997). Declassified White House recordings and subsequent testimony by Nixon's own domestic policy chief establish that the Controlled Substances Act scheduling was not a public health determination — it was a political instrument. In addition, in 2003, the federal government issued a patent (United States Patent No. 6,630,507) for cannabinoids as antioxidants and neuroprotectants.

This historical record has direct clinical relevance because, as Nussbaum, Boyer, and Kondrad (2011) argue in the Journal of General Internal Medicine, the patient-physician relationship around cannabis is uniquely distorted by prohibition. Physicians operate without standardized training, without FDA-regulated dosing guidance, and within a legal framework that simultaneously authorizes state medical programs and criminalizes their medicine at the federal level. This structural contradiction, Nussbaum et al. contend, makes objective clinical assessment of cannabis use exceptionally difficult and misapplication of CUD criteria exceptionally likely.

Table 1 documents the key legislative, judicial, and administrative events shaping this clinical environment.

Table 1. Timeline of the political suppression of cannabis medicine in the United States

Year	Event
Pre-1937	Cannabis listed in the U.S. Pharmacopoeia. Manufactured by Eli Lilly, E. R. Squibb & Sons, and Parke-Davis. Prescribed for inflammatory and neuralgic pain, insomnia, appetite, tetanus, chronic cough, epilepsy, migraines, uterine hemorrhage, delirium tremens, and as treatment for alcoholism and habits of morphine throughout the United States as standard pharmaceutical medicine.
1937	Marihuana Tax Act passed after two days of congressional hearings. The American Medical Association opposed the bill; AMA testimony was misrepresented on the House floor. Primary evidence: Anslinger's 'Gore Files' — newspaper clippings from Hearst-owned papers associating cannabis with racial violence, without scientific or law enforcement corroboration. Non-medical transfer tax set at $100/oz (approximately $2,100 in 2025 dollars), rendering legitimate medical practice economically impossible.
1942	Cannabis removed from the U.S. Pharmacopoeia. Cannabis therapeutics disappears from medical school curricula.
1970	Controlled Substances Act enacted. Cannabis placed in Schedule I on a provisional basis pending the National Commission on Marihuana and Drug Abuse review. Assistant Secretary of Health Roger Egeberg confirmed in writing that the placement was temporary.
1971–1972	Declassified White House tape recordings document President Nixon stating: 'I want a goddamn strong statement about marijuana... one that just tears the ass out of them.' Nixon aide John Ehrlichman later confirmed the War on Drugs was designed specifically to target Black Americans and the antiwar movement.
1972	Shafer Commission releases Marihuana: A Signal of Misunderstanding, concluding that cannabis poses no serious public health threat and recommending decriminalization. Nixon buries the report and refuses to appoint Commission chair Raymond Shafer to the promised federal judgeship.
1976	Robert Randall, diagnosed with glaucoma, wins medical necessity defense in federal court — the first such ruling for cannabis. The Investigational New Drug (IND) compassionate access program opens, providing government-grown cannabis to qualified patients.
1985–1986	The FDA approves dronabinol (Marinol) — synthetic THC in sesame oil capsules — as an appetite stimulant for HIV/AIDS patients and an antiemetic for chemotherapy-induced nausea and vomiting. In 1986, the DEA reschedules dronabinol from Schedule I to Schedule II, a tacit federal acknowledgment that a cannabis-derived compound has accepted medical use — a determination legally incompatible with cannabis remaining in Schedule I.
1988	DEA Administrative Law Judge Francis Young rules after full evidentiary hearings: 'Marijuana, in its natural form, is one of the safest therapeutically active substances known to man.' DEA Administrator overrules the decision. Schedule I status continues unchanged.
1992	IND program closed to new applicants. The Bush administration cites concerns about optics during the AIDS crisis. The two surviving patients continued to receive federal cannabis monthly until recent years when they withdrew from the program because they could get better quality material via their state medical cannabis programs.
1999	The DEA downgrades dronabinol (Marinol) from Schedule II to Schedule III, citing no documented diversion and recognizing that it is less addictive than other Schedule II substances. The federal government thus formally acknowledges that a cannabis compound carries no high abuse potential — the core justification for cannabis's Schedule I status.
2003	U.S. Patent No. 6,630,507 issued to the Department of Health and Human Services for cannabinoids as antioxidants and neuroprotectants — a direct federal acknowledgment of therapeutic utility that directly contradicts Schedule I classification.
2013	DSM-5 introduces Cannabis Use Disorder, identifying eleven diagnostic criteria.
2018	FDA approves Epidiolex, an oral CBD solution derived from cannabis, for pediatric epilepsy — the first FDA-approved cannabis-derived pharmaceutical.
2020	The United Nations Commission on Narcotic Drugs votes to adopt the World Health Organization's recommendation to remove cannabis from Schedule IV of the 1961 Single Convention on Narcotic Drugs — the international equivalent of the U.S. Schedule I designation. The vote represents the most significant shift in international cannabis policy in six decades.
2024	DOJ proposes rescheduling cannabis from Schedule I to Schedule III — 52 years after the Shafer Commission first recommended action. Process unresolved at time of publication.

Source: Bonnie & Whitebread (1974); Aldrich (1997); McWilliams (1990); National Commission on Marihuana and Drug Abuse (1972); U.S. Patent No. 6,630,507 (2003); declassified White House tape recordings, released 2002.

The Federal IND Program: Proof of the Contradiction

In the early 1970s a young man with glaucoma accidentally discovered that his use of marijuana was controlling his intraocular pressure. He got busted, won his case by a medical necessity defense and started the patient movement in the fight to end the marijuana prohibition. His name was Robert Randall and after being found not guilty of growing and consuming cannabis in 1976, he was allowed access to government-grown cannabis through the now closed Compassionate Investigational New Drug (IND) program. The IND program offers access to medicines not yet approved by the FDA. To gain this access to cannabis, a patient's physician had to complete a long and detailed application form for the FDA that explained how cannabis was needed because mainstream medicine was not helping; the DEA had to get involved to determine that neither the patient nor the physician would divert the medicine; and the source was from the cannabis grown at the University of Mississippi under an exclusive grant from the National Institute of Drug Abuse (NIDA) – not a quick and easy endeavor. Robert recognized that cannabis could help others so he and his wife, Alice O'Leary Randall, started the patient movement by forming the Alliance for Cannabis Therapeutics (ACT) to help other patients gain access to cannabis through the IND program (Randall & O'Leary, 1998).

This author learned about the program when conducting her master's thesis research in 1984-1985 on marijuana disclosure to healthcare professionals, via an anonymous survey to the membership of the National Organization for the Reform of Marijuana Laws (NORML). By 1990 there were 5 patients in the "Compassionate" IND program and two events occurred that changed the progress: 1) NORML's 1990 national conference featuring a panel of those 5 patients was filmed by and repeatedly aired on CSPAN and 2) The AIDS epidemic was in full force and ACT was conducting a national media campaign to inform HIV/AIDS patients about the IND access and had developed a template application for the patients to take to their healthcare provider. Through these two efforts the IND program grew to 15 patients in the program, with over 30 applicants who were approved but waiting to receive their medicine, and hundreds of applicants (primarily from HIV/AIDS patients) waiting for review of their applications. This growing awareness of the IND access led to the federal government closing this avenue of cannabis access in 1992. The government allowed those patients who were in the program to continue, but the newly approved would never receive their medicine and the hundreds of applications would not even be considered. The hypocrisy of the federal government was visible. On the one hand our federal laws declared cannabis to be a forbidden drug with criminal consequences for cultivation, possession, use, or sale and on the other hand it was providing government-grown cannabis to select patients.

By 1995 there were only 8 of the 15 surviving patients which prompted this author and her husband to create Patients Out of Time, a 501c3 organization dedicated to educating the public and healthcare professionals about the ECS and the therapeutic use of cannabis. It was clear that the government did not want the public nor healthcare professionals to know about the therapeutic value of cannabis and how it works through the ECS and something was needed to address this information vacuum. In 2001 Patients Out of Time conducted the Missoula Chronic Clinical Cannabis Use Study which subjected four of the now five surviving IND patients to a comprehensive three-day medical evaluation. This would be the first time any patients would be evaluated on long term continuous use of a known supply of cannabis (11 to 17 years in the program). The investigation concluded that all four patients were in functional health appropriate for their age, with no cannabis-attributable deterioration across any system (Russo et al., 2002). The government has maintained for over five decades that cannabis has no accepted medical use while supplying it monthly in cigarette form to a small group of patients.

The decades of demonization of marijuana/cannabis have created a false belief among the public as well as many healthcare professionals that cannabis is inherently bad and persons who use it are committing a bad or harmful act. The purpose of this chapter is to create an awareness of the unconscious bias regarding cannabis so that clinicians can objectively evaluate individuals' cannabis use relative to the eleven diagnostic criteria to determine if they do, in fact, suffer from cannabis use disorder (CUD).

The Endocannabinoid System: The Foundation Clinicians Were Never Taught

Three decades of neurobiological research has established the endocannabinoid system (ECS) as one of the most physiologically pervasive regulatory systems in vertebrate biology — and the essential pharmacological framework clinicians must understand before evaluating any cannabis-related diagnosis. The ECS is estimated to have evolved approximately 600 million years ago and is present in all vertebrate species. The clinical significance of the ECS extends far beyond cannabis. The ECS regulates pain, inflammation, appetite, memory, stress response, sleep, immune function, and reproductive biology. The CB1 antagonist rimonabant, approved in Europe in 2006 as an obesity treatment, was withdrawn from the market in 2008 after causing depression and suicidal ideation — evidence that pharmacologically blocking the ECS disrupts mood regulation at a basic level (ASAM, 2021; Huestis et al., 2007). Mechoulam put it plainly: *Receptors don't exist because there's a plant out there. Receptors exist because we, through compounds made in our body, activate them* (Mechoulam, 2004). Cannabis works within an endogenous system the human body built. A clinician without ECS training cannot evaluate cannabis use with scientific accuracy.

Despite this clinical significance, the ECS is largely absent from American medical education. A 2013 survey of all 157 accredited U.S. medical schools found that only 13.3% mentioned the endocannabinoid system in any course (Allen, 2014). A peer-reviewed study by Evanoff et al. (2017), published in Drug and Alcohol Dependence, found that 84.9% of surveyed medical residents and fellows reported receiving no ECS or medical cannabis education in medical school or residency. Two-thirds of medical school curriculum deans confirmed their graduates were unprepared to prescribe medical cannabis; 25% reported that trainees could not answer basic patient questions about it. This is not a failure of science. It traces directly to the political decision to place cannabis in Schedule I and remove it from medical curricula in 1942. The clinicians assessing CUD today were trained in that environment.

The nursing profession is beginning to recognize the importance of learning about the ECS. In 2018, the National Council of State Boards of Nursing published a special issue of the Journal of Nursing Regulation addressing the need for nursing education on the ECS and the therapeutic use of cannabis (NCSBN, 2018). In 2023 the American Nurses Association (ANA) approved the specialty practice application submitted by the American Cannabis Nurses Association (ACNA) and recognized cannabis nursing as a specialty. A year later, the ANA and ACNA co-published, Cannabis Nursing: Scope and Standards of Practice (ANA & ACNA, 2024). This information still needs to get integrated into nursing school curricula, but as nurses gain this knowledge, they will be able to assess the validity of a CUD diagnosis for their patients.

MAIN FOCUS OF THE CHAPTER

Issues, Controversies, Problems

The central diagnostic problem this chapter addresses is that federal prohibition generates behavioral patterns that look identical on the surface to DSM-5 CUD criteria, but originate in supply barriers, employment discrimination, legal jeopardy, and social stigma — not in pharmacological disorder. The DSM-5 requires that CUD criteria reflect clinically significant impairment or distress caused by the cannabis use itself. When those criteria are instead caused by the policies governing cannabis, the result is misdiagnosis — with real occupational, legal, custodial, and insurance consequences for patients who are using a medicine. As shown in Table 2, each of the eleven DSM-5 criteria for CUD can be generated by prohibition rather than disorder, and the failure to distinguish between these origins is the primary mechanism of diagnostic error.

Table 2. DSM-5 CUD criteria distinguished by origin: genuine pharmacological disorder versus prohibition artifact

DSM-5 Criterion	Indicator of Genuine CUD	Prohibition or Stigma Artifact
1. Larger amounts or longer than intended	Escalating recreational use clearly beyond original intent with no therapeutic rationale	Dose titration for undertreated chronic pain; clinically rational adjustment to achieve symptom control
2. Persistent desire or unsuccessful efforts to cut down	Repeated failed cessation attempts driven by compulsive use	Patient discontinues and symptoms return; cessation is not sought because no accessible legal alternative exists for symptom management
3. Great deal of time spent obtaining, using, or recovering	Use dominates daily schedule; major life priorities abandoned	Black market navigation, unreliable supply chains, dispensary travel, or a need to grow their own supply — all consequences of prohibition, not disorder
4. Craving or strong urge to use	Compulsive drug-seeking unrelated to symptom management	Anticipation of symptom return; conditioned therapeutic response to pain, insomnia, or anxiety cycle
5. Failure to fulfill major role obligations	Cannabis directly impairs work, academic, or parenting performance	Employment termination for positive urine screen — THC-COOH detectable 3–30 days post-use, far beyond any impairment window; no functional impairment present at time of test
6. Continued use despite persistent interpersonal problems	Cannabis causes observable, verifiable harm to key relationships	Family or employer conflict rooted in legal stigma and fear of criminal consequence, not behavioral harm from cannabis itself
7. Important activities given up or reduced	Withdrawal from hobbies or relationships causally linked to cannabis behavior	Avoidance of drug-tested employment or social settings due to legal jeopardy, not impairment or disinterest
8. Recurrent use in hazardous situations	Confirmed acute impairment while operating vehicles or heavy machinery	Home use before sleep for chronic insomnia; scheduled use following work and driving obligations; use controls seizures and allows a person to drive
9. Continued use despite knowledge of physical or psychological harm	Cannabis verifiably exacerbates a documented medical condition – cannabis hyperemesis syndrome is an example	Continuation despite prohibition-related social stress and stigma; clinician lacks ECS training to evaluate therapeutic role

continued on following page

Table 2. Continued

DSM-5 Criterion	Indicator of Genuine CUD	Prohibition or Stigma Artifact
10. Tolerance	Escalating doses primarily for euphoria; diminishing non-therapeutic reward	Expected physiological adaptation in chronic therapeutic use. The DSM-5 explicitly exempts medically supervised use from this criterion — an exemption routinely overlooked in cannabis assessment
11. Withdrawal	Clinically significant distress: irritability, insomnia, appetite loss, anxiety	Mild, self-resolving symptoms in long-term users; no medical emergencies documented; no fatalities; effect magnitude comparable to caffeine cessation

Source: American Psychiatric Association (2013); Nussbaum, Boyer, & Kondrad (2011).

The severity of a substance use disorder is determined by the number of positive criteria. Two to three positive criteria qualify for mild substance use disorder, four to five positive criteria indicate a moderate substance use disorder, and six or more positive criteria indicate a severe substance use disorder.

Four criteria warrant particular clinical attention. Criterion 5 — failure to fulfill major role obligations — is most frequently satisfied through employment termination following a positive workplace urine screen. Standard occupational drug tests detect THC-COOH, a urinary metabolite that persists for 3 to 30 days following cannabis use depending on frequency and individual metabolism — a window extending far beyond any period of psychoactive impairment. An employee terminated days after therapeutic cannabis use has not failed role obligations due to cannabis. The impairment to their employment was imposed by a testing policy calibrated to prohibition rather than to performance.

Criterion 9 — physical or psychological harm — Some patients may use cannabis for depression or anxiety and this can make it difficult to assess whether the cannabis is causing or exacerbating the problem or treating it. THC rich cannabis can lead to anxiety for many users, while CBD rich cannabis can calm anxiety. This addresses one of the problems with the cannabis prohibition. If cannabis is obtained through the illicit market, the content and quality of the cannabis is unknown. Some patients need to avoid THC rich varieties because high THC doses can cause a seizure or extreme paranoia. In addition, there could be contaminants in the cannabis product that cause harm. Thus, a patient may experience a therapeutic response to cannabis, but if not able to maintain a consistent and safe supply, the lack of the appropriate cannabis product or contaminants may cause unexpected physical or psychological problems for the patient.

Criteria 10 and 11 — tolerance and withdrawal — require careful clinical attention in medical cannabis populations. The DSM-5 states that tolerance and withdrawal should not be counted toward a substance use disorder diagnosis when they occur solely from appropriately prescribed, medically supervised treatment.

This guidance was written for opioids and benzodiazepines. The same reasoning applies to cannabis. Tolerance is an expected physiological adaptation to chronic medication use. Cannabis withdrawal — characterized by irritability, sleep disturbance, decreased appetite, and anxiety — is mild, resolves within one to two weeks, and carries none of the medically dangerous physiological consequences associated with opioid, alcohol, or benzodiazepine cessation. The DSM-5 protection that applies to every other chronically prescribed medication is routinely not applied when that medication is cannabis.

For a social user, or one who uses cannabis to experience the "high", tolerance may develop when used on a daily basis. If using a full spectrum cannabis (whole flower or a full spectrum extract product), tolerance will develop more slowly if the user alters the variety of cannabis rather than using a specific variety exclusively. In addition, tolerance to isolated cannabinoid products (such as dronabinol or THC isolates) will develop much sooner, than with whole plant material.

Case report from a patient in the IND program: Robert Randall received a steady supply of cannabis in cigarette form from the federal government to manage his glaucoma as noted previously. His prescription was for 10 cigarettes a day and he would receive them in a canister containing 300 cigarettes. For years he was able to control his intraocular pressure. However, there came a time when he ran out of his supply before his scheduled time, which led to inquiries. It was discovered that unbeknown to Robert or his physician, the federal government had decreased the amount of cannabis in each cigarette from 1 gram to 0.8 gram, thus shorting his supply. Upon this discovery, they were able to correct the change and he was once again given his correct amount of his medicine. Robert would report that over the years he didn't experience any high, but he never developed a tolerance to its ability to control his intraocular pressure.

Prevalence: Methodological Inflation and Its Clinical Consequences

Survey-based estimates of CUD prevalence range from approximately 9% to over 30% of lifetime cannabis users (Compton et al, 2019, SAMHSA, 2025, Baldwin et al, 2024, Ayers et al, 2025). This variation does not reflect genuine population differences. It reflects methodological inconsistency. Studies applying full DSM-5 diagnostic criteria through structured clinical interviews consistently produce lower estimates than studies relying on abbreviated screening instruments such as the Cannabis Use Disorders Identification Test — Revised (CUDIT-R) or the Cannabis Abuse Screening Test (CAST). These tools were designed and validated in recreational cannabis user populations. They have not been validated in medical cannabis populations, they are not diagnostic instruments, and their positive results cannot constitute a CUD diagnosis. Treating a positive CUDIT-R as diagnostic is methodologically equivalent to treating a positive PHQ-2 as a diagnosis of major depressive disorder.

The foundational population-level data, drawn from the National Comorbidity Survey by Anthony, Warner, and Kessler (1994), estimated that approximately 9% of lifetime cannabis users developed dependence — the lowest rate among all commonly studied psychoactive substances other than psychedelics, as shown in Table 3. Tobacco dependence formed in 32% of lifetime users; heroin in 23%; cocaine in 17%; alcohol in 15%. Cannabis's rate was comparable to anxiolytics and sedatives — prescription medications for which tolerance and withdrawal are treated as expected pharmacological phenomena rather than diagnostic criteria. The differential treatment of cannabis tolerance and withdrawal versus those same phenomena in prescription medications with comparable or higher risk profiles reflects prohibition's distortion of clinical judgment, not pharmacological science.

Table 3. Comparative dependence rates among lifetime users of common psychoactive substances

Substance	Dependence Rate Among Lifetime Users	Clinical and Regulatory Context
Tobacco	32%	3.6× higher than cannabis; dependence treated as expected pharmacological outcome
Heroin	23%	2.6× higher than cannabis; Schedule I
Cocaine	17%	1.9× higher than cannabis; Schedule II
Alcohol	15%	1.7× higher than cannabis; not scheduled
Anxiolytics / Sedatives	9%	Comparable to cannabis; tolerance and withdrawal treated as expected pharmacological adaptation; typically Schedule IV
Cannabis	9%	Reference; lowest dependence rate among all Schedule I substances
Classic psychedelics (LSD, psilocybin)	< 1%	Also Schedule I; lowest dependence risk among all commonly studied psychoactive substances

Source: Anthony, Warner, & Kessler (1994). Experimental and Clinical Psychopharmacology, 2(3), 244–268.

Persons with substance use disorders with drugs such as opioids or alcohol are often easily diagnosed due to the potential and serious harm from abuse of these drugs. Cannabis, on the other hand, is a plant with numerous constituents, with delta-9-tetrahydrocannabinol (THC) being the primary intoxicating cannabinoid. Other cannabinoids present in the plant, such as cannabidiol (CBD) actually help dampen down the intoxicating effects of THC. To be more precise, the DSM-5 diagnosis of CUD would be more appropriate to be called THC Use Disorder. Cannabis as an herbal medicine has a remarkably wide margin of safety and broad variety of therapeutic applications due to its interaction with the endocannabinoid system, which plays a significant role in most physiological activities in the human body. While CUD may become a problem for some cannabis users, the severity related to the consequences of CUD are fairly minor compared to other substance abuse disorders.

As a patient advocate it is important to recognize the problems facing patients who choose to use this plant because of its beneficial effects, while it is a plant that is prohibited by the federal government, and for many it is also prohibited under their state laws. Where do they get a safe and consistent supply - from an unknown dealer, grow their own, an expensive dispensary, or where else? Has it been tested for contents and contaminants? Does it have the best ratios of cannabinoids? Does it have the helpful terpenes? How do they afford cannabis when insurance won't cover it? Who can they tell about their use or their child's use of cannabis without getting busted? If they are drug tested at work, will they be fired or forced into drug treatment? If caught growing the plant or in possession of the plant, will they have to get a lawyer and go to court, will their property be forfeited, will they lose custody of their children, will they lose their driver's license, will they go to jail or worse get sent to prison? These are serious concerns and cause some changes in behavior to keep their cannabis use or the use of cannabis for a loved one a secret. When interacting with healthcare professionals, the cannabis user may wonder whether or not they can be honest regarding their cannabis use. Will the clinician understand, respect and support the patient's choice to use cannabis or will the person be judged negatively?

Cannabis as a Harm Reduction Agent

There is a dimension of the cannabis-disorder relationship that receives far less attention than it warrants: cannabis as a harm reduction agent for substances that can cause serious health problems, including death. The clinical stakes are real. A clinician who removes a patient's cannabis access on the basis of misapplied diagnostic criteria, without first evaluating whether that cannabis is displacing a more dangerous substance, may be removing the patient's most effective protection. Table 4 summarizes some of the key evidence.

Table 4. Cannabis as a harm reduction agent: summary of key peer-reviewed evidence

Target Substance	Key Research Finding	Source
Opioids — mortality	States with medical cannabis laws reported 24.8% lower mean annual opioid overdose mortality from 1999–2010, with the protective association strengthening to 33% by year five. A subsequent analysis extending data through 2017 found this association reversed as illicit fentanyl entered the supply — an essential methodological update demonstrating that cannabis access cannot substitute for comprehensive opioid policy in the presence of adulterated supply.	Bachhuber et al. (2014), JAMA Internal Medicine; Shover et al. (2019), PNAS
Opioids — cue-induced craving	In a double-blind RCT, CBD (400mg and 800mg) produced a 2–3 fold reduction in cue-induced heroin craving versus placebo at 7 days post-dosing. Reductions in salivary cortisol and heart rate confirmed objective physiological mechanism, ruling out placebo effect. Effect size calculated at Cohen's d = 2.0–3.0 — exceptionally large by clinical trial standards. No serious adverse events observed.	Hurd et al. (2019), American Journal of Psychiatry
Alcohol	92 of his patients reported using cannabis as an alternative to alcohol (Mikuriya, 2008). 40% of medical cannabis patients reported substituting cannabis for alcohol; 75% found cannabis more effective for their condition than alcohol had been (Lucas, 2012).	Mikuriya,(2008). Journal of Cannabis Therapeutics. Lucas et al. (2013), Harm Reduction Journal
Tobacco	CBD inhaler reduced cigarette consumption 40% over one week versus 0% in placebo group in a randomized controlled trial. Proposed mechanism: 5-HT1A receptor modulation of nicotine-cue anxiety.	Morgan et al. (2013), Addictive Behaviors
Benzodiazepines	45% of medical cannabis patients eliminated benzodiazepine use entirely following initiation of cannabis access. No withdrawal seizures reported.	Turna et al. (2017), Journal of Psychiatric Research

Source: Bachhuber et al. (2014); Shover et al. (2019); Hurd et al. (2019); Mikuriya (2008;) Lucas et al. (2013); Morgan et al. (2013); Turna et al. (2017).

A French group reviewed studies on the use of CBD for alcohol related problems. Their conclusions were that CBD could directly reduce the intake of alcohol. In addition, CBD could improve both hepatic and neurocognitive outcomes in persons with alcohol use disorder (AUD) by reducing alcohol-related steatosis processes in the liver and alcohol-related brain damage (De Ternay et al., 2019). A German double-blind placebo-controlled trial looked at the use of CBD as a potential treatment for AUD. A dose of 800mg CBD was used against a placebo on 28 subjects with AUD. They found that CBD reduced cue-induced nucleus accumbens (NAc) activity and alcohol craving, supporting the use of CBD for AUD (Zimmermann et al., 2025). An animal study (rats) found that chronic administration of cannabidiol (CBD) can mitigate alcohol dependence by reducing alcohol intake and withdrawal symptoms, lowering relapse-like behaviors, normalizing neuronal excitability in the basolateral amygdala (BLA) and preventing alcohol-induced neurodegeneration. In addition, CBD did not potentiate alcohol's sedative effects, but seemed to provide anxiolytic effects (Dirik et al., 2025).

Cannabis can play an important role with opioids. When cannabis is used in conjunction with opioids for management of chronic pain, it can help prevent Opioid Use Disorder (OUD) by reducing the amount of opioids needed because of the synergy in pain management when the two are used (Cichewicz, 2004). Cannabis also helps slow down tolerance to opioids, thus slowing the need for higher doses. Cannabis has been shown to be effective in alleviating opioid withdrawal symptoms when patients want to decrease or eliminate their use of opioids. Additionally, opioids may help to prevent relapse of OUD by decreasing the craving for opioids. (Wiese & Wilson-Poe, 2018).

An economist at the University of Georgia and his daughter, a sociologist, looked at Medicare spending from 2010-2013 for the use of prescription drugs for conditions in which cannabis could serve as an alternative. When comparing states with medical cannabis laws with states without such laws, they found a significant decrease in the spending on prescription drugs in states with medical cannabis laws. A year later, they reported their findings in a similar review of Medicaid spending from 2007-2014 and found a lower use of prescription drugs in states with medical cannabis laws. The authors conclude that there will be fewer Medicare and Medicaid prescriptions in states that allow the medical use of cannabis, which has a wider margin of safety (Bradford & Bradford, 2016, 2017). In 2018 two studies reported a decrease in opioid prescriptions for Medicaid enrollees from 2011-2016 (Wen & Hockenberry) and Medicare enrollees from 2010-2015 (Bradford et al., 2018) in states with medical cannabis laws compared to states where cannabis remains illegal under the federal prohibition.

Several studies have shown that cannabis can help decrease or eliminate the use of other drugs of abuse. Reiman and Lucas each conducted surveys of cannabis patients in California and Canada dispensaries respectively. A significant number of patients reported that they were able to decrease or eliminate their use of alcohol, opioids, prescription drugs and other substances because of their cannabis use. An anonymous survey of 350 patients at a cannabis dispensary in Berkeley, CA included 68% males, 54% single and 66% White, with a mean age of 39. Reasons for cannabis use included having a chronic medical condition (71%), managing pain (52%), or for a mental health issue (75%). Forty percent of the respondents used cannabis as a substitute for alcohol, 26% as a substitute for illicit drugs and 66% as a substitute for prescription drugs. Their top reasons for substituting included less adverse side effects (65%), better symptom management (57%), and less withdrawal potential (34%) (Reiman, 2009).

A later study by Lucas and others conducted a larger survey including 2032 Canadian cannabis patients. Respondents were primarily (91%) Caucasian and 62.6%

male with a mean age of 40 years, with 83.7% using cannabis for pain or mental health conditions. Cannabis was used as a substitute for prescription drugs (69.1%), alcohol (44.5%), tobacco (31/1%) and illicit substances (26.6%). Of the prescription drugs 35.3% were for opioids and 21.5% were for antidepressants; with 59.3% of the opioid using patients reporting total cessation of opioids (Lucas, Baron & Jikomes, 2019). Three main reasons the patients cited for cannabis substitution were Less withdrawal, fewer side effects, and better symptom management. (Lucas et al., 2013)

A small study that followed 25 male crack cocaine addicts in Brazil found that 68% used cannabis to overcome their crack addiction (Labigalini et al., 1999). A study of 122 crack cocaine addicts were able to decrease their frequency of crack with the use of cannabis (Socias et al., 2017). Melanie Dreher, PhD, RN conducted an ethnographic study of 33 female crack addicts in Jamaica for nine months. They used cannabis or "ganja" (smoking "spliffs") to counter negative effects of cocaine, specifically paranoia and weight loss and many found cannabis was the cheapest and most effective and readily available treatment for cessation of crack use (Dreher, 2002).

A study out of Philadelphia found that cannabis can be helpful during induction of methadone treatment for OUD. Methadone treatment occurs on an out-patient basis. Patients are assessed daily for withdrawal symptoms from opioids as they are started on methadone. Per law, during induction to methadone, an opioid treatment program must start at a low dose of methadone due to the risk of overdose of this long-acting substance and gradually increase the dose at each visit according to the individual's withdrawal symptoms. This induction period can be difficult for the patient due to the discomfort of the withdrawal symptoms as the patient gradually reaches his/her maintenance dose. Since this is done on an outpatient basis, some patients will self-medicate with other illicit drugs such as benzodiazepines or other opioids to help reduce their discomfort. This can be quite dangerous because the added drug(s) may peak at the same time the methadone's effect peaks resulting in an overdose and death. This study found via urine drug tests that for those patients who supplemented their induction period with cannabis, that the patients experienced a decrease in withdrawal symptoms and were able to get through the induction of methadone until they reached their maintenance dosage. The authors concluded that there is a potential role for cannabis during methadone induction (Scavone et al, 2013)

Adolescent Risk: Where Genuine Clinical Caution Is Warranted

The evidence does support clinical concern in one area: adolescent use during active neurodevelopment. CB1 receptors are expressed at elevated density during adolescence, and the ECS plays a significant role in synaptic pruning and neural circuit formation. Longitudinal data from the Dunedin cohort associated heavy adolescent cannabis use with neuropsychological decline into midlife (Meier et al., 2012), though subsequent analyses found that socioeconomic differences and pre-existing cognitive variation account for a substantial portion of the observed association (Rogeberg, 2013; Jackson et al., 2016). The evidence warrants clinical caution in adolescent populations specifically — not categorical conclusions that are then misapplied to adult therapeutic populations where the evidence base is different.

Missed Opportunities to Learn

The misdiagnosis of CUD can result in negative attitudes by health care clinicians, along with efforts to encourage drug treatment for patients when misdiagnosed. For those using cannabis as medicine, a CUD diagnosis is not only insulting, but decreases the patient's trust in the clinician and/or healthcare system. If clinicians demonstrate a judgmental attitude about the use of cannabis, patients will be reluctant to discuss their use of cannabis. This silence leads to a missed opportunity for the clinician to observe, document, and learn more about the therapeutic benefits of this therapeutic substance.

Another more important issue with the misdiagnosis of CUD is that by not recognizing the health benefits of cannabis, clinicians are missing opportunities to help guide the patient in safe and effective use of this herbal remedy as well as education on how to maintain a healthy ECS. The intoxicating effect of THC is the primary reason for the social use of cannabis and nurses can help advise individuals about safer use such as using a clean pipe rather than cigarette form, not holding their breath when smoking, vaping instead of smoking, or consuming infused beverages. When it comes to medical use, nurses can help patients find the most appropriate variety of cannabis products, which may include varieties lower in THC, but higher in other non-intoxicating cannabinoids. Terpene and flavonoid content should also be considered according to the desired effect. Guidance on dosage and routes of administration are additional areas for patient education.

Persons who develop a substance use disorder (SUD) often seek drug use as a means to cope with uncomfortable feelings or health problems (self-medicating). Hemp hearts and hemp seed oil (cannabis products) are highly nutritious and can help maintain the ECS. Cannabis medicinal and food products used appropriately can help supplement the ECS. Used in this manner, cannabis can help prevent substance use disorders.

The greatest harm related to the use of cannabis is the prohibition of this plant. Because of the decades-long prohibition, persons have suffered legal consequences including loss of property, loss of professional license to work, loss of child custody, court costs, arrests and possible incarceration, and more. Because of the prohibition there is lack of quality control of cannabis products resulting in unknown chemovar make-up, inconsistency in the products, and potential contamination. Many patients aren't aware of or able to access products and have limited their use to smoking plant material, when an alternative route of administration would be more appropriate. There is little to no medical supervision. Patients also suffer because clinicians (out of ignorance or intimidation) don't recommend the use of cannabis when it could be a safer alternative to more dangerous or expensive medications. State legislation has allowed for medical use in many states, but the laws vary from state to state and they are determined by politicians rather than healthcare professionals resulting in confusion and at times nonsensical regulations that put limits on what conditions would be allowed or limits related to dosage. Although some states may allow for cannabis use, patients cannot legally take their medicine across state lines due to the federal prohibition.

SOLUTIONS & RECOMMENDATIONS

A Framework for Objective Clinical Assessment

Every CUD evaluation conducted with a patient who uses or has recently used medical cannabis must establish four foundational domains before any criterion is applied: (1) the purpose, history, and clinical context of cannabis use, including the condition being managed, the patient's own assessment of therapeutic response, and any documentation of prior conventional treatment; (2) a criterion-by-criterion evaluation distinguishing pharmacological behavior from prohibition-generated behavioral consequence — including supply barriers, employment jeopardy, and interpersonal conflict rooted in legal stigma rather than observable harm from cannabis; (3) the patient's occupational, legal, and insurance environment, which shapes the behavioral expression of nearly every DSM-5 criterion; and (4) whether cannabis is functioning as a harm reduction agent for a more acutely dangerous substance use disorder, making withdrawal of cannabis access a patient safety question as well as a diagnostic one.

A positive urine toxicology screen is not a diagnosis. THC-COOH detection confirms cannabis use within a broad metabolic window. It does not establish impairment, frequency of use, therapeutic intent, or any DSM-5 diagnostic criterion. Tolerance and withdrawal must not be counted toward CUD when they occur in the context of ongoing therapeutic use without clinically significant distress beyond expected physiological adaptation — consistent with the DSM-5's existing guidance for all other chronically used medications. Screening instruments must be used only as their validation intended: to initiate clinical inquiry. No CUD diagnosis should rest on a screening score alone. A full structured diagnostic interview applying all eleven criteria, with attention to the patient's clinical and legal context, is required.

Integrating Endocannabinoid System Education Into Clinical Training

The majority of practicing U.S. clinicians received no instruction on the endocannabinoid system during their training. This needs to change. The ECS regulates core physiological processes regardless of cannabis policy — pain, inflammation, stress, immunity, metabolism — and its dysfunction appears in conditions every clinician sees. Patients Out of Time has addressed this gap through its national accredited conference series on cannabis therapeutics since 2000, providing continuing education for physicians, nurses, pharmacists, and attorneys. That work should not be necessary as a substitute for foundational medical education. The ECS belongs in standard pharmacology and physiology curricula with the same depth given to the adrenergic, serotonergic, and opioid systems. Continuing medical education programs must provide targeted training in criteria-based CUD assessment, cannabis pharmacokinetics and detection windows, the validation limits of screening instruments, and the current evidence base for therapeutic cannabis applications and drug interactions.

Regulatory Reform and Product Standardization

Cannabis does not satisfy the legal criteria for Schedule I classification under 21 U.S.C. §812. The FDA has approved a cannabis-derived medication. The federal government holds a neuroprotectant patent for cannabinoids. Synthetic THC is Schedule III. Schedule I legally requires no currently accepted medical use — a standard cannabis cannot meet when the federal government simultaneously patents its therapeutic applications, supplied it to patients through a compassionate access program, and licenses its derivatives as prescription drugs. Rescheduling to Schedule III or lower would enable FDA-regulated research, standard medical prescribing, insurance coverage, and resolution of the contradiction between federal prohibition and state medical programs that distorts clinical practice. Product standardization — verified cannabinoid and terpene profiles, contaminant testing, and therapeutic use labeling — is the prerequisite for cannabis medicine to function safely and for CUD assessment to be grounded in reliable dosing information rather than black market guesswork.

This author maintains that the plant cannabis must be de-scheduled rather than moved to a less restrictive schedule. The Schedule III status will allow for FDA approved formulations of cannabis, but will not allow home growing that allows for unlimited varieties. Schedule III will not allow personal adult use - it would still require a prescription. Cannabis therapeutic products for sale must be standardized and regulated, but the plant should be available for anyone to grow and enjoy its many benefits beyond its medicinal applications.

Research Priorities

Three research needs are most urgent. First, large-scale chart reviews applying full DSM-5 structured diagnostic interviews to medical cannabis patients would determine the actual prevalence of CUD misdiagnosis in therapeutic populations — data that do not currently exist. Second, validation studies comparing structured interview results against abbreviated screening tool results in the same medical cannabis populations would quantify the diagnostic inflation produced by methodological conflation and provide the empirical basis for corrected clinical guidance. Third, randomized controlled trials examining cannabinoids as adjuncts to buprenorphine and methadone maintenance therapy would test whether the craving-reduction effects demonstrated by Hurd et al. (2019) translate into reduced relapse rates in standard addiction treatment — addressing the most clinically urgent application of existing harm reduction evidence.

A glaring problem with CUD is that cannabis is not a drug, it is a plant. There are numerous varieties of the cannabis plant and countless products can be made from the plant. The effects will vary according to the constituents in the plant/product, whether it contains a single isolate, or various combinations of cannabinoids, terpenes and flavonoids. Delta-9-THC is the intoxicating cannabinoid and predictably THC rich cannabis products are of concern regarding the development of CUD. A priority in cannabis research should focus more on determining the therapeutic effectiveness of specific varieties for various conditions.

FUTURE RESEARCH DIRECTIONS

The science of the endocannabinoid system is approximately three decades old within a receptor system that evolved 600 million years ago and that has been pharmacologically active in human medicine for millennia. Research frontiers include characterization of additional receptor subtypes — including GPR55, GPR18, and GPR119 — and mapping of individual ECS tone variation across psychiatric, neurological, and metabolic conditions. The identification of pathological ECS states may eventually yield diagnostic biomarkers for conditions currently assessed only by behavioral report.

Research into minor phytocannabinoids — cannabigerol (CBG), cannabichromene (CBC), cannabinol (CBN), and tetrahydrocannabivarin (THCV) — has accelerated but remains early stage. The entourage effect hypothesis — that whole-plant cannabis preparations produce clinical outcomes distinct from isolated compounds through interaction among phytocannabinoids, terpenes, and flavonoids — was first described by Mechoulam and Ben-Shabat (1998) and developed further by Russo (2007). Adequately powered trials comparing whole-plant and isolated cannabinoid preparations in standardized therapeutic applications have not yet been conducted.

Longitudinal cohort studies prospectively tracking medical cannabis patients with structured DSM-5 assessments, validated functional outcome measures, and concurrent documentation of other substance use would generate the first population-level data needed to distinguish therapeutic use from disorder in clinical populations. The Bachhuber-to-Shover study arc — in which an early protective association between medical cannabis laws and opioid mortality later reversed with fentanyl supply expansion — shows both the methodological rigor cannabis research requires and what is at stake when it is absent. The regulatory barriers that have blocked such studies are a research ethics problem, not just a policy inconvenience.

CONCLUSION

Cannabis Use Disorder is a legitimate clinical diagnosis when DSM-5 criteria are met in the context of non-therapeutic, pattern-disordered use producing genuine, cannabis-attributable impairment or distress. This chapter does not dispute that. What it documents — with primary sources, peer-reviewed evidence, and the federal government's own internal record — is that the conditions under which CUD assessment currently occurs have been shaped by eighty years of prohibition in ways that produce diagnoses aimed at patients rather than at the policies driving their behavior.

The endocannabinoid system is not a pharmacological footnote. It is the system through which the body regulates pain, inflammation, memory, stress, immune function, and metabolism. A clinician who has never been taught it cannot accurately evaluate cannabis use. The reason most practicing clinicians were never taught it is a federal classification that was acknowledged as provisional in 1970, rejected by the Commission appointed to evaluate it in 1972, and held in place for more than five decades despite the contradictory evidence from the federal government's own programs, courts, and patent office.

The Shafer Commission told the federal government in 1972, based on the best available evidence, that cannabis should not be criminal. That report was buried. The DEA's own administrative law judge reached the same conclusion in 1988. That ruling was overruled. The federal IND patients — people the author of this chapter met in 1985 when they were using government cannabis to manage their conditions — are proof that the Schedule I classification was never a scientific finding.

Fifty-two years after the Shafer Commission, the patients harmed by those decisions are still in clinicians' offices. They deserve practitioners who understand the endocannabinoid system, who apply diagnostic criteria with contextual precision, and who can distinguish between the pharmacology of a medicine and the politics of its prohibition. That distinction matters. For patients still navigating a clinical landscape shaped by the choices made in 1937 and 1970, it may be the most important thing their provider gets right.

After decades of demonizing this plant as a dangerous drug, the negative stigma is hard to erase and interferes with the recognition of the overall safety and healing aspects of this ancient herb. The late Tod Mikuriya, MD resurrected the knowledge of cannabis therapeutics with his early publication, *Marijuana: Medical Papers 1839-1972* (1973). As a psychiatrist, he dedicated his life to educating others about the safety and efficacy of cannabis and treating numerous patients with this herb. This chapter ends with a quotation from Dr. Mikuriya:

> *We should be thinking of cannabis as a medicine first that happens to have some psychoactive properties, as many medicines do, rather than as an intoxicant that happens to have a few therapeutic properties on the side.*

REFERENCES

Aldrich, M. (1997). The history of medical cannabis. In Mathre, M. L. (Ed.), *Cannabis in medical practice: A legal, historical and pharmacological overview of the therapeutic use of marijuana* (pp. 35–55). McFarland & Company, Inc.

Allen, D. (2014). Survey of endocannabinoid system instruction at U.S. medical schools. Presented at *The Seventh National Clinical Conference on Cannabis Therapeutics, Patients Out of Time*. Portland, OR.

American Nurses Association & American Cannabis Nurses Association. (2024). *Cannabis Nursing: Scope and Standards of Practice*. ANA.

American Psychiatric Association. (2013). *Diagnostic and Statistical Manual on Mental Disorders* (5th ed.). American Psychiatric Association.

American Society of Addiction Medicine (ASAM). (Aug. 9, 2021). A Review of Potential Pharmacological Treatments for Cannabis Abuse. https://www.asam.org/blog-details/article/2021/08/09/a-review-of-potential-pharmacological-treatments-for-cannabis-abuse

Anthony, J. C., Warner, L. A., & Kessler, R. C. (1994). Comparative epidemiology of dependence upon alcohol, controlled substances, and inhalants: Basic findings from the National Comorbidity Survey. *Experimental and Clinical Psychopharmacology*, *2*(3), 244–268. DOI: 10.1037/1064-1297.2.3.244

Ayers, C., Robalino, S., Shaw, B., Ward, R., & Kansagara, D. (2025). *Prevalence and Risk of Developing Cannabis Use Disorder in Adults Who Use Cannabis, Living Systematic Review: Update 1*. Portland, OR: Systematically Testing the Evidence on Marijuana (STEM) Project;2022; updated Feb. 2025. https://www.cannabisevidence.org/evidence-syntheses/adult-cannabis-use-disorder/

Bachhuber, M. A., Saloner, B., Cunningham, C. O., & Barry, C. L. (2014). Medical cannabis laws and opioid analgesic overdose mortality in the United States, 1999-2010. *JAMA Internal Medicine*, *174*(10), 1668–1673. DOI: 10.1001/jamainternmed.2014.4005 PMID: 25154332

Baldwin, G. T., Vivolo, A., Hoots, B., Roehler, D. R., & Ko, J. Y. (2024). Current cannabis use in the United States: Implications for public health research. *American Journal of Public Health*, *114*(58), 5624–5627. DOI: 10.2105/AJPH.2024.307823 PMID: 39442034

Bonnie, R. J., & Whitebread, C. H. (1974). *The marijuana conviction: A history of marijuana prohibition in the United States*. University of Virginia.

Booth, M. (2004). *Cannabis: A History*. Thomas Dunne Books/St. Martin's Press.

Bradford, A. C., & Bradford, W. D. (2016). Medical marijuana laws reduce prescription medication use in Medicare Part D. *Health Affairs*, *35*(7), 1230–1236. Advance online publication. DOI: 10.1377/hlthaff.2015.1661 PMID: 27385238

Bradford, A. C., & Bradford, W. D. (2017). Medical marijuana laws may be associated with a decline in the number of prescriptions for Medicaid enrollees. *Health Affairs*, *36*(5), 945–951. DOI: 10.1377/hlthaff.2016.1135 PMID: 28424215

Bradford, A. C., Bradford, W. D., Abraham, A., & Adams, G. B. (2018). Association between US state medical cannabis laws and opioid prescribing in the Medicare Part D population. *JAMA Internal Medicine*, *178*(5), 667–672. DOI: 10.1001/jamainternmed.2018.0266 PMID: 29610897

Cichewicz, D. L. (2004). Synergistic interactions between cannabinoid and opioid analgesics. *Life Sciences*, *74*(11), 1317–1324. DOI: 10.1016/j.lfs.2003.09.038 PMID: 14706563

Compton, W. M., Han, B., Jones, C. M., & Blanco, C. (2019). Cannabis use disorders among adults in the United States during a time of increasing use of cannabis. *Drug and Alcohol Dependence*, *204*, 107468. DOI: 10.1016/j.drugalcdep.2019.05.008 PMID: 31586809

De Ternay, J., Naassila, M., Nourredine, M., Louvet, A., Bailly, F., Sescousse, G., Maurage, P., Cottencin, O., Carrioeri, P. M., & Rolland, B. (2019). Therapeutic prospects of cannabidiol for alcohol use disorder and alcohol-related damages on the liver and the brain. *Frontiers in Pharmacology*, *10*, 627. DOI: 10.3389/fphar.2019.00627 PMID: 31214036

Dirik, S., Doyle, M. R., Wood, C. P., Campo, P., Martinez, A. R., Fannon, M., Balaguer, M. G., Seely, S., Montoya, B. A., Cook, G. M. R., Palermo, G. M., Lin, J., Sist, M. D., Naghshineh, P. K., Lan, Z., Rahman, S. R. M. U., Suhandynata, R., Schweitzer, P., Kallupi, M., & de Guglielmo, G. (2025). Cannabidiol mitigates alcohol dependence and withdrawal with neuroprotective effects in the basolateral amygdala and striatum. *Neuropsychopharmacology : Official Publication of the American College of Neuropsychopharmacology*, *51*(3), 691–702. DOI: 10.1038/s41386-025-02164-6 PMID: 40640509

Dreher, M. (2002). Crack heads and roots daughters: The therapeutic use of cannabis in Jamaica. *Journal of Cannabis Therapeutics*, *2*(3/4), 121–133. DOI: 10.1300/J175v02n03_08

Huestis, M. A., Boyd, S. J., Heishman, S. J., Preston, K. L., Bonnet, D., LeFur, G., & Gorelick, D. A. (2007). Single and multiple doses of rimonabant antagonize acute effects of smoked cannabis in male cannabis users. *Psychopharmacology, 194*(4), 505–515. DOI: 10.1007/s00213-007-0861-5 PMID: 17619859

Hurd, Y. L., Spriggs, S., Alishayev, J., Winkel, G., Gurgov, K., Kudrich, C., Oprescu, A. M., & Salsitz, E. (2019). Cannabidiol for the reduction of cue-induced craving and anxiety in drug-abstinent individuals with heroin use disorder: A double-blind randomized placebo-controlled trial. *The American Journal of Psychiatry, 176*(11), 911–922. Advance online publication. DOI: 10.1176/appi.ajp.2019.18101191 PMID: 31109198

Jackson, N. J., Isen, J. D., Khoddam, R., Irons, D., Tuvblad, C., Iacono, W. G., McGue, M., Raine, A., & Baker, L. A. (2016). Impact of adolescent marijuana use on intelligence: Results from two longitudinal twin studies. *Proceedings of the National Academy of Sciences of the United States of America, 113*(5), E500–E508. DOI: 10.1073/pnas.1516648113 PMID: 26787878

Labigalini, E.Jr, Rodrigues, L. R., & Da Silveira, D. X. (1999). Therapeutic use of cannabis by crack addicts in Brazil. *Journal of Psychoactive Drugs, 31*(4), 451–455. DOI: 10.1080/02791072.1999.10471776 PMID: 10681113

Lucas, P. (2012). Cannabis as an adjunct to or substitute for opiates in the treatment of chronic pain. *Journal of Psychoactive Drugs, 44*(2), 125–133. DOI: 10.1080/02791072.2012.684624 PMID: 22880540

Lucas, P., Reiman, A., Earleywine, M., McGowan, S. K., Oleson, M., Coward, M. P., & Thomas, B. (2013). Cannabis as a substitute for alcohol and other drugs: A dispensary-based survey of substitution effect in Canadian medical cannabis patients. *Addiction Research and Theory, 21*(5), 435–442. DOI: 10.3109/16066359.2012.733465

Lucas, P., Baron, E. P., & Jikomes, N. (2019). Medical cannabis patterns of use and substitution for opioids & other pharmaceutical drugs, alcohol, tobacco, and other illicit substances: Results from a cross-sectional survey of authorized patients. *Harm Reduction Journal, 16*(9), 9. Advance online publication. DOI: 10.1186/s12954-019-0278-6 PMID: 30691503

McWilliams, J. C. (1990). *The protectors: Harry J. Anslinger and the Federal Bureau of Narcotics, 1930-1962*. University of Delaware Press.

Mechoulam, R., & Ben-Shabat, S. (1998). From gan-zi nu to anandamide and 2-arachidonoylglycerop: The ongoing story of cannabis. *Natural Product Reports, 16*(2), 131–143. DOI: 10.1039/a703973e PMID: 10331283

Mechoulam, R. (2004, May). *The Cannabinoid System in Neuroprotection*. Presented at *The Third National Clinical Conference on Cannabis Therapeutics, Patients Out of Time*. Charlottesville, VA.

Meier, M. H., Caspi, A., Ambler, A., Harrington, H., Houts, R., Keefe, R. S. E., McDonald, K., Ward, A., Poulton, R., & Moffit, T. E. (2012). Persistent cannabis users show neuropsychological decline from childhood to midlife. *Proceedings of the National Academy of Sciences of the United States of America, 109*(40), E2657–E2664. DOI: 10.1073/pnas.1206820109 PMID: 22927402

Mikuriya, T. H. (2008). Cannabis as a substitute for alcohol: A harm reduction approach. *Journal of Cannabis Therapeutics, 4*(1), 79–93. DOI: 10.1300/J175v04n01_04

Morgan, C. J. A., Das, R. K., Joye, A., Curran, H. V., & Kamboj, S. K. (2013). Cannabidiol reduces cigarette consumption in tobacco smokers: Preliminary findings. *Addictive Behaviors, 38*(9), 2433–2436. DOI: 10.1016/j.addbeh.2013.03.011 PMID: 23685330

National Commission on Marihuana and Drug Abuse. (1972). *Marihuana: A Signal of Misunderstanding*. U.S. Government Printing Office.

National Council of State Boards of Nursing. (2018, July). The NCSBN national nursing guidelines for medical marijuana. *Journal of Nursing Regulation, 9*(2).

Nussbaum, A. M., Boyer, J. A., & Kondrad, E. C. (2011). "But my doctor recommended pot": Medical marijuana and the patient-physician relationship. *Journal of General Internal Medicine, 26*(11), 1364–1367. DOI: 10.1007/s11606-011-1840-4 PMID: 21863349

Randall, R. C., & O'Leary, A. M. (1998). *Marijuana Rx: The Patients Fight for Medicinal Pot*. Thunder's Mouth Press.

Reiman, A. (2009). Cannabis as a substitute for alcohol and other drugs. *Harm Reduction Journal, 6*(1), 35. DOI: 10.1186/1477-7517-6-35 PMID: 19958538

Robinson, V. (1912). *An Essay on Hashish*. New York: Medical Review of Reviews, E.H. Ringer.

Rogeberg, O. (2013). Correlations between cannabis use and IQ change in the Dunedin cohort are consistent with confounding from socioeconomic status. *Proceedings of the National Academy of Sciences of the United States of America, 110*(11), 425–4254. DOI: 10.1073/pnas.1215678110 PMID: 23319626

Russo, E. B., Mathre, M. L., Byrne, A., Velin, R., Bach, P. J., Sanchez-Ramos, J., & Kirlin, K. A. (2002). Chronic cannabis use in the Compassionate Investigational New Drug Program: An examination of benefits and adverse effects of legal clinical cannabis. *Journal of Cannabis Therapeutics*, *2*(1), 3–57. DOI: 10.1300/J175v02n01_02

Russo, E. B. (2007). History of cannabis and its preparations in saga, science, and sobriquet. *Chemistry & Biodiversity*, *4*(8), 1614–1648. DOI: 10.1002/cbdv.200790144 PMID: 17712811

Scavone, J. L., Sterling, R. C., Weinstein, S. P., & Van Bockstaele, E. J. (2013). Impact of cannabis use during stabilization on methadone maintenance treatment. *The American Journal on Addictions*, *22*(4), 344–31. DOI: 10.1111/j.1521-0391.2013.12044.x PMID: 23795873

Shover, C. L., Davis, C. S., Gordon, S. C., & Humphreys, K. (2019). Association between medical cannabis laws and opioid overdose mortality has reversed over time. *Proceedings of the National Academy of Sciences of the United States of America*, *116*(26), 12624–12626. DOI: 10.1073/pnas.1903434116 PMID: 31182592

Socias, M. E., Kerr, T., Wood, E., Dong, H., Lake, S., Hayashi, K., DeBeck, K., Jutras-Aswad, D., Montaner, J., & Milloy, M. J. (2017). Intentional cannabis use to reduce crack cocaine use in a Canadian setting: A longitudinal analysis. *Addictive Behaviors*, *72*, 138–143. DOI: 10.1016/j.addbeh.2017.04.006 PMID: 28399488

Substance Abuse and Mental Health Services Administration. (2025). *Key substance use and mental health indicators in the United States: Results from the 2024 national Survey on Drug Use and Health* (HHS Publication No. PeP25-07-007, NSDUH Series H-60). Center for Behavioral Health Statistics and Quality, Substance Abuse and Mental Health Services Administration. https://www.samhsa.gov/data/data-we-collect/nsduh-national-survey-drug-use-and-health/national-releases

Turna, J., Patterson, B., & Van Ameringen, M. (2017). Is cannabis treatment for anxiety, mood, and related disorders ready for prime time? *Depression and Anxiety*, *34*(11), 1006–1017. DOI: 10.1002/da.22664 PMID: 28636769

U.S. Department of Health and Human Services, Food and Drug Administration. (2018, June 25). *FDA approves first drug comprised of an active ingredient derived from marijuana* (Press release). Retrieved from https://www.fda.gov

United States Patent No. 6,630,507. 2003. *Cannabinoids as antioxidants and neuroprotectants*. Inventors: Hampson, A. J., Grimaldi, M., Axelrod, J., & Wink, D. United States Patent and Trademark Office.

Wen, H., & Hockenberry, J. M. (2018). Association of medical and adult-use marijuana laws with opioid prescribing for Medicaid enrollees. *JAMA Internal Medicine, 178*(5), 673–679. DOI: 10.1001/jamainternmed.2018.1007 PMID: 29610827

Wiese, B., & Wilson-Poe, A. R. (2018). Emerging evidence for cannabis' role in opioid use disorder. *Cannabis and Cannabinoid Research, 3*(1), 179–189. DOI: 10.1089/can.2018.0022 PMID: 30221197

Zimmermann, S., Teetzmann, A., Baeßler, J., Schreckenberger, L., Zaiser, J., Pfisterer, M., Stenger, M., & Bach, P. (2025). Acute cannabidiol administration reduces alcohol craving and cue-induced nucleus accumbens activation in individuals with alcohol use disorder: The double-blind randomized controlled ICONIC trial. *Molecular Psychiatry, 30*(6), 2612–2619. DOI: 10.1038/s41380-024-02869-y PMID: 39668256

Evanoff, A. B., Quan, T., Dufault, C., Awad, M., & Bierut, L. J. (2017). Physicians-in-training are not prepared to prescribe medical marijuana. *Drug and Alcohol Dependence, 180*, 151–155. DOI: 10.1016/j.drugalcdep.2017.08.010 PMID: 28892720

KEY TERMS AND DEFINITIONS

Addiction: A primary, chronic, neurobiologic disease, with genetic, psychosocial, and environmental factors influencing its development and manifestations. It is characterized by behaviors that include one or more of the following: impaired control over drug use, compulsive use, continued use despite harm, and craving.

Controlled Substances Act: A federal law enacted October 27, 1970 that created 5 levels (Schedules) of potentially addictive drugs. The Schedules go from I (forbidden) down to 5 (least addictive).

Drug Dependence: A state of adaptation that is manifested by a drug class specific withdrawal syndrome that can be produced by abrupt cessation, rapid dose reduction, decreasing blood level of the drug, and/or administration of an antagonist.

Harm Reduction DSM-5: The abbreviation for the American Psychiatric Association's text, Diagnostic and Statistical Manual of Mental Disorders, Fifth Edition (2013). The primary diagnostic reference for mental health and substance use disorders in the United States.

Harm Reduction: A public health philosophy and clinical practice framework that seeks to reduce the negative consequences of drug use without requiring abstinence as a precondition for care. Encompasses naloxone distribution, needle exchange, medication-assisted treatment, and — as a growing body of peer-reviewed evidence supports — cannabis substitution therapy for more acutely dangerous substances.

IND Program: The Investigational New Drug Program allows approved patients to use a drug/medicine that has not yet been approved by the FDA. To gain access a patient's physician must complete an application that justifies the request, noting that current FDA approved medications have failed. In the case of cannabis, this access was referred to as the "Compassionate IND Program" and the program was closed to new applicants in 1992.

Missoula Chronic Clinical Cannabis Use Study: A 2001 study conducted by Patients Out of Time examining four surviving federal IND patients after 11 to 27 years of continuous government-supplied cannabis use. Investigators performed comprehensive three-day medical evaluations across all body systems. Conclusions: all four patients demonstrated functional health appropriate for their age, with no cannabis-attributable deterioration. Published in the Journal of Cannabis Therapeutics (Russo et al., 2002).

Patients Out of Time.: A national 501(c)(3) nonprofit organization co-founded in 1995 by the author of this chapter and her husband Al Byrne, both U.S. Navy veterans. Mission: to educate healthcare professionals and the public about the therapeutic use of cannabis and the endocannabinoid system. Known for its accredited National Clinical Conference on Cannabis Therapeutics series, which began in 2000 and has provided continuing education credits for physicians, nurses, pharmacists, and attorneys.

Schedule I: The most restricted level of psychoactive drug placement in the U.S. under the Controlled Substances Act. To belong in Schedule I a drug must meet 3 criteria: be highly addictive, have no approved medical value, and is not safe for medical use.

Substance Use Disorder: A general term for a cluster of cognitive, behavioral and physiological symptoms indicating that the individual continues using the substance despite significant substance-related problems. Substance use disorders are specified by the specific drug or class of drugs such as alcohol use disorder, opioid use disorder, cannabis use disorder, etc.

THC-COOH: The primary urinary metabolite of delta-9-tetrahydrocannabinol (THC). Detectable in urine for 3 to 30 days following cannabis use depending on frequency and individual metabolism — a window substantially exceeding any period of psychoactive impairment. Detection confirms cannabis use within this window. It does not establish impairment, frequency of use, therapeutic intent, or satisfaction of any DSM-5 criterion.

Tolerance: The body's physical adaptation to a drug: greater amounts of the drug are required over time to achieve the initial effects as the body "gets used to" and adapts to the intake.

Withdrawal Syndrome: A constellation of physiological and psychological symptoms following reduction or cessation of a substance after prolonged use. Cannabis withdrawal — characterized by irritability, sleep disturbance, decreased appetite, and anxiety — is mild, self-resolving within one to two weeks, produces no medically dangerous physiological derangement, and has no documented fatalities. Substantially less severe than withdrawal from opioids, alcohol, or benzodiazepines.

APPENDIX

The CAST questionnaire is a screening tool that clinicians have used to assess for a cannabis use problem.

CAST

1. Have you smoked cannabis before midday?
2. Have you smoked cannabis when you were alone?
3. Have you had memory problems when you smoked cannabis?
4. Have friends or members of your family told you that you ought to reduce your cannabis use?
5. Have you tried to reduce or stop your cannabis use without succeeding?
6. Have you had problems because of your use of cannabis (argument, fight, accident, bad result at school, etc.)?

Scoring: Coded 0-4 scale from never to very often, scores ranging from 0-24. Less than 3 indicates no addiction risk; 3-6 low risk; >7 high risk.

The CUDIT-R is a more specific screening tool to determine the level of severity of a problem with the use of cannabis.

Figure 1.

The Cannabis Use Disorder Identification Test - Revised (CUDIT-R)

Have you used any cannabis over the past six months? Yes________ No ________

If you answered "Yes" to the previous question, please answer the following questions about your cannabis use. Circle the response that is most correct for you in relation to your cannabis use over the *past six months*.

1. How often do you use cannabis?

Never	Monthly or less	2-4 times a month	2-3 times a week	4+ times a week
0	1	2	3	4

2. How many hours were you "stoned" on a typical day when you had been using cannabis?

Less than 1	1 or 2	3 or 4	5 or 6	7 or more
0	1	2	3	4

3. How often during the past 6 months did you find that you were not able to stop using cannabis once you had started?

Never	Less than monthly	Monthly	Weekly	Daily/almost daily
0	1	2	3	4

4. How often during the past 6 months did you fail to do what was normally expected from you because of using cannabis?

Never	Less than monthly	Monthly	Weekly	Daily or almost daily
0	1	2	3	4

5. How often in the past 6 months have you devoted a great deal of your time to getting, using, or recovering from cannabis?

Never	Less than monthly	Monthly	Weekly	Daily/almost daily
0	1	2	3	4

6. How often in the past 6 months have you had a problem with your memory or concentration after using cannabis?

Never	Less than monthly	Monthly	Weekly	Daily or almost daily
0	1	2	3	4

7. How often do you use cannabis in situations that could be physically hazardous, such as driving, operating machinery, or caring for children?

Never	Less than monthly	Monthly	Weekly	Daily/almost daily
0	1	2	3	4

8. Have you ever thought about cutting down, or stopping, your use of cannabis?

Never	Yes, but not in the past 6 months	Yes, during the past 6 months
0	2	4

This questionnaire was designed for self-administration and is scored by adding each of the 8 items:

Question 1-7 are scored on a 0-4 scale
Question 8 is scored 0,2, or 4

Score: ________

Scores of 8 or more indicate hazardous cannabis use, while scores of 12 or more indicate a possible cannabis use disorder for which further intervention may be required.

Adamson SJ, Kay-Lambkin FJ, Baker AL, Lewin TJ, Thornton L, Kelly BJ, and Sellman JD. (2010). An Improved Brief Measure of Cannabis Misuse: The Cannabis Use Disorders Identification Test – Revised (CUDIT-R). *Drug and Alcohol Dependence* 110:137-143.

Chapter 5

Cannabis and Anesthesia: Considerations for Anesthesia Providers

Christopher Giberson
http://orcid.org/0009-0009-7865-3478
Atlanticare Regional Medical Center, USA

ABSTRACT

Cannabis use in the United States has increased over the past several decades. This rise in prevalence parallels expanded legalization, increased societal acceptance, and the proliferation of commercially available cannabis products. These evolving patterns of use present unique and increasingly complex challenges for anesthesia providers. Cannabis has been shown to exert clinically significant effects across multiple organ systems, including the pulmonary, cardiovascular, and neurologic systems. Moreover, cannabinoids interact with numerous anesthetic agents. Although the body of literature examining cannabis use and anesthesia is expanding, evidence-based perioperative management guidelines remain in early stages of development. Anesthesia providers must therefore rely on a growing evidence base to guide clinical decision-making for patients using cannabis. This chapter examines historical and contemporary patterns of cannabis use, routes of administration, physiologic effects relevant to anesthesia, and the implications for perioperative assessment and anesthetic management.

DOI: 10.4018/979-8-2600-2035-7.ch005

INTRODUCTION

Historical Context of Cannabis Use in Medicine and Society

Cannabis is among the oldest cultivated plants in human history, with documented use spanning thousands of years across diverse geographic regions and cultural traditions. Archaeological and historical evidence suggests that cannabis cultivation originated as early as 4,000 BCE in ancient China, where the plant was initially valued for its industrial utility rather than its psychoactive or medicinal properties. Early Chinese societies used cannabis fibers extensively for textile production, rope making, and paper manufacturing, underscoring its economic and practical importance long before its therapeutic applications were widely recognized (Wishart et al., 2024). In addition to its industrial role, cannabis seeds were incorporated into dietary practices, providing a source of protein, essential fatty acids, and micronutrients. These nutritional uses reinforced the plant's value as a staple agricultural commodity, contributing to its widespread cultivation and dissemination along early trade routes. Even in contemporary settings, cannabis-derived oils and seeds continue to be used for nutritional and culinary purposes in various regions of the world, reflecting continuity between ancient and modern applications.

Beyond these early industrial and nutritional applications, cannabis gradually emerged as a medicinal agent in several ancient civilizations. In traditional Chinese medicine, early pharmacopeias documented the use of cannabis preparations to manage pain, gastrointestinal disorders such as constipation, infectious conditions including malaria, and gynecologic ailments (Zuardi, 2006). These early medical texts reflect an empirical understanding of cannabis as a therapeutic substance with broad physiological effects, even in the absence of modern pharmacologic frameworks or molecular explanations. Cannabis-based remedies were often administered in combination with other botanical agents, suggesting an early appreciation for synergistic effects within herbal medicine. Such practices laid the conceptual groundwork for later polypharmacy approaches in medicine, wherein multiple agents are used to target different symptoms or physiologic pathways.

Similarly, in ancient India, cannabis held a prominent role in both medical and religious traditions. Early Hindu texts and Ayurvedic writings described cannabis as a substance capable of alleviating suffering, improving appetite, reducing anxiety, and enhancing spiritual awareness. Often referred to as a "donator of joy," cannabis was believed to possess both healing and transcendental properties (Touw, 1981). Preparations such as bhang (a beverage made from cannabis leaves), ganja (dried flowering tops), and charas (resin) were consumed for medicinal, ritualistic, and recreational purposes. This culturally integrated approach to cannabis use blurred distinctions between therapeutic, spiritual, and social domains, illustrating how perceptions of cannabis were shaped by broader belief systems rather than narrowly defined medical indications. Such integration also contributed to normalization of use within these societies, a factor that contrasts sharply with later Western prohibitionist frameworks.

Cannabis also appeared in the medical traditions of the Middle East, Africa, and the Greco-Roman world. In ancient Egypt, cannabis was reportedly used in topical preparations for inflammation and ocular conditions. African cultures employed cannabis for analgesia, childbirth-related pain, and appetite stimulation. In the Greco-Roman tradition, physicians such as Dioscorides and Galen described cannabis seed preparations for their purported analgesic, anti-inflammatory, and antiemetic properties (Zuardi, 2006). Galen, in particular, noted the psychoactive effects of cannabis when consumed in excess, indicating early recognition of dose-dependent outcomes. In medieval Islamic medicine, cannabis extracts were employed for their sedative, anxiolytic, and anticonvulsant properties, despite religious debates surrounding intoxicating substances. These historical accounts collectively demonstrate that cannabis has long been recognized as a biologically active substance with diverse applications across civilizations, often occupying a complex position at the intersection of medicine, culture, and morality.

The transition of cannabis into Western medicine accelerated during the nineteenth century, particularly following British colonial exposure to Indian cannabis practices. Physicians and colonial administrators observed the widespread use of cannabis in South Asia and began to document its effects systematically. Cannabis tinctures and extracts subsequently entered European and North American pharmacopeias, where they were prescribed for conditions such as migraines, neuropathic pain, muscle spasms, insomnia, and menstrual disorders. During this period, cannabis was considered a legitimate therapeutic agent, comparable to other botanical medicines such as opium and digitalis (Zuardi, 2006). However, variability in plant potency, lack of standardized dosing, and the emergence of synthetic pharmaceuticals contributed to inconsistent clinical outcomes.

The early twentieth century marked a significant shift in the perception and regulation of cannabis. A convergence of sociopolitical forces, including concerns about recreational misuse, racialized narratives, and international drug control treaties, led to the gradual prohibition of cannabis in many countries. In the United States, the Marihuana Tax Act of 1937 effectively criminalized cannabis, and subsequent legislation classified it as a Schedule I substance, defined as having high abuse potential and no accepted medical use. This classification imposed substantial barriers to scientific research, resulting in a prolonged gap in rigorous clinical investigation (Zuardi, 2006). The stigmatization of cannabis during this era profoundly influenced medical education, public policy, and societal attitudes, effects that persist to varying degrees in contemporary discourse.

Despite these historical fluctuations, cannabis has reemerged in modern medical and societal discussions. Renewed interest in its therapeutic potential has been driven by patient advocacy, evolving scientific evidence, and shifting sociocultural attitudes toward substance use. Advances in molecular biology and neuroscience led to the discovery of the endocannabinoid system in the late twentieth century, providing a mechanistic framework for understanding the physiologic effects of cannabinoids. This discovery catalyzed a resurgence of research into cannabis and its constituents, including delta-9-tetrahydrocannabinol (THC), cannabidiol (CBD), and numerous minor cannabinoids. The reappraisal of cannabis within healthcare has profound implications for contemporary clinical practice, particularly in perioperative and anesthesia settings where cannabis use may influence physiologic responses, anesthetic requirements, and postoperative outcomes.

Legalization Trends and Implications for Perioperative Care

Over the past several decades, legalization trends in the United States have fundamentally altered the landscape of cannabis use. Beginning in the latter half of the twentieth century, public attitudes toward cannabis shifted as perceptions of harm diminished and comparisons to legal substances such as alcohol and tobacco became more common. Media portrayals increasingly framed cannabis as a relatively benign recreational substance, contributing to growing public support for decriminalization and legalization initiatives (Chiu et al., 2022). Concurrently, medical professionals and advocacy groups argued for cannabis access for patients with chronic pain, chemotherapy-induced nausea and vomiting, epilepsy, and other conditions resistant to conventional therapies. These arguments emphasized patient autonomy, harm reduction, and the limitations of existing pharmacologic options.

These evolving attitudes translated into legislative change. Early medical marijuana laws enacted in the 1990s represented incremental steps toward broader reform. Over time, these policies expanded in scope, culminating in widespread legalization of both medical and recreational cannabis at the state level. In 2012, Colorado and Washington became the first U.S. state to legalize recreational cannabis. Vermont did also legalize marijuana within a few short years later through legislative action rather than voter referendum, signaling increasing political acceptance of cannabis (Zvonarev et al., 2019). Currently, numerous states and the District of Columbia permit medical and/or recreational cannabis use. Although federal prohibition remains in place, the divergence between state and federal law has created a complex regulatory environment that shapes access, distribution, and research.

The motivations underlying legalization efforts are multifaceted. Proponents frequently cite economic benefits, including tax revenue generation, job creation, and reduced costs associated with cannabis-related arrests and incarceration. Others argue that legalization allows for regulation of product potency, quality control, and labeling, thereby improving public health oversight and consumer safety. Additional arguments include the potential for reducing illicit market activity and reallocating law enforcement resources toward more serious public safety concerns (Zvonarev et al., 2019). Regardless of the rationale, legalization has resulted in unprecedented access to cannabis products with increasingly diverse formulations and higher concentrations of THC than were historically available.

For anesthesia providers, these trends carry significant clinical implications. The normalization of cannabis use means that a growing proportion of surgical patients may present with acute or chronic exposure to cannabis. Patterns of use vary widely based on regional legislation, availability of dispensaries, cultural norms, and socioeconomic factors, creating substantial heterogeneity in patient populations. Legalization has also driven rapid innovation in cannabis delivery systems, including smoking, vaping, edibles, tinctures, transdermal preparations, and high-potency concentrates. Each of these modalities exhibits distinct pharmacokinetic and pharmacodynamic profiles, complicating perioperative assessment and management.

Understanding both national and regional legalization frameworks is therefore essential for perioperative clinicians. Legal status influences patient disclosure, frequency of use, and perceived safety, all of which affect preoperative evaluation. Patients may underestimate the relevance of cannabis use to anesthesia care or may not disclose use unless specifically prompted. In some cases, patients may fear judgment or legal consequences, particularly in jurisdictions where cannabis remains restricted. As a result, anesthesia providers must adopt a nonjudgmental, systematic approach to cannabis screening, integrating it into routine preoperative assessments alongside alcohol, tobacco, and prescription medication use. Key assessment elements include frequency of use, route of administration, timing of last exposure, product potency, and concomitant substance use. These factors directly inform anesthetic planning, risk stratification, and patient counseling.

Patterns of Cannabis Use

Modern patterns of cannabis use are characterized by increasing prevalence, diversification of products, and frequent co-use with other psychoactive substances. Epidemiologic data consistently demonstrate that cannabis is rarely used in isolation. Instead, it is commonly consumed in conjunction with alcohol, opioids, benzodiazepines, stimulants, and other substances. This pattern of polysubstance use presents significant challenges for perioperative management, as these agents may interact synergistically with anesthetic drugs and alter physiologic responses to surgery and anesthesia.

Among young adults aged 18 to 25 years, cannabis use is particularly prevalent. Carlini and Schauer (2022) reported that cannabis-only use accounts for approximately 2.0% of individuals in this age group, whereas cannabis use combined with other substances reaches 20.2%, representing the highest prevalence of polysubstance use across all age cohorts. Among adults overall, approximately 9% report cannabis use in combination with other substances, compared with only 0.9% reporting cannabis-only use. These findings underscore the relative rarity of isolated cannabis exposure and highlight the importance of comprehensive substance use assessment in the perioperative setting.

Gender differences further complicate these patterns. Males are more likely than females to report both cannabis-only use and polysubstance use, whereas females are more likely to report cannabis use in conjunction with prescription medications, including anxiolytics and antidepressants. Socioeconomic factors, mental health conditions, and chronic pain diagnoses also influence patterns of cannabis consumption, contributing to heterogeneity in patient presentations (Carlini & Schauer, 2022). These demographic trends intersect with surgical populations in meaningful ways, particularly in orthopedic, trauma, ambulatory, and pain-related procedures.

From an anesthesia perspective, polysubstance use involving cannabis has critical implications. Concurrent use of cannabis with alcohol, opioids, or benzodiazepines may potentiate central nervous system depression, impair airway reflexes, and increase the risk of perioperative respiratory compromise (Carlini & Schauer, 2022). Chronic cannabis use has been associated with pharmacologic tolerance, which may increase anesthetic and analgesic requirements, whereas acute use may exacerbate sympathetic stimulation, anxiety, or dysphoria. Additionally, withdrawal symptoms in chronic users, such as irritability, insomnia, and nausea, may complicate postoperative recovery and pain management.

Given these complexities, anesthesia providers must evaluate cannabis use within the broader context of substance use behaviors rather than as an isolated exposure. Detailed preoperative screening enables risk stratification, anticipatory planning, and individualized anesthetic management. As cannabis use continues to rise in parallel with legalization and commercialization, its relevance to perioperative care will only intensify, necessitating ongoing education and evidence-based practice among anesthesiologists and nurse anesthesiologists alike.

FORMS OF CANNABIS AND ROUTES OF ADMINISTRATION

The diversity of cannabis products available today necessitates a nuanced understanding of routes of administration and their physiologic implications. Cannabis can be consumed through multiple forms, each exhibiting distinct pharmacokinetic and pharmacodynamic profiles that influence anesthetic management. Leal and Moscrop-Blake (2024) identified eight primary methods of cannabis use: smoking, vaping, eating or drinking, dabbing, drops or lozenges, topical application, oral pills, and other less common routes such as rectal administration or inhalation via specialized devices. The pharmacokinetic distinctions among these routes are clinically significant, as they affect onset of action, peak plasma concentration, bioavailability, and duration of effect.

Inhalation

Inhaled routes, including both smoking and vaping, result in rapid absorption of cannabinoids into the systemic circulation via the alveolar-capillary interface. Peak plasma concentrations of THC are typically achieved within minutes, producing acute psychoactive and physiologic effects. Bioavailability varies widely, often ranging from 10% to 35%, depending on inhalation technique, depth, and product potency (Leal & Moscrop-Blake, 2024). These rapid-onset effects pose challenges for anesthesia providers, particularly when patients present with recent use or acute intoxication. Clinical manifestations may include tachycardia, anxiety, impaired judgment, and altered pain perception, all of which can complicate induction, airway management, and hemodynamic control.

Smoking cannabis also introduces combustion byproducts, including carbon monoxide, tar, and particulate matter, which contribute to airway irritation and systemic hypoxemia. Vaping, while often perceived as a safer alternative, involves aerosolization of concentrated cannabinoid liquids and additives that may carry their own risks. The variability in devices, temperatures, and formulations further complicates risk assessment, as patients may be unable to accurately describe product composition or exposure levels (Leal & Moscrop-Blake, 2024).

Oral Ingestion

Oral ingestion, encompassing edibles, beverages, and capsules, results in slower and more variable absorption due to first-pass hepatic metabolism. Peak plasma concentrations are typically delayed for one to three hours post-consumption, and bioavailability is lower, generally between 4% and 12% (Leal & Moscrop-Blake, 2024). The hepatic conversion of THC to the active metabolite 11-hydroxy-THC contributes to prolonged and sometimes unpredictable psychoactive effects. These delayed effects can extend into the postoperative period, influencing recovery times, sedation levels, and analgesic requirements. Patients may inadvertently consume excessive doses due to delayed onset, increasing the risk of perioperative complications.

Dabbing and Concentrates

Dabbing involves vaporizing highly concentrated cannabis extracts, which may contain 70% to 90% THC. This method delivers large quantities of cannabinoids rapidly, producing intense psychoactive and physiologic effects. Acute cardiovascular responses, including marked tachycardia and hypertension, have been reported, as well as neurologic symptoms such as agitation and altered consciousness (Inman & Cservenka, 2026). From an anesthetic perspective, these effects necessitate careful preoperative screening and may warrant postponement of elective procedures if recent use is suspected.

Topical and Transdermal Routes

Topical creams, ointments, and transdermal patches are generally associated with localized effects and minimal systemic absorption. However, the pharmacologic activity of cannabinoids, particularly CBD, may still influence hepatic enzyme systems involved in drug metabolism. Transdermal preparations provide slow, sustained absorption, which may contribute to baseline cannabinoid levels in chronic users (Inman & Cservenka, 2026). These effects, while subtle, may influence perioperative analgesia and interact with anesthetic agents.

Other Routes

Less common routes of administration include sublingual drops, lozenges, and rectal suppositories. Sublingual administration partially bypasses first-pass metabolism, resulting in more rapid onset than oral ingestion but less predictability than inhalation. Rectal absorption remains inconsistent and poorly studied but may be relevant in patients with gastrointestinal limitations. The unpredictability associated with these routes further underscores the importance of detailed preoperative assessment.

CANNABIS AND ITS EFFECTS ON DIFFERENT BODY SYSTEMS

Cannabis exerts systemic effects that are highly dependent on dose, chronicity of use, and route of administration. These effects span multiple organ systems, including pulmonary, cardiovascular, neurologic, gastrointestinal, and hepatic systems, all of which have direct relevance to anesthetic care.

Pulmonary Effects

Inhaled cannabis use through smoking or vaping has distinct pulmonary consequences. Acute inhalation has been associated with transient bronchodilation lasting one to two hours, mediated by β-adrenergic stimulation and smooth muscle relaxation. Despite this transient effect, chronic inhalation leads to airway irritation, increased sputum production, cough, and wheezing, contributing to airway hyperreactivity (Dahan et al., 2024). For anesthetized patients, hyperreactivity increases the risk of bronchospasm, laryngospasm, and difficulty with airway instrumentation.

Structural airway changes associated with chronic inhalation include bronchial epithelial inflammation and increased mucus secretion, which can complicate intubation and postoperative pulmonary care. Co-use of cannabis and tobacco further exacerbates these risks. Oster et al. (2023) reported higher rates of postoperative wound infections, pulmonary complications, and delayed healing in patients who used both substances compared with non-users or single-substance users. These findings highlight the importance of integrated screening and perioperative optimization.

Vaping-associated lung injury has emerged as a significant concern. E-cigarette or vaping use–associated lung injury (EVALI) presents with hypoxemia, impaired gas exchange, and radiographic abnormalities. THC has been detected in a majority of EVALI cases, implicating cannabis vaping products in disease pathogenesis (Khoj et al., 2024). Patients with a history of vaping-related lung injury pose substantial anesthetic challenges due to reduced pulmonary reserve and unpredictable airway responses.

Cardiovascular Effects

Cannabis exerts complex, dose-dependent effects on the cardiovascular system. Acute, low-dose use typically results in sympathetic stimulation, manifesting as tachycardia, hypertension, and increased cardiac output. These effects can complicate anesthetic induction and increase myocardial oxygen demand, particularly in patients with underlying cardiovascular disease. In contrast, high-dose or chronic use may shift autonomic balance toward parasympathetic predominance, resulting in bradycardia and hypotension.

Cannabis use has been associated with a range of cardiac dysrhythmias, including atrial fibrillation, supraventricular tachycardia, and ventricular arrhythmias. Acute use may precipitate coronary vasospasm, further increasing the risk of myocardial ischemia. Epidemiologic studies suggest a markedly increased risk of myocardial infarction within the first hour following cannabis consumption, particularly in younger adults without traditional cardiovascular risk factors (Lee et al., 2024; Ladha et al., 2021). These findings underscore the need for vigilant perioperative monitoring and risk assessment.

For anesthesia providers, the cardiovascular effects of cannabis necessitate careful consideration of anesthetic technique, agent selection, and intraoperative monitoring. Strategies may include avoidance of excessive sympathetic stimulation, readiness to manage dysrhythmias, and individualized approaches to fluid and vasoactive therapy. In select cases, regional anesthesia may offer advantages by minimizing hemodynamic stress, although potential interactions with systemic cannabinoids must still be considered.

Neurological Effects

Cannabis use has significant neurologic implications that are directly relevant to anesthesia practice and the safe delivery of anesthetic care. The majority of these effects are mediated through cannabinoid type 1 (CB1) receptors, which are densely distributed throughout the cerebral cortex, hippocampus, basal ganglia, cerebellum, and midbrain. CB1 receptors are G-protein–coupled receptors that inhibit adenylate cyclase activity and modulate intracellular calcium and potassium channels, ultimately reducing presynaptic neurotransmitter release. Through these mechanisms, activation of CB1 receptors alters the release of gamma-aminobutyric acid (GABA), glutamate, dopamine, serotonin, and norepinephrine, resulting in widespread effects on cortical processing, perception, mood, and arousal (Zuardi, 2006; Lee et al., 2024).

Clinically, these neurochemical changes manifest as alterations in consciousness, attention, working memory, executive function, and sensorimotor integration. From an anesthetic perspective, these alterations may influence preoperative assessment, patient cooperation, informed consent, and baseline neurologic status, particularly when cannabis has been used acutely or in high doses. Acute intoxication may impair the patient's ability to accurately report symptoms, comprehend perioperative risks, or provide valid informed consent. Furthermore, altered perception of time, dissociation, and impaired short-term memory can complicate communication and cooperation during regional anesthesia procedures or monitored anesthesia care.

Cannabis is frequently selected by users for its desired psychoactive effects, including euphoria, relaxation, sedation, and anxiolysis. These effects may superficially resemble those produced by commonly used anesthetic and sedative agents, such as benzodiazepines, propofol, and volatile anesthetics. This perceived similarity has led some patients to assume that cannabis use may enhance or substitute for perioperative anxiolysis. However, cannabis is not a predictable sedative-hypnotic agent, and its neurologic effects vary substantially based on dose, route of administration, cannabinoid composition, and individual susceptibility.

Paradoxical neurologic responses are well described, particularly in cannabis-naïve or infrequent users. Instead of sedation or relaxation, these individuals may experience heightened anxiety, panic, paranoia, dysphoria, hallucinations, or depersonalization. Such effects are believed to arise from dysregulated CB1 receptor signaling within limbic and prefrontal cortical circuits, leading to exaggerated emotional responses and impaired top-down cognitive control. High-potency THC products and concentrates are especially associated with these adverse effects. In the perioperative environment, paradoxical responses can complicate anxiolysis, increase sympathetic activation, and heighten the risk of agitation during anesthetic induction or emergence. Agitation at emergence poses safety risks to both patients and staff, particularly in the presence of airway devices, intravenous lines, or surgical wounds.

Both acute and chronic cannabis use have been associated with measurable changes in central nervous system function, particularly in cognition, attention, psychomotor performance, and motor coordination (Lee et al., 2024). Acute intoxication impairs reaction time, divided attention, executive function, and visuospatial processing. These deficits are relevant not only intraoperatively but also during postoperative recovery, when patients are expected to follow instructions, ambulate safely, and recognize complications. Chronic cannabis use has been linked to more persistent alterations in cognitive processing, including deficits in attention and memory, although the extent to which these changes are reversible remains an area of ongoing investigation.

Tolerance is another important neurologic phenomenon associated with chronic cannabis use. Repeated exposure to THC leads to downregulation and desensitization of CB1 receptors, resulting in diminished psychoactive effects over time. From an anesthetic standpoint, tolerance may extend beyond cannabis itself, potentially altering responsiveness to other central nervous system depressants. Some studies suggest that chronic cannabis users may require higher doses of anesthetic agents to achieve comparable levels of hypnosis or sedation, although findings remain inconsistent. Nonetheless, anesthesiologists and nurse anesthesiologists should be aware of the potential for altered anesthetic requirements and delayed emergence in chronic users.

Cannabis use has also been implicated in postoperative neurologic complications, including delirium and postoperative cognitive dysfunction (POCD). Although direct causal relationships have not been definitively established, cannabis-related alterations in neurotransmitter balance, sleep architecture, and circadian rhythms may predispose vulnerable patients—particularly older adults—to delirium. Acute withdrawal in chronic users, characterized by irritability, insomnia, anxiety, and nausea, may further exacerbate postoperative neurologic instability. Careful postoperative monitoring and early recognition of withdrawal symptoms are therefore essential components of perioperative care in this population.

CANNABIS USE AND PAIN MODULATION

Cannabis use in pain modulation has been increasingly examined within the scientific literature, and this body of knowledge continues to expand as legalization and medical utilization become more widespread. Cannabinoids exert analgesic effects through multiple mechanisms, including modulation of nociceptive signaling at the spinal cord level, alteration of supraspinal pain perception, and interaction with inflammatory pathways. CB1 receptors located in the dorsal horn of the spinal cord inhibit nociceptive transmission, while CB2 receptors expressed on immune cells modulate inflammatory mediator release. These mechanisms provide a biologic rationale for the use of cannabinoids in chronic pain conditions.

Despite this mechanistic plausibility, the clinical literature examining the impact of preoperative cannabis exposure on postoperative pain outcomes remains equivocal. In a comprehensive narrative review, King et al. (2025) initially identified 2,983 articles examining the relationship between cannabinoid exposure and postoperative pain. Following rigorous screening and application of predefined inclusion criteria, only 42 studies were deemed suitable for final analysis. This attrition highlights significant limitations in study quality, heterogeneity, and methodological rigor within the existing literature.

Findings from this review demonstrated substantial variability across surgical populations, cannabis exposure patterns, and outcome measures. Orthopedic procedures, particularly spine surgery, were associated with the highest reported levels of postoperative pain among cannabis users when compared with non-users. Of the 42 studies included, 18 reported increased postoperative pain in patients with preoperative cannabis exposure, 17 found no statistically significant difference in pain outcomes, and only 3 reported decreased postoperative pain among cannabis users. These findings suggest that, while cannabis may provide analgesic benefit in certain chronic pain contexts, its role in the perioperative period is complex and may differ substantially from its role in non-surgical pain management.

One proposed explanation for increased postoperative pain among cannabis users is the phenomenon of cannabis-induced hyperalgesia. Analogous to opioid-induced hyperalgesia, chronic exposure to cannabinoids may paradoxically increase pain sensitivity through central sensitization mechanisms. Animal models suggest that prolonged CB1 receptor activation may alter nociceptive processing and diminish endogenous pain inhibitory pathways. However, clinical evidence supporting cannabis-induced hyperalgesia remains limited, and further prospective research is required to clarify this relationship.

In recognition of the growing prevalence of cannabis use among surgical patients, the American Society of Regional Anesthesia and Pain Medicine (ASRA) published consensus guidelines addressing the perioperative management of patients using cannabis and cannabinoid products (Shah et al., 2023). These guidelines synthesize available evidence and expert opinion to provide practical recommendations for perioperative clinicians. Chronic pain is identified as one of the most common indications for medical cannabis use, underscoring the frequent intersection between cannabis exposure and surgical care.

The ASRA consensus guidelines also examine the relationship between cannabis use and opioid consumption. Some observational studies suggest that, in chronic pain populations, cannabis use may be associated with reduced opioid requirements, potentially reflecting an opioid-sparing effect (Shah et al., 2023). However, in the postoperative setting, cannabis users have often been observed to require higher opioid doses to achieve adequate analgesia. This apparent contradiction may reflect differences between chronic baseline pain management and acute postoperative pain, as well as the influence of tolerance, hyperalgesia, and psychosocial factors. Importantly, the overall quality of evidence supporting both opioid-sparing and opioid-augmenting effects remains low, limiting the strength of clinical recommendations.

From an anesthetic perspective, these findings underscore the importance of individualized, multimodal pain management strategies. Routine assumptions regarding reduced opioid requirements in cannabis users are not supported by current evidence. Instead, clinicians should anticipate the possibility of increased analgesic needs and incorporate non-opioid adjuncts, regional anesthesia techniques, and careful postoperative monitoring to optimize pain control while minimizing adverse effects.

INTERACTIONS BETWEEN CANNABIS AND ANESTHETIC AGENTS

Cannabis and Pharmacology

When considering the interactions between anesthesia and cannabis, understanding the pharmacological properties of cannabis is essential. Cannabis contains multiple active compounds, most notably tetrahydrocannabinol (THC) and cannabidiol (CBD), which can influence the pharmacokinetics of various medications. CBD, in particular, has been shown to interact with the cytochrome P450 (CYP450) enzyme system, specifically CYP3A4. This enzyme is responsible for the metabolism of a wide range of anesthetic agents, analgesics, and sedatives commonly used perioperatively. As a result, cannabis use may alter the metabolism of these drugs, potentially leading to either increased drug levels and toxicity or reduced therapeutic efficacy, depending on the interaction and dosing (Lee et al., 2024).

In addition to its effects on drug metabolism, cannabis has been implicated in modulating ion channel function, particularly voltage-gated calcium channels. These channels play a critical role in neuronal excitability, neurotransmitter release, and synaptic signaling, which are important processes during anesthesia. Inhibition of these channels by cannabinoids may influence anesthetic depth, neuromuscular blockade, and analgesic requirements. For example, altered calcium channel function could potentially modify responses to volatile anesthetics, intravenous sedatives, or opioid analgesics, making anesthetic management more challenging in cannabis users (Lee et al., 2024).

Furthermore, the complexity of cannabis interactions extends beyond pharmacokinetics and ion channel modulation. Chronic cannabis use may induce adaptive physiological changes, such as upregulation or downregulation of cannabinoid receptors, alterations in cardiovascular response, and modifications in pain perception. These adaptations may impact anesthetic planning, particularly in terms of hemodynamic stability, analgesic dosing, and postoperative recovery. Understanding both the acute and chronic effects of cannabis is therefore critical for nurse anesthesiologists, as individualized anesthetic management may be required to ensure patient safety and optimal perioperative outcomes.

Volatile Anesthetics

Cannabis' effect on volatile anesthetic agents can be examined through multiple pharmacologic, physiologic, and clinical lenses. With the increasing prevalence of cannabis use across diverse age groups in the United States, it is imperative that the nurse anesthesiologist remains vigilant when caring for patients who use cannabis in the perioperative period. Cannabis is not a benign substance in the context of anesthesia; rather, it can significantly influence anesthetic requirements, patient responses to anesthetic agents, and perioperative safety. While a growing body of literature has examined cannabis interactions with intravenous anesthetic agents through known metabolic pathways, the interaction between cannabis and volatile anesthetics warrants focused consideration, as these agents are influenced by distinct mechanisms unrelated to hepatic metabolism.

Volatile anesthetics such as sevoflurane, isoflurane, and desflurane exert their effects primarily through modulation of central nervous system activity, including gamma-aminobutyric acid (GABA) receptors, potassium channels, and other neuronal membrane targets. Unlike intravenous agents that rely heavily on hepatic metabolism via cytochrome P450 pathways, volatile anesthetics are largely eliminated through pulmonary exhalation (Lee et al., 2024). As such, cannabis-related alterations in anesthetic response to volatile agents are unlikely to be explained solely by metabolic interactions. Instead, the relationship may reflect cannabis-induced changes in central nervous system tolerance, receptor modulation, pulmonary physiology, or chronic neuroadaptation from repeated cannabinoid exposure.

The respiratory effects of cannabis are particularly relevant when discussing volatile anesthesia. Cannabis inhalation has been associated with airway inflammation, increased mucus production, cough, and bronchial hyperreactivity, especially in chronic users. These changes can influence anesthetic uptake, distribution, and elimination of inhaled agents. Volatile anesthetics depend on alveolar ventilation and effective gas exchange to achieve and maintain anesthetic depth. Any alteration in pulmonary mechanics—such as airway resistance or ventilation–perfusion mismatch—may impact anesthetic delivery and complicate titration. Consequently, cannabis use introduces an additional variable that must be considered when administering volatile anesthetics.

Beyond pulmonary considerations, cannabis may influence anesthetic requirements through its effects on neurophysiology. Chronic exposure to cannabinoids, particularly tetrahydrocannabinol (THC), can lead to receptor desensitization and downregulation of cannabinoid type 1 (CB1) receptors in the central nervous system. These adaptive changes may produce cross-tolerance to other centrally acting agents, including volatile anesthetics (Lee et al., 2024). This hypothesis has gained traction in the anesthesia literature, as several studies have suggested that cannabis users may require higher doses of anesthetic agents to achieve equivalent hypnotic effects.

Davidson, Raz, and Eyal (2020) were among the early authors to highlight the potential for increased volatile anesthetic requirements in cannabis users. Their review described how chronic cannabis exposure may alter anesthetic sensitivity, resulting in a higher minimum alveolar concentration (MAC) requirement to maintain adequate anesthesia. MAC is a standardized measure of anesthetic potency, defined as the alveolar concentration of an inhaled anesthetic that prevents movement in response to surgical stimulus in 50% of patients. An increase in MAC implies a need for higher anesthetic concentrations to achieve the same depth of anesthesia, which carries important implications for anesthetic planning and intraoperative management.

The findings reported by Davidson et al. (2020) suggested that cannabis users may demonstrate increased anesthetic tolerance, though much of the early literature relied on observational data or extrapolations from pharmacologic principles. Nevertheless, their work underscored the importance of individualized anesthetic care and raised awareness among anesthesia providers regarding the potential for altered anesthetic requirements in this growing patient population.

More robust evidence supporting increased volatile anesthetic requirements in cannabis users emerged in subsequent studies, including the work of Sajdeya et al. (2024). This propensity-matched retrospective cohort study focused specifically on older adults, a population already known to exhibit altered anesthetic pharmacodynamics due to age-related physiologic changes. By narrowing the study population to adults aged 65 years and older, Sajdeya et al. (2024) addressed an important gap in the literature, as older patients may be particularly vulnerable to both under- and over-anesthetization.

In their study, Sajdeya et al. (2024) examined minimal alveolar concentration requirements for isoflurane and sevoflurane at one-minute intervals during general anesthesia. Cannabis use was defined within a 60-day window prior to surgery, allowing the researchers to capture relatively recent exposure while minimizing recall bias. The use of a propensity-matched design strengthened the validity of the findings by reducing confounding variables such as comorbid conditions, surgical type, and baseline demographic differences between cannabis users and non-users.

One of the notable findings of the study was that cannabis users required significantly higher MAC levels of volatile anesthetics compared to non-cannabis users within the same age group. This finding aligns with earlier observations described by Davidson et al. (2020) and provides stronger empirical support for the concept of increased anesthetic tolerance in cannabis users. Importantly, the increased MAC requirements were observed despite the advanced age of the population, which typically correlates with decreased anesthetic needs due to reduced central nervous system sensitivity. The fact that cannabis users still demonstrated higher anesthetic requirements suggests that the effects of cannabis may counteract age-related reductions in anesthetic dose requirements.

An interesting ad hoc finding reported by Sajdeya et al. (2024) was the lack of a significant difference in bispectral index (BIS) scores between cannabis users and non-users. BIS monitoring is commonly used to assess hypnotic depth during general anesthesia by analyzing electroencephalographic activity. The absence of BIS differences despite increased MAC requirements raises important clinical considerations. It suggests that while cannabis users may require higher concentrations of volatile anesthetics to suppress motor response, the cortical hypnotic effect—as measured by BIS—may not differ substantially between groups. This discrepancy highlights the complexity of anesthetic depth and reinforces the need for multimodal monitoring rather than reliance on a single parameter.

From a clinical perspective, these findings emphasize the importance of vigilant anesthetic titration in cannabis users, particularly older adults. Nurse anesthesiologists must be prepared for the possibility that standard age-adjusted MAC values may underestimate anesthetic requirements in this population. Failure to recognize increased anesthetic needs could result in intraoperative awareness, patient movement, or sympathetic responses to surgical stimuli. Conversely, aggressive dosing without careful monitoring may increase the risk of hemodynamic instability, delayed emergence, or postoperative cognitive dysfunction, especially in older patients.

The implications of increased volatile anesthetic requirements extend beyond the intraoperative period. Higher anesthetic concentrations may contribute to prolonged recovery times, increased postoperative nausea and vomiting, and greater exposure to anesthetic-related side effects. Additionally, older adults are at increased risk for postoperative delirium and cognitive impairment, and the relationship between anesthetic depth, cannabis use, and neurocognitive outcomes remains an area requiring further investigation.

Taken together, the literature supports the conclusion that cannabis use is associated with increased volatile anesthetic requirements, particularly in older adults. The findings reported by Davidson et al. (2020) and Sajdeya et al. (2024) collectively reinforce the need for individualized anesthetic management and heightened vigilance when caring for cannabis-using patients. These studies also underscore the importance of thorough preoperative assessment, including explicit inquiry about cannabis use, frequency, and timing of last exposure.

As cannabis legalization continues to expand and usage rates rise, anesthesia providers must remain informed about its perioperative implications. Ongoing research is needed to further elucidate the mechanisms underlying increased anesthetic requirements, differentiate the effects of acute versus chronic cannabis use, and establish evidence-based guidelines for anesthetic management. Until such guidelines are available, nurse anesthesiologists should approach cannabis-using patients with careful assessment, dynamic anesthetic titration, and comprehensive monitoring to ensure patient safety and optimal outcomes.

Intravenous Anesthetics

Intravenous anesthetic agents may present a significant clinical challenge in patients who use cannabis, largely due to the complex pharmacokinetic and pharmacodynamic interactions associated with cannabinoid exposure. A primary mechanism underlying these interactions is cannabis' effect on hepatic metabolism, particularly its influence on the cytochrome P450 (CYP450) enzyme system. Cannabinoids, most notably cannabidiol (CBD) and tetrahydrocannabinol (THC), have been shown to modulate several CYP450 isoenzymes, including CYP3A4, CYP2C9, and CYP2C19 (Lee et al., 2024). Many intravenous medications routinely used in anesthesia practice rely on these metabolic pathways for clearance. Alterations in enzyme activity caused by cannabis use can therefore result in unpredictable drug concentrations, delayed metabolism, or altered duration of action, complicating anesthetic management and increasing the risk of adverse events.

In addition to anesthetic agents themselves, patients presenting for anesthesia often take medications for coexisting medical conditions that are also metabolized through CYP450 pathways. These may include anticoagulants, antidepressants, antiepileptic medications, beta-blockers, and opioids. Cannabis-induced modulation of hepatic metabolism may therefore create a cascade of drug–drug interactions that extend beyond anesthesia induction and maintenance. For the nurse anesthesiologist, this necessitates a comprehensive preoperative medication review and heightened awareness of how cannabis use may alter both anesthetic requirements and responses to adjunctive medications administered perioperatively.

Among intravenous anesthetic agents, propofol remains the most commonly used medication for induction of general anesthesia and for procedural sedation. Propofol is favored for its rapid onset, short duration of action, and favorable recovery profile. It is widely used in operating rooms, procedural suites, endoscopy centers, and intensive care units worldwide. Propofol produces unconsciousness primarily through potentiation of gamma-aminobutyric acid (GABA)–mediated inhibitory neurotransmission within the central nervous system. Although propofol undergoes hepatic metabolism, its clinical effects are also influenced by redistribution kinetics and central nervous system sensitivity, making it particularly susceptible to variability in patients with altered neurophysiology, including those who use cannabis.

The relationship between cannabis use and propofol dosing has been increasingly examined in the literature. Bornemann-Cimenti et al. (2025) conducted a systematic review and meta-analysis to evaluate propofol dosing requirements in cannabis users compared to non-cannabis users. This study represents one of the most comprehensive evaluations of the topic to date. The authors analyzed available data across multiple clinical settings, including surgical and procedural sedation environments, and found a statistically significant increase in propofol requirements among cannabis users. These findings support the growing body of evidence suggesting that chronic cannabis exposure may induce a degree of anesthetic tolerance, necessitating higher doses to achieve equivalent levels of sedation or unconsciousness.

Despite the statistical significance of these findings, Bornemann-Cimenti et al. (2025) also emphasized that the magnitude of increased propofol requirements may be modest and not always clinically meaningful. This distinction is important for anesthesia providers, as it underscores the need to balance statistical outcomes with real-world clinical relevance. While nurse anesthesiologists should anticipate the possibility of increased propofol dosing in cannabis users, the findings suggest that dramatic dose escalations may not be universally required. Instead, careful titration guided by patient response and physiologic monitoring remains the cornerstone of safe anesthetic care.

The clinical implications of this meta-analysis are particularly relevant for certified registered nurse anesthetists (CRNAs), who frequently manage anesthetics across a wide range of patient populations and procedural settings. Awareness of the potential for increased propofol requirements allows the CRNA to anticipate dosing needs, avoid under-sedation, and reduce the risk of patient movement or awareness during procedures. At the same time, recognition that the increased requirements may be relatively small helps prevent unnecessary over-administration, which could increase the risk of hypotension, respiratory depression, or delayed recovery.

Additional insight into the interaction between cannabis use and propofol has been provided by Imasogie et al. (2021), who conducted a study focusing specifically on patients undergoing endoscopic procedures. This investigation evaluated propofol requirements during colonoscopies and esophagogastroduodenoscopies (EGD) in cannabis users and non-cannabis users. The endoscopy setting offers a unique context for examining anesthetic requirements, as sedation must balance patient comfort with preservation of spontaneous ventilation and airway reflexes.

Imasogie et al. (2021) found that cannabis users required significantly higher doses of propofol to achieve adequate sedation compared to non-cannabis users. These findings are consistent with those reported in broader anesthetic contexts and further reinforce the association between cannabis use and increased propofol requirements. However, the study also identified additional clinically relevant observations. Notably, three patients in the cannabis-exposed group required supplemental oxygenation via bag-valve-mask ventilation during the procedure, suggesting an increased incidence of respiratory compromise in this population.

The authors explored several potential explanations for these findings. One important consideration was the age disparity between the two groups studied. Cannabis users in the study had a significantly lower mean age (43.76 years) compared to non-cannabis users (53.8 years). Younger patients often require higher doses of propofol due to increased metabolic activity and central nervous system responsiveness. Therefore, some portion of the increased propofol requirement observed in cannabis users may be attributable to age rather than cannabis use alone. This highlights the importance of controlling for demographic variables when interpreting anesthetic dosing studies (Imasogie et al., 2021).

Another factor that may contribute to increased propofol requirements and respiratory events in cannabis users is airway reactivity. Chronic cannabis smoking has been associated with airway inflammation, increased secretions, and bronchial hyperresponsiveness. These changes may predispose patients to coughing, laryngospasm, or hypoventilation during sedation, prompting the need for deeper anesthetic planes to suppress airway reflexes. In the endoscopy setting, where airway instrumentation is minimal and patient positioning may compromise ventilation, these effects can be particularly pronounced.

While the study by Imasogie et al. (2021) provides valuable insights, it also illustrates the complexity of interpreting anesthetic requirements in cannabis users. Multiple variables including age, route of cannabis administration, frequency of use, airway physiology, and procedural factors—may influence anesthetic dosing. As such, the findings reinforce the need for individualized anesthetic care rather than reliance on standardized dosing algorithms.

Beyond propofol, other intravenous anesthetic agents may also be affected by cannabis use. Ketamine, in particular, warrants careful consideration due to its unique pharmacologic profile. Ketamine is a dissociative anesthetic that produces analgesia, amnesia, and sedation primarily through antagonism of N-methyl-D-aspartate (NMDA) receptors. It also stimulates the sympathetic nervous system and has well-documented psychomimetic effects, including hallucinations and dissociation.

Interestingly, ketamine has been shown to induce the release of endogenous cannabinoids, which may partially mediate its analgesic and psychoactive effects. In patients who use cannabis, this interaction may be amplified, leading to exaggerated psychomotor and perceptual effects when ketamine is administered. Lee et al. (2024) note that concomitant use of cannabis and ketamine may result in increased psychomotor agitation, altered perception, and prolonged recovery times.

For the nurse anesthesiologist, these interactions necessitate cautious use of ketamine in patients with known cannabis use. While ketamine may still be an appropriate choice in certain clinical scenarios, such as in hemodynamically unstable patients or those requiring analgesia without respiratory depression, close monitoring for adverse psychomotor effects is essential. Adjunctive medications, such as benzodiazepines, may be considered to mitigate emergence reactions, though these agents introduce additional considerations related to respiratory depression and delayed recovery.

The cumulative evidence regarding intravenous anesthetic agents and cannabis use underscores the importance of vigilant perioperative management. Cannabis use introduces variability into anesthetic care that may not be immediately apparent through standard preoperative assessment. As legalization and social acceptance of cannabis continue to expand, anesthesia providers are increasingly likely to encounter patients with both acute and chronic exposure. Clear communication, thorough history-taking, and nonjudgmental inquiry about cannabis use are critical components of preoperative evaluation.

In clinical practice, the nurse anesthesiologist must rely on continuous physiologic monitoring to guide anesthetic delivery in cannabis users. Rather than assuming fixed dose requirements, anesthetic agents should be titrated carefully to effect, with attention to hemodynamics, respiratory status, and depth of anesthesia. The use of processed electroencephalographic monitors, when appropriate, may provide additional insight into hypnotic depth, though these tools should be interpreted in conjunction with clinical signs.

In conclusion, intravenous anesthetic agents, particularly propofol and ketamine, present unique challenges in patients who use cannabis. The existing literature suggests that cannabis users may require higher doses of propofol, though the clinical significance of this increase varies depending on patient characteristics and procedural context. Ketamine use in cannabis users may be associated with enhanced psychomotor effects, necessitating cautious administration and close monitoring. Collectively, these findings highlight the need for individualized anesthetic care, informed by an understanding of cannabis pharmacology and its potential interactions. As research in this area continues to evolve, nurse anesthesiologists must remain adaptable, evidence-informed, and vigilant to ensure safe and effective anesthesia care for this growing patient population.

Opioids and Analgesics

Opioids and their interaction with cannabis have been examined more extensively than many other anesthetic adjuncts, largely due to the central role both substances play in pain modulation. Cannabinoids exert their analgesic effects primarily through cannabinoid type 1 (CB1) and type 2 (CB2) receptors, which are widely distributed throughout the central and peripheral nervous systems. These receptors are closely integrated with endogenous opioid pathways, suggesting a biologically plausible interaction between cannabis and opioid analgesia. King et al. (2025) describes how activation of CB1 receptors can influence μ-opioid receptor signaling, potentially altering nociceptive processing and modifying opioid efficacy. This shared neuroanatomical and molecular framework has prompted significant interest in whether cannabis use enhances, diminishes, or otherwise alters opioid analgesic requirements in the perioperative setting.

Despite this theoretical framework suggesting potential opioid-sparing effects of cannabinoids, clinical findings have been inconsistent. Some studies have reported increased opioid requirements among cannabis users, while others suggest no significant difference or even reduced opioid consumption. The variability in these findings likely reflects differences in study design, patient populations, patterns of cannabis use, and the timing of exposure relative to surgery. Lee et al. (2024) argue that chronic cannabis users may demonstrate increased opioid consumption postoperatively and experience greater difficulty achieving adequate pain control. This observation may be explained by cannabinoid-induced tolerance, central sensitization, or altered pain perception resulting from long-term cannabis exposure.

Further complicating interpretation is the heterogeneity of cannabis products and routes of administration. Smoked, vaporized, edible, and concentrated forms of cannabis produce distinct pharmacokinetic profiles, which may differentially affect pain pathways and opioid responsiveness. Additionally, the ratio of THC to cannabidiol (CBD) may influence analgesic outcomes, as THC is primarily responsible for psychoactive effects while CBD may modulate inflammation and nociception through non-opioid mechanisms. These factors contribute to the lack of consensus in the literature regarding whether cannabis use is associated with improved or worsened pain scores. As a result, the relationship between cannabis use and postoperative pain remains nebulous, with no definitive conclusions regarding analgesic efficacy or opioid-sparing potential.

Given the current state of evidence, it is imperative for the nurse anesthesiologist to maintain heightened vigilance when managing analgesia in patients who use cannabis. While the literature remains inconclusive regarding definitive changes in pain scores, multiple studies suggest that cannabis users may require increased opioid dosing and may present greater challenges in achieving effective analgesia (Lee et al., 2024). This underscores the importance of individualized pain management strategies, multimodal analgesia, and careful opioid titration in this population. By anticipating the potential for increased analgesic requirements and closely monitoring patient response, nurse anesthesiologists can optimize pain control while minimizing opioid-related adverse effects in the cannabis-using patient.

Drug–Drug Interactions

A fundamental responsibility of the nurse anesthesiologist is the comprehensive understanding of medication interactions involving anesthetic agents and patients' existing pharmacologic therapies. This responsibility is magnified in the context of cannabis use, given the growing prevalence of both medical and recreational cannabis consumption. Cannabis exerts clinically meaningful effects on drug metabolism pathways, most notably the cytochrome P450 (CYP450) enzyme system. Cannabinoids such as tetrahydrocannabinol (THC) and cannabidiol (CBD) have been shown to inhibit or induce several CYP450 isoenzymes, including CYP3A4, CYP2C9, and CYP2C19, which are responsible for the metabolism of many anesthetic and non-anesthetic medications (Lee et al., 2024; Lopera et al., 2022). As a result, cannabis use introduces a significant layer of complexity into perioperative pharmacologic management, necessitating heightened caution and clinical vigilance by the nurse anesthesiologist.

The scope of potential cannabis–drug interactions is broad and includes numerous medication classes commonly encountered in anesthesia practice. These include antidepressants, opioids, anticonvulsants, benzodiazepines, nonsteroidal anti-inflammatory drugs (NSAIDs), muscle relaxants, antiarrhythmics, beta blockers, antiplatelet agents, anticoagulants, and select antibiotics. Alterations in CYP450 activity can lead to subtherapeutic drug levels or, conversely, toxic accumulation depending on whether enzyme inhibition or induction predominates. Consequently, preoperative assessment should include detailed screening for cannabis use, including frequency, route of administration, and timing of last exposure. Intraoperatively and postoperatively, close monitoring for signs of inadequate therapeutic effect or drug toxicity is essential to ensure patient safety and optimize outcomes (Lopera et al., 2022).

Antiplatelet therapy represents a particularly important area of concern in cannabis-using patients. Clopidogrel, a prodrug requiring metabolic activation via CYP2C19, may be affected by cannabinoid-mediated enzyme inhibition. Shah et al. (2023) highlight the potential for reduced antiplatelet efficacy or altered bleeding risk when clopidogrel is used concomitantly with cannabis. In patients with known cannabis use, consideration may be given, when clinically appropriate, to alternative antiplatelet agents that do not rely on the same metabolic pathways. For the nurse anesthesiologist, this consideration is especially relevant during perioperative planning, where balancing thrombotic and hemorrhagic risks is critical.

Neuromuscular blocking agents also warrant careful consideration in cannabis users. Emerging evidence suggests that cannabis use may influence neuromuscular blockade through cannabinoid receptor type 1 (CB1) activation, which has been associated with increased acetylcholine release at the neuromuscular junction. This mechanism may result in shortened duration or reduced efficacy of non-depolarizing neuromuscular blocking agents. Although the clinical significance of this interaction is not yet fully defined, it underscores the importance of quantitative neuromuscular monitoring and individualized dosing strategies. Failure to recognize altered responses to neuromuscular blockers could result in inadequate paralysis during surgery or residual neuromuscular blockade postoperatively, both of which carry significant patient safety implications.

Anticoagulant therapy, particularly with warfarin, presents another high-risk interaction in cannabis-using patients. Warfarin is primarily metabolized via CYP2C9, an enzyme known to be affected by cannabinoid exposure. Cannabis use may inhibit warfarin metabolism, leading to elevated plasma concentrations and an increased risk of hemorrhagic complications (Lee et al., 2024). For patients receiving warfarin, close monitoring of international normalized ratio (INR) values is essential, and perioperative bleeding risk should be carefully assessed. In this context, the nurse anesthesiologist plays a critical role in coordinating care with surgical and medical teams to ensure appropriate monitoring, dose adjustments, and risk mitigation strategies.

Cannabis use introduces a wide array of clinically significant drug–drug interactions that directly impact anesthesia care. Through its effects on CYP450 metabolism, cannabis can alter the pharmacokinetics and pharmacodynamics of numerous medications commonly encountered in the perioperative setting. The nurse anesthesiologist must therefore approach the cannabis-using patient with a high degree of pharmacologic awareness, employing thorough assessment, vigilant monitoring, and individualized anesthetic planning. As cannabis use continues to rise, mastery of these interactions will remain an essential component of safe, evidence-informed anesthesia practice.

SPECIAL POPULATION

Cannabis and the Parturient

A particularly vulnerable population affected by cannabis use in the perioperative setting is the parturient patient. Cannabis is one of the most commonly used psychoactive substances among pregnant individuals, with reported prevalence rates as high as 5.4%, making it one of the most frequently encountered substances of misuse during pregnancy (Shah et al., 2023). From an anesthetic perspective, this prevalence has significant implications, as cannabinoids readily cross the placental barrier. Studies estimate that approximately 10% of maternal cannabinoid exposure is transferred to the fetus, resulting in direct fetal exposure to psychoactive compounds. Prenatal cannabis exposure has been associated with adverse fetal outcomes, including impaired neurodevelopment, potential disruptions in glucose metabolism, and reduced birth weight, all of which may influence both immediate neonatal outcomes and long-term developmental trajectories (Shah et al., 2023).

Additional concerns related to cannabis use in the parturient include maternal and neonatal complications that extend beyond fetal development alone. Cannabis hyperemesis syndrome may complicate pregnancy by contributing to dehydration, electrolyte imbalance, and nutritional deficiencies, all of which pose anesthetic and obstetric risks. Emerging literature also suggests an association between cannabis use and an increased risk of hypertensive disorders of pregnancy, including cannabis-associated preeclampsia, further complicating peripartum management (Shah et al.,

2023). Postnatally, cannabinoids may be transferred to the neonate through breast milk, raising concerns regarding ongoing neurodevelopmental exposure during early infancy. In light of these risks, authoritative regulatory and professional organizations, including the Food and Drug Administration (FDA) and the American College of Obstetricians and Gynecologists (ACOG), uniformly recommend abstinence from cannabis use during pregnancy and lactation. For the nurse anesthesiologist, these recommendations underscore the importance of thorough screening, patient education, and multidisciplinary collaboration to optimize maternal and fetal outcomes in the cannabis-using parturient (Shah et al., 2023).

Preoperative Assessment of the Cannabis User

The preoperative assessment and physical examination is a foundational component of safe anesthesia practice and serves as a critical opportunity to identify factors that may influence anesthetic management and patient outcomes. In patients who use cannabis, the preoperative evaluation assumes heightened importance due to the complex pharmacologic and physiologic effects associated with cannabinoid exposure. The American Society of Regional Anesthesia and Pain Medicine (ASRA) recommends that all patients presenting for procedures requiring anesthesia be routinely screened for cannabis use during the preoperative interview (Shah et al., 2023). These recommendations are supported with a moderate level of evidence and are consistent with guidance from other professional organizations involved in perioperative care. Routine screening allows the anesthesia provider to anticipate potential alterations in anesthetic requirements, hemodynamic responses, and perioperative complications, thereby enhancing patient safety.

Beyond simple identification of cannabis use, the preoperative assessment should include a detailed exploration of usage patterns. Davidson et al. (2020) emphasize the importance of assessing frequency of use, timing of last exposure, route of administration, and the possibility of acute intoxication at the time of surgery. Acute cannabis intoxication may increase the risk of cardiovascular instability, airway reactivity, and altered mental status, making anesthesia administration more hazardous. Additionally, the potential for cannabis withdrawal must be considered, particularly in chronic users. Withdrawal symptoms may occur within one to two days of cessation and can include irritability, anxiety, insomnia, nausea, and autonomic instability. Davidson et al. (2020) note that in select cases, resumption of cannabis use may be considered to mitigate withdrawal symptoms, though such decisions require careful clinical judgment and interdisciplinary collaboration.

Once cannabis use has been confirmed, the nurse anesthesiologist must engage in a comprehensive evaluation of how cannabis may impact perioperative care. This includes consideration of cannabis-related effects on individual organ systems, interactions with anesthetic agents, and potential drug–drug interactions with the patient's existing medication regimen. Cannabis-induced alterations in cardiovascular, respiratory, neurologic, and gastrointestinal function may influence anesthetic planning and monitoring strategies. Furthermore, as discussed throughout this chapter, cannabis can significantly affect the metabolism and efficacy of anesthetic medications and other commonly prescribed drugs, increasing the risk of adverse sequelae. A thorough, cannabis-informed preoperative assessment therefore enables the nurse anesthesiologist to develop an individualized anesthetic plan that accounts for these complexities and promotes optimal perioperative outcomes.

CONCLUSION

In conclusion, the nurse anesthesiologist must possess a comprehensive understanding of the complex interactions between cannabis and anesthetic medications to ensure safe and effective perioperative care. This responsibility begins with a thorough and systematic preoperative assessment, during which cannabis use is identified and evaluated in detail. By synthesizing information from the patient's current clinical status, past medical and surgical history, medication profile, and patterns of cannabis use, the nurse anesthesiologist can develop a patient-specific anesthetic plan of care. Consideration of potential anesthetic drug interactions, altered pharmacokinetics, and organ system involvement is essential, as cannabis use has been shown to influence cardiovascular, respiratory, neurologic, and metabolic function (Davidson et al., 2020; Shah et al., 2023). A holistic, individualized approach to anesthetic planning allows the nurse anesthesiologist to anticipate challenges and mitigate perioperative risks associated with cannabis exposure.

As cannabis use continues to rise in prevalence across diverse patient populations, it is critical to recognize that cannabis is not a benign substance in the context of anesthesia. Its effects on anesthetic requirements, pain management, and medication metabolism underscore the need for ongoing vigilance and evidence-informed practice. The nurse anesthesiologist must remain engaged with the evolving body of literature and professional guidelines to refine clinical decision-making and optimize patient outcomes. Through continued education, critical appraisal of emerging research, and adherence to professional standards, nurse anesthesiologists are well positioned to provide safe, compassionate, and effective anesthesia care for patients who use cannabis (Davidson et al., 2020; Shah et al., 2023).

REFERENCES

Bornemann-Cimenti, H., Lang-Illievich, K., Neuwersch-Sommeregger, S., Lang, J., Danninger, T., Hammer, S., Szilagyi, I. S., & Klivinyi, C. (2025). Effect of cannabinoid consumption on propofol dosage: A systematic review and meta-analysis. *British Journal of Anaesthesia*, *134*(3), 875–878. DOI: 10.1016/j.bja.2024.12.015 PMID: 39855936

Carlini, B. H., & Schauer, G. L. (2022). Cannabis-only use in the USA: Prevalence, demographics, use patterns, and health indicators. *Drug and Alcohol Dependence*, *212*, 108–115. DOI: 10.1016/j.drugalcdep.2020.108115 PMID: 35864553

Chiu, V., Hall, W., Chan, G., Hides, L., & Leung, J. (2022). A Systematic Review of Trends in US Attitudes toward Cannabis Legalization. *Substance Use & Misuse*, *57*(7), 1052–1061. DOI: 10.1080/10826084.2022.2063893 PMID: 35435131

Dahan, A., Hooten, W. M., & Furnish, T. (2024). Cannabis use and anesthesia. *Advances in Anesthesia*, *42*(1), 85–96. DOI: 10.1016/j.aan.2024.07.007 PMID: 39443052

Davidson, E. M., Raz, N., & Eyal, A. M. (2020). Anesthetic considerations in medical cannabis patients. *Current Opinion in Anaesthesiology*, *33*(6), 832–840. DOI: 10.1097/ACO.0000000000000932 PMID: 33093301

Imasogie, N., Rose, R. V., & Wilson, A. (2021). High quantities: Evaluating the association between cannabis use and propofol anesthesia during endoscopy. *PLoS One*, *16*(3), e0248062. DOI: 10.1371/journal.pone.0248062 PMID: 33661987

Inman, A., & Cservenka, A. (2026). Cannabis flower, concentrates, and edibles: A narrative review comparing prevalence of use, methods of consumption, and cannabis use disorder outcomes. *Journal of Addictive Diseases*, *44*(1), 3–13. DOI: 10.1080/10550887.2024.2418225 PMID: 39460749

Khoj, L., Zagà, V., Amram, D. L., Hosein, K., Pistone, G., Bisconti, M., Serafini, A., Cammarata, L. M., Cattaruzza, M. S., & Mura, M. (2024). Effects of cannabis smoking on the respiratory system: A state-of-the-art review. *Respiratory Medicine*, *221*, 107494. DOI: 10.1016/j.rmed.2023.107494 PMID: 38056532

King, D. D., Temmermand, R., & Greenwood, J. E. (2025). Preoperative cannabinoid exposure and postoperative pain: A narrative review. *Journal of Clinical Anesthesia*, *109*, 112097. Advance online publication. DOI: 10.1016/j.jclinane.2025.112097 PMID: 41406677

Ladha, K. S., Mistry, N., Wijeysundera, D. N., Clarke, H., Verma, S., Hare, G. M. T., & Mazer, C. D. (2021). Recent cannabis use and myocardial infarction in young adults: A cross-sectional study. *Canadian Medical Association Journal, 193*(35), E1377–E1384. DOI: 10.1503/cmaj.202392 PMID: 34493564

Leal, W. E., & Moscrop-Blake, K. (2024). The many forms of cannabis use: Prevalence and correlates of routes of administration among nationally representative samples of U.S. adult and adolescent cannabis users. *Addictive Behaviors, 159*, 108146. Advance online publication. DOI: 10.1016/j.addbeh.2024.108146 PMID: 39222559

Lee, B. H., Sideris, A., Ladha, K. S., Johnson, R. L., & Wu, C. L. (2024). Cannabis and cannabinoids in the perioperative period. *Anesthesia and Analgesia, 138*(1), 16–30. DOI: 10.1213/ANE.0000000000006070 PMID: 35551150

Lopera, V., Rodríguez, A., & Amariles, P. (2022). Clinical relevance of drug interactions with cannabis: A systematic review. *Journal of Clinical Medicine, 11*(5), 1154. DOI: 10.3390/jcm11051154 PMID: 35268245

Oster, B., Hameed, D., Bains, S. S., Johnson, A. J., Nace, J., & Mont, M. A. (2023). Tobacco and cannabis use have a synergistic association on infection risk following total knee arthroplasty. *The Journal of Arthroplasty*, *38*(10), 2137–2141. DOI: 10.1016/j.arth.2023.04.053 PMID: 37142070

Sajdeya, R., Rouhizadeh, M., Cook, R. L., Ison, R. L., Bai, C., Jugl, S., Gao, H., Mardini, M. T., Zandbiglari, K., Adiba, F. I., Dasa, O., Winterstein, A. G., Price, C. C., Pearson, T. A., Seubert, C. N., & Tighe, P. J. (2024). Cannabis use and inhalational anesthesia administration in older adults: A propensity-matched retrospective cohort study. *Anesthesiology*, *141*(5), 870–880. DOI: 10.1097/ALN.0000000000005146 PMID: 38980341

Shah, S., Schwenk, E. S., Sondekoppam, R. V., Clarke, H., Zakowski, M., Rzasa-Lynn, R. S., Yeung, B., Nicholson, K., Schwartz, G., Hooten, W. M., Wallace, M., Viscusi, E. R., & Narouze, S. (2023). ASRA Pain Medicine consensus guidelines on the management of the perioperative patient on cannabis and cannabinoids. *Regional Anesthesia and Pain Medicine*, *48*(3), 97–117. DOI: 10.1136/rapm-2022-104013 PMID: 36596580

Touw, M. (1981). The religious and medicinal uses of cannabis in China, India and Tibet. *Journal of Psychoactive Drugs*, *13*(1), 23–34. DOI: 10.1080/02791072.1981.10471447 PMID: 7024492

Wishart, D. S., Hiebert-Giesbrecht, M., Inchehborouni, G., Cao, X., Guo, A. C., LeVatte, M. A., Torres-Calzada, C., Gautam, V., Johnson, M., Liigand, J., Wang, F., Zahraei, S., Bhumireddy, S., Wang, Y., Zheng, J., Mandal, R., & Dyck, J. R. B. (2024). Chemical composition of commercial cannabis. Journal of Agricultural and Environmental Chemistry. Advance online publication. https://doi.org/DOI: 10.1021/acs.jafc.3c08552

Zuardi, A. W. (2006). History of cannabis as a medicine: A review. *Revista Brasileira de Psiquiatria : Orgão Oficial da Associação Brasileira de Psiquiatria, Asociación Psiqui´trica de la América Latina*, *28*(2), 153–157. DOI: 10.1590/S1516-44462006000200015 PMID: 16810401

Zvonarev, V., Fatuki, T. A., & Tregubenko, P. (2019). The public health concerns of marijuana legalization: An overview of current trends. *Cureus*, *11*(9), e5806. DOI: 10.7759/cureus.5806 PMID: 31723545

Chapter 6
The Perioperative Period: Assessment and Anesthesia for Surgery and Procedures

Daniel D. King
http://orcid.org/0000-0002-6427-9480
Rosalind Franklin University of Medicine and Science, USA

ABSTRACT

This chapter explores anesthetic and perioperative implications of cannabinoids and the endocannabinoid system (ECS), emphasizing nursing roles in assessment, risk mitigation, and communication. It aims to translate cannabis science into practical guidance for nurse anesthesiologists, perianesthesia nurses, and care partners, amid rising use and inconsistent disclosure. Content covers ECS mechanisms, pharmacokinetics (including CYP450 interactions and tolerance), and relevant anesthesia considerations affecting depth, dosing, and recovery. It highlights perioperative risks from research, focusing on cardiovascular, respiratory, gastrointestinal, pain pathways, TRPV1, and cannabinoid hyperalgesia. The chapter recommends structured screening with the CUBAT framework and aligns practice with existing professional, societal, evidence-based, educational, and policy guidance.

CHAPTER OVERVIEW

The growing integration of cannabis into contemporary healthcare requires perioperative nursing professionals to develop competency in cannabis-informed anesthesiology and surgical or procedural care. Nurse anesthesiologists (Certified Registered Nurse Anesthetists [CRNAs]), perianesthesia nurses, and the broader community of anesthesia providers, perioperative clinicians, researchers, educators, and interdisciplinary healthcare professionals work at the intersection of anesthesia

DOI: 10.4018/979-8-2600-2035-7.ch006

science, patient advocacy, and education—roles that position them as essential contributors to cannabis-informed perioperative practice. As cannabis normalization advances, all clinicians must adapt traditional frameworks to a new era of patient disclosure, medical and pharmacologic complexity, and evidence-based care while maintaining ethical responsibility.

Cannabis is known to be among the most used substances worldwide, and despite emerging guidance, such as the American Society for Regional Anesthesia (ASRA) Pain Medicine consensus (SAMHSA, 2025; Shah et al., 2023), perioperative recommendations remain unevenly implemented and often nonspecific across settings. This reality poses both a clinical and safety gap: patients who use cannabis may experience unpredictable anesthetic responses, altered hemodynamics and cardiorespiratory risk, and increased postoperative pain, while clinicians often lack the education, validated tools, and clinical guidance to assess or mitigate these risks. More broadly, the perioperative continuum can unintentionally reduce cannabis to a risk variable, eclipsing its role for many patients in symptom relief, coping, function, and overall well-being, especially when histories are incomplete, and care is constrained by stigma, production pressure, and protocolized medicine.

This chapter addresses these gaps by translating emerging science and integrating holistic care into clinical practice. Drawing on the ASRA Pain Medicine consensus guidelines (Shah et al., 2023), the American Association of Nurse Anesthesiology (AANA) practice recommendations (King et al., 2023b), and the Cannabis Use and Behaviors Assessment Tool (CUBAT) framework (Sladkey et al., 2025), the chapter proposes a structured, stigma-free approach to preoperative cannabis assessment and subsequent perioperative management. These frameworks are part of the broader mission of comprehensive cannabis nursing. Cannabis nurses operate within a model that integrates evidence, empathy, and education to improve patient outcomes and promote equity in healthcare.

How to Use This Chapter (Quick Guide for Clinicians)

- Use Table 3 (CUBAT) for preanesthesia screening and documentation
- Use the Perioperative Risks section to identify airway/aspiration/hemodynamic risk modifiers.
- Use the Pain/Opioid Stewardship section to guide multimodal planning and patient messaging.
- Use the Communication/Stigma section to improve disclosure reliability and reduce fear of punishment.

Purpose and Scope

While other chapters address foundational concepts such as pharmacology, the endocannabinoid system (ECS), and sociocultural determinants of cannabis use, this chapter focuses on the perioperative and anesthetic aspects of care, where the science of cannabis meets the realities of the operating room and procedural suites. It applies cannabinoid pharmacology to perioperative decision-making, integrates disclosure dynamics into anesthesia safety, and elevates nursing leadership in policy, research, and interprofessional collaboration. Specifically, this chapter will:

1. **Integrate current evidence** on how cannabis use affects anesthetic and analgesic management across the preoperative, intraoperative, and postoperative phases of care.
2. **Examine disclosure behavior and stigma** as clinical variables that influence perioperative safety and outcomes.
3. **Identify physiologic and pharmacologic mechanisms** relevant to anesthetic and medication dosing, airway responsiveness, and hemodynamic stability.
4. **Highlight nursing leadership roles** in patient education, interdisciplinary communication, and development of informed, institutional cannabis policies.
5. **Outline future directions** for nursing research, relevant curriculum design, and quality improvement in cannabis-informed anesthesia care.

INTRODUCTION: CANNABIS EVOLUTION IN ANESTHESIOLOGY

Cannabis has been embedded in human medicine for millennia, with ancient Chinese, Egyptian, Indian, and Persian texts describing its use for pain relief, including labor pain, inflammation, and respiratory issues, as well as for anesthesia (Brand & Zhao, 2017; Dave et al., 2024; Smith, 2021). Around 200 CE, the Chinese surgeon Hua Tuo pioneered the use of powdered cannabis mixed with wine (*máfèisan*) to induce surgical anesthesia. Some authors speculate that this anesthetic formula, *mafei* powder, may have contained *mafen* (the cannabis inflorescence), given the shared pronunciation of the characters in the formula name (Brand & Zhao, 2017). The Chinese term for anesthesia, *mázui*, literally combines 'hemp/cannabis' and 'intoxication/anesthesia,' underscoring the plant's historical association with analgesia and sedation. By 600 CE, the *Sushruta Samhita*, a foundational text on surgery, advised the use of preparations of wine, as well as incense made from Indian hemp (*Cannabis indica*) to be inhaled, and potentially as an oral or topical application, for sedation and analgesia during procedures, setting a standard for the requisite analgesia for complex surgical procedures (Dave et al., 2024) (Figure 1).

Figure 1. Statue of Sushruta, revered as the "Father of Plastic Surgery," located at Patanjali Yogpeeth, Haridwar, India

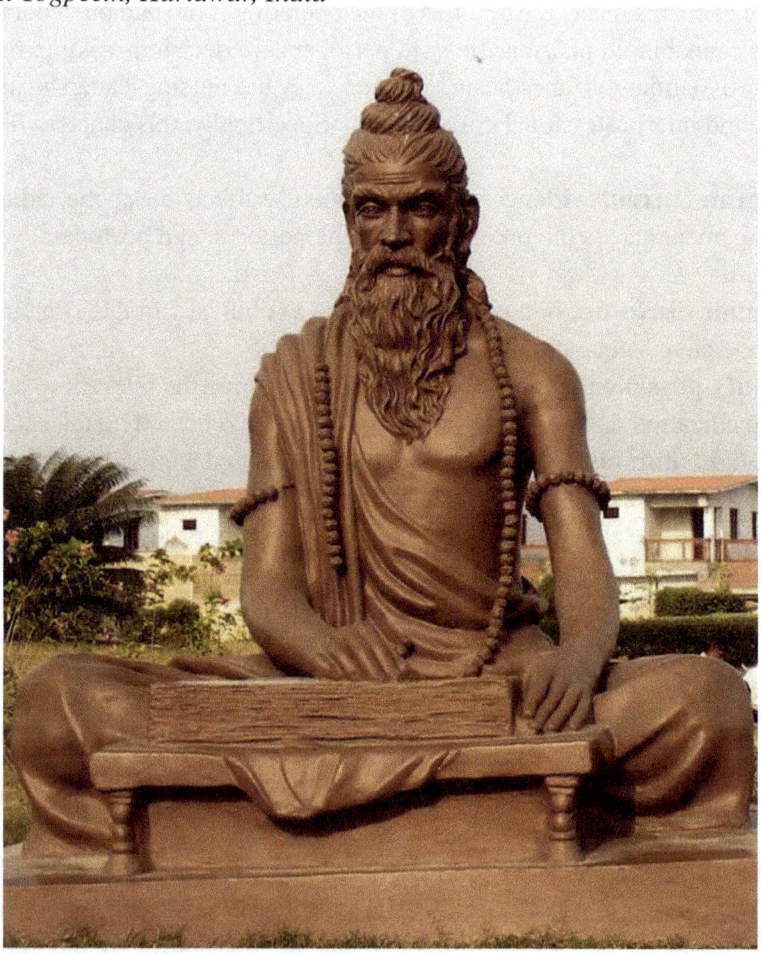

Source: Original image by Alokprasad, uploaded by Ibolya Horváth, published on January 11, 2018, by the copyright holder under the Creative Commons attribution (https://commons.wikimedia.org/wiki/File:Shushrut_statue.jpg)

Modern legalization has reignited clinical interest while simultaneously expanding the population of surgical patients presenting with active cannabis use – and with it, the perioperative safety questions this chapter addresses. Prevalence persists among surgical populations, arguably to a greater degree, to control symptomatology that may overlap with surgical indicators; yet routine screening and collaborative approaches that inform care plan development remain rare. The perioperative setting, with its critical nature and emphasis on airway management, drug titration, and dynamic physiologic shifts, reflects the importance of recognizing cannabis use as a meaningful variable in patient safety (King et al., 2021).

Recent research points to the urgent perioperative relevance. A growing body of literature suggests that patients who use cannabis may require higher induction doses of the hypnotic agent propofol, experience altered sympathetic tone, and exhibit concerning postoperative pain thresholds (Baker et al., 2025; King et al., 2021; Shah et al., 2023). However, findings vary by population, procedure type, and use pattern. Observational studies in some surgical cohorts (notably orthopedics/spine) associate cannabis use or cannabis use disorder (CUD) with an increased risk of perioperative complications, including deep vein thrombosis, surgical site infections, and delayed wound healing (Hoveidaei et al., 2024; Turan et al., 2024; Yang et al., 2024). However, findings to date are mixed, and confounding (tobacco, comorbidity, CUD severity) remains a limitation. Conversely, certain cannabinoids demonstrate anti-inflammatory and opioid-sparing effects, implying possible benefits in postoperative pain management when appropriately characterized and monitored (Abdallah et al., 2020; Nielsen et al., 2017). This duality of cannabis—therapeutic potential versus physiological unpredictability—demands a nuanced, evidence-informed approach.

Evidence Limitations and Confounders

Interpreting the perioperative cannabis evidence base necessitates explicit recognition of four prevalent confounders. First, tobacco co-use represents the most significant confounding variable in research on respiratory and cardiovascular outcomes. Failure to account for tobacco use often leads to an overestimation of cannabis-associated risks. Second, substantial variability in product potency and composition is rarely addressed in primary studies, which frequently categorize cannabis exposure dichotomously. This approach obscures critical distinctions among high-THC flower, CBD-dominant oils, and low-potency edibles. Third, self-reported data on timing, dosage, and frequency of cannabis use are often unreliable. Underreporting may occur due to stigma, and accurate dose estimation is challenging without standardized labeling. Fourth, many large-scale administrative database studies conflate cannabis use disorder (CUD) with non-dependent, recreational, or medical cannabis use. These populations exhibit markedly different exposure patterns, health profiles, and risk levels. Therefore, caution is warranted when extrapolating findings from CUD-coded cohorts to non-dependent users (Shah et al., 2023; King et al., 2026). Table 1 summarizes the current state of perioperative cannabis evidence across established, probable, and unresolved domains

Table 1. Evidence synthesis: perioperative cannabis evidence across established, probable, and unresolved clinical domains

Established (Guideline/Consensus-Level)	Probable/Directional (Observational Evidence)	Unresolved / Uncertain (Mechanistic or Absent Data)
Universal structured cannabis screening (history-based, not toxicology) is recommended pre-procedure (ASRA; AANA)	Frequent/daily cannabis use is directionally associated with higher propofol requirements in some cohorts; not universal	Dose-response relationship between cannabis use frequency and anesthetic requirement in humans (direct causal evidence absent)
Elective surgery should be postponed when acute intoxication/ impaired consent capacity is present (ASRA; AANA)	Regular cannabis use is associated with higher acute postoperative pain and opioid consumption in spine and mixed surgical cohorts	Optimal preoperative tapering window and whether tapering reduces perioperative risk (no RCT evidence)
Delay elective surgery ≥2 hours after smoking cannabis due to cardiovascular risk window (ASRA)	CUD is associated with approximately 2x increased odds of postoperative MI in large propensity-matched cohorts; confounding by baseline cardiovascular risk is present	Safe delay period for non-smoked cannabinoid products before elective surgery (insufficient data)
Cannabis withdrawal syndrome (CWS) is a foreseeable perioperative risk in daily users and should be anticipated, monitored, and managed (DSM-5 criteria; ASRA)	Daily cannabis use is associated with approximately 20% relative increase in PONV risk vs. non-daily use in some analyses; effect is heterogeneous across studies	Cannabinoid-induced hyperalgesia mechanism in perioperative humans (proposed TRPV1 mechanism lacks direct clinical confirmation)
Routine urine toxicology is not recommended for universal preanesthesia screening; history-based assessment is preferred (ASRA)	Chronic inhalational use is associated with obstructive airway patterns, chronic bronchitis symptoms, and increased bronchospasm risk; confounded by tobacco in many studies	Interactive effects of cannabinoids and neuraxial opioids on thermoregulation; whether cannabis modifies malignant hyperthermia risk in clinical settings

Note. *Evidence classifications reflect the level of support in the published literature as of the chapter writing date. 'Established' reflects consensus-guideline-level support; 'Probable/Directional' reflects consistent observational signals subject to confounding; 'Unresolved' reflects areas where mechanistic hypotheses exist but human evidence is absent or insufficient to inform practice. All claims remain subject to revision as the perioperative cannabis evidence base matures.*

The Disclosure Divide

Despite increasing normalization and social acceptance of cannabis, patient disclosure and clinical capture of cannabis use remain inconsistent, and this inconsistency is the most significant barrier to clinical knowledge gains and to strengthening the evidence base for care delivery. In a recent U.S. national exploratory survey of adults in healthcare settings, only 46.1% reported *always* disclosing cannabis use to providers, 32.7% *sometimes*, and 21.2% *never* did (King et al., 2024). Importantly, most disclosures (57%) came from patients rather than clinicians (15%), indicating that patients often lead clinicians across this communication chasm. Anticipated stigma, a persistent fear of judgment or being treated differently if a healthcare provider learns of cannabis use, and uncertainty about clinical relevance, contribute significantly to underreporting (King et al., 2024).

For perianesthesia professionals, nondisclosure creates a blind spot in essential safety management and holistic patient care. One cannot even begin to prepare an informed plan of anesthesia delivery and perioperative management without essential knowledge of an underlying cannabinoid-based mechanism. Furthermore, unrecognized cannabis exposure can alter anesthetic requirements, hemodynamic stability, and recovery trajectories. Then, the ability to conduct research and correlate clinical outcomes is often missing or severely limited. These gaps are not merely informational—they are ethical. As the American Association of Nurse Anesthesiology (2018) practice considerations for promoting a culture of safety and the American Nurses Association (2025) code of ethics emphasize, nurses have a duty to foster open, nonjudgmental dialogue that supports informed, collaborative decision-making. Reframing cannabis disclosure as a safety-critical component of whole-person, goal-concordant care, rather than a moral admission, is essential to equitable perioperative practice.

Advancing Quality and Safety in Perioperative Cannabis Care

Perioperative clinicians, particularly anesthesia providers and perianesthesia nurses, are well-positioned to advance safer and more consistent cannabis-informed surgical care. Structured approaches, such as the Cannabis Use and Behaviors Assessment Tool (CUBAT), facilitate standardized assessment of product type, route, frequency, timing, and effects (Sladkey et al., 2025). These factors can influence airway reactivity, cardiovascular responses, anesthetic depth, drug metabolism, and recovery. Integrating evidence-based screening with patient education on preoperative withholding, tapering, and postoperative resumption enables clinicians to identify risks such as additive sedation, optimize anesthetic planning, and foster trust through nonjudgmental communication. Cannabis care thus represents a frontier in quality and safety, challenging perioperative systems to anticipate variation, standardize assessment, and adapt with evidence, empathy, and vigilance rather than avoidance or stigma.

THE ENDOCANNABINOID SYSTEM AND ANESTHETIC IMPLICATIONS

Established across basic and translational science, the ECS is widely expressed in tissues central to perioperative care, including the brain, heart, lungs, spinal cord, autonomic nervous system, gastrointestinal tract, immune system, and liver. This broad distribution helps explain why cannabis use can alter anesthetic requirements, hemodynamic responses, and postoperative pain, among other effects.

CB1 and CB2 Receptors in the Perioperative Context

Cannabinoid type 1 (CB1) receptors are highly expressed throughout the central nervous system, especially in the cerebral cortex, hippocampus, amygdala, basal ganglia, and cerebellum. CB1 functions as a presynaptic inhibitory modulator. When activated, these Gi/o-coupled receptors:

- reduce cyclic adenosine monophosphate (cAMP),
- inhibit voltage-gated Ca^{2+} channels, and
- increase K^+ efflux,

shortening the duration of pre-synaptic action potentials in a now hyperpolarized neuron that is much less likely to be depolarized, or fire, in the future. The result is diminished neurotransmitter release across a synapse, including both excitatory (e.g., glutamate) and inhibitory (e.g., GABA) neurotransmitters. Because CB1 can suppress the release of both glutamate and GABA, the net effect may be inhibitory or disinhibitory depending on circuit location and baseline tone. Accordingly, CB1 signaling can either enhance or limit analgesia depending on the network engaged and clinical context. In the cortex and basal ganglia, this modulates arousal, motor control, and cognition; in the hippocampus, it influences memory and learning; and in the amygdala, it shapes fear, anxiety, and the stress response. Because CB1 signaling intersects with many of the same neurobehavioral and autonomic networks influenced by anesthetics, sedatives, and opioids, perioperative effects can vary meaningfully by exposure pattern. This is particularly important when stratifying the timing of last use and whether cannabis exposure leading up to the anesthetic course is acute, chronic, or recently discontinued. In general terms, acute exposure may be more associated with altered attention, anxiety, and impaired psychomotor function (particularly with tetrahydrocannabinol), whereas chronic, frequent exposure may be associated with physiologic adaptation (tolerance) and more heterogeneous medication responses. These considerations become clinically relevant during anesthesia induction, emergence, and early recovery (Allsop et al., 2016; Echeverria-Villalobos et al., 2025; Flanagan, 2021; Health Canada, 2018).

Cannabinoid type 2 (CB2) receptors were once thought to be restricted to immune cells but are now recognized in peripheral organs (spleen, tonsils, thymus, bone marrow, gastrointestinal (GI) tract) and, at lower density, in glial and some neuronal populations. CB2 activation is largely immunomodulatory and anti-inflammatory, dampening cytokine release and leukocyte activation and contributing to analgesia in inflammatory and neuropathic pain models. From a perioperative perspective, this immune and inflammatory signaling framework helps explain why cannabinoids are often discussed in relation to postoperative pain management, symptom burden, and recovery trajectories, while also underscoring that clinical effects may be variable and patient-specific. CB2 signaling has also been linked to tissue repair and remodeling in the musculoskeletal system, with theoretical implications for postoperative recovery and chronic pain. CB2 is associated with a variety of responses and regulatory functions. However, perhaps most interesting to perioperative and anesthesia providers is that this receptor is a major focus of pain and neuroinflammation research, including glial signaling and peripheral immune pathways, with interest in achieving analgesia without CB1-mediated psychotropic effects. At a high level, this CB1/CB2 contrast is a useful organizing principle for the chapter: CB1 is more closely associated with central neurobehavioral effects (e.g., cognition, anxiety, sedation), whereas CB2 is more closely associated with immunomodulation and inflammatory pain mechanisms. Both are highly relevant in surgical care (Allsop et al., 2016; Echeverria-Villalobos et al., 2025; Flanagan, 2021; Goyal et al., 2017; Health Canada, 2018).

In the GI tract, CB1 and CB2 receptors modulate enteric cholinergic tone and smooth muscle activity. Activation of these receptors can inhibit acetylcholine release, slow peristalsis, and reduce secretions, thereby contributing to delayed gastric emptying and constipation. For anesthesia providers, this may raise concern about "full-stomach" physiology, particularly in heavy, chronic, or acutely intoxicated cannabis patients and in those with cannabinoid hyperemesis syndrome (CHS). Aspiration precautions and rapid-sequence induction may be considered based on overall risk assessment. This GI physiology also creates an important perioperative paradox worth noting upfront: cannabinoid signaling is often discussed in relation to nausea and appetite regulation, yet a subset of patients (e.g., those with chronic, heavy exposure), may present with severe, recurrent vomiting (CHS), dehydration, and electrolyte disturbances, which can amplify aspiration risk and complicate postoperative nausea and vomiting (PONV) management. Accordingly, perioperative nursing assessments should explicitly include timing of last use, route and frequency of use, and any history of CHS episodes or prolonged vomiting – details that later sections of this chapter will translate into practical screening and management considerations (Allsop et al., 2016; Health Canada, 2018; Flanagan, 2021; King et al., 2021; Shah et al., 2023).

Enzymatic Regulation: FAAH, MAGL, and CYP450

Endocannabinoid signals are short-lived because specific enzymes rapidly degrade them. Fatty acid amide hydrolase (FAAH) breaks down anandamide, while monoacylglycerol lipase (MAGL) hydrolyzes most (~85%) 2-arachidonylglycerol (2-AG), thereby shaping signal duration and strength. Importantly, FAAH hydrolyzes anandamide primarily into arachidonic acid and ethanolamine, and MAGL hydrolyzes 2-AG primarily into arachidonic acid and glycerol. This links to broader arachidonic acid (eicosanoid) signaling relevant to inflammation and pain. MAGL is present at a significant fraction of brain synapses, particularly those involved in glutamatergic and GABAergic transmission, thereby strongly shaping mood, cognition, and nociception. Although MAGL accounts for most of the brain's 2-AG hydrolysis, other enzymes (notably ABHD6 and ABHD12) contribute meaningfully and may regulate distinct pools of 2-AG based on subcellular localization, an organizational concept that helps explain why endocannabinoid tone can vary across brain regions and physiologic states. Inhibition of MAGL or FAAH increases endocannabinoid tone, as demonstrated in experimental models, thereby reducing neuroinflammation and enhancing analgesia. In certain disease states, MAGL inhibition is associated with reduced neuroinflammation. At a high level, endocannabinoid signal duration is not governed solely by FAAH and MAGL. 2-AG and related lipids can also be oxygenated by COX-2, lipoxygenases, and even CYP pathways, producing additional (non-CB1/CB2) bioactive metabolites that may influence perioperative inflammation and nociception (Allsop et al., 2016; Echeverria-Villalobos et al., 2025; Flanagan, 2021; Health Canada, 2018; Hasckel Gewehr et al., 2024; Murataeva et al., 2014).

Supported by experimental but not large-scale human data, propofol appears to inhibit FAAH and increase brain anandamide concentrations, thereby enhancing CB1-mediated signaling in a dose-dependent manner. Experimental studies have shown increased brain anandamide after propofol exposure and inhibition of anandamide hydrolysis via FAAH. This mechanistic overlap may contribute to propofol's unique psychotropic profile and its interaction with chronic cannabinoid exposure. Comparable FAAH modulation has not been consistently demonstrated for other commonly used agents. The clinical significance of this interaction is evident in differential endocannabinoid profiles during intravenous or inhalational general anesthesia. For instance, inhaled sevoflurane has been associated with decreased anandamide levels, whereas intravenous propofol preserves these endocannabinoids. While such human studies suggest general anesthesia may alter circulating endocannabinoid levels, patterns may differ by technique (volatile vs total intravenous anesthesia [TIVA]), though clinical significance remains uncertain (Allsop et al., 2016; Echeverria-Villalobos et al., 2025; Flanagan, 2021; Health Canada, 2018; Hasckel Gewehr et al., 2024; Patel et al., 2003; Schelling et al., 2006).

Phase I metabolism of phytocannabinoids is primarily mediated by the hepatic mixed-function oxidase cytochrome P450 (CYP450) system. These enzymes add an oxygen atom to substrate molecules (from cannabis or anesthetic drugs), often yielding dealkylated and hydroxylated metabolites via oxidation. This process aims to detoxify and facilitate metabolism. There are at least 50 isoenzyme subtypes, each of which can be inhibited, induced, or otherwise affected by exposure to various drugs or genetic factors. For Δ^9-THC specifically, CYP2C9 is a major driver of conversion to the psychoactive metabolite 11-hydroxy-THC (11-OH-THC), which is further oxidized to inactive 11-nor-9-carboxy-THC (THC-COOH). These metabolites then undergo substantial Phase II conjugation (glucuronidation), with UGT2B7 and UGT1A9 among important contributors. For CBD, CYP2C19 and CYP2C9 contribute to the formation of 7-hydroxy-CBD (7-OH-CBD), while CYP3A4 contributes to additional oxidative pathways. This provides important context for why CBD is frequently implicated in drug-drug interactions (Allsop et al., 2016; Beers et al., 2021; Echeverria-Villalobos et al., 2025; Hassenberg et al., 2020; Health Canada, 2018; Nasrin et al., 2021; Patilea-Vrana et al., 2019; Sharma et al., 2012). The general mechanism of liver enzymes is illustrated in Figure 2.

Figure 2. Cytochrome P450–mediated metabolism and drug–drug interaction pathways relevant to perioperative care

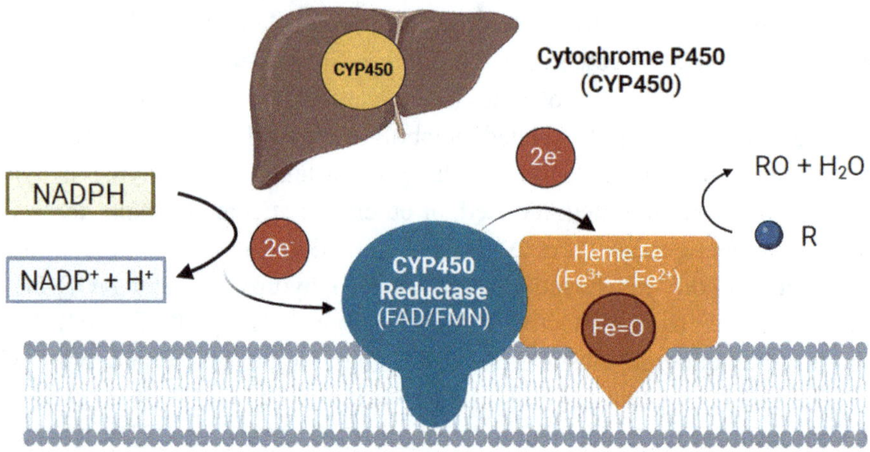

Note. *This figure illustrates the hepatic cytochrome P450 (CYP450) monooxygenase system, a primary pathway for the metabolism of many anesthetic agents, analgesics, sedatives, and cannabinoids. Electrons derived from nicotinamide adenine dinucleotide phosphate (NADPH) are transferred via CYP450 reductase (containing flavin adenine dinucleotide and flavin mononucleotide) to the heme iron of the membrane-bound CYP450 enzyme within the endoplasmic reticulum. Sequential electron transfer reduces heme iron from Fe^{3+} to Fe^{2+}, thereby enabling the activation of molecular oxygen and the oxidative biotransformation of lipophilic substrates (R) into more water-soluble metabolites (RO), with water as a byproduct. In the perioperative context, cannabinoids—particularly Δ9-tetrahydrocannabinol (THC) and cannabidiol (CBD)—share CYP450 metabolic pathways with commonly administered anesthetic and analgesic medications, creating the potential for altered drug metabolism through enzyme inhibition or induction. This shared metabolic framework provides a mechanistic basis for interindividual variability in anesthetic and analgesic responses and calls attention to the importance of medication reconciliation and cannabis use assessment prior to surgery. Source: Created in BioRender. King, D. (2026) https://BioRender.com/r6l2e75*

The CYP450 family serves as the cleanup crew for cannabinoids and many anesthetic drugs, regulating how long they remain active and how they interact with other medications. Delta-9-tetrahydrocannabinol (Δ^9-THC) is primarily metabolized by CYP2C9, CYP3A4, and CYP2C19, while cannabidiol (CBD) is primarily metabolized by CYP3A4 and CYP2C19, with variable involvement of CYP2C9. Many anesthetic and analgesic agents, such as propofol (CYP2C9), ketamine (CYP3A4/2C9), midazolam (CYP3A4), and fentanyl (CYP3A4), are also metabolized by these pathways. Overall, CYP and UGT enzymes govern cannabinoid clearance and metabolite formation, contributing to interindividual variability in exposure and drug-drug interaction potential. A key nuance for perioperative clinicians and practitioners is that cannabis exposure is not uniform across contexts. For example, inhaled or smoked products can introduce polycyclic aromatic hydrocarbons that induce CYP1A2, whereas oral/high-dose CBD products are more commonly discussed as inhibitors (and sometimes inducers) of multiple CYP enzymes (Echeverria-Villalobos et al., 2025; Health Canada, 2018; King et al., 2021; Shah et al., 2023).

When cannabis and anesthetic drugs share demand for CYP isoenzymes, chronic exposure may drive enzyme up-regulation (induction) and faster clearance. In contrast, acute high-dose exposure, particularly with CBD, can inhibit these enzymes and increase drug levels. CBD has documented inhibitory potential across several CYP isoenzymes (including CYP2C19, CYP2C9, and CYP3A4), and some data suggest time-dependent inhibition of CYP3A4. These features help explain why CBD is disproportionately represented in clinically relevant drug–drug interaction reports. Cannabinoids and their metabolites may inhibit multiple UGT enzymes, including UGT1A9 and UGT2B7 in experimental models, potentially altering the glucuronidation of substrates such as morphine. Finally, common genetic variability (e.g., CYP2C9 intermediate- or poor-metabolizer status) can meaningfully alter cannabinoid exposure and metabolite profiles, adding another layer of interindividual variability that becomes relevant when perioperative medications share these pathways (Echeverria-Villalobos et al., 2025; Herdegen & Cascorbi, 2023; King et al., 2021; Nasrin et al., 2021; Shah et al., 2023; Smith & Gruber, 2023).

Cross-Tolerance and Anesthetic Drug Requirements

Mechanistic hypotheses propose that shared metabolic and receptor pathways may explain altered anesthetic and sedative dose requirements in some cannabis-exposed patients. However, human evidence supporting this relationship is of low certainty and remains heterogeneous. Table 2 presents a proposed enzymatic mechanism for cross-tolerance (Herdegen & Cascorbi, 2023; King et al., 2021; Thomas et al., 2022). However, this display should be interpreted as a high-level summary of shared metabolic pathways that may contribute to variable drug exposure; it does not, by itself, establish cross-tolerance. Clinically observed differences in anesthetic requirements likely reflect a combination of pharmacokinetic (exposure-related) and pharmacodynamic (receptor- and network-level) adaptations, with the relative contribution varying by agent, dose, timing of last use, route, and exposure pattern (Shah et al., 2023).

Table 2. Primary shared Phase I CYP/Phase II UGT pathways that may contribute to drug-drug interactions and variable anesthetic requirements

Drug/substance	CYP2C9	CYP3A4	CYP2C19	CYP2B6	UGT1A9	UGT2B7
Δ⁹- THC	X	X	?			
CBD		X	X		X	X
Propofol	X			X	X	
Ketamine	X	X		X		
Fentanyl		X				
Midazolam		X				
Oxycodone		X				
NSAIDs	X					
Warfarin	X					
Clopidogrel			X	X		

Note. *X indicates a major or clinically relevant metabolic pathway for the listed drug/substance; blank cells indicate no major pathway shown in this simplified overview. "?" indicates variable or less consistently reported involvement across sources. This table is intended as a high-level summary of shared CYP/UGT pathways that may contribute to drug–drug interactions and variability in anesthetic requirements; it is not an exhaustive mapping of all metabolic routes or transporter effects and is not intended to represent enzyme inhibition/induction. Additional CYP isoenzymes and UGT pathways may contribute depending on formulation, route of administration, dose, duration of exposure, comorbid hepatic dysfunction, and genetic variability.*

Human studies evaluating dose requirements in cannabis-exposed patients are often heterogeneous and confounded by factors such as patient history, procedure duration, co-medications, and provider dosing variability. Findings should be interpreted cautiously (King et al., 2021; Shah et al., 2023). Case series, cohort studies, and limited comparative data suggest that some regular users may require higher propofol (and adjunct) dosing, but the clinical significance varies and is not uniform across all patients (Baker et al., 2025; Flisberg et al., 2009; Imasogie et al., 2021; Shah et al., 2023). One of the most hazardous assumptions is that a patient encountered in the preoperative area with a positive cannabis history inherently requires higher concentrations and doses of anesthetic drugs.

Early findings from a randomized, single-blinded study showed that participants who regularly consume cannabis required higher propofol doses for successful laryngeal mask airway insertion than nonusers (314.0 ± 109.3 mg vs 263.2 ± 69.5 mg, $p < .04$). However, the timing of cannabis use relative to induction was unclear, and all participants were male (Flisberg et al., 2009). In a later retrospective study of 250 endoscopy patients, the cannabis group (n=25) received higher midazolam, fentanyl, and propofol doses; however, the authors identified multiple confounders (including procedure duration and potential provider-level dosing differences), and the absolute dose differences were small and of uncertain clinical significance (Twardowski et al., 2019). In a separate study of 635 upper endoscopy patients, when matched with cannabis use (n=23), no differences in midazolam, fentanyl, ketamine, or propofol dose requirements were observed, with similar study limitations (King et al., 2021).

Frequency-response relationships (e.g., daily vs. intermittent use) are plausible but inconsistently measured across studies, leaving a significant evidence gap (Imasogie et al., 2021; Shah et al., 2023). These relationships are thought to reflect CB1 receptor downregulation and desensitization from chronic THC exposure (Yeung et al., 2022) and broader neuroadaptations in overlapping GABAergic and glutamatergic networks. However, direct causal evidence in humans linking CB1 changes to anesthetic dose requirements remains limited (Shah et al., 2023). Research is needed to correlate specific cannabis history, including dose patterns, with clinical responses.

Consistent with the extant literature, repeated THC exposure is associated with CB1 receptor down-regulation and desensitization across relevant brain regions, which may reduce responsiveness to neuromodulatory effects and contribute to cross-tolerance hypotheses (Yeung et al., 2022; Shah et al., 2023). Similar, though limited, patterns have been observed with potent inhalational (volatile) anesthetics. For instance, a retrospective analysis of patients undergoing isolated tibial fracture repair reported higher sevoflurane minimum alveolar concentration (MAC) requirements among patients who used cannabis within the month before surgery ($p = .023$), with no statistically significant difference in desflurane MAC; there were no statistically significant differences observed in cumulative propofol dosing (Holmen et al., 2020). Mechanistic hypotheses (e.g., CB1 downregulation with chronic THC exposure and broader network-level neuroadaptation) offer a plausible rationale for why some long-term cannabis patients have higher anesthetic needs, but they do not justify automatic dose escalation. Current recommendations caution against implementing a practice change given the inconsistent and limited findings (Shah et al., 2023).

Acute exposure provides additional, important insights. In an early animal, double-blind, randomized controlled trial (RCT) in which nabiximols (Sativex®) was administered 20 minutes before induction, the mean bispectral index (BIS) during sevoflurane anesthesia was significantly higher in the high-dose cannabis group after controlling for MAC (Ibera et al., 2018). These findings suggest altered hypnotic depth signals during volatile anesthetic administration, although BIS differences are highly debated and do not necessarily reflect definitive changes in anesthetic dose requirements. Furthermore, the investigators did not provide data showing that higher BIS reflected a lighter plane of anesthetic depth, and it remains unclear how cannabis-related changes in neural oscillations affect processed EEG measures. Accordingly, BIS differences should be interpreted cautiously and should not be treated as a direct surrogate for anesthetic requirement in this patient population (Shah et al., 2023).

Further rodent studies build on these findings, noting dose-dependent bidirectional relationships. For instance, pretreatment with 20 mg/kg CBD significantly shortened the isoflurane anesthesia induction time, whereas 100 mg/kg CBD paradoxically prolonged induction time and delayed recovery, suggesting that complex interactions between cannabinoids and volatile agents may differ significantly from those observed with intravenous agents (Uršič et al., 2022). The important takeaway is that cannabinoid-volatile anesthetic interactions are complex and, at this point, not directly generalizable to clinical dosing decisions.

Acute cannabinoid administration, particularly in naïve subjects, can transiently reduce anesthetic requirements via CB1 activation and increased endocannabinoid tone. Experimental models have indicated that CBD-rich extracts lower propofol induction doses, and THC potentiates barbiturate or etomidate sedation, possibly through CB1 but not CB2 activation. However, these effects are not reliably replicated in chronically exposed human patients.

Given the low certainty of evidence, consensus recommendations emphasize individualized titration and dose adjustment based on clinical presentation and the timing of the last cannabis use. The safest inference is variability: cannabis exposure should prompt careful titration to effect, attention to the timing of the last use, and readiness for either increased or decreased sensitivity, depending on pharmacogenomic profile, acute exposure, exposure pattern, and comedications. In other words, cannabis history is a signal to individualize care, not a reliable predictor of the direction or magnitude of anesthetic requirements (King et al., 2023b; Shah et al., 2023).

Taken together, the direction and magnitude of cannabinoid-anesthetic interactions appear highly dependent on timing (acute vs. chronic), dose, route, and baseline tolerance, all of which are addressed in the later perioperative assessment and management sections. Ketamine shows a unique profile, with limited human data suggesting THC ingestion can enhance ketamine's hypnotic effects, contrasting with the tolerance observed for GABAergic agents (Echeverria-Villalobos et al., 2025). However, evidence remains limited and should be interpreted cautiously.

Pharmacodynamic Interactions and Safety Considerations

Beyond metabolism, cannabis and anesthetic agents share overlapping pharmacodynamic effects that can influence perioperative safety and drug titration – particularly as a function of the timing of the last use, route (inhaled versus ingested), and whether the patient has acutely used or regularly uses cannabis. As an overview, these considerations include:

- **Neurocognitive impairment and consent capacity:** Acute cannabis use can produce altered mental status and impaired decision-making capacity; therefore, the frequency and timing of last use are clinically important. Elective procedures should be postponed when impairment is present (Alexander & Joshi, 2019; King et al., 2023b; Shah et al., 2023; Sladkey et al., 2025).
- **Central nervous system and respiratory depression:** Cannabinoids can produce clinically meaningful additive effects with sedatives and analgesics, increasing risk for impaired arousal and ventilation, especially in the presence of opioids. In a controlled volunteer study with administered THC intravenously (a research route to standardize dosing), co-administration with opioids was associated with lower oxygen saturation and greater sedation with further reductions in ventilation and carbon dioxide-mediated ventilatory responses. A nonjudgmental and complete preoperative medication history can help clinicians anticipate cumulative sedative burden and monitor closely for compromise (Flanagan, 2021; Goyal et al., 2017; Shah et al., 2023).
- **Cardiovascular effects:** THC commonly causes dose-related tachycardia, modest vasodilation in the awake state, and increases cardiac index. Smoking cannabis can elevate heart rate and blood pressure, most prominently within the first 1-2 hours, and may be temporally associated with a higher risk of perioperative acute myocardial infarction, with guidelines recommending delaying elective surgery for at least 2 hours after smoking (Goyal et al., 2017; Health Canada, 2018; King et al., 2023b; Shah et al., 2023). In broader literature, CUD has been associated with higher odds of postoperative MI and stroke, and acute postoperative cardiovascular events (MI, arrhythmias, stroke, cardiac arrest, cardiomyopathy) have been reported (Huson et al., 2018; Jeffers et al., 2024; Shah et al., 2023). At the same time, chronic users under general anesthesia may exhibit relative hemodynamic stability and reduced vasopressor requirements, likely due to vascular CB1 down-regulation and altered autonomic tone (Yeung et al., 2022). Still, hemodynamic effects are not uniformly protective, as one systematic review and meta-analysis of perioperative cannabinoid compounds used as adjuncts for acute postoperative pain found that cannabinoids were associated with increased odds of postoperative hypotension (Abdallah et al., 2020).
- **Pulmonary/airway effects and respiratory adverse events:** Cannabis smoking may have deleterious effects on airway resistance and a moderate impact on perioperative respiratory adverse events. Long-term exposure can be associated with alterations in pulmonary function and respiratory physiology relevant to intraoperative and postoperative ventilation planning. Cannabis smoke raises similar concerns for airway and ventilatory management as tobacco (Shah et al., 2023; Tetrault et al., 2007).

From a practical perspective, acute THC effects that alter neurobehavioral and cognitive status should prompt postponement of elective procedures until autonomous decision-making capacity is fully restored, if possible. For patients who have smoked cannabis, elective surgery should be delayed for a minimum of 2 hours, given the temporal association with increased cardiovascular risk. If surgery is unavoidable (emergent), consideration should be given to adjusting induction and maintenance dosing based on clinical presentation and the timing of the last use, and maintaining heightened vigilance in hemodynamic and respiratory monitoring, with readiness to secure the airway and effectively manage ventilatory patterns and ensuing complications. In contrast, chronic daily users often require higher induction and maintenance doses of GABAergic agents in the absence of acute use, though evidence remains limited; dose titration should be individualized rather than protocolized (King et al., 2023b; Shah et al., 2023).

PREANESTHESIA AND PREPROCEDURAL CANNABIS SCREENING AND ASSESSMENT

Preanesthesia assessment is often the first—and sometimes the only—opportunity to understand a patient's cannabis history and its potential impact, if any, on anesthesia care. Although stigma and communication barriers (addressed later in this chapter) can limit disclosure, a structured, nonjudgmental assessment improves the completeness and clinical usefulness of the history. To date, efforts to link preoperative cannabinoid exposure with perioperative outcomes have been limited by inconsistent documentation of product type, THC/CBD composition (when known), chemovar profile, dose, route, frequency, and timing of last use. This is further complicated by variability in product labeling and the use of unregulated products, where cannabinoid content may be uncertain. Without a structured assessment approach, key details are often missing or reduced to a nonspecific "substance use: yes/no" entry in the medical record.

Both the American Society for Regional Anesthesia and Pain Medicine (ASRA) (Shah et al., 2023) and the American Association of Nurse Anesthesiology (AANA) (King et al., 2023b) now recommend universal, standardized preanesthesia screening for cannabinoids based on patient history for all patients undergoing procedures under anesthesia. Importantly, this recommendation is not synonymous with universal toxicology testing. ASRA advises that preanesthesia clinicians routinely ask about the type of cannabis or cannabinoid product, time of last use, route of administration, amount, and frequency of use (Shah et al., 2023). AANA's clinical practice considerations similarly recommend documenting the pattern of substance use (dose, frequency, route, duration), time of last use, and related pain experiences as part of a complete preanesthesia evaluation (King et al., 2023b). These guidance documents promote a clinical shift that supports better risk stratification and documentation while remaining patient-centric.

Cannabis Use and Behaviors Assessment Tool (CUBAT)

To implement these recommendations, Sladkey, King, and Reede (2025) developed the Cannabis Use and Behaviors Assessment Tool (CUBAT; Table 3), an evidence-informed preanesthesia cannabis assessment tool developed through a multistage modified Delphi consensus process to establish content validity, with psychometric validation as a future direction. The process distilled the tool into seven core assessment items, along with instructions for use and a glossary of terms. The tool is designed to serve as a conversational guide, not a checklist handed to the patient. Before asking about cannabis, clinicians are instructed to briefly explain – in neutral, nonjudgmental language – that the information is protected under usual health privacy practices and used to develop the safest possible anesthesia and analgesia plan.

Table 3. Cannabis Use and Behaviors Assessment Tool (CUBAT).

CUBAT Domain	Clinical Question	Anesthesia Relevance
Recent Use	"Have you used cannabis, in any form, within the last month?"	Establishes current exposure risk and aligns with ASRA/AANA universal screening recommendations
Frequency of Use	"How often do you typically use cannabis?"	Higher frequency is associated with tolerance, withdrawal risk, and altered anesthetic requirements
Route of Administration	"What are primary ways you consume cannabis?"	Helps anticipate airway/pulmonary considerations (smoked/vaped) and delayed/prolonged effects (oral)
Timing of Last Use	"When was the last time you used cannabis?"	Critical for identifying possible acute impairment, myocardial risk, and planning timing/ appropriateness of elective anesthesia
Potency/THC-CBD Content (if known)	"Can you describe the concentration/contents of the cannabis you consume?"	High-potency THC may increase cardiovascular and psychotropic risks; unknown composition increases uncertainty in perioperative planning
Reason for Use	"Are there any specific reasons you use cannabis? If so, what are they?"	Identifies underlying symptom burden and guides perioperative analgesia planning; may identify patients at higher risk for postoperative pain and opioid needs
Adverse Effects or Withdrawal	"Have you ever experienced a bad reaction/withdrawal from cannabis?"	Screens for withdrawal risk and CHS; supports planning for postoperative monitoring and management

Note. *Content has been refined for perioperative relevance; tool domains preserved. Source: Sladkey et al., 2025.*

The seven CUBAT items are presented in a table and systematically cover: (1) any cannabis use in the past month; (2) frequency of use; (3) primary routes of administration; (4) timing of last use; (5) THC/CBD content or potency; (6) reasons for use (medical, recreational, or both); and (7) previous adverse reactions or withdrawal. Collectively, these items encompass the aspects of cannabis exposure most likely to influence airway reactivity, hemodynamics, anesthetic and analgesic needs, PONV, and the risk of cannabis withdrawal or cannabinoid hyperemesis in the perioperative period. In addition to exposure history, clinicians should assess for acute impairment of the patient's decision-making capacity as part of routine perioperative safety and informed consent considerations.

Importantly, how clinicians ask questions may be as important as what they ask. Stigma—encompassing anticipated, perceived, enacted, and internalized stigma—is linked to nondisclosure of cannabis use (King et al., 2024). Patients may withhold information out of fear of judgment, documentation or labeling, legal consequences, or cancellation of procedures. The CUBAT was intentionally written in neutral, non-stigmatizing language and emphasizes a collaborative approach ("help me understand how you're using cannabis so we can keep you safe") rather than a policing approach ("you aren't using any drugs, are you?"). Expert panel feedback during CUBAT development stressed the importance of pairing the tool with provider education and broader stigma-reduction strategies to encourage disclosure and build trust.

In practice, a brief preanesthesia interview might begin with a normalizing opener such as, "Many people use cannabis or CBD products for pain, sleep, or other reasons. I'm going to ask a few questions so we can plan our anesthesia as safely as possible." The clinician then walks through the CUBAT items, using open-ended prompts and clarifying follow-up questions, and records responses in the preanesthesia record. Objective toxicology testing is not recommended for routine screening and is used only when acute intoxication is suspected, the history is unreliable, and the results will immediately alter or influence the anesthesia plan. This is consistent with ASRA's guidance that universal toxicology testing is not necessary.

Because CUBAT was developed through expert consensus, its primary value is to standardize the minimal essential dataset for perioperative cannabis assessment, disclosure, workflow burden, and patient-centered outcomes (Sladkey et al., 2025). The chapter can therefore present CUBAT as a first-of-its-kind, consensus-based framework that operationalizes ASRA and AANA recommendations and represents a promising yet evolving best practice for cannabis assessment in anesthesia care.

Minimum Preanesthesia Documentation Fields

To ensure comprehensive preanesthesia assessment and individualized anesthesia care planning, in accordance with AANA Standards 2 and 5 (American Association of Nurse Anesthesiology, 2019), AANA practice considerations for patients with substance use disorders (American Association of Nurse Anesthesiology, 2023), and ASRA Pain Medicine consensus guidance (Shah et al., 2023), the following seven fields should be documented in the preanesthesia record when cannabis use is disclosed: (1) product type and primary cannabinoid (THC-dominant, CBD-dominant, balanced, or unknown); (2) primary route(s) of administration (smoked, vaped, oral/edible, sublingual, topical); (3) frequency of use (daily, several times per week, weekly or less, occasional); (4) timing of last use (hours or days since last use, by route if multiple); (5) approximate dose or potency, if known (e.g., mg THC per edible dose, percentage THC in flower); (6) stated reason for use (medical symptom management, recreational use, or both, and, if medical, the symptom(s) being treated); (7) impairment assessment result (capacity intact, capacity impaired, or assessment deferred, with rationale documented). These fields correspond directly to the CUBAT domains and align with ASRA and AANA documentation guidance (American Association of Nurse Anesthesiology, 2019, 2023; Shah et al., 2023; Sladkey et al., 2025).

Drug Screening

Urine (and most serum) cannabinoid testing is not recommended for routine preanesthesia screening. These tests primarily detect THC or carboxy-THC, and a positive result does not indicate dose, route, timing of use, or clinical impairment. Detection can persist for days to weeks, depending on frequency of use and individual factors, so results often remain positive long after clinically meaningful impairment has resolved. Additionally, available toxicology tests do not reliably determine current intoxication or decision-making capacity, further limiting their perioperative utility unless results will immediately change management. More importantly, routine screening should be history-based, with toxicology testing reserved for clinical concerns. Recent perioperative work also shows that preoperative THC urine testing is common in some systems despite evidence-based guidance, reinforcing the need to prioritize structured history over default testing with unsubstantiated costs, time, and documentation. In short: a positive THC test is evidence of exposure, not directly a perioperative risk score, and not routinely an important test; the history and bedside clinical assessment remain the most actionable tools for anesthetic planning and consent (Connors et al., 2020; Raghunathan et al., 2025; Shah et al., 2023).

An important clinical distinction is frequently obscured in the perioperative literature: administrative CUD coding and self-reported cannabis use are often treated as interchangeable exposure variables, yet they represent meaningfully different patient populations. CUD involves a threshold that the majority of medicinal and recreational consumers do not meet. Because this distinction carries real consequences for withdrawal risk stratification, analgesic planning, and the interpretation of published outcomes data, clinicians should document which category applies when the history supports it (American Psychiatric Association, 2022; Shah et al., 2023).

Informed Consent

Informed consent should be guided by decision-making capacity and not by cannabis use alone. Before obtaining informed consent, the patient's neurocognitive status should be evaluated and documented as part of routine practice. Acute cannabis effects can include alterations in cognition, perception, and psychomotor performance, which may impair the ability to provide informed consent. When patients demonstrate altered mental status or impaired decision-making capacity consistent with acute intoxication, elective procedures should be postponed when feasible, and consent deferred until capacity is restored. Clinically, cues that may raise concern for acute cannabis intoxication or impairment include marked anxiety or agitation, paranoia, hallucinations or psychosis, impaired attention or short-term memory, disorganized thinking, and psychomotor slowing. These findings should prompt a focused capacity assessment and clear documentation of decision-making ability (Shah et al., 2023). Documentation of impairment assessment should use neutral, clinically descriptive language. For example: 'Patient demonstrates altered attention and impaired short-term recall consistent with acute cannabis effect; decision-making capacity deferred per clinical assessment. Elective procedure postponed pending capacity reassessment.' Avoid inferential or pejorative labels such as 'intoxicated,' 'high,' or 'altered' without paired clinical observations.

As a cannabis-specific addition to routine consent discussions, clinicians should incorporate the patient's reported exposure pattern (especially the timing of the last use and product potency, when known) into perioperative risk communication – particularly when it may influence anesthetic or analgesic requirements, postoperative pain and opioid requirements, and PONV risk, among others (Ekrami et al., 2024; Shah et al., 2023; Suhre et al., 2020).

Clinical Scenario Framework

Because cannabis-related perioperative risk varies substantially by recency, route, and pattern of use, clinical decision-making is best anchored in the patient's specific exposure scenario rather than a generalized 'cannabis user' designation. The framework in Table 4 organizes key management considerations by scenario. This is intended to be a decision-support tool rather than a rigid protocol and should be applied alongside individualized clinical judgment.

Table 4. Perioperative management considerations by clinical scenario

Clinical Scenario	Key Perioperative Considerations	Primary Actions
Acute intoxication at time of scheduled procedure	Impaired consent capacity; unpredictable anesthetic interaction; hemodynamic instability risk	Postpone elective procedure. Document capacity assessment. If emergent: heightened hemodynamic and airway vigilance; titrate carefully to effect.
Recent smoked (within 2 hours)	Elevated perioperative MI risk window; airway irritability; tachycardia possible	Delay elective surgery at least 2 hours per ASRA guidance. If emergent: continuous cardiac monitoring; readiness for bronchospasm.
Chronic daily use, no acute intoxication	Possible CB1 downregulation/cross-tolerance; CWS risk with inpatient abstinence; sensitized pain phenotype risk; PONV modifier	Individualized dose titration — do not assume higher requirements; proactive multimodal analgesia; CWS monitoring scale; deliberate PONV prophylaxis.
Cannabis withdrawal state at presentation	Irritability, insomnia, anxiety, restlessness, nausea may amplify pain perception and complicate recovery; may mimic or worsen surgical pain	Validate withdrawal with Cannabis Withdrawal Scale. Mild-moderate: supportive care. Severe: consider dronabinol per consensus guidance. Consult addiction medicine or psychiatry for refractory cases.
Edible/oral use only (no inhalation)	No acute airway irritant concern; delayed and prolonged absorption; delayed gastric emptying possible even with NPO compliance	Lower aspiration threshold in heavy daily edible users; avoid stacking doses; no airway-specific precautions beyond standard practice.

Note. *Scenarios are not mutually exclusive; patients may present with combinations (e.g., chronic daily inhalational use currently in withdrawal). Apply individualized clinical judgment. Actions are consistent with ASRA Pain Medicine consensus guidance (Shah et al., 2023) and PAIN Consensus Recommendations (Ladha et al., 2021).*

PERIOPERATIVE RISKS AND ANESTHETIC CONSIDERATIONS

Cardiovascular

The cardiovascular effects of THC are dose- and time-dependent, often biphasic: acute exposure tends to produce sympathetic predominance (tachycardia ± increased blood pressure), whereas chronic exposure or tolerance may shift toward less pronounced sympathetic responses and, in some contexts, greater parasympathetic influence. Clinically, the perioperative relevance is greatest in the immediate post-use window, when smoked cannabis can produce tachycardia and increased cardiac workload within minutes, peaking over the first 1–2 hours and persisting for several hours in some individuals. This period has also been associated with an increased risk of myocardial infarction shortly after use in observational data (Latif & Garg, 2020; Mittleman et al., 2001).

Older controlled human data help illustrate the "ends" of this physiologic spectrum. In an oral surgery cohort receiving IV Δ9-THC, Gregg et al. (1976) reported dose-related tachycardia and a predisposition to syncopal hypotension shortly after administration, highlighting that acute THC can produce both tachycardia and hemodynamic instability in susceptible patients. In contrast, more contemporary procedural-sedation cohorts have not consistently revealed meaningful differences in mean arterial pressure between those who use cannabis and those who do not (King et al., 2021; Gangwani et al., 2023; Shah et al., 2023).

In the perioperative setting, surgical stress elicits sympathetic nervous system responses, including selective beta-adrenergic stimulation. Increased circulating catecholamines, heightened myocardial demand, and compounded surgical stress can predispose patients to myocardial events. Potential contributors include sympathetic stimulation, increased myocardial oxygen demand, and (when smoked) combustion-related factors (e.g., carboxyhemoglobin) that may worsen oxygen supply-demand mismatch. Case-crossover data suggest a transiently increased risk of MI onset shortly after cannabis use, with the highest relative risk in the first hour and rapid decline thereafter (Mittleman et al., 2001). Consensus guidance similarly notes that within one hour after smoking, MI onset risk is elevated, and that the relative risk declines in the second hour (though it does not vanish completely), supporting time-sensitive perioperative decision-making (Shah et al., 2023).

In a large propensity-matched cohort (Goel et al., 2020), CUD was associated with nearly a twofold increase in the odds of postoperative myocardial infarction (aOR 1.88), and meta-analytic data from arthroplasty populations report a similar magnitude of increased risk of cardiac complications (Cheng et al., 2024). Notably, the risk signal appears to be modified by baseline cardiac risk. Recreational cannabis use accompanied by low baseline risk did not show an increased incidence of major adverse cardiac and cerebrovascular events, whereas those with higher baseline cardiac risk did (Ashrafian et al., 2025).

A more recent matched cohort study of major elective inpatient noncardiac surgery likewise found that CUD was associated with increased perioperative morbidity and mortality (Potnuru et al., 2023), reinforcing the value of identifying higher-risk use patterns during perioperative assessment. Meta-analytic and procedure-specific studies (including arthroplasty and other surgical cohorts) suggest a similar magnitude of increased risk of cardiac complications in some populations, though findings remain vulnerable to confounding. There is also evidence linking CUD to higher adjusted odds of postoperative acute cerebrovascular events, perioperative myocardial infarction (MI), and stroke (Shah et al., 2023). In vulnerable patients, the risk of death from myocardial infarction may be increased 2.5-4-fold (Pacher et al.,

2018). Contemporary cardiovascular epidemiology continues to report associations between cannabis use and myocardial infarction and stroke risk at the population level, supporting continued caution in surgical candidates with elevated baseline cardiovascular risk (Jeffers et al., 2024).

From an intraoperative management perspective, arrhythmia data are generally reassuring when confounding factors (especially tobacco) are accounted for (Barkay et al., 2023; Kumar et al., 2024; Shanthanna et al., 2021; Zhang et al., 2021). Limited studies assessing vasopressor or inotropic requirements have not found significant differences between participants who use cannabis and controls (Kumar et al., 2024; Sohail et al., 2025). Short-duration, low-stress procedures (including endoscopy) similarly report low rates of major cardiovascular complications regardless of cannabis status (Gangwani et al., 2023; King et al., 2021).

Because acute inhalation can transiently increase heart rate and blood pressure, and has been linked to perioperative MI risk soon after use, the ASRA Pain Medicine perioperative cannabis guidelines and the AANA recommend delaying elective surgery for at least two hours after smoking and postponing elective procedures when patients have an altered mental status from intoxication (King et al., 2023b; Shah et al., 2023). There are insufficient data to recommend a specific delay period for non-smoked cannabinoid use, and a risk-benefit analysis should be conducted alongside risk counseling.

In addition to myocardial risk, thromboembolic signals have been reported across several surgical populations (e.g., increased deep vein thrombosis (DVT) after total hip/knee arthroplasty; higher thromboembolism odds in spine surgery cohorts), and a post-percutaneous coronary intervention dataset reported elevated stroke risk. Surgery and general anesthesia induce a procoagulatory state, and emerging evidence suggests that cannabis use may further modify thrombotic risk in specific perioperative populations. These findings remain vulnerable to confounding but are difficult to ignore when caring for high-risk patients. Such thromboembolic and cardiovascular risk deserves explicit consideration during preoperative risk stratification, particularly for surgical candidates with known vascular disease or multiple cardiovascular risk factors (Barkay et al., 2023; Chiu et al., 2021; Hoveidaei et al., 2024; Lu et al., 2023; Shah et al., 2023; Yoo et al., 2020).

Respiratory

Rare but high-stakes respiratory complications related to inhaled cannabis include diffuse alveolar hemorrhage (DAH) and uvular edema, both of which warrant a lower threshold for postoperative vigilance – particularly when the exposure history includes smoking/vaping or very recent use. The broader perioperative respiratory theme in the literature is more familiar: airway irritation, bronchial hyperreactivity, and obstruction, with bronchospasm repeatedly flagged as a recognized concern in narrative reviews and clinical guidance. This pattern persists even though primary perioperative studies have not produced clean incidence estimates for bronchospasm, laryngospasm, difficult ventilation, intubation, or other discrete airway events attributable to cannabis alone. To add nuance, acute THC exposure may cause bronchodilation, but cannabis smoking or aerosolized THC can also irritate airways and trigger bronchoconstriction in susceptible patients (e.g., those with reactive airway disease), and the evidence remains low quality overall (Echeverria-Villalobos et al., 2019; Scheuerman et al., 2025; Shah et al., 2023).

Isolated case reports describe DAH after cannabis smoking and, less commonly, in the perioperative period, presenting with dyspnea, hemoptysis, hypoxemia, and acute respiratory failure. Published studies often describe acute shortness of breath and hemoptysis within hours of cannabis use and include DAH among severe pulmonary complications, including in the context of vaping-associated lung injury. Proposed mechanisms include injury at the alveolar–capillary interface (with increased permeability and bleeding), sometimes in the setting of intense coughing or airway irritation after heavy smoking or vaping. In postoperative patients, clinicians should also consider whether upper-airway obstruction events (e.g., biting, laryngospasm/partial obstruction) could contribute via negative-pressure phenomena that may complicate presentation. Primary case findings support DAH as a rare but potentially life-threatening condition. Treatment is primarily supportive and diagnostic: oxygenation and ventilation as needed, early imaging, and consideration of bronchoscopy with bronchoalveolar lavage to establish a diagnosis and exclude alternative etiologies. Steroids are reported in case management, but evidence is limited to case-level data; therefore, escalation should be individualized and coordinated with colleagues in pulmonology and critical care. Importantly, DAH can be fatal, and early recognition during the early postoperative care period is essential (Alqahtani et al., 2019; Shafi et al., 2018; Shah et al., 2023).

Multiple isolated case reports describe uvular edema (uvulitis) after cannabis inhalation, including perioperative airway compromise. Classic anesthesia literature highlights cannabis-related uvular edema as a postoperative airway concern (Mallat et al., 1996; Boyce & Quigley, 2002). In the immediate postoperative period, the practical fear is clear: partial or complete airway obstruction that may require urgent airway support, including intubation. Onset ranges from soon after smoking to several hours later, though the risk appears greatest after heavy inhalational exposure. If obstruction or irritation precipitates bronchospasm, treatment with bronchodilation (e.g., an inhaled beta-agonist) and systemic steroids is reasonable. Dosing strategies in the case literature include dexamethasone (0.1 mg/kg every 6-12 hours for 1-2 days) for the uvular edema component. Case reports also describe the use of antihistamines with symptom resolution. Because the evidence base is case level, no universal prophylactic regimen can be recommended. Instead, emphasis is on anticipation (recent heavy smoking), early recognition (muffled voice, drooling, stridor, dysphagia), and readiness for airway intervention (Mallat et al., 1996; Boyce & Quigley, 2002).

Vaped cannabis products introduce an additional hazard profile, with multiple reports of vaping-related lung injury, including among THC-containing products. E-cigarette or vaping product use-associated lung injury (EVALI) has been linked to severe pathologies such as acute eosinophilic pneumonia, diffuse alveolar hemorrhage, lipoid pneumonia, and respiratory bronchiolitis (interstitial lung disease), often attributed to additives or contaminants (e.g., vitamin E acetate) rather than cannabinoids alone. Obliterative (or constrictive) bronchiolitis, also known as "popcorn lung," is classically associated with inhalational exposure to diacetyl (buttery flavoring) in occupational settings. E-cigarette research has detected diacetyl and related flavoring chemicals in many flavored vaping liquids, raising concern about potential risk, though confirmed clinical cases attributable specifically to vaping exposures remain uncommon. In the perioperative period, this should be considered a high-stakes, low-frequency consideration, particularly in patients with chronic vaping histories, unexplained obstructive symptoms, or prior vaping-related lung injury (Allen et al., 2016; Landman et al., 2019; Shah et al., 2023).

In broader, heterogeneous perioperative studies, the evidence is mixed and heavily context-dependent. Chronic inhalational cannabis exposure is associated with obstructive lung disease patterns, including chronic bronchitis symptoms and airflow obstruction in large airways. Increased airway resistance is also observed, even when classic spirometric obstruction is not clearly demonstrated (Huson et al., 2018; Shah et al., 2023).

In high-risk surgical populations (e.g., aortic surgery, spine surgery, burn care), CUD has been associated with approximately 1.2- to 2.4-fold higher odds of respiratory complications, including respiratory failure and pneumonia (Bernal et al., 2024; Chiu et al., 2021). In contrast, shorter or lower-risk procedures (e.g., gastroscopy) often do not result in adverse respiratory events (Ekrami et al., 2024; King et al., 2021). The primary interpretive challenge is tobacco co-use. When analyses control for tobacco, previously observed increases in hypoxia are attenuated or no longer significant, making it difficult to isolate cannabis-only risk (Barkay et al., 2023; Stefani et al., 2020). An exception is Chiu et al. (2021), who explicitly controlled for comorbid tobacco use and still found increased respiratory complications (OR 2.0).

Careful assessment and clinical preparedness are the first steps to safe airway management. Limited outcomes evidence still supports vigilance. At a high level, patients using only oral cannabinoids generally do not require ventilatory setting adjustments. Consider ventilatory adjustments in the setting of chronic inhalational use, especially those with comorbid pulmonary risk, because obstructive patterns may be present. Currently, insufficient evidence exists to guide changes in ventilation after acute inhalational exposure (Shah et al., 2023).

Bullae and pneumothorax have been reported in association with cannabis smoking, though causality remains uncertain. Combined cannabis and tobacco use increases the risk of pneumothorax. Chronic inhalational cannabis use is repeatedly associated with chronic bronchitis symptoms (cough, sputum, wheeze), airway obstruction, and bronchial hyperreactivity (Shah et al., 2023). Thus, some reviews advise avoiding cannabis for 72 hours of general anesthesia or longer (Huson et al., 2018). However, this is a pragmatic recommendation, as timing data are rarely captured in primary studies.

Ensuring an adequate plane of anesthesia before airway instrumentation is essential, with consideration of drug cross-tolerance and measures to mitigate airway reactivity (Flisberg et al., 2009). Although increased propofol doses may be required, a case series describes propofol-associated hypersalivation in participants with chronic cannabis exposure, which is an intuitive setup for secretion burden, laryngospasm, and aspiration risk dynamics (Derise et al., 2022). Given the inhalational airway-irritant profile, this chapter can explicitly recommend: (1) documenting smoked vs vaped vs oral route; (2) clarifying the timing of the last inhalation; (3) heightened readiness for bronchospasm or airway obstruction in the setting of chronic inhalational use and for those with reactive airway disease; and (4) post-anesthesia care unit (PACU) vigilance for hemoptysis, hypoxemia, stridor, or rapidly evolving upper-airway obstruction in patients with very recent heavy inhalational exposure (Shah et al., 2023).

Gastrointestinal

For patients who smoke (including cannabis), clinicians should anticipate oral findings, such as nicotinic stomatitis and gingival enlargement, which may have implications for airway management and may predispose to bleeding during oropharyngeal manipulation or instrumentation. This supports a practical nursing approach that includes documenting baseline dentition, using atraumatic suctioning, and maintaining a low threshold for protecting vulnerable teeth or inflamed mucosa, especially when approaching laryngoscopy (Liu et al., 2020; Shah et al., 2023).

Gastric emptying and motility are clinically relevant because the gut has extensive CB1 receptor regulation; when cannabinoids bind to these receptors, acetylcholine release is inhibited. Clinically, this can manifest as delayed gastric emptying and intestinal motility. Clinical evidence suggests delayed gastric emptying of approximately 30 minutes to 2 hours beyond the normal range, although perioperative, procedure-specific evidence remains limited. Clinical signals indicate that delayed gastric emptying can be clinically meaningful and may be present even when patients are asymptomatic. This may warrant aspiration precautions, even when patients are compliant with nil per os (NPO) guidelines. In the perioperative literature, direct evidence is limited largely to case reports, but it is meaningful: one report described a patient who used cannabis daily, fasted overnight, yet had substantial gastric contents encountered immediately after airway placement during induction, despite denying preoperative symptoms of hyperemesis (Cammarano & Villaluz, 2021). Taken together, this does not revise fasting guidelines but supports a lower threshold for aspiration precautions in patients reporting heavy daily use, particularly when other risk factors are present. In higher-risk patients, consider standard aspiration-risk mitigation consistent with standard practice (e.g., nonparticulate antacid and/or H2 blocker per protocol) and a protected airway approach (including rapid sequence intubation when indicated) based on overall risk assessment rather than cannabis exposure alone. Gastric point-of-care ultrasound (POCUS) may be used to stratify the presence of gastric contents (Shah et al., 2023).

Although some patients use cannabis for nausea because of its antiemetic properties, it has not been proven reliably effective in preventing PONV. In fact, daily cannabis use has been associated with a modest increase in PONV of approximately 20% (relative increase risk) in some analyses, whereas non-daily use shows a smaller, less convincing association (Suhre et al., 2020). Importantly, these findings are heterogeneous across studies: some show no difference, while others show the opposite trend. Accordingly, the most defensible takeaway is to avoid assuming cannabis will cover PONV risk and instead plan prophylaxis deliberately when daily use is known.

Overuse and/or abrupt withdrawal of cannabis have also been associated with a hyperemesis syndrome. CHS is a unique phenomenon characterized by abrupt withdrawal or, more commonly, long-term, high-frequency cannabis use. It typically occurs in patients younger than fifty years of age, and symptoms include severe, cyclical nausea and vomiting, flushing, diaphoresis, and weight loss. Perioperatively, CHS matters because it can present as refractory, unresponsive to standard antiemetic therapy, with features such as compulsory relief with hot bathing and clinical resolution tied to cannabis cessation rather than escalating medication strategies. This association may relieve symptoms because heat activates transient receptor potential vanilloid 1 (TRPV1) receptors and triggers the release of substance P, which may modulate nausea pathways (Shah et al., 2023). It is also described as underrecognized in perioperative settings because symptoms may be misattributed to anesthetic effects, opioids, or surgical complications, delaying appropriate management and leading to unnecessary workups (Atkins et al., 2025). The vague symptomatology of nausea and vomiting may prompt gastroscopy studies, though cannabinoid use may not be well-stratified during the workup. When CHS is suspected perioperatively, recent systematic reviews support considering therapies beyond traditional antiemetics (e.g., topical capsaicin and dopamine antagonists such as droperidol or haloperidol), alongside IV fluids, electrolyte correction, and counseling that cessation is definitive treatment (Pourmand et al., 2021; Sabbineni et al., 2024).

Finally, in endoscopy populations, where gastrointestinal symptoms intersect most directly, several studies have evaluated whether cannabis exposure alters sedation requirements (Baker et al., 2025; King et al., 2021; Twardowski et al., 2019). Recent meta-analytic evidence indicates a directional trend toward higher propofol requirements, with a frequency-related pattern in which daily cannabis use is associated with higher requirements than weekly or monthly use, while emphasizing heterogeneity in exposure definitions (Bornemann-Cimenti et al., 2025). Other studies found no significant differences (King et al., 2021) or reported that differences attenuated after adjusting for procedural duration (Imasogie et al., 2021; Loeb et al., 2025). Mixed human evidence warrants caution, as observed differences may be confounded by procedural sedation and variability in provider dosing. Given this variability and inconsistent exposure definitions across studies, the bedside implication is less about a singular dosing strategy and more about properly identifying cannabis-exposed patients, assessing for daily use, and anticipating that sedation needs may require increased titration and persistent vigilance.

Thermoregulation

General anesthesia is well known to alter hypothalamic regulation of body temperature and contribute to vasodilation, necessitating active warming strategies, particularly within the first 30-60 minutes after induction. Heat loss in the standard operating room occurs primarily through radiation, followed by convection, with contributions from evaporation and conduction. Limited studies have evaluated the role of cannabis use in perioperative thermoregulation, with limited comparator data and heterogeneous exposure across studies. Based on the available evidence, cannabis use appears to be associated with a trend toward increased postoperative hypothermia (Echeverria-Villalobos et al., 2019) and increased postoperative shivering incidence and severity (Sankar-Maharaj et al., 2018). However, when it comes to postoperative shivering, there is an overall paucity of high-quality perioperative data, and statistical analyses to evaluate these findings are further limited (Shah et al., 2023). For example, a prospective observational study reported higher shivering incidence and intensity among patients who use cannabis but did not establish a statistically significant difference (Sankar-Maharaj et al., 2018).

The ECS regulates temperature through central control via CB1 receptors in the hypothalamus. The ECS fine-tunes neuronal communication and feedback loops to regulate temperature (Wenger & Moldrich, 2002). The mechanistic basis for altered temperature regulation in patients who use cannabis involves CB1 receptor agonism-mediated changes in central thermoregulatory set points and autonomic output, with potential amplification by anesthetic-induced vasodilation and redistribution hypothermia (Echeverria-Villalobos et al., 2019; Shah et al., 2023). High-dose cannabinoids often decrease heat production, whereas low doses can sometimes increase body temperature (Wenger & Moldrich, 2002). Furthermore, temperature effects related to CB1 agonism, particularly with chronic, high-quantity use, may be reversible in preclinical models through CB1 receptor antagonism and inverse agonism (Pryce & Baker, 2017; Shah et al., 2023). The clinical significance of these temperature-related findings remains uncertain, though given the higher incidence and severity of postoperative shivering in cannabis-exposed patients, additional clinical vigilance is suggested alongside routine core temperature monitoring and active warming strategies.

Of additional note, neuraxial opioids can lower the thermoregulatory set point and contribute to hypothermia. The combined effects of neuraxial opioids and systemic cannabinoids remain an evidence gap, and their interactive effects are unknown, warranting careful monitoring rather than assumptions of protection or harm. In addition, CBD may influence thermoregulation via TRPV1 activation (thermal sensing), although the perioperative implications remain unclear (Shah et al., 2023).

Emerging literature further links thermoregulation, skeletal muscle calcium homeostasis, and the ECS in the context of malignant hyperthermia (MH). MH is a pharmacogenetic disorder, most commonly caused by mutations in the ryanodine receptor 1 (RYR1), characterized by uncontrolled calcium release from the sarcoplasmic reticulum. This leads to hypermetabolism, muscle rigidity, and profound, life-threatening hyperthermia following exposure to triggering anesthetic agents (e.g., volatile anesthetics, succinylcholine). Preclinical and mechanistic data suggest that CB1 receptor activation modulates intracellular calcium dynamics by inhibiting protein kinase A-mediated phosphorylation of RYR1 and L-type calcium channels, thereby reducing myoplasmic calcium concentrations and muscle contractility. Additional ECS-mediated effects, including modulation of transient receptor potential vanilloid 1 (TRPV1) channels, may further attenuate calcium release and heat generation. Although these findings do not establish cannabinoids as protective or therapeutic agents in MH, they show a biologically plausible connection between cannabinoid signaling, calcium regulation, and temperature control. These scientific observations should not be interpreted as clinical prevention or treatment of MH, nor do they change standard MH preparedness or management, such as early recognition and prompt treatment with dantrolene (Dalle & Dalle, 2025).

SPECIAL PERIOPERATIVE POPULATIONS

Obstetric Care

Pregnancy and the peripartum period are times when cannabis use often shifts from a background behavior to a clinically central issue because symptoms and physiology change, and the care pathway can rapidly include procedures (labor analgesia, cesarean birth, postpartum interventions) in which cannabis exposure affects safety planning. In the peripartum literature, pregnant and postpartum patients frequently describe cannabis use as symptom-driven, most commonly for nausea and vomiting of pregnancy (NVP), sleep disruption, anxiety, and pain (Michel & King, 2025). Concerningly, cannabis smoking has been linked to intrauterine growth restriction, preterm delivery, and small-for-gestational-age status (Michel & King, 2025). Because many studies rely heavily on self-report, underreporting is common and often driven by stigma and fear of punitive consequences; clinicians also fail to ask because of limited education and training (King et al., 2024; Michel & King, 2025).

Perinatal settings are uniquely vulnerable to variability in surveillance, testing, and reporting across states and facilities (Daniels et al., 2023; Greene et al., 2023). Nurses should understand local requirements and be prepared to explain confidentiality, legal rights, and why disclosure improves safety planning (Bureau of Justice Assistance, 2023; English & Greyson, 2022; Michel & King, 2025). As nurses, the peripartum task is not to shame symptoms or minimize distress; it is to keep counseling anchored in what we know (and what we do not yet know), while supporting safer choices and coordinated care during a time of heightened vulnerability for both the pregnant person and the fetus or newborn (American College of Obstetricians and Gynecologists [ACOG], 2017; Michel & King, 2025).

A central clinical tension in obstetric care is that cannabis is commonly used for nausea, yet vomiting in pregnancy can also be the setting where cannabis-related harms are missed. A critical emerging finding is the reported association between cannabis use and NVP, which complicates the standard understanding of cannabis's antiemetic properties (Metz et al., 2022). In addition, CHS can masquerade as refractory hyperemesis in pregnant patients with chronic use, creating a cycle in which escalating cannabis use worsens symptoms rather than relieving them (Flament et al., 2020; Michel & King, 2025). In obstetric settings, CHS is not just a diagnostic nuance but a safety issue, because repeated severe vomiting increases dehydration, electrolyte imbalance risk, and urgent care utilization, and can lead to repeated exposure to medications and procedures without addressing the underlying driver. A cannabis-informed nursing assessment should explicitly ask about hot-shower/bath relief, chronicity and frequency, and prior unexplained cyclic vomiting episodes, and should avoid anchoring on cannabis as a reliable antiemetic for pregnancy-related nausea.

Mental health and sleep symptom relief are also common reasons patients report peripartum cannabis use (Michel & King, 2025). In this context, nursing care benefits from a "both/and" stance: validate what the patient is trying to manage while maintaining evidence-based honesty that perceived benefit is not equivalent to established peripartum mental health treatment. When cannabis use is heavy, escalating, or clearly functioning as a primary coping strategy, the nurse's role broadens to include screening for problematic use patterns and supporting referrals to appropriate behavioral health or substance use disorder resources, without framing the patient as irresponsible or morally failing (Holland et al., 2016; Michel & King, 2025). Importantly, best-practice screening distinguishes cannabis use from CUD and favors structured, nonjudgmental verbal screening (rather than reflexive urine or serum testing) with informed consent when testing is used (Michel & King, 2025).

The peripartum period often becomes perioperative: labor neuraxial analgesia, emergent conversion to cesarean birth, postpartum procedures, and unplanned surgery can occur rapidly. In that context, it is clinically important to recognize that neuraxial techniques (epidural/spinal anesthesia) are not automatically contraindicated solely because a patient uses cannabis; instead, the focus shifts to physiologic stability, current impairment, and coordinated planning with the anesthesia team (Michel & King, 2025; Shah et al., 2023). Consensus perioperative guidance also emphasizes structured management of patients using cannabis and cannabinoids, reinforcing that obstetric patients should be approached through a safety-planning lens rather than a punitive one (Shah et al., 2023). This includes routine assessment of bleeding risk. For nurses counseling patients who may undergo labor analgesia or cesarean birth, the practical educational message is direct: the anesthesia provider asks about cannabis use to prevent avoidable complications and optimize nausea control, hemodynamics, and postoperative pain planning, not to label or punish.

Postpartum counseling, especially during lactation, is where many patients encounter the most conflicting and stigmatized messages. Nursing care is most effective when it pairs clear, safety-forward recommendations with trauma-informed, nonjudgmental support that considers the realities of the postpartum period (e.g., sleep deprivation, pain, anxiety/depression, stress, and limited resources). Evidence shows that cannabinoids can transfer not only via the placenta but also into breast milk, raising clinical concern even as the field continues to refine understanding of downstream neurodevelopmental effects (Bertrand et al., 2018; Grant et al., 2018). THC's lipophilicity supports prolonged retention and release; persistence in breast milk can extend for days after maternal use, with exposure estimates varying by product, dose, route, and chronicity (Bertrand et al., 2018; Grant et al., 2018; Harris et al., 2023; Ryan et al., 2018). Professional guidance discourages cannabis use during lactation while emphasizing structured, compassionate counseling within the broader context of perinatal health, mental health, and individualized risk assessment (ACOG, 2017; Harris et al., 2023). Further, the Academy of Breastfeeding Medicine recommends discontinuation or reduction and emphasizes shared decision-making when patients do not stop immediately (ACOG, 2017; Ryan et al., 2018; Harris et al., 2023). In practice, the most effective nursing approach is to clearly state the safest recommendation (avoid cannabis while breastfeeding) while staying engaged with patients who are not ready or able to stop immediately, because disengagement increases risk. This sustained therapeutic alliance reduces risk and supports follow-up. This is where cannabis nursing can be most impactful: helping patients reduce exposure (e.g., avoiding smoke exposure in the infant's environment), avoid caregiving if impaired, and connect to lactation, mental health, and nonpunitive treatment and social supports, all while preserving dignity and continuity of care (Harris et al., 2023; Michel & King, 2025).

Older Adults

Older adults constitute a rapidly expanding segment of cannabis users in the United States and are disproportionately represented among surgical patients. Perioperative risk is increased by age-related pharmacokinetic changes, including reduced hepatic CYP450 activity and renal clearance, lower albumin levels affecting drug protein binding, and decreased lean body mass. These factors can prolong the duration and intensify the effects of cannabinoids and their metabolites. Polypharmacy is a significant concern, as older adults are more likely to use anticoagulants (notably warfarin, which shares CYP2C9 metabolism with THC and CBD), sedative-hypnotics, opioids, and cardiovascular medications that interact with cannabinoids. The risk of falls is heightened due to the additive cognitive and vestibular effects of cannabis combined with other central nervous system agents in the perioperative period. Disclosure barriers are also distinct in this population: older adults are more likely to use cannabis without informing healthcare providers, to seek information from dispensaries or peers rather than clinicians, and to modify or substitute prescription medications with cannabis without coordinated oversight (Abu Baker et al., 2024). Screening should be normalized and non-presumptive. Presenting cannabis as a substance commonly used by older adults for sleep, pain, or anxiety before inquiring about use helps avoid the assumption that cannabis use is primarily associated with younger individuals.

Patients with Significant Cardiovascular Comorbidity

Perioperative cardiovascular risk associated with cannabis use varies among surgical candidates. Recent evidence indicates that baseline cardiovascular risk influences the extent of cannabis-associated perioperative cardiac complications: patients with low baseline risk do not exhibit significantly increased rates of major adverse cardiac and cerebrovascular events, whereas those with preexisting coronary artery disease, atrial fibrillation, prior stroke, or multiple cardiovascular risk factors are at greater risk (Ashrafian et al., 2025). Preoperative risk stratification is essential. Patients with known cardiovascular disease or elevated Revised Cardiac Risk Index (RCRI) scores require explicit discussion of cannabis-specific cardiac risk, thorough documentation of recent use patterns, and a lower threshold for extended cardiac monitoring during and after surgery. The recommendation to delay surgery for at least two hours after cannabis smoking is particularly important in this population, as the relative risk of myocardial infarction onset is highest within the first hour after smoking (Shah et al., 2023; Mittleman et al., 2001).

Patients with Chronic Pain

Patients with chronic pain constitute one of the highest-risk groups for analgesic complexity in the perioperative setting, and cannabis use is prevalent in this population. Use is frequently medicinal, often involves high doses, and is sometimes combined with opioids or gabapentinoids. The perioperative challenge is multifactorial: preexisting central sensitization may exacerbate the proposed cannabinoid-induced hyperalgesia mechanism, resulting in additive upregulation of nociceptive signaling and amplifying acute postoperative pain beyond procedural expectations. Coexisting opioid tolerance may further narrow the therapeutic window. Preoperative cannabis use patterns should be carefully documented in chronic pain patients, including route, frequency, THC/CBD composition, and whether cannabis is used to manage the condition for which surgery is planned. Early involvement of the acute pain service or a chronic pain specialist is recommended for surgical candidates with chronic pain, daily high-THC cannabis use, and baseline opioid exposure, as this combination presents the greatest analgesic complexity in the postoperative period (King et al., 2026; Shah et al., 2023).

Cannabis and Tobacco Co-Use

Tobacco co-use occurs in a substantial minority of cannabis users and is the most significant confounding variable in the perioperative cannabis literature. Many studies associating cannabis with increased respiratory complications, hypoxia, or airway events do not adequately control for tobacco use. When tobacco co-use is considered, cannabis-attributable respiratory risk is often reduced or no longer statistically significant (Barkay et al., 2023; Stefani et al., 2020). An exception is Chiu et al. (2021), who explicitly controlled for tobacco co-use and still observed elevated odds of respiratory complications (OR 2.0), providing stronger evidence for an independent cannabis effect. In clinical practice, patients who co-use cannabis and tobacco should be assessed for cumulative airway risk, as combined inhalational exposure increases chronic bronchitis symptoms, airway hyperreactivity, and mucociliary dysfunction beyond the effects of either substance alone. Airway management planning and PACU monitoring should address this additive risk. When interpreting published findings for patient counseling, clinicians should determine whether the source study accounted for tobacco use, as this significantly influences the attribution of risk to cannabis versus combined inhalational exposure.

POSTOPERATIVE PAIN AND OPIOID STEWARDSHIP

While cannabis is widely accepted by patients and many clinical advocates for its analgesic properties, perioperative evidence increasingly points to a paradoxical outcome: potentially worse acute postoperative pain and variable (often higher) opioid requirements among those who regularly use cannabis. ASRA Pain Medicine consensus guidance similarly provides evidence of increased postoperative pain and opioid requirements, although of low certainty (Shah et al., 2023). Together, these findings may reflect a sensitized pain phenotype and/or proposed cannabis-induced hyperalgesia in some patients who use cannabis frequently or at high-THC doses or concentrations, particularly in the acute postoperative window (King et al., 2026). This section integrates basic receptor pharmacology, translational data from preclinical models, and perioperative clinical outcomes to explain why some cannabis-exposed patients experience this phenomenon, while others do not (King et al., 2026).

Cannabis engages multiple receptor systems, including the canonical CB1/CB2 G-protein-coupled receptors (GPCRs) and ionotropic TRP channels. In acute exposure, CB1 signaling predominates, producing analgesia by inhibiting adenylyl cyclase and reducing neurotransmitter release, including glutamate signaling. In chronic cannabis use, however, receptor desensitization, internalization, and altered crosstalk (interaction between signaling pathways) with TRPV receptors can disrupt this balance (King et al., 2026). The perioperative setting magnifies the problem: surgical injury, inflammatory mediators, and anesthetic drugs converge on sensitized nociceptive pathways. Thus, the paradox may reflect neuroadaptations in cannabinoid-related signaling that interact with surgical inflammation and perioperative pharmacology;

however, causal pathways in humans remain incompletely defined, and available perioperative data are heterogeneous and often confounded by baseline differences (e.g., chronic pain, opioid use) (Shah et al., 2023).

Cannabinoid-Opioid Interactions

Regarding analgesic synergy, preclinical evidence supports cannabinoid-opioid interactions, with cannabinoid exposure shifting opioid dose. In preclinical models, THC has shifted opioid dose-response curves (e.g., reducing morphine ED50), supporting biologic plausibility for cannabinoid-opioid interactions; however, this has not translated into a consistent opioid-sparing effect in acute perioperative human studies (Echeverria-Villalobos et al., 2019, 2025; Nielsen et al., 2017). However, a synthesis of the evidence indicates that any opioid-sparing signal described in chronic pain contexts is not apparent in acute pain settings, and perioperative human data do not reliably demonstrate an opioid-sparing effect (Shah et al., 2023). Specific mechanistic hypotheses include cannabinoid-induced dynorphin release at the spinal level, as intrathecal THC induced immunoreactive dynorphin release has been attenuated by CB1 antagonism. Clinical translation remains inconsistent, with perioperative human studies frequently showing no opioid-sparing effect and, in some cohorts, increased postoperative opioid needs among patients with preoperative cannabinoid exposure (Shah et al., 2023).

Context matters. Endogenous endocannabinoid tone appears to influence opioid responsiveness in surgical patients, suggesting that perioperative analgesic requirements are shaped not only by exogenous exposure (THC/CBD) but also by baseline variability in inhibitory systems. For instance, a prospective cohort study of cesarean delivery patients found significant multiplicative interactions between preoperative beta-endorphin concentrations and endocannabinoids on postoperative opioid use. Higher preoperative plasma and cerebrospinal fluid (CSF) levels of 2-arachidonoylglycerol were linked to reduced outpatient opioid analgesic use, particularly in patients with low CSF beta-endorphin. Conversely, higher preoperative beta-endorphin levels were associated with lower pain in individuals with low plasma anandamide levels, suggesting a compensatory relationship between endogenous inhibitory systems (Stone et al., 2024). This understanding corresponds to the broader observation that cannabis exposure is rarely an isolated variable; it intersects with baseline pain phenotypes, anxiety and sleep disturbances, co-use of other substances, and preoperative opioid exposure, which are all factors that routinely drive postoperative analgesic trajectories (King et al., 2026).

TRPV1 as a Theoretical Mechanistic Fulcrum

Transient receptor potential vanilloid channels—especially TRPV1—are part of a larger TRP superfamily that function as molecular signal integrators at the interface of pain and inflammation. They are nonselective cation channels, also known as non-canonical targets, modulated by certain endocannabinoids and phytocannabinoids. TRPV1 is a classic polymodal nociceptor. It responds to multiple stimuli: noxious heat (approximately 42 °C and above), acidic pH in inflammatory or ischemic tissue, and vanilloids such as capsaicin. These channels are highly expressed in peripheral sensory neurons (e.g., dorsal root ganglia), where their activation triggers neurogenic inflammation and the release of neuropeptides, including calcitonin gene-related peptide (CGRP) and substance P.

Importantly, TRPV channels also interact with endocannabinoids and certain phytocannabinoids. Anandamide and other cannabinoids, including CBD, can activate TRPV1 and related channels. With sustained agonist exposure, TRPV1 can desensitize, a mechanism often invoked to explain cannabinoid-associated analgesia in select contexts. At the same time, TRPV1 frequently co-localizes with CB1/CB2 in primary sensory neurons, enabling bidirectional crosstalk between the endocannabinoid and nociceptive systems. This dual role—sensor and modulator—helps explain why TRPV1 is central to both cannabinoid-induced analgesia and, paradoxically, cannabinoid-associated hyperalgesia under chronic stimulation (proposed) (King et al., 2026).

Cannabinoid-induced Hyperalgesia (CIH)

Cannabinoid-Induced Hyperalgesia, or CIH, is a proposed paradoxical state of heightened pain sensitivity that emerges with sustained cannabinoid exposure. It differs fundamentally from:

- **Tolerance**, which reflects diminished drug effect with repeated exposure, and
- **Withdrawal**, which reflects transient rebound symptoms after cessation.

CIH, as a clinical construct, denotes a sensitized nociceptive state characterized by lowered pain thresholds and exaggerated responses to noxious stimuli. Proposed mechanisms implicate the TRPV1 receptor as a key mediator, but the molecular basis remains incompletely elucidated (King et al., 2026). In essence, chronic cannabinoid exposure, particularly THC, can downregulate CB1 receptors (receptor desensitization/internalization) and alter downstream signaling, potentially facilitating phosphorylation-dependent TRPV1 sensitization, increased calcium influx, and neuropeptide release, thereby producing both peripheral and central sensitization, or "wind-up," in which spinal neurons respond excessively to repeated input (King et al., 2026). Clinically, this manifests as lowered pain thresholds and exaggerated responses to noxious stimuli (mechanical, thermal, and inflammatory surgical stimuli)—the opposite of the intended analgesic effect—and complicates postoperative pain management.

Although studies demonstrating a direct link between CIH and a specific molecular target in humans remain lacking, TRPV1 has emerged as a therapeutic target (King et al., 2026). TRPV1 antagonists and other TRPV1-targeting strategies have been explored in analgesic development, but early antagonists were limited by clinically relevant thermoregulatory adverse effects (often hyperthermia), pointing to the complexity of translating TRPV1 blockade into safe pain therapeutics (Garami et al., 2020). Awareness of CIH and these emerging strategies allows perioperative professionals to anticipate paradoxical pain patterns and plan multimodal, mechanism-based interventions. A practical perioperative implication precedes abrupt peri-hospitalization cessation, which can precipitate withdrawal symptoms that may be misinterpreted as uncontrolled surgical pain, potentially escalating opioid administration (King et al., 2026). Cannabis withdrawal syndrome (CWS) may also occur in the postoperative period. At the same time, chronic exposure may coexist with baseline central sensitization that lowers pain thresholds and amplifies nociceptive signaling.

Perioperative Outcomes

When the mechanism is applied to the perioperative setting, data show that patients who regularly use cannabis—especially high-THC products—tend to have higher postoperative pain scores and may require higher opioid doses in the *immediate* postoperative period (including up to ~twofold higher opioid needs in some studies), compared with non-users (King et al., 2026). Although TRPV1 modulation is suggested, the exact mechanism remains incompletely understood. Interestingly, these same patients can demonstrate lower *outpatient* opioid use and may be *less likely* to become persistent opioid users, making the picture complex (Hedge et al., 2022). Evidence is currently limited and of low certainty, and should be individualized (King et al., 2026).

A recent integrative review of the current literature supports directional trends rather than definitive causal inference (King et al., 2026). Across 42 observational studies, postoperative pain outcomes were reported inconsistently, limiting certainty. Overall, 14/42 (33.3%) reported increased pain, 10/42 (24%) reported no change, 2/42 (5%) reported reduced pain, and 16/42 (38%) did not report pain outcomes. When stratified by surgical specialty, mixed/broad cohorts and spine populations showed the strongest directional trend toward higher postoperative pain, whereas arthroplasty and minor orthopedic cohorts reported no differences more frequently.

Opioid consumption data are similarly heterogeneous. With frequent or daily cannabis use, increased postoperative opioid requirements are commonly reported but not universal, consistent with an upregulated hyperalgesic state (King et al., 2026). By contrast, occasional or therapeutic cannabis use sometimes shows neutral or even reduced requirements. One plausible explanation is differential TRPV1 desensitization: low-dose CBD can induce receptor desensitization and anti-hyperalgesic effects, whereas sustained THC-dominant exposure can promote sensitization. This dichotomy accentuates the translational challenge that not all cannabis exposures are equivalent at the receptor level. Observed variability likely reflects heterogeneous exposure patterns (route, recency, frequency/chronicity, THC: CBD composition) that are not commonly captured, as well as baseline pain and comorbidity differences. Formulation-level detail is grossly absent and should be stratified in future research.

Across the same 42 studies, 18/42 (42.9%) reported higher postoperative opioid consumption among preoperative cannabinoid exposed patients, 17/42 (40%) found no difference, 3/42 (7%) indicated decreased use, and 4/42 (9.5%) did not report opioid outcomes. When grouped by specialty, the most consistent evidence for increased opioid requirements was again seen in mixed cohorts and spine populations; arthroplasty and other orthopedic studies more often reported no differences (King et al., 2026).

Methodological constraints include frequent limitations in exposure ascertainment (e.g., self-report or administrative coding), exposure windows that vary widely (e.g., 24-72 hours, 30-60 days, or 6-12 months), and a lack of formulation-level detail in studies (e.g., dose, route, frequency, chronicity, THC: CBD). These issues constrain inference and render a simple "yes/no cannabis exposure" variable biologically blunt (King et al., 2026).

Cannabis as a Postoperative Opioid Substitute

Amid many clinical controversies and safety concerns, a portion of the broader literature and public narrative supports the plausibility of cannabis as a primary postoperative adjunct to minimize or substitute for conventional opioids. Cannabis is well established as a therapy for chronic pain and is promoted for opioid reduction and elimination. However, the collective evidence does not currently support cannabis as a routine postoperative analgesic substitute, particularly when the outcomes of interest are immediate postoperative pain control and opioid requirements. This conclusion is not an argument against patient-reported benefit in selected individuals; rather, it reflects that the perioperative evidence base is predominantly observational, confounded by baseline pain and indication, and inconsistent in demonstrating an opioid-sparing effect in the acute postoperative window (King et al., 2026).

Limited, low-certainty evidence suggests that for patients with postoperative hyperalgesia, improvement may be observed with the resumption or administration of low-dose CBD. Additionally, resuming a patient's personal cannabis use after discharge may be associated with lower persistent opioid use in some contexts. However, counseling should be individualized and should not replace guideline-based analgesic care (King et al., 2026).

Opioid Stewardship and Multimodal Analgesia

The clinically defensible position is not that all patients who use cannabis will always require more opioids, but that cannabis exposure – particularly frequent, high-THC use – may act as a risk modifier for analgesic variability, including the potential for higher early pain and opioid needs in some settings. The response ought to be individualized, mechanism-informed, and anchored in opioid stewardship principles. Clinically, multimodal analgesia remains the most evidence-supported perioperative strategy across populations. In cannabis-exposed patients with suspected sensitized phenotypes (high baseline pain burden, daily high-THC exposure, preoperative opioid exposure, or peri-hospitalization abstinence), the mechanistic rationale is poly-pathway inhibition: disrupting multiple sensitization cascades rather than escalating a single class of analgesic. Core opioid-sparing foundations and adjunctive modalities are outlined in Table 5. This is consistent with ASRA guidance that opioids may be administered when indicated for perioperative pain in patients who use cannabis, with increased vigilance, and that there is insufficient evidence to recommend for or against adjusting postoperative opioid prescriptions solely based on cannabinoid use (King et al., 2026; Shah et al., 2023).

Table 5. Core opioid-sparing foundations and adjunctive modalities

Core opioid-sparing foundation (when not contraindicated): • Acetaminophen and NSAIDs/COX-2 inhibitors as foundational non-opioid analgesics (procedure- and patient-specific) • Regional/neuraxial anesthesia when feasible to reduce afferent nociceptive input and blunt central sensitization • Nonpharmacologic adjuncts embedded in perioperative recovery pathways (e.g., expectation setting, sleep support, mobilization)
Adjunctive modalities (selected patients, pathway dependent): • NMDA modulating strategies (e.g., ketamine and/or magnesium in appropriate settings) to counter central "wind-up" physiology • α2-agonists (e.g. dexmedetomidine) and systemic lidocaine within safe monitoring parameters and supported practice environments • Procedure-specific local anesthetic techniques and long-acting local anesthetic strategies

Acute cannabis exposure produces CB1-dominant analgesia and is thought to be concurrent with TRPV1 activation, permitting cation influx (including Ca^{2+}). With sustained agonism, TRPV1 may desensitize, a proposed mechanism for analgesia in certain contexts. With chronic exposure, however, TRPV1 may become sensitized: phosphorylation increases channel open probability, CB1 receptors are downregulated, and excitatory TRPV1 signaling predominates. This receptor-level shift could manifest as hyperalgesia. Crosstalk with transient receptor potential ankyrin 1 (TRPA1) further amplifies this cycle, while the absence of CB1 inhibitory tone leaves TRPV1 unopposed. The result is persistent nociceptive amplification despite ongoing cannabinoid intake. Clinically, multimodal analgesia remains the most evidence-supported strategy. Regional anesthesia circumvents central sensitization by blocking afferent input. NMDA antagonists, such as ketamine and magnesium, inhibit central wind-up and directly counteract TRPV1-driven sensitization. Additional classes such as NSAIDs, acetaminophen, gabapentinoids, α2 agonists, and systemic lidocaine target complementary pathways. The sound rationale is poly-pathway inhibition, which disrupts multiple sensitization cascades to offset the dominant TRPV1 excitatory drive (King et al., 2026).

Current CIH treatment options include high-dose capsaicin (the 8% patch), a prototypical TRPV1 agonist. It produces a paradoxical analgesic effect through receptor activation followed by desensitization: a large calcium influx that leads to channel inactivation or internalization. In the perioperative setting, clinicians may also consider preoperative cannabis tapering to reduce TRPV1 sensitization and lidocaine infusions to block sodium channels downstream of nociceptive transmission. Researchers are also testing selective TRPV1 antagonists in clinical trials, although first-generation agents were limited by hyperthermia due to disruption of TRPV1's thermoregulatory role. Newer strategies include combined TRPV1/TRPA1 modulators and CBD, which acts as a TRPV1 modulator. In the future, TRPV1 is expected to gain recognition as a biomarker of pain sensitization, with upregulation and phosphorylation observed in conditions such as inflammatory pain and diabetic neuropathy (King et al., 2026).

This opens the door to personalized analgesic protocols informed by cannabis use patterns and perioperative cannabinoid receptor modulation strategies. Screening is clinical, not moral, and patient education is central. Frank discussions about potential perioperative challenges and postoperative pain expectations improve outcomes. Furthermore, opioid stewardship does not imply undertreatment but rather entails prescribing only what is needed for the expected duration of severe pain, pairing opioids with a clear taper plan, and reassessing when pain does not align with expected recovery. This conforms to CDC guidance on prescribing for acute pain (quantity and duration matched to expected need) (Dowell et al., 2022; King et al., 2026).

Preoperative Dose Tapering

Perioperative concerns, particularly those related to hyperalgesia, may prompt consideration of tapering the cannabis dose in the preoperative period. For medicinal cannabis patients, a legitimate concern is that if asked to abstain, treated conditions may re-emerge or worsen, and that abrupt cessation during the peri-hospitalization period can precipitate CWS symptoms, potentially complicating perioperative symptom interpretation and analgesic planning (Shah et al., 2023).

Limited safety data further complicates concerns about preoperative dose tapering. ASRA notes that few studies have examined the benefits and risks of preoperative cannabinoid tapering and concludes that the overall benefit is of low certainty, and therefore cannot be recommended (Shah et al., 2023). Accordingly, abrupt cessation, particularly close to surgery, should be avoided when it risks destabilizing the treated condition and/or provoking withdrawal symptoms (Ladha et al., 2021).

In limited cases where tapering may be desirable, some methods have been proposed. For example, the Perioperative Pain and Addiction Interdisciplinary Network (PAIN) Consensus Recommendations (2021) recommend considering weaning high-dose users for more than seven days before surgery and caution against attempting to wean within seven days. High dose is defined as greater than: 1.5 grams per day (smoked), 300 milligrams per day of CBD oil, 20 milligrams per day of THC, or an unknown dose taken greater than 2-3 times per day. Notably, PAIN reports no consensus on tapering 1-6 days preoperatively and specifically advises against weaning or cessation 24 hours before surgery due to concerns about CWS and possible exacerbation of underlying conditions (e.g., chronic pain, anxiety) (Ladha et al., 2021).

A key practical limitation raised by clinicians, and echoed in the literature, is that real-world cannabis applications rarely fit neatly into discrete categories (e.g., "smoked" vs "THC oil" vs "CBD oil"). Cannabis formulations and CBD: THC ratios are highly integrative, often holistic, and patients commonly trial or use multiple products and routes throughout their health journey, making it difficult to develop or apply strictly separate recommendations (Ladha et al., 2021). This realization further stresses the needs surrounding preoperative guidance and situational understanding.

This is also a space where cannabis nurses can lead: by operationalizing structured, informative histories that capture combined routes and products, collaborating with the authorizing clinician when tapering is considered (particularly for medical cannabis), and providing patient-centered counseling that focuses on safety (e.g., anticipating withdrawal risk) while advocating against stigma or punitive messaging. As the evidence base evolves, nursing-led standardization of perioperative cannabis assessment and supportive workflows can directly address current gaps in guidance and improve perioperative risk stratification (Ladha et al., 2021; Shah et al., 2023).

POSTOPERATIVE MANAGEMENT AND DISCHARGE CONSIDERATIONS

PACU and Early Recovery Monitoring

Perioperative clinicians must maintain heightened vigilance for cannabis-specific recovery complications in PACU. Core monitoring priorities are as follows: (1) Respiratory status: For patients with chronic inhalational exposure, monitor for bronchospasm, hemoptysis, stridor, or upper-airway obstruction. In patients with very recent heavy inhalational exposure, maintain a low threshold for oxygen supplementation and ensure bedside airway equipment is available. (2) Cardiovascular monitoring: Given the association between cannabis use disorder (CUD) and postoperative myocardial infarction (MI) and arrhythmia risk in higher-risk patients, standard continuous cardiac monitoring is indicated, with heightened awareness in those with preexisting cardiovascular risk factors. (3) Pain assessment: In daily high-THC users, higher initial pain scores, neuropathic pain descriptors (burning, shooting, allodynia), or pain extending beyond the immediate surgical site may indicate a sensitized or neuropathic pain component rather than purely nociceptive pain. Escalate multimodal strategies before increasing opioid doses. (4) Temperature monitoring: Apply routine active warming. In daily cannabis users, the potential for increased hypothermia and shivering incidence supports attentive core temperature monitoring and a low threshold for augmenting warming measures (Shah et al., 2023; Echeverria-Villalobos et al., 2019).

Cannabis Withdrawal Syndrome

Cannabis withdrawal syndrome (CWS) should be treated as a foreseeable perioperative risk for patients who regularly use THC-containing products and are likely to experience abrupt interruption of exposure during hospitalization (e.g., inpatient admission, restricted access, prolonged NPO periods). In this context, screening should prompt the development of a monitoring and management plan rather than merely documenting cannabis use (Shah et al., 2023; Sladkey et al., 2025).

Risk stratification depends on exposure magnitude and THC content. Patients consuming high quantities or products with unknown THC concentrations appear to be at greatest risk. CBD-dominant products (>10:1 CBD: THC) may confer lower risk. A high index of suspicion is warranted when patients report > 1.5 g/day of inhaled cannabis, > 20 mg/day of THC-dominant oil, or unknown phytocannabinoid content > 2-3 times daily (Ladha et al., 2021; Shah et al., 2023).

DSM-5 criteria should guide recognition and documentation (American Psychiatric Association, 2022). CWS is diagnosed when the abrupt cessation of prolonged or heavy cannabis use is followed by ≥3 core symptoms (e.g., irritability, anger, anxiety, insomnia, decreased appetite, restlessness, depressed mood) and ≥1 physical symptom causing significant discomfort (e.g., abdominal pain, tremors, sweating, fever, chills, headache). Symptoms typically begin 24-72 hours after cessation, peak in the first week, and may persist for up to 2 weeks, a timeline highly relevant to postoperative inpatient care (Shah et al., 2023).

In hospitalized patients, CWS may present with disrupted sleep, agitation or restlessness, changes in opioid requirements, and/or unexpectedly poor pain control, and can be misattributed if not anticipated. Because perioperative cannabis exposure is also associated with higher postoperative pain and opioid consumption across several cohorts, clinicians should avoid assuming that increased subjective pain reports are purely surgical and should consider CWS in the differential when symptoms cluster with insomnia, irritability, or restlessness (Ekrami et al., 2024; King et al., 2026).

Patients who use cannabis regularly should be counseled about CWS risk and monitored postoperatively with a validated, reliable withdrawal scale. The Cannabis Withdrawal Scale is one validated option (Allsop et al., 2011; Shah et al., 2023). Pharmacologic management is still off-label, and evidence is evolving; however, a perioperative, stepwise approach is presented below. For

- **Mild-moderate CWS:** prioritize supportive care (sleep hygiene, reassurance, mobilization, hydration, and nutrition as appropriate) and address symptom drivers (pain control, nausea, and anxiety). Maintain a structured reassessment cadence using the same scale to track trajectory (Shah et al., 2023).
- **Severe postoperative CWS:** consensus recommendations are to initiate a low-dose cannabinoid agonist (e.g., dronabinol) as the preferred treatment strategy (Shah et al., 2023). Evidence supporting agonist replacement includes RCTs and experimental medicine studies showing reduced withdrawal with dronabinol and attenuated withdrawal/relapse measures with nabilone. In an inpatient RCT, nabiximols reduced overall withdrawal severity and irritability, depression, and craving (Levin et al., 2011; Haney et al., 2013; Allsop et al., 2014). As a regulatory safety note, dronabinol and nabilone are not FDA-approved for the treatment of CWS. Therefore, institutions should align their use with pharmacy policy and local regulations (Shah et al., 2023).

Adjuncts are supported by trial evidence, though not perioperative-specific. These include N-acetylcysteine and gabapentin (1200 mg/day), which reduced withdrawal symptoms in a proof-of-concept RCT (Mason et al., 2012; Shah et al., 2023). Other investigational approaches (e.g., FAAH inhibition) have shown signal in phase 2 work but are not standard perioperative therapies (D'Souza et al., 2019; Shah et al., 2023). For insomnia specifically, agents such as mirtazapine or zolpidem have been discussed. Quetiapine may improve sleep or appetite but can worsen cravings in some patients.

For high-risk patients or those with a clinically significant symptom burden, consider consultation (e.g., addiction medicine, psychiatry, acute pain service), especially when withdrawal may compromise postoperative recovery, participation in care, or discharge readiness (Allsop et al., 2016; Bonnet & Preuss, 2017; King et al., 2023b; Ladha et al., 2021; Shah et al., 2023).

Ambulatory Anesthesia and Same-Day Discharge Considerations

In patients undergoing ambulatory procedures, cannabis exposure introduces specific discharge readiness considerations not typically encountered in the inpatient setting. First, discharge to home following recent cannabis resumption, particularly when combined with opioids, benzodiazepines, or other central nervous system depressants, increases the risk of impairment and falls. Patients should be counseled prior to discharge that combining cannabis with any remaining postoperative sedating medications is unsafe, and that driving or operating machinery is contraindicated during this period, regardless of subjective perception of impairment. Second, patients with daily high-THC use patterns should be assessed for CWS risk before discharge. If the procedure requires inpatient NPO status and the patient is discharged the same day, they may enter the CWS onset window at home without support or monitoring. Brief education regarding symptoms to monitor (such as irritability, insomnia, and nausea by postoperative day 1 to 2) and guidance on when to contact the care team can reduce the risk of unplanned readmission or self-escalation of cannabis or opioid use. Third, PACU length-of-stay criteria should not be modified specifically for cannabis use, but the threshold for extending observation should be lower in patients with very recent heavy inhalational use (due to airway concerns) or those at high risk for CWS (Shah et al., 2023; Ladha et al., 2021).

Discharge Planning and Cannabis Resumption Counseling

Safe discharge planning for cannabis-exposed patients should include a structured discussion regarding postoperative cannabis resumption. Although there is currently no evidence-based prohibition on cannabis resumption after surgery, the timing and context of resumption have important safety implications. The following guidance is recommended: (1) Cannabis should be avoided while the patient is receiving moderate-to-high dose opioids, benzodiazepines, or other central nervous system depressants due to the risk of additive sedation, impaired coordination, and respiratory depression. (2) If cannabis is to be resumed for symptom management, particularly for pain or sleep, shared decision-making should emphasize a 'start low, go slow' approach. Patients should return at a fraction of the preoperative dose, initially prefer non-inhaled routes to avoid airway irritation, and avoid escalating the dose to manage breakthrough pain without first contacting the care team. (3) For patients at high risk for CWS, early cannabis resumption may be therapeutically appropriate to prevent or resolve postoperative withdrawal symptoms. In these cases, resumption should be integrated into the analgesic and recovery plan. (4) Patients should be instructed to contact the care team rather than self-escalate cannabis or opioid use if pain is not controlled, withdrawal symptoms emerge, or if sedation, confusion, or chest or respiratory symptoms develop. For patients with complex pain phenotypes, a history of CUD, or those at high risk for CWS, referral to the acute pain service, addiction medicine, or outpatient cannabis nurse follow-up should be considered before discharge (Shah et al., 2023; King et al., 2026).

COMMUNICATION, EDUCATION, AND STIGMA REDUCTION

Cannabis nurses work in uniquely powerful cannabis contexts, often hearing the authentic stories of cannabis use – why a patient started, what it helps with, what they fear, and what they will not say to other clinicians. That unsaid space is where stigma lives and where safety risks accumulate. Across the cannabis nursing evidence, anticipated stigma has recently been better understood and explored as a primary barrier to honest disclosure in healthcare settings and subsequent collaborative care. Anticipated stigma is the future-oriented expectation of negative treatment upon disclosing cannabis use, often shaped by social norms, prior discrimination, and structural policy realities (Earnshaw et al., 2013; King et al., 2024; Quinn & Chaudoir, 2009). In a national exploratory study of U.S. adults using cannabis, this stigma framework was intentionally operationalized alongside perceived, internalized, and enacted stigma to reflect the multidimensional nature of cannabis stigma in healthcare encounters (King et al., 2024).

Stigma Mechanisms that Shape Preoperative Disclosure

For patients who use cannabis, the most actionable stigma mechanism at the point of care is thought to be anticipated stigma, which is directly influenced by the patient's appraisal of how healthcare workers will respond to knowledge of their cannabis use (Quinn & Chaudoir, 2009; Earnshaw et al., 2013; King et al., 2024, 2026). Defining attributes include:

- Future-oriented expectation of negative treatment if revealed (Earnshaw et al., 2012; Quinn et al., 2014; Tsai et al., 2021).
- Social and interpersonal focus, with concern about reactions from family, clinicians, employers, and the community (Amarante et al., 2024; Oga et al., 2022; Peltzer & Pengpid, 2016; Rice et al., 2019).
- Emotional and cognitive anticipation (worry, fear, concern about devaluation/rejection) (Chaudoir & Quinn, 2015).
- Multidimensionality (varies by source, identity, and setting) (Aslam & Sarwat, 2021; Chaudoir & Quinn, 2015; Moore & Tangney, 2017).

In clinical care, anticipated stigma often co-occurs with perceived stigma (belief others hold negative attitudes), internalized stigma (absorbing stereotypes into self-concept), and enacted stigma (actual discriminatory treatment) (King et al., 2024, 2026). These types of stigma are presented in Table 6.

Table 6. Commonly encountered stigma subtypes

Stigma Type	Manifestations	Impact on Care
Anticipated stigma	• Fear of judgment from providers • Fear of legal consequences • Concern about being treated differently	Statistically significant association with nondisclosure
Internalized (felt) stigma	• Personal shame and guilt • Reluctance to discuss use	• Delayed treatment onset • Concealment strategies • Guilt • Shame
Enacted stigma	• Overt discrimination • Labeling • Directing to addiction services	• Barriers to accessing information and support • Dismissal • Reduced care
Perceived stigma	• Beliefs about provider opposition • Stereotypes about cannabis use	Reluctance to disclose and seeking non-medical sources for information/education

Sources: King et al., 2024, 2026

Cultural Safety and Intersectional Stigma

Cultural safety is not optional in these conversations, especially for people facing intersectional stigma. Black patients, for example, have described unique concerns about racial bias, and patients of color can face disproportionate punitive consequences for disclosing cannabis use (King et al., 2026; Walters et al., 2023). An example may include being directed toward addiction services rather than receiving the support they sought. Consequently, it is recommended that people with lived experience be involved in developing resources and implementing anti-oppressive training. Nurses must work to separate their roles from surveillance whenever possible. Acknowledging that disclosure risk is not evenly distributed drives adjustments to the nursing approach, with greater clarity and transparency. These dynamics are especially salient in perinatal contexts, where stigma and surveillance shape disclosure and engagement in care (Daniels et al., 2023; Greene et al., 2023; Walters et al., 2023).

Communication

When cannabis history is absent from the perioperative record, the clinical consequences include unrecognized medication interactions, incomplete hemodynamic and airway planning, and missed withdrawal risk – all of which are addressable through the communication practices that follow. Yet, conversation gaps are common. As established in the 'Disclosure Divide' subsection, provider-initiated cannabis conversations remain rare, and patients shoulder the majority of disclosure responsibility (King et al., 2024). This lack of initiative shifts decision-making to informal, nonmedical sources. In older adults, nondisclosure and self-directed information seeking (e.g., from friends, dispensaries, or the internet) are common, and some older adults alter or substitute medication doses without coordinated oversight as a result (Abu Baker et al., 2024). When providers are not prepared to partner, dispensaries and websites may supplant the healthcare team as the trusted authority on cannabis (Dahlke et al., 2024).

Communication practices that reduce stigma and improve disclosure and collaboration at the point of care include:

1) Leading with a universal, normalized invitation: The simplest reduction move is to universalize the topic, so that cannabis becomes a routine part of the health history rather than a special or pointed interrogation. Emphasis should be on nursing-initiated, patient-centered communication that validates patients' experiences, incorporates shared decision-making, and uses a harm-reduction orientation. In perioperative language, this may sound like:
    - "Cannabis can change how anesthesia and pain medicine work, and through knowing more, I can better keep you safe."
    - "Some people do not mention cannabis to their surgical team because they're not sure if it matters. It *does* matter for anesthesia planning."
2) Ask the clinically relevant questions without moral framing: Perioperative teams need details that patients may not recognize as clinically appropriate, including recency, route, potency, frequency, and reason for use. When patients are asked

neutrally about these, a signal is sent that this is about pharmacology and safety rather than character judgment. This matters because patients report discomfort when they perceive clinicians lack cannabis knowledge, and providers themselves report knowledge gaps that undermine their ability to counsel or even initiate discussions. This pattern has also been described in nurse populations caring for patients with chemotherapy-related nausea, where knowledge gaps and low confidence constrain cannabis-related communication (Xiao et al., 2023).

3) Use harm reduction as your counseling default stance: It appears across the evidence as a practical communication approach, with nonjudgmental support paired with risk-mitigation discussions. In perioperative care, harm reduction is precise rather than permissive. Some harm-reduction perioperative messaging examples include:
    - "Here's what increases anesthesia risk,"
    - "Here are safe alternatives in this window,"
    - "Here's how we should manage your cannabis during this time,"
    - "Here's how to avoid withdrawal, severe anxiety, or unmanaged pain."
4) Close the loop with teach-back and shared planning: Shared decision-making is repeatedly identified as a preferred model for cannabis counseling because it promotes open conversation, values clarification, information exchange, and decision support. In perioperative settings, shared planning might include agreements on preoperative tapering plans when relevant, symptom (e.g., sleep, nausea, anxiety) substitution options, postoperative pain expectations and monitoring, and documentation preferences and privacy concerns.

To make this practical, a simple pathway model helps explain why disclosure breaks down in perioperative settings and where cannabis nurses can intervene. Figure 3 shows how structural forces and stigma mechanisms shape disclosure behaviors, which then determine the quality of the perioperative cannabis history, and ultimately, safety and symptom outcomes.

Figure 3. The disclosure-to-safety pathway in perioperative cannabis care (conceptual model)

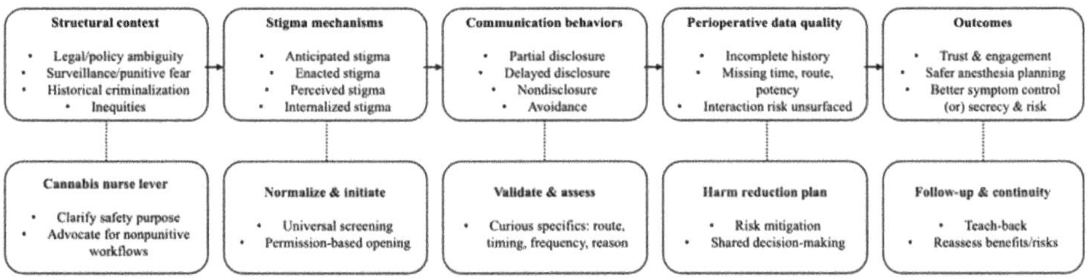

Note. *A conceptual model illustrating how structural context (policy ambiguity, surveillance fears, and inequities) influences stigma mechanisms (perceived, internalized, enacted, anticipated), which shape disclosure behaviors (partial disclosure, delayed disclosure, nondisclosure). Disclosure quality determines perioperative data quality and downstream safety outcomes. The lower row highlights nursing leverage points: normalize/initiate, validate/assess, harm-reduction planning, and follow-up/continuity.*

Education

Despite increasing social acceptance and legislation that normalize cannabis use, knowledge gaps persist among healthcare practitioners, undermining communication quality. In a recent oncology nursing study, only 47.8% answered questions correctly about cannabis effectiveness for chemotherapy-induced nausea, and 60.9% were not confident in providing related guidance (Xiao et al., 2023). This pattern also applies in perioperative care. When nurses feel uncertain, the easiest response is avoidance, which is precisely the pattern patients experience. Competence, as guided by the National Council of State Boards of Nursing [NCSBN] (2018) framework and the cannabis nursing scope and standards (American Nurses Association & American Cannabis Nurses Association, 2024), is part of stigma reduction. In the disclosure literature, increased provider knowledge and education may be associated with more positive perceptions (King et al., 2024).

Pre-licensure and advanced practice nursing education programs should promote product literacy that fosters understanding of the ECS, cannabinoid ratios, routes of administration, onset, and duration. Continuing education programs for perioperative clinicians should emphasize unique considerations aligned with the anesthetic period. In addition, medication reconciliation practices should be promoted to ensure reliable documentation. Interaction counseling is a third educational area highlighted as relevant in settings with high polypharmacy risk. Thus, awareness of potential drug interactions, particularly with sedatives and analgesics used in the perioperative course, improves interaction counseling strategies. Finally, communication skill-building through educational initiatives ensures proficiency in nonjudgmental language. The incorporation of teach-back and shared planning methods should also be considered. In doing so, it should not be overlooked that patients may have rational fears about the consequences, and that punitive frameworks create barriers that can be overcome through improved ethical and legal understanding.

Organizational-level Stigma Reduction

Importantly for nurses, their environment must align with their values. Even skilled nurses are constrained by the systems in which they work. Organizational barriers, such as a lack of workplace guidance, time constraints, and punitive policies that structurally impede nonjudgmental dialogue, are common. For nursing leaders, three system-level changes can have positive effects. First, non-stigmatized cannabis assessment prompts embedded in preoperative workflows lift the burden of individual courage. The CUBAT is an implementation-ready tool for integration into the electronic health record (Sladkey et al., 2025). Additionally, written workplace guidance and continuing education are essential. Nurses should know what to ask, how to document accurately, and how to make appropriate referrals, all of which are central to patient safety and improving care. Finally, an explicit harm-reduction orientation in policies and patient education materials is needed, as patients seek information through both conversations and educational materials.

CURRICULUM AND COMPETENCY DEVELOPMENT

One of the most explicit messages in nursing, especially for those educating perioperative and nurse anesthesiology learners, is that knowledge gaps are tangible, measurable, and fixable. In pilot testing of a focused cannabis curriculum with doctoral nurse anesthesia residents, findings revealed only 23.5% reported any prior cannabis education at baseline, and pre-intervention comfort with "ideal knowledge" for caring for patients who use cannabis was low (median 2/5) (King et al., 2023a). After a single synchronous educational session, both perceived and tested knowledge improved significantly (self-assessed knowledge increased from 8/20 to 16/20, and tested knowledge from 3/5 to 5/5; both $p < .001$). Just as importantly, learners strongly agreed that the content should be formally integrated into the curriculum and described its immediate practice relevance. This was especially true regarding drug interactions with anesthetic agents, ECS fundamentals, and feeling more prepared to ask patients about cannabis use. For competency development, that combination (documented gaps → rapid, measurable gains → strong learner-perceived practice impact) is precisely the evidence base needed to justify formally placing cannabis science in perioperative education rather than treating it as an elective or novelty topic. In perioperative settings, this is not optional knowledge. Cannabis exposure can shape airway and respiratory risks, hemodynamics, aspiration physiology, anesthetic and sedation variability, withdrawal risk, and postoperative pain trajectories, all of which require competent assessment and documentation. More importantly, for many patients, it is part of their identity, health journey, and healing, warranting a greater understanding of the patient as a whole person.

From a curriculum-design standpoint, the pilot also provides a practical blueprint: build competencies using nationally recognized nursing guidance as scaffolding, then contextualize them for anesthesia and perioperative realities. The aforementioned curriculum (King et al., 2023a) used national guidelines (NCSBN, 2018) as the conceptual framework and covered cannabis pharmacology, ECS, and physiology. The program-level must include elements that fit well with competency-based education: legalization status; medical cannabis program fundamentals; ECS dynamics (receptors/cannabinoids/interactions); pharmacology; safety considerations; stigma; and administration considerations (NCSBN, 2018). These guidelines are especially important in perioperative care because cannabis lacks the usual FDA-style standardization of indication, dosing, and efficacy, requiring nurses to apply more nuanced clinical judgment during medication reconciliation, preoperative screening, and patient teaching (NCSBN, 2018).

In practice, it is recommended to embed these competencies longitudinally across the nurse anesthesiology and perioperative sequence: integrating foundational cannabis science into pharmacology, physiology, and pathophysiology courses (where it naturally belongs), reinforcing application through case-based perioperative seminars (e.g., "cannabis + airway reactivity," "cannabis + anesthetic dosing variability," "cannabis + post-op pain trajectories"), and finally validating performance with explicit evaluations (objective structured clinical examination (OSCE)-style patient interviews, simulation debrief checklists, and documentation rubrics). Because many patients use multiple products and routes, competency checks should require learners to assess and document route(s), frequency, recency, approximate potency/THC: CBD ratio when known, co-use, and symptom-driven reasons for use—then translate that history into a perioperative plan (risk counseling, safety precautions, communication with anesthesia/surgical teams). By approaching cannabis education this way, it transforms into a collection of observable competencies (what the learner can explain, ask, document, anticipate, and teach) rather than a single lecture that fails to leave a lasting impression.

POLICY, LEGAL, AND ETHICAL ASPECTS

Cannabis nursing exists within a complex policy landscape. Cannabis may be legal in a state, yet patients still fear criminalization, judgment, or downstream consequences, especially when documentation seems permanent. This tension is heightened by contemporary market dynamics, including the rise of high-concentration/potency THC products, which point to the need for targeted, competency-based education that includes risk mitigation and safer-use counseling within time-limited perioperative windows (National Academies of Sciences, Engineering, and Medicine [NASEM], 2024).

In perioperative care, the conversation should be structured so that cannabis history is treated as protected health information (PHI), and the Health Insurance Portability and Accountability Act (HIPAA) supports confidential communication among the care team for treatment and safety planning (U.S. Department of Health & Human Services [HHS], 2025). Patient-facing education should reassure patients that it is generally legally safe to tell their anesthesia provider and perioperative team about cannabis and frame disclosure as a safety issue rather than a moral one (Enochs, 2021). This approach is also equity relevant. For example, punitive prenatal drug use policies and inequitable testing practices can deter people from seeking care, further highlighting the need for nonjudgmental, clinically focused counseling rather than surveillance framing (NASEM, 2024).

Legally speaking, HIPAA does not give healthcare workers an open door to disclose cannabis use to law enforcement. Such disclosures are limited and typically tied to specific legal processes (e.g., a court order or certain subpoenas) (HHS, 2022a; HHS, 2020). HIPAA permits disclosure in narrow safety situations, such as when a clinician has a good-faith belief that disclosure is needed to prevent or lessen a serious and imminent threat (HHS, 2022b). Beyond imminent harm, another primary exception nurses must understand is that HIPAA permits disclosures required by law, including reporting known or suspected abuse or neglect to authorized authorities (HHS, 2013). Thus, limited disclosures may occur when legally required or narrowly permitted under HIPAA's "serious and imminent threat" standard, but that is not the only pathway. Mandatory reporting laws and institutional policies can create additional obligations depending on the setting and state.

Ethically, nursing works to keep patients safe without turning healthcare into surveillance. This is especially important in perinatal settings, where pregnant and parenting patients have documented concerns about stigma and surveillance, and where fear of Child Protective Services (CPS) involvement can shape engagement with care (Daniels et al., 2023; Greene et al., 2023). Nursing should document clinically relevant facts in neutral language, avoid speculative or stigmatizing labels, and be transparent about confidentiality limits within one's institution. Importantly, this includes when nurses are required to report or refer, and when a consult with leadership/risk management is appropriate. In quality improvement initiatives, nurses should not rely solely on individual bedside judgment. Standardized perioperative cannabis workflows, universal screening practices, documentation templates, and referral pathways reduce bias-driven variability and support safer anesthesia planning.

Clinically, patient-facing messages in consumer-facing educational resources should be consistent with perioperative professional guidance. Patients should disclose cannabis use because it can affect cardiovascular/respiratory physiology, airway reactivity, anesthetic dosing requirements, and postoperative pain/nausea management. Furthermore, nurses should foster an environment in which patients feel safe and understand that knowledge of cannabis within a nurse-patient relationship is mutually empowering (Enochs, 2021; American Association of Nurse Anesthesiology, 2025; Shah et al., 2023).

ILLUSTRATIVE CASE STUDY

A 28-year-old male presents for elective lumbar fusion for spondylolisthesis with radicular pain. During the preoperative nursing assessment, he reports daily cannabis use for >5 years, primarily for sleep and chronic back pain. His pattern includes multiple products and routes: high-THC flower (smoked most evenings), occasional vape cartridges on weekends, and a nightly edible ("10 mg, sometimes 20 mg if pain is bad"). His last inhaled use was "late last night," and his last edible was "around midnight." He denies alcohol use and reports intermittent nicotine vaping. He has no prior anesthetic complications. He reports episodic reflux symptoms but no current nausea or vomiting. On exam, he appears calm, oriented, and neurocognitively intact with no evidence of impaired judgment.

Preoperative Nursing Assessment and Safety Planning

The cannabis nurse obtains the cannabis history using a normalized, nonjudgmental script and documents it in clinically actionable terms (route(s), frequency, dose range, recency, approximate THC/CBD content when known, and reason for use) consistent with perioperative consensus recommendations for screening and structured documentation (Shah et al., 2023; Sladkey et al., 2025). The nurse explicitly clarifies that disclosure is for safe anesthesia and recovery planning, not punishment. Because the patient uses multiple routes and variable dosing, the nurse avoids overly simplistic categories (e.g., "smoker" vs. "edible user") and instead summarizes total exposure in a form immediately useful to the perioperative team. Action and decision points should include:

1. **Assess acute impairment and capacity:** The nurse screens for evidence of acute impairment in judgment (attention, short-term memory, timeline reliability, and ability to participate in consent and postoperative instructions). The patient demonstrates intact capacity. The nurse documents: "No clinical signs of acute impairment; reliable historian." If impairment were present, the nurse would recommend deferring elective surgery, consistent with consensus guidance (Shah et al., 2023).
2. **Screen for aspiration/PONV modifiers:** The nurse notes reflux symptoms and recent edible exposure and communicates that oral cannabis (edibles) may be associated with delayed gastric emptying and aspiration risk in some patients; the team considers a lower threshold for aspiration precautions and proactive PONV prophylaxis (Shah et al., 2023).
3. **Anticipate withdrawal-related contributors:** Given daily long-term use and anticipated inpatient abstinence, the nurse screens for baseline sleep disturbance and anxiety and flags potential postoperative withdrawal symptoms (insomnia, irritability, restlessness, anxiety, decreased appetite, nausea) that can mimic or amplify pain-related distress (Shah et al., 2023).
4. **Set expectations without stigma:** The nurse frames cannabis exposure as a physiologic variable that can affect anesthetic and analgesic response, not a moral issue. The nurse explains: "Some patients with chronic daily use experience higher acute pain or require different combinations of medications after surgery. Our goal is to control pain safely and minimize opioids."

To reduce miscommunication, the nurse provides a concise, structured handoff summary to the anesthesia and surgical teams:

"Daily high-THC exposure >5 years; mixed routes; last smoked late last night; last edible ~midnight (10–20 mg typical); intermittent nicotine vaping; episodic reflux; no clinical impairment today; higher risk for withdrawal-related insomnia/anxiety and for higher postoperative pain/opioid needs in some cohorts; recommend proactive multimodal plan and withdrawal-aware recovery support." (Shah et al., 2023; King et al., 2026)

Key preoperative considerations communicated to the team include:

- **Acute use/capacity:** Elective surgery should be deferred if the patient shows evidence of acutely impaired judgment or inability to provide informed consent (Shah et al., 2023).
- **Aspiration risk modifiers:** Reflux symptoms + edible exposure support a lower threshold for aspiration precautions and deliberate PONV prophylaxis planning (Shah et al., 2023).

- **Pain phenotype and expectations:** Chronic daily high-THC patterns may be associated with higher acute postoperative pain and higher early opioid requirements in some cohorts; proactive multimodal planning and expectation-setting are emphasized (Shah et al., 2023; King et al., 2026).
- **Tapering/resumption conversation:** The nurse explains that evidence for preoperative tapering is limited and individualized; abrupt cessation may worsen symptom control and can precipitate withdrawal. If tapering is considered, it should be planned with adequate lead time and shared decision-making. The nurse explicitly adds: "We will also make a postoperative plan for if/when cannabis is resumed so it supports opioid stewardship and safety rather than undermining it." (Shah et al., 2023; King et al., 2026)

Intraoperative Decision-making

The anesthesia plan prioritizes opioid-sparing multimodal analgesia given potential analgesic variability and the procedure's high nociceptive burden. Preoperative medications include acetaminophen and gabapentin (or an equivalent per institutional protocol and considering respiratory/sedation risk), with consideration of intraoperative ketamine and magnesium infusions to reduce central sensitization and local anesthetic infiltration at the surgical site. The team prepares for analgesic variability without reflexively escalating opioids early, instead escalating multimodal options first. PONV prophylaxis is planned deliberately; the team does not assume cannabis is protective against PONV. Airway and hemodynamic management follow standard practice, with situational awareness that smoking/vaping (and nicotine co-use) may add airway/respiratory considerations.

PACU and Early Recovery Course

Despite multimodal analgesia, the patient reports PACU pain scores 6–8/10 with a "burning, electric" quality and intermittent spread beyond the immediate incision area—features that may reflect a neuropathic/sensitized pain pattern rather than purely nociceptive pain. Over the first 48 postoperative hours, he requires moderately higher-than-average opioid exposure (e.g., ~110–140 mg oral morphine equivalents, compared with an institutional average of ~90 mg for similar cases), mobilizes later than planned, and remains hospitalized ~2 days rather than 1.5. Interventions in PACU/early recovery should include:

1. **Phenotype the pain before escalating opioids:** The nurse assesses pain quality (burning/shooting), allodynia, and distribution. Recognizing neuropathic/sensitization features, the nurse communicates to the team that the pain quality

suggests a neuropathic/sensitized component; recommends optimizing multimodal/neuropathic strategy and anti-sensitization measures before further opioid escalation.

2. **Screen for withdrawal-related amplification:** The nurse assesses for irritability, anxiety, insomnia, restlessness, nausea, and appetite changes, which are symptoms that can amplify perceived pain and drive opioid demand. When the patient reports poor sleep and restlessness on night one, the nurse treats these as physiologic and expected, not as behavioral noncompliance, and communicates findings to the team for targeted support.
3. **Maintain stigma-reducing communication:** The nurse reinforces that symptoms reflect neurobiology and recovery stress, not character. The nurse avoids labeling the patient as "drug-seeking" and instead frames management around function (sleep, mobilization, participation in PT, and safe analgesia).

This course is consistent with a mild-to-moderate sensitized nociceptive state rather than dramatic, unexplained hyperalgesia. Surgical inflammation releases mediators (e.g., prostaglandins, bradykinin, NGF) that sensitize nociceptive signaling, and chronic cannabinoid exposure may contribute to variable receptor network signaling and altered pain modulation in some patients. The neuropathic descriptors and pain spread support a sensitization or neuropathic contribution, prompting the team to optimize multimodal strategies rather than rely on opioid escalation alone.

Discharge and Recovery Education

Before discharge, the cannabis nurse provides brief, structured education and documents a shared plan, highlighting safety, function, and opioid stewardship:

1. **Shared plan for cannabis during recovery (timing + strategy)**
   - o **Immediate postoperative window:** The nurse advises avoiding cannabis while opioids are still required at moderate doses, because combining cannabinoids with opioids, benzodiazepines, or other sedatives can increase sedation, dizziness, impaired coordination, and fall/respiratory risk. The nurse emphasizes this as a safety issue, not a moral rule.
   - o **If resuming cannabis is considered:** The nurse uses shared decision-making and recommends a stepwise resumption strategy:
     - ▪ Prefer delaying THC resumption until opioids are minimal or discontinued when feasible to support safe opioid tapering and reduce additive impairment risk.

        - If resuming after opioids are stopped or near-zero, *start low and go slow* (return at a fraction of usual dose; avoid high-potency products initially).
        - Prefer non-inhaled routes early (to avoid airway irritation/coughing) and avoid "stacking" edibles due to delayed onset.
        - If the primary goal is sleep, consider lower-THC strategies and avoid escalating the dose to chase analgesia.
    - The nurse documents the patient-specific plan and instructs the patient to discuss timing with the surgical/anesthesia team and the cannabis nurse follow-up.
2. **Opioid stewardship and multimodal foundation**
    - The nurse reinforces scheduled nonopioid foundations (acetaminophen ± NSAID if allowed, neuropathic adjuncts as prescribed) and non-pharmacologic supports (mobility plan, ice/heat as appropriate, sleep hygiene).
    - The nurse sets expectations for pain trajectory after lumbar fusion and emphasizes that improved function (sleep, walking, PT participation) is a key outcome, not just pain score.
3. **Withdrawal vs pain monitoring**
    - The nurse educates on withdrawal symptoms (insomnia, irritability, anxiety, restlessness, nausea, appetite change) that may appear with abrupt cessation and can be mistaken for uncontrolled surgical pain.
    - The nurse advises early contact if symptoms escalate rather than self-escalating opioids or cannabis.
4. **Red flags and when to seek urgent evaluation**
    - Severe sedation, confusion, falls/dizziness, uncontrolled vomiting (including concern for CHS if pattern fits), chest pain, or shortness of breath prompt urgent evaluation.
    - The nurse reiterates not to combine cannabis with opioids or other sedatives without a shared plan; instead, call the team first.

This case illustrates where cannabis nurses directly support improved outcomes as they relate to: (a) obtaining a high-quality, stigma-reducing cannabis history that reflects real-world mixed product use, (b) translating that exposure pattern into actionable perioperative risk communication, (c) differentiating sensitization/neuropathic pain from withdrawal-related distress to guide safer analgesic escalation, and (d) providing a concrete, opioid-stewardship–aligned plan for postoperative cannabis resumption which prioritizes function and safety.

FUTURE DIRECTIONS AND RESEARCH PRIORITIES

Although perioperative cannabis guidance is advancing, the evidence base remains limited by heterogeneity in exposure definitions and reliance on observational designs. Three priorities stand out:

1. **Standardize cannabis exposure measurement for perioperative research and clinical workflows.** Current studies often treat cannabis exposure as binary, but real-world use is multidimensional (route(s), frequency, recency, potency, THC: CBD ratio, and co-use). Developing a pragmatic perioperative cannabis exposure index that captures combined patterns (not single-route categories) would improve both research comparability and bedside risk stratification.
2. **Clarify the effectiveness and safety of preoperative tapering or abstinence strategies.** Evidence for dose tapering remains sparse, and one-size thresholds are difficult to apply when patients use mixed products. Pragmatic trials and implementation studies are needed to determine (a) who benefits from tapering, (b) feasible time windows, and (c) how to prevent withdrawal and symptom rebound, which is an area where cannabis nurses can lead through protocol development, education, and patient-centered monitoring.
3. **Advance perioperative pain science.** Research should test whether biomarkers or phenotyping tools can identify patients at risk for cannabinoid-associated hyperalgesia and postoperative analgesic variability, and whether tailored multimodal strategies improve outcomes. Translational work linking receptor/network mechanisms to surgical pain trajectories is needed, including studies that evaluate adjunct strategies without worsening thermoregulation or other physiologic safeguards.

Across all priorities, nursing-led implementation research is essential. Integrating standardized screening (e.g., EHR prompts), building communication competencies, evaluating stigma-reduction interventions, and measuring downstream outcomes, including disclosure rates, complications, pain control, opioid utilization, and patient-reported experience.

CONCLUSION

Cannabis use is now a routine perioperative reality, and cannabis nursing provides a safety-critical bridge between patient disclosure and clinical decision-making. Across the perioperative continuum, nurses can reduce stigma, obtain accurate exposure histories that reflect real-world mixed products and routes, and translate cannabis pharmacology into practical risk mitigation, such as aspiration and PONV planning, hemodynamic and airway awareness, withdrawal recognition, and multimodal pain strategies grounded in opioid stewardship. While evidence gaps persist, consensus guidance supports a clear nursing mandate to normalize cannabis use as a clinical variable, personalize perioperative planning, and deliver patient-centered education that protects safety, dignity, and continuity of care.

The findings presented in this chapter have implications that extend beyond individual clinical practice. Regarding perioperative standards, the evidence supports the formalization of cannabis screening as a required component of the preanesthesia evaluation, to be conducted alongside medication reconciliation and allergy review. In research, urgent priorities include the development of standardized exposure measurements that account for route, frequency, recency, and THC/CBD composition, as well as pragmatic trials on preoperative tapering and studies that identify patients at highest risk for cannabis-induced hyperemesis (CIH) and cannabis withdrawal syndrome (CWS) prior to surgery. In the context of education, pilot curriculum data reviewed in this chapter indicate that knowledge deficits in anesthesia training programs are both measurable and rapidly correctable. This supports the intentional integration of cannabis science into pharmacology, physiology, and clinical decision-making curricula, rather than reliance on self-directed learning. For patient safety strategy, cannabis-informed perioperative practice is consistent with high-reliability organization principles by anticipating variation, standardizing assessment, and ensuring that safety information is visible. The perioperative encounter represents, for many cannabis-using patients, a critical point of contact with the healthcare system, where accurate history-taking, stigma-free communication, and individualized care planning can significantly influence outcomes. Cannabis nursing is particularly well positioned to lead these initiatives.

REFERENCES

Abdallah, F. W., Hussain, N., Weaver, T., & Brull, R. (2020). Analgesic efficacy of cannabinoids for acute pain management after surgery: A systematic review and meta-analysis. *Regional Anesthesia and Pain Medicine*, *45*(7), 509–519. DOI: 10.1136/rapm-2020-101340 PMID: 32471924

Abu Baker, D., Cruz Rivera, P. N., Narasimhan, R., Nguyen, N., Tibiriçá, L., Kepner, W. E., O'Malley, P., Nguyen, A. L., & Moore, A. A. (2024). Older adults' use of cannabis and attitudes around disclosing medical cannabis use to their healthcare providers in California: A mixed methods study. *Drugs - Real World Outcomes*, *11*(4), 647–658. DOI: 10.1007/s40801-024-00451-0 PMID: 39294485

Alexander, J. C., & Joshi, G. P. (2019). A review of the anesthetic implications of marijuana use. *Proceedings - Baylor University. Medical Center*, *32*(3), 364–371. DOI: 10.1080/08998280.2019.1603034 PMID: 31384188

Allen, J. G., Flanigan, S. S., LeBlanc, M., Vallarino, J., MacNaughton, P., Stewart, J. H., & Christiani, D. C. (2016). Flavoring Chemicals in e-cigarettes: Diacetyl, 2,3-pentanedione, and acetoin in a sample of 51 products, including fruit-, candy-, and cocktail-flavored e-cigarettes. *Environmental Health Perspectives*, *124*(6), 733–739. DOI: 10.1289/ehp.1510185 PMID: 26642857

Allsop, D., Norberg, M., Copeland, J., Fu, S., & Budney, A. J. (2011). The Cannabis Withdrawal Scale development: Patterns and predictors of cannabis withdrawal and distress. *Drug and Alcohol Dependence*, *119*(1-2), 123–129. DOI: 10.1016/j.drugalcdep.2011.06.003 PMID: 21724338

Allsop, D. J., Copeland, J., Lintzeris, N., Dunlop, A. J., Montebello, M., Sadler, C., Rivas, G. R., Holland, R. M., Muhleisen, P., Norberg, M. M., Booth, J., & McGregor, I. S. (2014). Nabiximols as an agonist replacement therapy during cannabis withdrawal: A randomized clinical trial. *JAMA Psychiatry*, *71*(3), 281–291. DOI: 10.1001/jamapsychiatry.2013.3947 PMID: 24430917

Allsop, D. J., Kevin, R. C., & Arnold, J. C. (2016). Cannabis: The pharmacokinetics and pharmacodynamics of recreational and medicinal cannabis. In Sher, K. J. (Ed.), *The SAGE handbook of drug and alcohol studies* (Vol. 2, pp. 194–210). SAGE Publications Ltd., https://sk.sagepub.com/reference/the-sage-handbook-of-drug-alcohol-studies-v2/i1737.xml DOI: 10.4135/9781473922143.n13

Alqahtani, A., Ammari, Z., Ramahi, A., Said Ahmed, T. S., & Klada, E. (2019). Cannabis smoking-induced diffuse alveolar hemorrhage. *Cureus*, *11*(7), e5089. DOI: 10.7759/cureus.5089 PMID: 31511809

Amarante, I. C. J., Lippman, S. A., Sevelius, J. M., Saggese, G. S. R., da Silva, A. A. M., & Veras, M. A. S. M. (2024). Anticipated stigma and social barriers to communication between transgender women newly diagnosed with HIV and health care providers: A mediation analysis. *LGBT Health*, *11*(3), 229–238. DOI: 10.1089/lgbt.2023.0041 PMID: 37910864

American Association of Nurse Anesthesiology. (2018). Promoting a culture of safety and healthy work environment. In *AANA Professional Practice Manual*. https://www.aana.com/practice-manual/aana-practice-manual-promoting-a-culture-of-safety-and-healthy-work-environment

American Association of Nurse Anesthesiology. (2019). *Standards for nurse anesthesia practice*. https://www.aana.com/docs/default-source/practice-aana-com-web-documents-(all)/standards-for-nurse-anesthesia-practice.pdf

American Association of Nurse Anesthesiology. (2023). *Analgesia and anesthesia for the substance use disorder patient: Practice considerations*. https://www.aana.com/docs/default-source/practice-aana-com-web-documents-(all)/analgesia-and-anesthesia-for-the-substance-use-disorder-patient.pdf

American Association of Nurse Anesthesiology. (2025). *Cannabis*. https://www.aana.com/practice/clinical-practice/clinical-practice-resources/cannabis/

American College of Obstetricians and Gynecologists. (2017). Committee Opinion No. 722: Marijuana use during pregnancy and lactation. *Obstetrics and Gynecology*, *130*(4), e205–e209. DOI: 10.1097/AOG.0000000000002354 PMID: 28937574

American Nurses Association. (2025). *Code of Ethics for Nurses*. American Nurses Association. https://www.nursingworld.org/coe-view-only

American Nurses Association & American Cannabis Nurses Association. (2024). *Cannabis nursing: Scope and standards of practice*. ANA.

American Psychiatric Association. (2022). Diagnostic and Statistical Manual of Mental Disorders (5th ed., text rev.). American Psychiatric Publishing., DSM-5-TR.

Ashrafian, S., Ahrens, E., Wachtendorf, L. J., Munoz-Acuna, R., Shay, D., Suleiman, A., Redaelli, S., von Wedel, D., Chen, G., Wolff, G., Hill, K. P., & Schaefer, M. S. (2025). Association of cannabis use with major cardiovascular and cerebrovascular events after surgery or interventional procedures. *The American Journal on Addictions*, *34*(5), 517–527. DOI: 10.1111/ajad.70029 PMID: 40204668

Aslam, M., & Sarwat, N. (2021). Linking anticipated stigma to psychological well-being: Mediating role of anxiety and depression. *International Journal of Business and Economic Affairs*, *6*(3), 201–212. DOI: 10.24088/IJBEA-2021-63008

Atkins, J. B., Levine, D., & Shaw, L. (2025). Cannabinoid hyperemesis syndrome presenting as postoperative nausea and vomiting in a chronic cannabis user: A case report. *Cureus*, *17*(7), e87990. DOI: 10.7759/cureus.87990 PMID: 40821157

Baker, M. B., Binda, D. D., Nozari, A., Kennedy, J. M., Dienes, E., & Baker, W. E. (2025). Quantitative analysis of propofol dosage in cannabis users: A systematic review and meta-analysis. *Journal of Clinical Medicine*, *14*(3), 858. DOI: 10.3390/jcm14030858 PMID: 39941531

Barkay, G., Solomito, M. J., Kostyun, R. O., Esmende, S., & Makanji, H. (2023). The effect of cannabis use on postoperative complications in patients undergoing spine surgery: A national database study. *North American Spine Society Journal*, *16*, 100265. DOI: 10.1016/j.xnsj.2023.100265 PMID: 37745195

Beers, J. L., Fu, D., & Jackson, K. D. (2021). Cytochrome P450-catalyzed metabolism of cannabidiol to the active metabolite 7-hydroxy-cannabidiol. *Drug Metabolism and Disposition: the Biological Fate of Chemicals*, *49*(10), 882–891. DOI: 10.1124/dmd.120.000350 PMID: 34330718

Bernal, L. R., Tanaka, A., Ikeno, Y., Afifi, R. O., Sandhu, H. K., Miller, C. C.III, & Estrera, A. L. (2024). Outcomes after open repair of aortic aneurysms and dissections in cannabis consumers. *JTCVS Open*, *22*, 107–113. DOI: 10.1016/j.xjon.2024.08.002 PMID: 39780794

Bertrand, K. A., Hanan, N. J., Honerkamp-Smith, G., Best, B. M., & Chambers, C. D. (2018). Marijuana use by breastfeeding mothers and cannabinoid concentrations in breast milk. *Pediatrics*, *142*(3), e20181076. Advance online publication. DOI: 10.1542/peds.2018-1076 PMID: 30150212

Bonnet, U., & Preuss, U. W. (2017). The cannabis withdrawal syndrome: Current insights. *Substance Abuse and Rehabilitation*, *8*, 9–37. DOI: 10.2147/SAR.S109576 PMID: 28490916

Bornemann-Cimenti, H., Lang-Illievich, K., Neuwersch-Sommeregger, S., Lang, J., Danninger, T., Hammer, S., Szilagyi, I. S., & Klivinyi, C. (2025). Effect of cannabinoid consumption on propofol dosage: A systematic review and meta-analysis. *British Journal of Anaesthesia*, *134*(3), 875–878. DOI: 10.1016/j.bja.2024.12.015 PMID: 39855936

Boyce, S. H., & Quigley, M. A. (2002). Uvulitis and partial upper airway obstruction following cannabis inhalation. *Emergency Medicine*, *14*(1), 106–108. DOI: 10.1046/j.1442-2026.2002.00294.x PMID: 11993827

Brand, E. J., & Zhao, Z. (2017). Cannabis in Chinese medicine: Are some traditional indications referenced in ancient literature related to cannabinoids? *Frontiers in Pharmacology*, *8*, 108. DOI: 10.3389/fphar.2017.00108 PMID: 28344554

Bureau of Justice Assistance. (2023, March 1). *Substance Use and Pregnancy - Part 1: Current State Policies on Mandatory Reporting of Substance Use during Pregnancy, and Their Implications (March 2023).* https://bja.ojp.gov/library/publications/substance-use-andpregnancy-part-1-current-state-policies-mandatory-0-

Cammarano, C. A., & Villaluz, J. E. (2021). A reason to rethink gasting guidelines? Marijuana-induced gastroparesis and the implications for aspiration risk in the nil per os (NPO) patient: A case report. *The American Journal of Case Reports*, *22*, e934187. DOI: 10.12659/AJCR.934187 PMID: 34840324

Chaudoir, S. R., & Quinn, D. M. (2015). Evidence that anticipated stigma predicts poorer depressive symptom trajectories among emerging adults living with concealable stigmatized identities. *Self and Identity*, *15*(2), 139–151. DOI: 10.1080/15298868.2015.1091378

Cheng, D., Dongdong, X., & Tao, C. (2024). Cannabis use disorder associated with increased risk of postoperative complications after hip or knee arthroplasties: A meta-analysis of observational studies. *The Journal of the American Academy of Orthopaedic Surgeons*, *32*(20), e1067–e1078. DOI: 10.5435/JAAOS-D-23-00407 PMID: 38759231

Chiu, R. G., Patel, S., Siddiqui, N., Nunna, R. S., & Mehta, A. I. (2021). Cannabis abuse and perioperative complications following inpatient spine surgery in the United States. *Spine*, *46*(11), 734–743. DOI: 10.1097/BRS.0000000000004035 PMID: 33769411

Connors, N., Kosnett, M. J., Kulig, K., Nelson, L. S., & Stolbach, A. I. (2020). ACMT Position Statement: Interpretation of urine for tetrahydrocannabinol metabolites. *Journal of Medical Toxicology; Official Journal of the American College of Medical Toxicology*, *16*(2), 240–242. DOI: 10.1007/s13181-019-00753-8 PMID: 31939053

D'Souza, D. C., Cortes-Briones, J., Creatura, G., Blucz, G., Thurnauer, H., Deaso, E., Bielen, K., Surti, T., Radhakrishnan, R., Gupta, A., Gupta, S., Cahill, J., Sherif, M. A., Makriyannis, A., Morgan, P. T., Ranganathan, M., & Skosnik, P. D. (2019). Efficacy and safety of a fatty acid amide hydrolase inhibitor (PF-04457845) in the treatment of cannabis withdrawal and dependence in men: A double-blind, placebo-controlled, parallel group, phase 2a single-site randomised controlled trial. *The Lancet. Psychiatry*, *6*(1), 35–45. DOI: 10.1016/S2215-0366(18)30427-9 PMID: 30528676

Dahlke, S., Butler, J. I., Hunter, K. F., Toubiana, M., Kalogirou, M. R., Shrestha, S., Devkota, R., Law, J., & Scheuerman, M. (2024). The effects of stigma: Older persons and medicinal cannabis. *Qualitative Health Research, 34*(8-9), 717–731. DOI: 10.1177/10497323241227419 PMID: 38305270

Dalle, S., & Dalle, S. (2025). The endocannabinoid system & malignant hyperthermia: From molecular signaling towards clinical implications. *Progress in Lipid Research, 99*, 101342. DOI: 10.1016/j.plipres.2025.101342 PMID: 40680894

Daniels, S., St. Pierre, M., Sanchez, T., & Walsh, Z. (2023). Physician communication and perceived stigma in prenatal cannabis use. *Journal of Psychoactive Drugs, 55*(3), 290–298. DOI: 10.1080/02791072.2022.2076179 PMID: 35580234

Dave, T., Habte, A., Vora, V., Sheikh, M. Q., Sanker, V., & Gopal, S. V. (2024). Sushruta: The father of Indian surgical history. *Plastic and Reconstructive Surgery. Global Open, 12*(4), e5715. DOI: 10.1097/GOX.0000000000005715 PMID: 38596573

Derise, A., Ford, C., Hafiz, N., Pandit, S., Vyas, A., Igbinedion, S., Morris, J., Jordan, P., Cai, Q., & Alexander, J. S. (2022). Chronic cannabis intoxication and propofol-induced salivation: Causes and considerations. *Pathophysiology : the Official Journal of the International Society for Pathophysiology, 29*(2), 223–232. DOI: 10.3390/pathophysiology29020018 PMID: 35736646

Dowell, D., Ragan, K. R., Jones, C. M., Baldwin, G. T., & Chou, R. (2022). CDC clinical practice guideline for prescribing opioids for pain—United States, 2022. *MMWR. Recommendations and Reports, 71*(3, No. RR-3), 1–95. DOI: 10.15585/mmwr.rr7103a1 PMID: 36327391

Earnshaw, V., Quinn, D. M., & Park, C. L. (2012). Anticipated stigma and quality of life among people living with chronic illnesses. *Chronic Illness, 8*(2), 79–88. Advance online publication. DOI: 10.1177/1742395311429393 PMID: 22080524

Earnshaw, V. A., Smith, L. R., Chaudoir, S. R., Amico, K. R., & Copenhaver, M. M. (2013). HIV stigma mechanisms and well-being among PLWH: A test of the HIV stigma framework. *AIDS and Behavior, 17*(5), 1785–1795. DOI: 10.1007/s10461-013-0437-9 PMID: 23456594

Echeverria-Villalobos, M., Fabian, C. A., Mitchell, J. G., Mazzotta, E., Fiorda Diaz, J., Noon, K., & Weaver, T. E. (2025). Cannabinoids and general anesthetics: Revisiting molecular mechanisms of their pharmacological interactions. *Anesthesia and Analgesia, 140*(6), 1401–1413. DOI: 10.1213/ANE.0000000000007313 PMID: 39504269

Echeverria-Villalobos, M., Todeschini, A. B., Stoicea, N., Fiorda-Diaz, J., Weaver, T., & Bergese, S. D. (2019). Perioperative care of cannabis users: A comprehensive review of pharmacological and anesthetic considerations. *Journal of Clinical Anesthesia, 57*, 41–49. DOI: 10.1016/j.jclinane.2019.03.011 PMID: 30852326

Ekrami, E., Sari, S., Kopac, O., Wang, D., Mascha, E. J., Stamper, S., Esa, W. A. S., Nair, H., Ruetzler, K., & Turan, A. (2024). Association between cannabis use and opioid consumption, pain, and respiratory complications after surgery: A retrospective cohort analysis. *Anesthesia and Analgesia, 139*(4), 724–733. DOI: 10.1213/ANE.0000000000006785 PMID: 38190341

English, F., & Greyson, D. (2022). "You still have that fear": Policy constraints on informed decision making about legalized cannabis use during pregnancy and lactation. *The International Journal on Drug Policy, 106*, 103774. Advance online publication. DOI: 10.1016/j.drugpo.2022.103774 PMID: 35772267

Enochs, E. (2021, June 10). *How cannabis can impact anesthesia and surgery*. Leafly. https://www.leafly.com/news/health/cannabis-surgery-anesthesia

Flament, J., Scius, N., & Thonon, H. (2020). Cannabinoid hyperemesis syndrome in the pregnant patient: Clinical case and literature review. *International Journal of Emergency Medicine, 13*(1), 52. DOI: 10.1186/s12245-020-00311-y PMID: 33115404

Flanagan, B. (2021). Harnessing the endocannabinoid system: What it means for the anesthesia provider. *AANA Journal, 89*(3), 261–268. PMID: 34042578

Flisberg, P., Paech, M. J., Shah, T., Ledowski, T., Kurowski, I., & Parsons, R. (2009). Induction dose of propofol in patients using cannabis. *European Journal of Anaesthesiology, 26*(3), 192–195. DOI: 10.1097/EJA.0b013e328319be59 PMID: 19237981

Gangwani, P., Lillian, D., Dobbins, J., Feng, C., Vorrasi, J., & Kolokythas, A. (2023). Is recreational marijuana use associated with changes in the vital signs or anesthetic requirements during intravenous sedation? *Journal of Oral and Maxillofacial Surgery, 81*(5), 527–535. DOI: 10.1016/j.joms.2023.01.007 PMID: 36746375

Garami, A., Shimansky, Y. P., Rumbus, Z., Vizin, R. C. L., Farkas, N., Hegyi, J., Szakacs, Z., Solymar, M., Csenkey, A., Chichc, D. A., Kapil, R., Kyle, D. J., Van Horn, W. D., Hegyi, P., & Romanovsky, A. A. (2020). Hyperthermia induced by transient receptor potential vanilloid-1 (TRPV1) antagonists in human clinical trials: Insights from mathematical modeling and meta-analysis. *Pharmacology & Therapeutics, 208*, 107474. DOI: 10.1016/j.pharmthera.2020.107474 PMID: 31926897

Goel, A., McGuinness, B., Jivraj, N. K., Wijeysundera, D. N., Mittleman, M. A., Bateman, B. T., Clarke, H., Ph, D., Kotra, L. P., & Ladha, K. (2020). Cannabis use disorder and perioperative outcomes in major elective surgeries: A retrospective cohort analysis. *Anesthesiology*, *132*(4), 625–635. DOI: 10.1097/ALN.0000000000003067 PMID: 31789638

Goyal, H., Awad, H. H., & Ghali, J. K. (2017). Role of cannabis in cardiovascular disorders. *Journal of Thoracic Disease*, *9*(7), 2079–2092. DOI: 10.21037/jtd.2017.06.104 PMID: 28840009

Grant, K. S., Petroff, R., Isoherranen, N., Stella, N., & Burbacher, T. M. (2018). Cannabis use during pregnancy: Pharmacokinetics and effects on child development. *Pharmacology & Therapeutics*, *182*, 133–151. DOI: 10.1016/j.pharmthera.2017.08.014 PMID: 28847562

Greene, S., Vaccaro, M., Bernier, A., Griffith, G., Ion, A., Maurice, R., Gabel, C., & Blake, M. (2023). "Digging in": Stigma and surveillance in the lives of pregnant and breastfeeding mothers who consume cannabis. *Critical Public Health*, *33*(5), 697–708. DOI: 10.1080/09581596.2023.2262739

Gregg, J. M., Campbell, R. L., Levin, K. J., Jawahar, G., & Elliott, R. A. (1976). Cardiovascular effects of cannabinol during oral surgery. *Anesthesia and Analgesia*, *55*(2), 202–213. DOI: 10.1213/00000539-197603000-00017 PMID: 769605

Haney, M., Cooper, Z. D., Bedi, G., Vosburg, S. K., Comer, S. D., & Foltin, R. W. (2013). Nabilone decreases marijuana withdrawal and a laboratory measure of marijuana relapse. *Neuropsychopharmacology : Official Publication of the American College of Neuropsychopharmacology*, *38*(8), 1557–1565. DOI: 10.1038/npp.2013.54 PMID: 23443718

Harris, M., Schiff, D. M., Saia, K., Muftu, S., Standish, K. R., & Wachman, E. M. (2023). Academy of Breastfeeding Medicine clinical protocol #21: Breastfeeding in the setting of substance use and substance use disorder (revised 2023). *Breastfeeding Medicine*, *18*(10), 715–733. DOI: 10.1089/bfm.2023.29256.abm PMID: 37856658

Hasckel Gewehr, J. L., Enzele, M. L., Freiria, L. M., Nunes, M. M., Spengler, J., Dondoerfer Teixeira, A. P., Amazonas, E., & Sesso Padilha, V. (2024). Full spectrum cannabidiol-rich extract reduced propofol dosage required for anesthetic induction in dogs – a pilot study. *Frontiers in Veterinary Science*, *11*, 1352314. Advance online publication. DOI: 10.3389/fvets.2024.1352314 PMID: 38645644

Hassenberg, C., Clausen, F., Hoffmann, G., Studer, A., & Schürenkamp, J. (2020). Investigation of phase II metabolism of 11-hydroxy-Δ-9-tetrahydrocannabinol and metabolite verification by chemical synthesis of 11-hydroxy-Δ-9-tetrahydro-cannabinol-glucuronide. *International Journal of Legal Medicine*, *134*(6), 2105–2119. DOI: 10.1007/s00414-020-02387-w PMID: 32808050

Health Canada. (2018). *Information for health care professionals: Cannabis and cannabinoids*. https://www.canada.ca/en/health-canada/services/drugs-medication/cannabis/information-medical-practitioners/information-health-care-professionals-cannabis-cannabinoids.html

Herdegen, T., & Cascorbi, I. (2023). Drug interactions of tetrahydrocannabinol and cannabidiol in cannabinoid drugs. *Deutsches Ärzteblatt International*, *120*(49), 833–840. DOI: 10.3238/arztebl.m2023.0223 PMID: 37874128

Holland, C. L., Nkumsah, M. A., Morrison, P., Tarr, J. A., Rubio, D., Rodriguez, K. L., Kraemer, K. L., Day, N., Arnold, R. M., & Chang, J. C. (2016). "Anything above marijuana takes priority": Obstetric providers' attitudes and counseling strategies regarding perinatal marijuana use. *Patient Education and Counseling*, *99*(9), 1446–1451. DOI: 10.1016/j.pec.2016.06.003 PMID: 27316326

Holmen, I. C., Beach, J. P., Kaizer, A. M., & Gumidyala, R. (2020). The association between preoperative cannabis use and intraoperative inhaled anesthetic consumption: A retrospective study. *Journal of Clinical Anesthesia*, *67*, 109980. DOI: 10.1016/j.jclinane.2020.109980 PMID: 32653758

Hoveidaei, A. H., Pouramini, A., Mousavi-Nasab, M. M., Taghavi, P., Miri, L., Saggar, R., & Conway, J. D. (2024). The role of cannabis on total hip and knee surgeries outcomes: A systematic review and meta-analysis. *International Orthopaedics*, *49*(2), 343–355. DOI: 10.1007/s00264-024-06359-2 PMID: 39562357

Huson, H. B., Granados, T. M., & Rasko, Y. (2018). Surgical considerations of marijuana use in elective procedures. *Heliyon*, *4*(9), e00779. DOI: 10.1016/j.heliyon.2018.e00779 PMID: 30225378

Ibera, C., Shalom, B., Saifi, F., Shrader, J., & Davidson, E. (2018). Effects of cannabis extract premedication on anesthetic depth. *Harefuah*, *157*(3), 162–166. PMID: 29582946

Imasogie, N., Rose, R. V., & Wilson, A. (2021). High quantities: Evaluating the association between cannabis use and propofol anesthesia during endoscopy. *PLoS One*, *16*(3), e0248062. DOI: 10.1371/journal.pone.0248062 PMID: 33661987

Jeffers, A. M., Glantz, S., Byers, A. L., & Keyhani, S. (2024). Association of cannabis use with cardiovascular outcomes among US adults. *Journal of the American Heart Association, 13*(5), e030178. DOI: 10.1161/JAHA.123.030178 PMID: 38415581

King, D., Greenier, E., Caballero, M., & Morgan, B. (2023b). Integrating the ASRA Pain Medicine Cannabis Consensus Guidelines into Certified Registered Nurse Anesthetist clinical practice. *AANA Journal, 91*(4), 28–30. PMID: 38809193

King, D. D. (2026). Anticipated stigma in nursing: A concept analysis informed by cannabis use disclosure. *Journal of Advanced Nursing*, jan.70499. Advance online publication. DOI: 10.1111/jan.70499 PMID: 41588830

King, D. D., DeCarlo, M., Mylott, L., & Yarossi, M. (2023a). Cannabis knowledge gaps in nursing education: Pilot testing cannabis curriculum. *Teaching and Learning in Nursing, 18*(4), 474–479. DOI: 10.1016/j.teln.2023.06.012

King, D. D., Gill, C. J., Cadieux, C. S., & Singh, N. (2024). The role of stigma in cannabis use disclosure: An exploratory study. *Harm Reduction Journal, 21*(21), 21. Advance online publication. DOI: 10.1186/s12954-024-00929-8 PMID: 38273362

King, D. D., Stewart, S. A., Collins-Yoder, A., Fleckner, T., & Price, L. L. (2021). Anesthesia for patients who self-report cannabis (marijuana) use before esophagogastroduodenoscopy: A retrospective review. *AANA Journal, 89*(3), 205–212. PMID: 34042571

King, D. D., Termmemand, R., & Greenwood, J. E. (2026). Preoperative cannabinoid exposure and postoperative pain: A narrative review. *Journal of Clinical Anesthesia, 109*, 112097. DOI: 10.1016/j.jclinane.2025.112097 PMID: 41406677

Kumar, U., Macko, A. R., Kang, N., Darian, N. G., Salek, F. O., & Khalpey, Z. (2024). Perioperative cannabinoids significantly reduce postoperative opioid requirements in patients undergoing coronary artery bypass graft surgery. *Cureus, 16*(4), e58566. DOI: 10.7759/cureus.58566 PMID: 38765405

Ladha, K. S., McLaren-Blades, A., Goel, A., Buys, M. J., Farquhar-Smith, P., Haroutounian, S., Kotteeswaran, Y., Kwofie, K., Le Foll, B., Lightfoot, N. J., Loiselle, J., Mace, H., Nicholls, J., Regev, A., Rosseland, L. A., Shanthanna, H., Sinha, A., Sutherland, A., Tanguay, R., & Clarke, H. (2021). Perioperative Pain and Addiction Interdisciplinary Network (PAIN): Consensus recommendations for perioperative management of cannabis and cannabinoid-based medicine users by a modified Delphi process. *British Journal of Anaesthesia, 126*(1), 304–318. DOI: 10.1016/j.bja.2020.09.026 PMID: 33129489

Landman, S. T., Dhaliwal, I., Mackenzie, C. A., Martinu, T., Steel, A., & Bosma, K. J. (2019). Life-threatening bronchiolitis related to electronic cigarette use in a Canadian youth. *Canadian Medical Association Journal*, *191*(48), E1321–E1331. DOI: 10.1503/cmaj.191402 PMID: 31753841

Latif, Z., & Garg, N. (2020). The impact of marijuana on the cardiovascular system: A review of the most common cardiovascular events associated with marijuana use. *Journal of Clinical Medicine*, *9*(6), 1925. DOI: 10.3390/jcm9061925 PMID: 32575540

Levin, F. R., Mariani, J. J., Brooks, D. J., Pavlicova, M., Cheng, W., & Nunes, E. V. (2011). Dronabinol for the treatment of cannabis dependence: A randomized, double-blind, placebo-controlled trial. *Drug and Alcohol Dependence*, *116*(1-3), 142–150. DOI: 10.1016/j.drugalcdep.2010.12.010 PMID: 21310551

Loeb, L., Hochwald, A., Picco, M. F., Chan, J. L., Hashash, J. G., Chadha, R., Farraye, F. A., & Kinnucan, J. A. (2025). Cannabis use in patients with inflammation is associated with longer endoscopic duration and inflammation. *Crohn's & Colitis 360*, *7*(3), otaf034. Advance online publication. DOI: 10.1093/crocol/otaf034 PMID: 40667460

Lu, Y., Mahajan, L., Rudy, H. L., Yan, Y., & Ricci, J. A. (2023). The impact of marijuana use on postoperative outcomes in abdominal-based free flap breast reconstruction. *Journal of Reconstructive Microsurgery*, *40*(9), 680–687. DOI: 10.1055/a-2277-0117 PMID: 38413008

Mallat, A., Roberson, J., & Brock-Utne, J. G. (1996). Preoperative marijuana inhalation — An airway concern. *Canadian Journal of Anaesthesia*, *43*(7), 691–693. DOI: 10.1007/BF03017953 PMID: 8807175

Mason, B. J., Crean, R., Goodell, V., Light, J. M., Quello, S., Shadan, F., Buffkins, K., Kyle, M., Adusumalli, M., Begovic, A., & Rao, S. (2012). A proof-of-concept randomized controlled study of gabapentin: Effects on cannabis use, withdrawal and executive function deficits in cannabis-dependent adults. *Neuropsychopharmacology : Official Publication of the American College of Neuropsychopharmacology*, *37*(7), 1689–1698. DOI: 10.1038/npp.2012.14 PMID: 22373942

Metz, T. D., Allshouse, A. A., McMillin, G. A., Silver, R. M., Smid, M. C., Haas, D. M., Simhan, H. N., Saade, G. R., Grobman, W. A., Parry, S., Chung, J. H., & Jarlenski, M. P. (2022). Association of cannabis use with nausea and vomiting of pregnancy. *Obstetrics and Gynecology*, *140*(2), 266–270. DOI: 10.1097/AOG.0000000000004850 PMID: 35852278

Michel, A., & King, D. D. (2025). Cannabis use in the peripartum period. *Nursing for Women's Health, 29*(5), 311–327. DOI: 10.1016/j.nwh.2025.04.005 PMID: 40912671

Mittleman, M. A., Lewis, R. A., Maclure, M., Sherwood, J. B., & Muller, J. E. (2001). Triggering myocardial infarction by marijuana. *Circulation, 103*(23), 2805–2809. DOI: 10.1161/01.CIR.103.23.2805 PMID: 11401936

Moore, K. E., & Tangney, J. P. (2017). Managing the concealable stigma of criminal justice system involvement: A longitudinal examination of anticipated stigma, social withdrawal, and post-release adjustment. *The Journal of Social Issues, 7*(2), 322–340. DOI: 10.1111/josi.12219 PMID: 34334814

Murataeva, N., Straiker, A., & Mackie, K. (2014). Parsing the players: 2-arachidonoyl-glycerol synthesis and degradation in the CNS. *British Journal of Pharmacology, 171*(6), 1379–1391. DOI: 10.1111/bph.12411 PMID: 24102242

Nasrin, S., Watson, C. J. W., Bardhi, K., Fort, G., Chen, G., & Lazarus, P. (2021). Inhibition of UDP-glucuronosyltransferase enzymes by major cannabinoids and their metabolites. *Drug Metabolism and Disposition: the Biological Fate of Chemicals, 49*(12), 1081–1089. DOI: 10.1124/dmd.121.000530 PMID: 34493601

National Academies of Sciences, Engineering, and Medicine [NASEM]. (2024). *Cannabis Policy Impacts Public Health and Health Equity*. The National Academies Press. https://doi.org/DOI: 10.17226/27766

National Council of State Boards of Nursing. (2018). The NCSBN national nursing guidelines for medical marijuana: Current legislation, scientific literature review, and nursing implications. *Journal of Nursing Regulation, 9*(2, Suppl.), S1–S60. DOI: 10.1016/S2155-8256(18)30003-0

Nielsen, S., Sabioni, P., Trigo, J., Ware, M. A., Betz-Stablein, B. D., Murnion, B., Lintzeris, N., Khor, K. E., Farrell, M., Smith, A., & Le Foll, B. (2017). Opioid-sparing effect of cannabinoids: A systematic review and meta-analysis. *Neuropsychopharmacology : Official Publication of the American College of Neuropsychopharmacology, 42*(9), 1752–1765. DOI: 10.1038/npp.2017.51 PMID: 28327548

Oga, E., Stockton, M. A., Stewart, C., Kraemer, J., Kimani, J., Mbote, D., Njuguna, S., & Nyblade, L. (2022). Validating a measure of anticipated sex work-related stigma among male and female sex workers in Kenya. *Global Public Health: An International Journal for Research, Policy and Practice, 17*(12), 3583–3595. DOI: 10.1080/17441692.2022.2105377 PMID: 35938397

Pacher, P., Steffens, S., Haskó, G., Schindler, T. H., & Kunos, G. (2018). Cardiovascular effects of marijuana and synthetic cannabinoids: The good, the bad, and the ugly. *Nature Reviews. Cardiology*, *15*(3), 151–166. DOI: 10.1038/nrcardio.2017.130 PMID: 28905873

Patel, S., Wohlfeil, E. R., Rademacher, D. J., Carrier, E. J., Perry, L. J., Kundu, A., Falck, J. R., Nithipatikom, K., Campbell, W. B., & Hillard, C. J. (2003). The general anesthetic propofol increases brain N-arachidonylethanolamine (anandamide) content and inhibits fatty acid amide hydrolase. *British Journal of Pharmacology*, *139*(5), 1005–1013. DOI: 10.1038/sj.bjp.0705334 PMID: 12839875

Patilea-Vrana, G. I., Anoshchenko, O., & Unadkat, J. D. (2019). Hepatic enzymes relevant to the disposition of (-)-Δ^9-Tetrahydrocannabinol (THC) and its psychoactive metabolite, 11-OH-THC. *Drug Metabolism and Disposition: the Biological Fate of Chemicals*, *47*(3), 249–256. DOI: 10.1124/dmd.118.085548 PMID: 30567877

Peltzer, K., & Pengpid, S. (2016). Anticipated stigma in chronic illness patients in Cambodia, Myanmar and Vietnam. *Nagoya Journal of Medical Science*, *78*(4), 423–435. DOI: 10.18999/nagjms.78.4.423 PMID: 28008198

Potnuru, P. P., Jonna, S., & Williams, G. W.II. (2023). Cannabis use disorder and perioperative complications. *JAMA Surgery*, *158*(9), 935–944. DOI: 10.1001/jamasurg.2023.2403 PMID: 37405729

Pourmand, A., Esmailian, G., Mazer-Amirshahi, M., Lee-Park, O., & Tran, Q. K. (2021). Topical capsaicin for the treatment of cannabinoid hyperemesis syndrome, a systematic review and meta-analysis. *The American Journal of Emergency Medicine*, *43*, 35–40. DOI: 10.1016/j.ajem.2021.01.004 PMID: 33493995

Pryce, G., & Baker, D. (2017). Antidote to cannabinoid intoxication: The CB_1 receptor inverse agonist, AM251, reverses hypothermic effects of the CB_1 receptor agonist, CB-13, in mice. *British Journal of Pharmacology*, *174*(21), 3790–3794. DOI: 10.1111/bph.13973 PMID: 28800377

Quinn, D. M., & Chaudoir, S. R. (2009). Living with a concealable stigmatized identity: The impact of anticipated stigma, centrality, salience, and cultural stigma on psychological distress and health. *Journal of Personality and Social Psychology*, *97*(4), 634–651. DOI: 10.1037/a0015815 PMID: 19785483

Quinn, D. M., Williams, M. K., Quintana, F., Gaskins, J. L., Overstreet, N. M., Pishori, A., Earnshaw, V. A., Perez, G., & Chaudoir, S. R. (2014). Examining effects of anticipated stigma, centrality, salience, internalization, and outness on psychological distress for people with concealable stigmatized identities. *PLoS One*, *9*(5), e96977. DOI: 10.1371/journal.pone.0096977 PMID: 24817189

Raghunathan, K., Pyati, S., Dunworth, S., Sajdeya, R., Costin, B., Blalock, D., Bartels, K., Pepin, M., & Bryan, W. (2025). Urine tests for THC in patients undergoing elective inpatient surgery: A nationwide longitudinal electronic health record study in US veterans. *British Journal of Anaesthesia*, *134*(4), 1244–1246. DOI: 10.1016/j.bja.2024.12.031 PMID: 39893066

Rice, W. S., Turan, B., Fletcher, F. E., Nápoles, T. M., Walcott, M., Batchelder, A., Kempf, M.-C., Konkle-Parker, D. J., Wilson, T. E., Tien, P. C., Wingood, G. M., Neilands, T. B., Johnson, M. O., Weiser, S. D., & Turan, J. M. (2019). A mixed methods study of anticipated and experienced stigma in health care settings among women living with HIV in the United States. *AIDS Patient Care and STDs*, *33*(4), 184–195. DOI: 10.1089/apc.2018.0282 PMID: 30932700

Ryan, S. A., Ammerman, S. D., O'Connor, M. E., Gonzalez, L., Patrick, S. W., Quigley, J., Walker, L. R., Meek, J. Y., Johnston, M., Stellwagen, L., Thomas, J., & Ware, J. (2018). Marijuana use during pregnancy and breastfeeding: Implications for neonatal and childhood outcomes. *Pediatrics*, *142*(3), e20181889. Advance online publication. DOI: 10.1542/peds.2018-1889 PMID: 30150209

Sabbineni, M., Scott, W., Punia, K., Manuja, K., Singh, A., Campbell, K., MacKillop, J., & Balodis, I. (2024). Dopamine antagonists and topical capsaicin for cannabis hyperemesis syndrome in the emergency department: A systematic review of direct evidence. *Academic Emergency Medicine*, *31*(5), 493–503. DOI: 10.1111/acem.14770 PMID: 37391387

Sankar-Maharaj, S., Chen, D., & Hariharan, S. (2018). Postoperative shivering among cannabis users at a public hospital in Trinidad, West Indies. *Journal of Perianesthesia Nursing*, *33*(1), 37–44. DOI: 10.1016/j.jopan.2016.03.010 PMID: 29362045

Schelling, G., Hauer, D., Azad, S. C., Schmoelz, M., Chouker, A., Schmidt, M., Hornuss, C., Rippberger, M., Briegel, J., Thiel, M., & Vogeser, M. (2006). Effects of general anesthesia on anandamide blood levels in humans. *Anesthesiology*, *104*(2), 273–277. DOI: 10.1097/00000542-200602000-00012 PMID: 16436846

Shafi, M. I., Liaquat, S., & Auckley, D. (2018). Up in smoke: An unusual case of diffuse alveolar hemorrhage from marijuana. *Respiratory Medicine Case Reports*, *25*, 22–24. DOI: 10.1016/j.rmcr.2018.05.028 PMID: 29998053

Shah, S., Schwenk, E. S., Sondekoppam, R. V., Clarke, H., Zakowski, M., Rzasa-Lynn, R. S., Yeung, B., Nicholson, K., Schwartz, G., Hooten, W. M., Wallace, M., Viscusi, E. R., & Narouze, S. (2023). ASRA Pain Medicine consensus guidelines on the management of the perioperative patient on cannabis and cannabinoids. *Regional Anesthesia and Pain Medicine*, *48*(3), 97–117. DOI: 10.1136/rapm-2022-104013 PMID: 36596580

Shanthanna, H., Zhang, B. H., Saud, H., Sengputa, N., Chen, M., Bakshi, D., Richardson, L., & Wang, L. (2021). Effect of self-reported cannabis use on postoperative outcomes: A propensity matched cohort analysis of non-cardiac surgery patients. *Regional Anesthesia and Pain Medicine*, *46*(8), 656. DOI: 10.1136/rapm-2021-102754 PMID: 33990441

Sharma, P., Murthy, P., & Bharath, M. M. (2012). Chemistry, metabolism, and toxicology of cannabis: Clinical implications. *Iranian Journal of Psychiatry*, *7*(4), 149–156. PMID: 23408483

Sladkey, N., King, D. D., & Reede, L. J. (2025). Enhancing the preanesthesia evaluation: Consensus development of the Cannabis Use and Behaviors Assessment Tool (CUBAT). *Journal of Perianesthesia Nursing*, *40*(1), 83–89. DOI: 10.1016/j.jopan.2024.03.011 PMID: 38935007

Smith, L. D. (2021). History of cannabis and prohibition. In Clark, C. S. (Ed.), *Cannabis: A handbook for nurses*. Wolters Kluwer.

Smith, R. T., & Gruber, S. A. (2023). Contemplating cannabis? The complex relationship between cannabinoids and hepatic metabolism resulting in the potential for drug-drug interactions. *Frontiers in Psychiatry*, *13*, 1055481. DOI: 10.3389/fpsyt.2022.1055481 PMID: 36704740

Sohail, A. H., Quazi, M. A., Sheikh, A. B., Greenbaum, A., Nir, I., & Hernandez, M. C. (2025). Impact of cannabis consumption on perioperative outcomes in patients undergoing hepatobiliary and pancreatic surgery: A nationwide analysis. *HPB : The Official Journal of the International Hepato Pancreato Biliary Association*, *27*(7), 981–987. DOI: 10.1016/j.hpb.2025.04.006 PMID: 40324909

Stefani, A., Aramini, B., Baraldi, C., Pellesi, L., Della Casa, G., Morandi, U., & Guerzoni, S. (2020). Secondary spontaneous pneumothorax and bullous lung disease in cannabis and tobacco smokers: A case-control study. *PLoS One*, *15*(3), e0230419. DOI: 10.1371/journal.pone.0230419 PMID: 32226050

Stone, A. L., Pham, A., Osmundson, S. S., Pedowitz, A., Kingsley, P. J., Marnett, L. J., Patel, S., Wickersham, N., Sorabella, L. L., & Bruehl, S. (2024). Interactions between endocannabinoid and endogenous opioid systems prospectively influence postoperative opioid use in pregnant patients undergoing cesarean delivery. *The Journal of Pain, 25*(9), 104548. DOI: 10.1016/j.jpain.2024.104548 PMID: 38663651

Substance Abuse and Mental Health Services Administration. [SAMHSA]. (2025). *Key Substance Use and Mental Health Indicators in the United States: Results from the 2024 National Survey on Drug Use and Health* (HHS Publication No. PEP25-07-007, NSDUH Series H-60). Center for Behavioral Health Statistics and Quality, Substance Abuse and Mental Health Services Administration. https://www.samhsa.gov/data/data-we-collect/nsduh-national-survey-drug-use-and-health/national-releases

Suhre, W., O'Reilly-Shah, V., & Van Cleve, W. (2020). Cannabis use is associated with a small increase in the risk of postoperative nausea and vomiting: A retrospective machine learning causal analysis. *BMC Anesthesiology, 20*(115), 115. Advance online publication. DOI: 10.1186/s12871-020-01036-4 PMID: 32423445

Tetrault, J. M., Crothers, K., Moore, B. A., Mehra, R., Concato, J., & Fiellin, D. A. (2007). Effects of marijuana smoking on pulmonary function and respiratory complications: A systematic review. *Archives of Internal Medicine, 167*(3), 221–228. DOI: 10.1001/archinte.167.3.221 PMID: 17296876

Thomas, T. F., Metaxas, E. S., Nguyen, T., Bennett, W., Skiendzielewski, K. V., Quinn, D. H., & Scaletta, A. L. (2022). Case report: Medical cannabis—warfarin drug-drug interaction. *Journal of Cannabis Research, 4*(1), 6. DOI: 10.1186/s42238-021-00112-x PMID: 35012687

Tsai, A. C., Kakuhikire, B., Perkins, J. M., Downey, J. M., Baguma, C., Satinsky, E. N., Gumisiriza, P., Kananura, J., & Bangsberg, D. R. (2021). Normative vs personal attitudes toward persons with HIV, and the mediating role of perceived HIV stigma in rural Uganda. *Journal of Global Health, 11*, 04056. DOI: 10.7189/jogh.11.04056 PMID: 34552725

Turan, O. A., Rullan, P. J., Pasqualini, I., Pumo, T. J., Surace, P. A., Murray, T. G., & Piuzzi, N. S. (2024). Cannabis use following total joint arthroplasty is associated with increased risks? A meta-analysis. *The Journal of Arthroplasty, 39*(2), 533–540. DOI: 10.1016/j.arth.2023.07.008 PMID: 37454951

Twardowski, M. A., Link, M. M., & Twardowski, N. M. (2019). Effects of cannabis use on sedation requirements for endoscopic procedures. *The Journal of the American Osteopathic Association*, *119*(5), 307–311. DOI: 10.7556/jaoa.2019.052 PMID: 30985870

Uršič, M., Babič, A., Vake, T., & Snoj, T. (2022). The impact of cannabidiol on the induction of isoflurane anesthesia and recovery in Wistar rats. *Cannabis and Cannabinoid Research*, *7*(3), 289–293. DOI: 10.1089/can.2021.0014 PMID: 33998903

U.S. Department of Health & Human Services [HHS]. (2025, March 14). *Summary of the HIPAA Privacy Rule*. https://www.hhs.gov/hipaa/for-professionals/privacy/laws-regulations/index.html

Walters, S. M., Kerr, J., Cano, M., Earnshaw, V., & Link, B. (2023). Intersectional Stigma as a Fundamental Cause of Health Disparities: A case study of how drug use stigma intersecting with racism and xenophobia creates health inequities for Black and Hispanic persons who use drugs over time. *Stigma and Health*, *8*(3), 325–343. DOI: 10.1037/sah0000426 PMID: 37744082

Wenger, T., & Moldrich, G. (2002). The role of endocannabinoids in the hypothalamic regulation of visceral function. *Prostaglandins, Leukotrienes, and Essential Fatty Acids*, *66*(2-3), 301–307. DOI: 10.1054/plef.2001.0353 PMID: 12052044

Xiao, T. T., Phillips, J. C., Macartney, G., & Stacey, D. (2023). Factors influencing Canadian oncology nurses discussing cannabis use with patients experiencing chemotherapy-induced nausea. *Canadian Oncology Nursing Journal = Revue Canadienne de Nursing Oncologique*, *33*(3), 300–309. DOI: 10.5737/23688076333 PMID: 38919903

Yang, G., Li, F., Wang, Q., Liu, Y., Guo, J., & Yue, C. (2024). Association between history of cannabis use and outcomes after total hip or knee arthroplasty: A systematic review and meta-analysis. *Frontiers in Public Health*, *12*, 1377688. Advance online publication. DOI: 10.3389/fpubh.2024.1377688 PMID: 38827608

Yeung, B. G., Ma, M. W., & Nelson, A. M. (2022). Cannabis exposure decreases need for blood pressure support during general anesthesia in orthopedic trauma surgery. *Cannabis and Cannabinoid Research*, *7*(3), 328–335. DOI: 10.1089/can.2021.0009 PMID: 34227872

Yoo, S.G., Seth, M., Earl, T.J., Ruwende, C., Karve, M., Shah, I., Hill, T., Gurm, H.S., & Sukul, D. (2020). Abstract 14449: Not so harmless: Marijuana use and in-hospital outcomes after percutaneous coronary intervention: Insights from the Blue Cross Blue Shield of Michigan Cardiovascular Consortium. *Circulation, 142*(Number Suppl_3). https://doi.org/DOI: 10.1161/circ.142.suppl_3.14449

Zhang, B. H., Saud, H., Sengupta, N., Chen, M., Bakshi, D., Richardson, L., Wang, L., & Shanthanna, H. (2021). Effect of preoperative cannabis use on perioperative outcomes: A retrospective cohort study. *Regional Anesthesia and Pain Medicine*, *46*(8), 650–655. DOI: 10.1136/rapm-2021-102479 PMID: 33990440

KEY TERMS AND DEFINITIONS

Acute Cannabis Intoxication: A clinically relevant state of recent cannabis exposure associated with impaired attention, altered perception, tachycardia or anxiety, and reduced ability to provide reliable history or consent, which may increase procedural risk.

Aspiration Risk Stratification: A perioperative assessment process that estimates the likelihood of aspiration of gastric contents during anesthesia based on patient factors, timing of intake, symptoms, and drug effects that may slow gastric emptying.

Cannabinoid-Induced Hyperalgesia: A pain-amplifying phenomenon in which frequent or high-dose cannabinoid exposure is associated with heightened pain sensitivity and greater analgesic needs despite ongoing use.

Cannabis Hyperemesis Syndrome (CHS): A syndrome characterized by recurrent nausea, vomiting, and abdominal discomfort in chronic cannabis users, often with symptom relief from hot showers and recurrence with continued cannabis use.

Cannabis Use and Behaviors Assessment Tool (CUBAT): A structured, preanesthesia screening framework that captures cannabis products, routes, dosing patterns, timing of last use, goals for use, and risk signals to support individualized anesthesia and recovery planning.

Cross-Tolerance: A reduction in response to one drug class that occurs after repeated exposure to another, such as altered anesthetic or analgesic requirements in patients with frequent, prolonged cannabinoid exposure.

Cytochrome P450 (CYP450) Interactions: Potential changes in medication effects caused by shared hepatic metabolic pathways between cannabinoids and perioperative drugs, leading to variability in drug levels, duration, or adverse effects.

Multimodal Analgesia: A pain management approach that combines medications and techniques with distinct mechanisms (e.g., acetaminophen, regional anesthesia, NSAIDs when appropriate, ketamine, gabapentinoids) to improve analgesia while reducing opioid exposure.

Opioid Stewardship: A deliberate strategy to minimize opioid-related harm through multimodal analgesia, functional goals, careful titration, and patient education, while still providing effective pain treatment.

Perioperative Cannabis Nursing: A specialized practice focus that integrates cannabis science, risk mitigation, education, and advocacy across the preoperative, intraoperative, and postoperative phases to support safety, equity, and continuity of care.

Stigma-Informed Communication: A patient-centered communication approach that normalizes cannabis as a clinical variable, uses nonjudgmental language, and reduces fear of punishment, enabling accurate disclosure and participation in shared decision-making.

Withdrawal Recognition: The identification of predictable symptom clusters that may occur after abrupt reduction or cessation of frequent cannabis use, such as irritability, sleep disturbances, appetite changes, anxiety, or autonomic symptoms, which can mimic other perioperative problems.

Chapter 7
Cannabinoid Therapeutics and Sexual Wellness

M'lissa A. Duncan
http://orcid.org/0009-0002-5828-8660
American Cannabis Nurses Association, USA

Christobal E. Mozingo-Goodwin
http://orcid.org/0009-0008-5674-1402
Linfield University, USA

ABSTRACT

This chapter aims to serve as a comprehensive guide to the benefits and risks associated with cannabinoid therapeutics in relation to sexual health issues. It seeks to inform readers about how cannabinoids might influence conditions such as sexual desire disorders, sexual pain disorders, orgasmic disorders, and sexual arousal disorders by exploring both potential therapeutic effects and side effects. In doing so, the chapter provides insights into how cannabinoid use could enhance or hinder sexual health and overall quality of life. Additionally, the chapter strives to raise awareness among consumers and providers about how cannabis interacts with different body systems, aiming to reduce adverse effects and promote wellness with cannabis, rather than harm.

INTRODUCTION

The endocannabinoid system (ECS) is a complex biological network comprised of enzymes, receptors, and signaling molecules. The ECS plays a crucial role in

DOI: 10.4018/979-8-2600-2035-7.ch007

maintaining the body's homeostasis, which is essential in its role as being protective against chronic illnesses. It involves regulating various bodily functions such as digestion, repair, restoration, and sleep. Additionally, the ECS influences behavioral mechanisms and oversees hormonal and chemical processes vital for the body's proper functioning. This includes its role in the male and female reproductive systems, ensuring they operate effectively.

Sexual wellness is often overlooked and not addressed in the current healthcare system. Sexual wellness, similar to mental health, significantly impacts our physical and overall well-being. Participating in consensual and enjoyable sexual activity provides numerous benefits, such as strengthening pelvic floor muscles, burning more calories, reducing joint stiffness, enhancing immunity, improving sleep quality, and decreasing the risk of heart disease and high blood pressure.

Unfortunately, sexual dysfunction includes, but is not limited to, the following disorders:

- Conception/infertility
- Premenstrual Syndrome (PMS/PMDD)
- Female Orgasmic Disorder (inability to obtain orgasm)
- Menopause (estrogen and androgen deficiencies)
- Endometriosis
- Libido
- Erectile dysfunction (inability to maintain an erection)
- Polycystic ovarian syndrome
- Post-coital pain (lubrication).

According to the World Health Organization (WHO), sexual dysfunction can be divided into four categories (Belau et al., 2022). These categories include sexual desire disorders, sexual pain disorders, orgasmic disorders, and sexual arousal disorders. These conditions may be associated with symptoms of anxiety and depression, potentially affecting a person's quality of life.

Research by Sun & Eisenberg (2017) found a positive correlation between cannabis use and sexual frequency. Their findings indicate that marijuana use is associated with higher sexual frequency among both men and women, across various demographic groups, and does not appear to affect sexual function adversely.

Other research, such as by Belau et al. (2022), notes exceptions. Their study found a connection between sexual dysfunction and **heavy** polysubstance use (including cannabis, tobacco, and alcohol), as well as the development of depression. The study suggests that both women and men with at least one sexual dysfunction may be more likely to experience depression than those without dysfunction. Psychological distress and complicated interpersonal relationships can also negatively impact sexual activity and relationships.

This chapter aims to serve as a comprehensive guide to the benefits and risks associated with cannabinoid therapeutics in relation to sexual health issues. The intent is to educate readers on the potential impact of cannabinoids on conditions like sexual desire disorders, sexual pain disorders, orgasmic disorders, and sexual arousal disorders. By examining both the possible therapeutic benefits and side effects, this chapter sheds light on how cannabinoid use might improve or impede sexual health and overall quality of life. Additionally, the chapter strives to raise awareness among consumers and providers about how cannabis interacts with different body systems, aiming to reduce adverse effects and promote wellness with cannabis while reducing undesirable side effects.

Historical Use of Cannabis for Sexual Outcomes

Since ancient times, cannabis has been used in Asia to either enhance or suppress sexual desire. In certain cultures, it acted as an aphrodisiac, possibly increasing sensory perception and intimacy. Traditional medical systems, such as Ayurveda in India, have recorded cannabis formulations designed to boost vitality and sexual health (Backes & Weil, 2017).

Conversely, historical records indicate that cannabis was also used to suppress sexual urges, particularly in religious contexts. Monks and ascetics relied on its sedative effects to aid in maintaining celibacy and concentrating on spiritual practices. This dual historical usage underscores cannabis's versatile effects and highlights how cultural attitudes have shaped its role in sexuality and medicine (Crocq, 2020).

Harm Reduction vs Traditional Healthcare

Women are more likely than men to experience sexual dysfunction due to both physiological and psychological factors. The female sexual response encompasses a broad array of elements, which can increase the chances of difficulties occurring at different stages, including desire, arousal, and orgasm. Significant hormonal changes throughout their lives—menstrual cycles, pregnancy, postpartum, menopause, and hormonal contraceptive use—can all impact sexual desire and function. Additionally, higher rates of stress, anxiety, depression, relationship issues, and a history of trauma or abuse may contribute to the problem.

Societal attitudes and cultural norms influence women's experiences of sexual dysfunction. Women may be more comfortable reporting these issues due to societal expectations about female sexuality and more frequent engagement with healthcare providers for reproductive health needs, increasing the likelihood of addressing sexual health concerns.

Sexual dysfunction in men may be underreported due to stigma or threats to masculinity, causing apparent lower reporting rates. Men may hesitate to discuss sexual health with providers and seek information from non-clinical sources.

Risk vs Reward

Chronic cannabinoid therapy has been shown to cause an increase in menstrual cycle length, altered female reproductive hormone levels, and ovarian dysfunction in women (Lo et al., 2022). LO et al. (2022) continue by stating that in males, chronic use can cause testicular atrophy, abnormal spermatogenesis, and erectile dysfunction.

When considering the use of cannabis for managing pain or other health issues, it is important to evaluate a variety of factors that can influence its safety and effectiveness. Education is essential for understanding how cannabis affects the body, as well as the potential benefits and risks involved, which is vital for making informed decisions. Personal experience with cannabis—or the absence of it—can influence one's expectations and comfort level. Clearly defining the motivation and goals for cannabis use, whether it's for pain relief, improved mobility, or other reasons, is important. For individuals with dexterity or mobility challenges, choosing a suitable method of consumption is crucial; for example, using edibles or tinctures might be more practical than smoking or vaping.

A holistic evaluation should be considered, as each person is unique, and genetic factors can affect how individuals metabolize cannabis. This can influence its effectiveness and potential for side effects. As well, considering drug-drug interactions is vital, particularly if other medications are being taken simultaneously, to avoid adverse effects and ensure safety. Good nutrition can impact overall health and may influence or modulate the effects of cannabis.

Additionally, having a strong social support system which can provide emotional backing and logistical support, such as access to transportation, often needed for obtaining cannabis, especially if it is only available at specific dispensaries. Lastly, financial considerations also come into play, as cannabis products can be costly and are rarely covered by insurance.

Diagnosis Disclaimer

This chapter should not be used to diagnose; it is intended only to guide healthcare consumers who already have a medical diagnosis from a healthcare professional. Currently, there is limited evidence regarding the safety of cannabinoid therapeutics in reproductive health.

Conception/Infertility

Infertility can be described as the inability to conceive after having one year of unsuccessful attempts by having regular, unprotected sex with the intent to get pregnant. Infertility is typically diagnosed when a couple has been actively trying to conceive for one year or more without success. For women over the age of 35, this timeframe is typically reduced to six months due to the decrease in fertility that can occur with age. Infertility can result from issues with the woman, the man, or a combination of both partners. Signs and symptoms may include, but are not limited to, pelvic pain, irregular vaginal bleeding, no menses, penile disorders, and ejaculation issues.

Some causes of infertility include ovulatory disorders, low testosterone, low sperm count, endometriosis, sexually transmitted diseases, radiation, chemotherapy, thyroid disorders, sickle cell anemia, autoimmune disorders, genetic disorders, physical injury, surgical traumas, eating disorders, excessive alcohol intake, environmental toxins, over-exercising, smoking, hormone dysregulation, and substance abuse.

Traditional infertility treatments include ovulation stimulants, such as clomiphene, menotropins, and choriogonadotropin alfa, and assisted reproductive technology, such as in vitro fertilization. Side effects of pharmaceutical management include, but are not limited to, tachycardia, deep vein thrombosis, dizziness, headaches, flushing, depression, anxiety, restlessness, nausea, bloating, constipation, vomiting, urticaria, and multiple pregnancies (Lilley et al., 2020). When these medications are taken with tricyclic antidepressants, antihypertensives, and phenothiazines, fertility may be impaired. Fertility drugs are contraindicated in those with uncontrolled thyroid or adrenal function, liver disease, pituitary tumor, abnormal uterine bleeding, or sex hormone-dependent tumors.

According to Lingegowda et al. (2022), long-term exposure to cannabis in females can cause menstrual cycle disruption, delay in maturation, and dysregulate sex hormones. For those trying to conceive, this may be contraindicated (Lingegowda et al., 2022). Fertility can be impaired by cannabis use by causing a decrease in LH serum levels, inhibiting prolactin secretion, increasing testosterone levels, and disturbing the menstrual cycle (Popescu-Spineni et al., 2022).

Although there is limited evidence regarding the safety of cannabinoid therapy during pregnancy, cannabis use can negatively affect fertility in both men and women. Abnormal embryo implantation and development can be associated with cannabis use (Lo et al., 2022). Lynn et al. (2020) showed that cannabis use in female rats decreased luteinizing hormone surges and inhibited ovulation. Sperm cells have a complete endocannabinoid system and are involved in sperm fertilization and oocyte recognition (Carvalho et al., 2018). CBD studies in rats found to reduce sexual activities in test animals, a reduction in the size of the testis, and the total number of sperm cells (Blesching, 2025).

The World Health Organization states that polycystic ovarian syndrome is one of the most common causes of infertility (*Polycystic Ovary Syndrome*, 2026). 1 in 5 women between 15 and 49 years old struggle with infertility in the United States, and about 1 in 20 women struggle with infertility after the first child. 48 million couples worldwide live with infertility (*Infertility*, 2023). Twenty-five percent of couples facing infertility experience more than one contributing factor.

Holistic treatment may include a diet high in avocados, which are rich in zinc and vitamin E and support sperm quality and testosterone levels. Figs can help stimulate fertility. Eating cheese can interfere with sperm morphology and motility, hindering conception. Processed baked goods can hinder conception. Fats reduce oxygen to the sex organs. Sperm and eggs have difficulty multiplying when nutrition is dampened from diets high in saturated fat. Medication tracking in a journal can be helpful for those trying to conceive.

Using cannabinoid therapeutics when attempting to conceive may impair the successful implantation of the egg in the uterus and can impact fertility (Backes & Weil, 2017).The preparation of the endometrium and embryo implantation relies on a balanced ECS (Popescu-Spineni et al., 2022). Suppression of LH, FSH, prolactin, and a 24-hour delay in ovulation have been shown in pre-clinical rat models with acute THC administration (Lo et al., 2022). THC (tetrahydrocannabinol) has been shown to blunt the activation of hormones that affect sexual function (Lynn et al., 2020). The absence of cannabinoids during periods when individuals are attempting to conceive may be best.

Premenstrual Syndrome (PMS)

Premenstrual Syndrome (PMS) includes a variety of physical and emotional symptoms that many people experience prior to their menstrual period. PMS involves a range of symptoms that can affect various parts of the body, though it does not directly affect specific organs as some other medical conditions do. Instead, PMS influences the function of certain body systems, often due to hormonal fluctuations. include mood swings, irritability, fatigue, bloating, breast tenderness, and cramps. With growing interest in alternative therapies, some have considered the use of cannabis to manage these symptoms.

PMS is a complex condition that reflects interactions between hormonal changes and various body systems, leading to physical, emotional, and behavioral symptoms. It is the most common women's health complaint, affecting up to 80 percent of younger female healthcare consumers (Malka, 2022).

While PMS is related to the menstrual cycle, The main changes are related to hormonal fluctuations, like those of estrogen and progesterone, rather than direct impacts on reproductive organs such as the ovaries or uterus. Mood swings, irritability, anxiety, and depression are common PMS symptoms that are associated with neurochemical changes in the brain caused by these hormonal shifts. Unfortunately, some women experience bloating, abdominal cramps, and changes in bowel habits related to PMS. Additionally, PMS may cause muscle and joint pain or a feeling of tiredness and fatigue. Many women report breast tenderness or swelling as part of PMS. During menstruation, pain regulation, inflammation, uterine tone, and emotional stress responses influence how cramps, pelvic discomfort, mood changes, and sensitivity are controlled by endocannabinoid system signaling (Blesching, 2026).

Traditional treatments for premenstrual syndrome (PMS) aim to relieve symptoms and may differ based on their severity and effect on daily activities. Over-the-counter pain relievers, such as non-steroidal anti-inflammatory drugs (NSAIDs) like acetaminophen, ibuprofen, or naproxen can help alleviate cramps and breast tenderness. Allopathic medical providers sometimes will use oral contraceptives, i.e., birth control pills, which regulate hormonal fluctuations and reduce PMS symptoms for some women. Additionally, antidepressants such as selective serotonin reuptake inhibitors (SSRIs) or serotonin-norepinephrine reuptake inhibitors (SNRIs) can be prescribed for severe mood-related symptoms of PMS.

Holistic treatment for Premenstrual Syndrome (PMS) focuses on addressing the whole person—body, mind, and spirit—rather than just alleviating symptoms. This approach often combines lifestyle changes, natural remedies, and alternative therapies.

Diet plays a crucial role in alleviating symptoms and supporting the body during this cycle of change. Encourage individuals to maintain a balanced diet and avoid excessive sugar, salt, refined carbohydrates, and caffeine. Research indicates that calcium and magnesium supplements may help alleviate PMS symptoms. Therefore, advise patients to include foods rich in these minerals, such as leafy greens, dairy products, nuts, and seeds, in their diet (Muthukumaran et al., 2025).

According to various studies and health resources, it is estimated that approximately 75% of women experience some form of premenstrual symptoms during their reproductive years. Symptoms can vary from mild to severe, but about 25% of women report moderate to severe symptoms that can affect daily functioning and may require medical attention or intervention (Zhu et al., 2024).

Women frequently utilize cannabis products containing cannabinoids for the management of both physical and emotional symptoms associated with menstruation. Female healthcare consumers often list menstrual cramps as the primary reason they seek out medical cannabis.

Cannabis is widely recognized for its pain-relieving properties, which can help ease cramps and other aches associated with PMS. The active compounds in cannabis, such as THC (tetrahydrocannabinol), CBD (cannabidiol), and CBG (cannabigerol), interact with the body's endocannabinoid system to influence pain perception and reduce inflammation. Non-intoxicating treatment alternatives include PEA, OEA, and terpenes like β-caryophyllene, eucalyptol, and linalool, which can help alleviate symptoms of premenstrual syndrome (Cannakeys, 2025).

While THC has not been specifically tested in controlled clinical trials for dysmenorrhea, its known effects on pain management, emotional regulation, and stress response suggest it could have a therapeutic impact. However, individual responses can vary significantly, and due to each person's unique tolerance and reaction to THC, a careful and comprehensive evaluation is necessary (Blesching, 2026). Research by Dahlgreen et al. (2024) confirmed that CBD-based vaginal suppositories (100 mg) were associated with reduced menstrual pain and good tolerability, supporting localized cannabinoid delivery as a potential dysmenorrhea treatment. Anecdotal evidence suggests that applying cannabinoids topically on the abdomen and using suppositories can effectively reduce inflammation and pain related to premenstrual cramping and discomfort. Many cannabis products are available for PMS sufferers, including suppositories, topicals, patches, edibles, full-spectrum oral preparations, and cannabis flowers.

The current evidence suggests that cannabis medicines should be carefully integrated alongside standard care, rather than replacing it. While existing data provide biological plausibility and early clinical indications, the results are still incomplete and diverse.

Female Orgasmic Disorder (FOD)

Female Orgasmic Disorder (FOD) is a common but frequently underestimated sexual disorder that impacts many women globally. According to the DSM-5 (Diagnostic and Statistical Manual of Mental Disorders, Fifth Edition), FOD is categorized as a sexual dysfunction. Multiple factors, such as stress, anxiety, past trauma, and cultural or religious factors, can influence the ability to achieve orgasm. Physical conditions such as hormonal imbalances, chronic illness, and pharmaceuticals may also impact sexual wellness. Psychological causes include anxiety, depression, stress, and trauma. Contributing factors may include relationship issues, lack of sexual knowledge, decreased sexual desire, religion, or culture. FOD can be a lifelong issue or acquired and situational.

Signs and Symptoms of Female Orgasm Disorder

Cannakeys (2025) describes FOD as:

- difficulty achieving orgasm despite adequate sexual stimulation,
- delayed or infrequent orgasms,
- poor quality orgasm,
- reduced intensity of orgasmic sensations,
- absence of orgasm (anorgasmia),
- frustration with sex,
- distress with sexual activities,
- or anxiety related to the inability to reach orgasm,
- decreased sexual satisfaction,
- changes in orgasm intensities,
- and significantly less intense orgasms.

In the most recent US study of female sexual dysfunction, from over 30,000 women, the prevalence of FOD was approximately 21% (American Sexual Health Association, 2018). About 3 out of 4 women say they cannot orgasm through vaginal penetration alone. Currently, conventional treatments offer little help in this area. Cannabinoid therapeutics (CT) are an emerging evidence-based treatment. Given the limitations of traditional therapy, research indicates that cannabis may provide a new avenue for managing this condition, along with other women's sexual health issues.

Female Orgasm Disorder and the Endocannabinoid System

The endocannabinoid system (ECS) plays a critical role in modulating sexual arousal, pleasure, and orgasm. The ECS comprises cannabinoid receptors (CB1 and CB2), endogenous ligands, and enzymatic pathways that regulate various physiological processes, including mood, pain perception, and sexual function (Backes & Weil, 2017). Research suggests that activating CB1 receptors is linked to heightened sexual desire and an improved orgasmic response (Lynn et al., 2019).

The interaction between endocannabinoids and neurotransmitters such as oxytocin boosts emotional connection and intensifies orgasms. Endocannabinoids assist in achieving the ideal balance between relaxation and arousal, aiding in orgasms for women. A study by Lynn et al. (2019) found that women who used cannabis before sex experienced increased sexual satisfaction, heightened libido, and more frequent orgasms compared to those who did not use cannabis. Additionally, a study by Moser et al. (2023) suggested that cannabis enhances sensory perception and reduces anxiety, which might indirectly help women with Female Orgasmic Disorder (FOD) achieve orgasms.

Additionally, cannabidiol (CBD), a non-psychoactive cannabinoid, has demonstrated anxiolytic and muscle-relaxant effects, which may help overcome certain psychological and physical obstacles to achieving orgasm. Tetrahydrocannabinol (THC), the main psychoactive component in cannabis, engages with CB1 receptors to elevate dopamine levels, essential for pleasure and reward pathways, potentially enhancing the likelihood of orgasm. According to Malka (2022), THC can improve a deficient endocannabinoid system (ECS) tone, often associated with hormonal changes in women, such as those occurring during menstruation, perimenopause, and menopause.

While the prevalence of FOD is significant and conventional treatments may have limitations, it is crucial to consider the potential benefits and risks associated with using cannabis as a treatment option. Here are some key considerations:

Limited Research: Although there is increasing interest in exploring the potential therapeutic effects of cannabis on sexual dysfunction, it is important to recognize that research in this area is still in its early stages and remains limited. More comprehensive scientific studies are needed to understand better the specific mechanisms of action, effectiveness, safety profile, and appropriate dosing of cannabis for managing FOD. It is believed that the CB1 receptors can enhance sexual response and function. Backes and Weil (2017) continue by stating that higher doses of cannabinoid therapeutics can, in fact, impair sexual response by activating the TRPV1 channels. A survey of 373 women found that the use of cannabis before sexual activity increased their sex drive and decreased pain. Malka (2022) also found research with confirmed studies indicates some women find cannabinoid therapeutics helpful to reduce anxiety and increased relaxation, which may facilitate orgasm for those struggling with FOD, specifically.

Individual Variability: This is a key consideration when it comes to using cannabis for any potential therapeutic purposes, including addressing FOD. Various factors, such as the specific type of cannabinoids (such as THC, CBD, etc.), the method of consumption (smoking, edibles, topical applications), dosage, and individual tolerance levels, can all influence how cannabis may affect individuals differently. Personalized and careful dosing is crucial not only to minimize potential side effects but also to optimize the potential therapeutic benefits of cannabis. It is essential for healthcare consumers considering cannabinoid therapeutics as a treatment option to work closely with healthcare professionals who can provide guidance on dosing, monitor any effects or changes, and help ensure a safe and effective approach. Women have reported a positive impact on sexual desire, pleasure, and orgasmic quality with moderate consumption of cannabis (Backes & Weil, 2017). Since every endocannabinoid system (ECS) is unique, what is effective for one person may not be effective for another. Aphrodisiac experiences should not be generalized across different biological sexes.

Legal and Ethical Considerations: The legal status of cannabis varies widely around the world, with some regions legalizing medical and/or recreational use, while others maintain strict restrictions or prohibit its use entirely. Healthcare providers and healthcare consumers need to be aware of and adhere to the local laws and regulations regarding the use of cannabis when considering it as a treatment option for any medical condition.

Before exploring cannabis as a potential treatment, healthcare consumers should research and understand the laws and regulations concerning its use in their specific region. It is important to acknowledge that the legal status of cannabis can change over time, so staying informed about any regulatory updates or changes is crucial for individuals considering cannabis as a treatment option.

How cannabinoid therapeutics work in the body (Cannakeys, 2025).

1. **THC Alters Mental State:** THC may temporarily shift mental patterns linked to FOD, helping break habitual barriers to orgasm. THC and CBD decrease anxiety, can help distinguish traumatic thoughts, and reduce stress (Malka, 2022).
2. **ECS-Based Neuroplasticity:** ECS-driven neuroplasticity might assist women in learning to achieve orgasm while using cannabis. Once they develop this ability, they may no longer need cannabis to reach orgasm.
3. **Multi-Modal Treatment:** Utilizing cannabis for other purposes might also reduce symptoms of female orgasmic disorder (FOD), indicating potential indirect benefits for sexual function.
4. **Amygdala Reduction Theory:** By reducing fear, stress, and trauma responses in the amygdala, cannabis may alleviate psychological factors that contribute to FOD.

Treatment Options: Traditional treatment methods include cognitive-behavioral therapy (CBT), hormonal therapy, and medications, although their success rates can vary widely. Pharmaceuticals often come with undesirable side effects and do not always provide a consumer-centered approach to healthcare. Additional treatment options can consist of education about plant medicine, sexual stimulation, sexual enhancement devices, and individual or couple therapy (Mayo Clinic, 2024). Trauma-informed care is instrumental in breaking the cycle of sexual trauma. Plant-based medicine can be a safe and effective adjunct in treating FOD, offering benefits without the adverse effects commonly associated with pharmaceuticals.

We can upregulate our ECS with lifestyle changes such as exercise, diet, massage, open communication, acupuncture, and aromatherapy. Our diet should include greens, beans, onions, mushrooms, berries, seeds, and omega-3 fatty acids (Konieczny, 2018). Additional holistic approaches focus on risk reduction, stress management, identifying underlying causes, bodywork, meditation, mindfulness, nutraceuticals, bio-identical hormone replacement, and overall wellness. Healthcare providers should take an informed, personalized approach when considering cannabis as a potential supplementary therapy for women experiencing difficulties with orgasm (Mulvehill & Tishler, 2024).

MENOPAUSE

Menopause is defined as the natural cessation of menses for 12 consecutive months. It comprises three stages: perimenopause, menopause, and post menopause. The mean age of natural menopause ranges from 48 to 52 (Gulanick & Myers, 2017). However, it can occur as early as 35 and as late as 60. Menopause is a normal and natural part of the biological aging process. Fluctuations in estrogen and progesterone cause it (Popescu-Spineni et al., 2022). Estrogen deficiency downregulates the endocannabinoid system and is associated with vasomotor symptoms (Dahlgren et al., 2022). Surgical trauma, cigarette smoking, chemotherapy, and epigenetics have also been linked to the onset (Gulanick & Myers, 2017). Menopause involves the endocrine, integumentary, and reproductive systems, affecting the uterus, vagina, ovaries, and endometrium.

Signs and symptoms of menopause include, but are not limited to, hot flashes, sleep disturbance, depression, anxiety, palpitations, vaginal atrophy, and urinary tract conditions. Menopause can cause ineffective coping, impaired memory, ineffective sexuality patterns, and emotional distress. Some women may experience economic and psychosocial burden, increased shame, loss of productivity, and lower quality of life. African-American menopausal individuals have a high risk for vasomotor symptoms, and Hispanics are at greater risk for mood changes compared to white menopausal individuals (Dahlgren et al., 2022)

Traditionally, HRT (hormone replacement therapy) is the most common pharmaceutical treatment for menopausal symptoms. Steroidal replacement, such as estrogen and progesterone, does not address the healthcare consumer's unique ECS. The most common side effects include nausea, vomiting, diarrhea, breast pain, depression, hypertension, edema, vaginal discharge, pain with intercourse, itching or pain in the vaginal region, difficulty urinating, photosensitivity, and pain in the back or side (*Conjugated Estrogens Topical Side Effects*, 2025). Most estrogen products contain a black-box warning to alert consumers that this product can increase their risk for breast, uterine, or endometrial cancers, thrombophlebitis, and coronary heart disease (Lilley et al., 2020). For healthcare consumers with a past medical history of these disorders, estrogen may be contraindicated. In consumers over the age of 65, it may increase the risk of dementia. These warnings often cause consumers to seek other, less harmful products for symptom management.

Other pharmaceutical treatments used for menopausal management include Osphena, used to treat painful intercourse in post-menopausal women, and Addyi, used to treat those with a hypoactive sexual desire. It is also contraindicated in those who drink alcohol, have hepatic impairment, or use CYP3A4 inhibitors. For individuals who cannot undergo hormone replacement therapy (HRT), options such as low-dose antidepressants, gabapentin, and antihypertensives are available. However, these medications may have side effects, including nausea and sexual dysfunction.

Although research is limited, the use of cannabinoid therapies to ease menopausal symptoms has been on the rise. (Lo et al., 2022). The number and severity of symptoms correlate with the frequency of cannabis use (Lo et al., 2022). Dahlgren et al. (2022) showed that cannabis, when taken with anandamide, may be a more effective nonhormone treatment option with possibly fewer side effects compared to existing treatments. Symptoms most relieved with cannabinoid therapeutics were joint/muscle discomfort, irritability, sleep disturbance, hot flashes, anxiety, and depression. One study of 258 menopausal women showed that those in post menopause reported a significantly worse sexual dysfunction (Dahlgren et al., 2022). The top three reasons menopausal healthcare consumers seek cannabinoid therapeutics are sleep disturbance, mood/anxiety, and libido.

Lifestyle modifications, such as boosting physical activity, quitting smoking, managing weight, and reducing or cutting out alcohol, are advised. A diet that is low in fat and rich in fruits, vegetables, fiber, and calcium supports overall health. Engaging exercises that incorporate strengthening, stretching, and weight-bearing activities can enhance bone growth and help lower risk of osteoporosis. Nutraceuticals, including bio-identical hormone replacement, soy, red clover, dong quai, evening primrose, ginseng, and black cohosh, are frequently used to alleviate hot flashes. Evidence for these options remains limited. However, some women find these helpful despite the evidence to the contrary. Soy in an oral preparation may interfere with thyroid hormone absorption (Lilley et al., 2020). Support groups can reduce a consumer's sense of isolation and anxiety and enhance coping skills.

During menopause, exposure to cannabinoids may have a differential effect on female reproductive health (Lo et al., 2022). Cannabinoids such as THC, CBD, and CBG can help reduce pain and inflammation. THCV can reduce anxiety without mind-altering properties. Acids like THCA and CBDA can also be beneficial without having mood-altering effects. To avoid drug-to-drug interactions, cannabinoids should be used two hours before or after oral pharmaceutical HRT therapy and any medications using CYP3 enzymes. CBD-rich cannabis offers an alternative option to hormone therapy for hot flashes and menopausal sleep disorder.

Cannabis appears to mitigate menopausal symptoms such as hot flashes, anxiety, depression, insomnia, irritability, and musculoskeletal discomfort (Lo et al.,

2022). Chronic use can inhibit hormone production. Product suggestions include suppositories, tinctures, patches, oral preparations, edibles, and full-spectrum flower.

ENDOMETRIOSIS

Endometriosis (EMS) is a chronic condition where tissue similar to the lining of the uterus grows outside the uterus, leading to pain, inflammation, abdominal bloating, nausea, fatigue, depression, anxiety, dysmenorrhea, and sometimes infertility. It can happen in the ovaries, uterus, endometrium, surrounding ligaments, and extrauterine locations.

Managing endometriosis can be challenging, and traditional treatments often include hormonal therapies, neuromodulators, pain management, and surgery. Traditional treatments limit fertility, have limited effectiveness, and result in the recurrence of symptoms. For healthcare consumers trying to conceive, pharmaceuticals may not be suitable. Surgical intervention provides only temporary relief and has a recurrence rate of 40-50% (Liang et al., 2022). EMS can lead to declines in social relationships, financial stability, mental health, and physical activity (Liang et al., 2022). Because EMS has a complex pathophysiology, delays in diagnosis and treatment may occur, thereby reducing the healthcare consumer's quality of life (Lingegowda et al., 2022). In recent years, there has been growing interest in the potential use of cannabis for symptom relief in endometriosis and as an option for harm reduction. Finding an economical and effective way to manage symptoms of EMS that do not affect fertility is a growing concern.

Endocannabinoids play a huge role in homeostasis, tissue repair, and immune response. Chronic inflammatory diseases such as endometriosis have been associated with endocannabinoid imbalances. According to Liang et al. (2022), chronic pelvic pain affects 26% of women worldwide. Pelvic pain accounts for 12% of hysterectomies, 40% of laparoscopies, and 10% of gynecological visits in the United States (Liang et al., 2022). The World Health Organization (WHO) estimates that EMS affects 10% (190 million) of reproductive-age women worldwide (*World Health Organization*, 2025).

According to research, the following endocannabinoid imbalances have been identified in healthcare consumers with EMS: AEA (arachidonoyl ethanolamide) and 2-AG (2-archidonoyl glycerol) is elevated, PEA (palmitoylethanolamide) and OEA (oleoylethanolamide) is elevated, CB1 (cannabinoid receptor 1) and CB2 (cannabinoid receptor 2) are decreased, TRPV1/TRPVA1 receptors are increased, FAAH (fatty acid amide hydrolase), NAPE (*N*-acyl phosphatidylethanolamine), MAGL (monoacylglycerol lipase), and DAGL (diacylglycerol lipase) enzymes are decreased (Lingegowda et al., 2022). This is termed clinical endocannabinoid deficiency (CED) (Russo, 2016). Russo (2016) continues to state that CED arises from multiple comorbidities and treatment-resistant pathophysiology. Ligands AEA, PEA, 2-AG, and OEA function in fertility, anti-inflammatory, immune modulation, and cell growth and survival. CB1 and CB2 receptors function in nociception, neuroprotection, inflammation, and autophagy. Enzymes NAPE, FAAH, DAGL, and MAGL function in AEA and PEA synthesis, AEA metabolism, 2-AG synthesis, and 2-AG metabolism. Non-classical receptors GPR and TRP function in leukocyte migration, hyperalgesia, and the cell cycle (Lingegowda et al., 2022).

Etiology of endometriosis has been suspected from retrograde menstruation, hormonal imbalances, immune system abnormalities, genetics, environmental issues, and metaplasia (Anvari Aliabad et al., 2024).

Some healthcare consumers find that exercise and dietary changes can help eliminate symptoms. Other holistic modalities include cognitive behavioral therapy (CBT), support groups, and nutraceuticals such as palmitoylethanolamide (PEA) and antioxidants.

Cannabis contains compounds like THC (tetrahydrocannabinol) and CBD (cannabidiol) that interact with the body's endocannabinoid system, which plays a role in the regulation of pain and inflammation. Other cannabinoids that may help with pain and inflammation include CBD and CBG. Some individuals report that cannabis use helps alleviate the chronic pelvic pain associated with endometriosis. Cannabis can help reduce the use of pharmaceuticals and help healthcare consumers improve pain management and quality of life.

While some individuals with endometriosis find relief through cannabis use, it is crucial to approach this treatment option with caution and consult healthcare professionals. They can offer guidance based on the latest research, take patient-specific factors into account, and monitor the safety and effectiveness of this therapy within a comprehensive treatment plan. The development of more explicit guidelines and additional research in controlled settings is needed to better understand the role of cannabis in managing endometriosis symptoms. Products such as cannabinoid suppositories, tinctures, topicals, oral preparations, patches, and whole-plant flower are great treatment options.

LIBIDO

Hormones and neurotransmitters that affect sexual behavior interact with the body's internal endocannabinoid system. Dopamine is the key sexual modulator in normal excitatory female sexual function. Dopamine is enhanced through the activation of cannabinoid receptors. Norepinephrine and dopamine play a role in the excitatory processes of sexual function. Serotonin plays a role in the loss of desire. Testosterone, estrogen, melanocortin, progesterone, prolactin, and oxytocin interact with neurotransmitters to modulate the female sexual response (Lynn et al., 2020). Oxytocin plays an essential role in sexual arousal, romantic attachment, trust, and recognition in both sexes. It improves social interactions and relaxation, and it increases sexual receptiveness. Signs and symptoms of libido include the lack of sexual desire and biological urges, sexual needs, apathy, and emotional distress. Cannabinoid receptors are found in the hypothalamus, prefrontal cortex, amygdala, hippocampus, and the sexual organs, which control sexual function.

Medical conditions, hormone deficiencies, thyroid dysfunction, anemia, pharmaceutical side effects, surgical trauma, pain with intercourse, emotional stress or trauma, loss of a family member or spouse, diet, weight, mobility issues, and use of alcohol and/or illicit drugs can cause problems with libido.

Traditional treatments for libido include pharmaceutical management, including the use of oxytocin. Oxytocin can increase sexual drive and function. It has been used to treat hypoactive sexual desire disorder, or absence of sexual desire, in women. PT-141 is an FDA-approved peptide that stimulates sexual pathways in the central nervous system and increases dopamine. It is specifically used to increase arousal and desire.

One cross-sectional study aimed to examine how women who consume cannabis perceive their sexual experiences, including sex drive. This study of 373 female cannabis participants found that the majority of them self-reported an increase or no change in desire, an increase in sexual enjoyment, and orgasm intensity (Lynn et al., 2019). Of the 373 participants, 197 were non-cannabis consumers, 127 used cannabis before sex, and 49 cannabis consumers did not. Sixty percent who used it before sex noted an increase in sex drive. Of the women who reported using cannabis prior to sexual activity, they had 2.13 times higher odds of having a satisfactory orgasm. Frequent female cannabis users had 2.10 times higher odds of reporting satisfactory orgasms regardless of whether they used cannabis prior to sex or not, versus females who did not use cannabis.

Lynn et al. (2020) showed that a comprehensive review of data has indicated that cannabinoid therapeutics have dose-dependent effects on female sexual desire and receptivity. High doses can inhibit these effects, while a low dose generally facilitates sexual desire. AEA also enhanced sexual desire in female rats. A survey reviewed by Lynn et al. (2020) of 200 cannabis consumers, 44 percent reported "definitely increases their sexual desire", with 50 percent of those being women. Seventy percent of consumers in this survey increased sexual pleasure with frequent but not daily use of cannabis compared to heavy everyday use.

A survey of 281 sexually active participants revealed that overall, participants had more positive sexual experiences on illicit drugs, including cannabis, compared to consuming alcohol. The most frequently used substances to improve sexual activity were cannabis and ecstasy. These drugs reported greater sexual pleasure, greater willingness to experiment sexually, and increased contact with their partner compared to alcohol (Lynn et al., 2020). A survey with 679 participants evaluated cannabis, ecstasy, and alcohol on self-reported sexual effects. This survey focused on cannabis consumers and reported an increase in sexual enjoyment by 53.5 percent of cannabis consumers.

The U.S. Commission on Marihuana and Drug Abuse (1972) showed in a study of 200 cannabis participants (male and female) that an increase in sexual desire occurred in 70 percent of consumers who used cannabis frequently compared to daily usage. Several million U.S. women are estimated to have female sexual arousal disorder by the American Medical Association (Delvin & Webber, 2014).

Several over-the-counter nutraceuticals claim to increase libido. Libido enhancers for women claim to support sexual response by improving vaginal blood flow, arousal, lubrication, and pleasure. These products claim to work by increasing nitric oxide and circulation; others claim to address hormone imbalances, the stress response, or mood. For men, libido enhancers claim to increase testosterone levels, improve blood circulation, heighten libido, reduce stress, and support cellular function to improve stamina.

Foods that may help an individual increase their libido and have aphrodisiac properties include chocolate, black raspberries, broccoli, cloves, figs, watermelon, ginger, lettuce, saffron, and avocados. Foods rich in zinc contribute to hormone production and increase clitoral sensitivity. High-vitamin C foods, such as broccoli, aid blood flow to organs and have been linked to enhanced female libido. Avocados are rich in phytonutrients, zinc, and vitamin E, all of which boost sexual pleasure and drive libido. Figs are known to enhance pheromone production. Lettuce contains a chemical signal that stimulates the activation of sex hormones. Watermelon contains citrulline, which relaxes blood vessels in a manner similar to how Viagra works.

Diet should include various healthy fats and calcium. Large amounts of saturated fats may lead to atherosclerosis, a factor in causing sexual dysfunction and poor blood circulation. Calcium is linked to sexual health by increasing circulation to the genitalia: soy milk, leafy greens, sprouted beans, cabbage, and wheatgrass juice. A diet high in processed baked goods can suppress libido by elevating blood sugar levels, thereby impeding circulation. Oysters contain high levels of zinc; however, the absorption of environmental toxins and parasites reduces their benefits.

Horny goat weed, saw palmetto, ginseng, and reishi are great non-intoxicating, nutraceutical options. There is some evidence that L-arginine, chasteberry, maca, and DHEA could help to improve sex for some women. Unconventional, off label options include psilocybin, ecstasy, and LSD,

THC (tetrahydrocannabinol) has been shown to affect female sexuality (Lynn et al., 2020). Overconsumption of cannabinoid therapeutics can cause individuals to become unmotivated, decreasing their desire for sexual intercourse. Other cannabinoids that may be beneficial include CBD, CBN (cannabinol), and β-caryophyllene.

Cannabis products such as infused bath products, edibles, capsules, tinctures, and full-spectrum flowers can help treat libido problems. Cannabinoid therapeutics may lower sexual inhibitions and increase willingness to experiment and confidence. Heightened sense of touch and increased physical intimacy have been noted with the female cannabis consumer. Higher doses of cannabis have been speculated to inhibit sexual activity due to the increased sedative effects.

ERECTILE DYSFUNCTION (ED)

Erectile dysfunction (ED) can be described as changes in the ability to have an erection, hold an erection, or ejaculate during partnered sexual activities not caused by a medical condition. Erectile dysfunction can lead to poor self-esteem, emotional distress, and poor quality of life. It is the most common sexual health concern for men. It affects the penis, testes, and the surrounding vascularity.

Medical conditions such as hypertension, diabetes, spinal or nerve damage, renal disorders, depression, side effects of prescription medications, atherosclerosis, and testosterone deficiencies. Physiological conditions like loss of a family member or spouse, preoccupation with work, family or marital conflict, cigarette smoking, heavy use of alcohol, poor nutrition, fatigue, surgical trauma, exposure to environmental hazards, or emotional distress. (Lilley et al., 2020). While low testosterone can contribute to erectile dysfunction (ED), it is not the most common cause. ED is typically the result of a combination of physical and psychological factors. Common physical causes include cardiovascular disease, diabetes, high blood pressure, and certain medications, all of which can affect blood flow and nerve function. Psychological factors can include stress, anxiety, and depression.

Pharmaceutical medications such as estrogen, antihypertensives, narcotics, antidepressants, antispasmodics, sedatives, and tranquilizers can have a direct effect on erectile dysfunction. Finasteride, a medication for benign prostatic hyperplasia (BPH), has been reported to cause loss of libido, loss of erection, and ejaculatory dysfunction, among others.

Pharmaceutical management of erectile dysfunction includes avanafil (Stendra), sildenafil (Viagra), tadalafil (Cialis), vardenafil (Levitra), and alprostadil (Caverject). These medications cause penile erection after sexual arousal by relaxing smooth muscle and increasing blood flow into the penis. Treatment may also include intraurethral and intracavernosal injections (Caverject).

Viagra, sildenafil, stays in the body longer and can increase the possibility of drug interactions and toxicity (Lilley et al., 2020). Negative effects can include, but are not limited to, headache, flushing, muscular pain, rash, heartburn, dry mouth, nausea, vomiting, priapism, unexplained vision loss, and diarrhea. These medications are contraindicated in cardiac individuals, especially if they are taken with nitrates, as they can cause hypotension and angina. Cialis is now being used off-label to treat sexual sensitivity in women. Apomorphine can increase dopamine levels and bind to receptors, triggering erections. PT-141 is also a viable treatment option, as it additionally increases dopamine levels.

Pharmaceuticals are the most effective treatment option, with a success rate of 60-80%. Vacuum erection devices, Intraurethral suppositories, and penile implants are highly effective for severe ED. Psychotherapy may be a treatment option, along with lifestyle modifications and changes. Surprisingly,

Low doses of cannabinoids can enhance sexual response and function by activating CB1 receptors; higher doses impair that response by activating the TRPV1 channel (Backes & Weil, 2017). Semen parameters, male fertility, and premature or delayed ejaculation can be affected by cannabis use (Lo et al., 2022). One study with male mice showed that exposure to cannabidiol (15-30mg for 34 days) delayed first mount and intromission, reduced the number of mounts and ejaculations, and reduced fertility by 30% (Carvalho et al., 2018). Another study found that cannabis lowers testosterone, decreases the weight of the testes, and affects spermatogenesis in male rats (Lynn et al., 2020).

Thirty million men in the United States are affected by erectile dysfunction. In men younger than 60, erectile dysfunction occurs in 12 percent. 2% are men aged 60 to 69, and 30% are men aged 70 or older (Lilley et al., 2020). Almost 65 percent of men over the age of 35 have experienced some form of erectile dysfunction in their lifetime (Lane, 2022). Psychological causes of ED are more common in younger men and can be the primary cause in 10-20% of cases.

The use of cannabinoid therapeutics for erectile dysfunction cannot be proven yet by researchers. Research provides limited insight into treatment. However, the use of cannabis to reduce stress and the ability to rewire the brain show a promising option. Historically, cannabis is believed to have aphrodisiac properties, increasing sexual pleasure. It should never be used as a sole treatment option, and determining the root cause is imperative.

A review in a Urology journal found that strengthening muscles in a man's pelvic floor can help diminish erectile dysfunction and premature ejaculation. When men have an erection, their pelvic muscles keep blood in the shaft. Squeezing these muscles can delay orgasm. This helps to enhance and maintain the rigidity of the erected tissue. Kegel exercises have been known to improve a male's ability to maintain a long, lasting erection. In one study, 75 percent of men experienced improvements in their erectile function after performing Kegel exercises. Additionally, research conducted by Italian scientists found that 61 percent of men overcame premature ejaculation by undergoing pelvic floor muscle rehabilitation.

Another exercise is to challenge the brain. Using one's mind to imagine overcome erectile dysfunction can be key to improving it. Research suggested that thinking thoughts regarding arousing imagery can help rewire your brain. Energy work has also been a holistic treatment for erectile dysfunction. Nutraceuticals like taurine and L-arginine help improve circulation.

Cannabinoids such as THCA, CBDA, and THC are helpful for symptom management. Sublingual preparations and suppositories are the recommended routes of administration. Whole-plant preparations should include the following terpenes: myrcene, limonene, beta-caryophyllene, and linalool (Backes & Weil, 2017).

POLYCYSTIC OVARIAN SYNDROME (PCOS)

Polycystic Ovarian Syndrome (PCOS) affects the female ovaries. It is characterized by amenorrhea for three months, difficulty conceiving, infertility, acne, hirsutism, hair loss, eating disorders, negative body image, weight gain, menstrual pain, cramps, pelvic pain, or infrequent menses. The pathophysiology of PCOS from angiogenic factor dysregulation may contribute to ovulatory dysfunction, subfertility, and ovarian hyperstimulation syndrome, which are commonly seen in women with PCOS. Polycystic ovarian syndrome is a chronic disease caused by an increase in luteinizing hormone (LH) and a decrease in follicle-stimulating hormone (FSH) (Konick-McMahan, 2007). These hormones stimulate the development of ovarian follicles and the onset of ovulation. This imbalance prevents the ovaries from releasing an egg each month. Benign cysts form on the ovaries related to the failure of the ovaries to release eggs. This inappropriate hormone signaling leads to elevated androgen levels. It can cause infertility, weight gain, and hirsutism in 6-15 percent of women who are reproductive-aged (Jarvis et al., 2020).

Polycystic ovary syndrome (PCOS) is frequently linked to insulin resistance and obesity. PCOS is usually diagnosed when women have difficulty conceiving. Those diagnosed with PCOS are at a higher risk of pregnancy complications.

Polycystic ovarian disorder affects the reproductive and endocrine systems are involved in PCOS, specifically including the ovaries. Dysregulation includes vascular endothelial growth factors, angiopoietins, platelet-derived growth factor, transforming growth factor-β, and basic fibroblast growth factor (Tal et al., 2015). Imbalances can also occur in the hypothalamus and pituitary gland.

Polycystic Ovarian Syndrome is thought to involve a combination of causes from genetic, environmental, and lifestyle factors. Obesity contributes to the problems associated with PCOS. Women with a family history or genetic risk factor of type 2 diabetes or PCOS are at a high risk of developing PCOS.

Polycystic ovarian syndrome (PCOS) is a common endocrine disorder in reproductive age, affecting 5 to 7% of women (Tal et al., 2015). The World Health Organization (WHO) has estimated that up 70% of women with PCOS worldwide do not know they have this condition (Polycystic Ovary Syndrome, 2026).

Traditional treatment includes diabetic medications (Metformin), hormonal regulation of menses (oral contraceptives), surgeries, and infertility specialists. Ovulation may be induced for women desiring pregnancy, using fertility drugs like Clomid. Surgeries can be performed to stimulate ovulation. Assisted reproductive technology, such as in vitro fertilization, is a common infertility treatment.

Oral contraceptives carry a black box warning, cautioning consumers that cardiovascular events, deep vein thrombosis, endometrial cancer, breast cancer, and dementia can occur. Consumers should discontinue smoking cigarettes. Antiepileptic drugs, antibiotics, beta blockers, hypnotics, antidiabetic drugs, warfarin, theophylline, tricyclic antidepressants, and vitamins may have decreased therapeutic effects when taken in conjunction with oral contraceptives. Oral contraceptive hormones must be taken at the same time every day.

Oral diabetic drugs like Metformin can cause abdominal bloating, nausea, cramping, a feeling of fullness, hyperventilation, cold and clammy skin, muscle pain, dizziness, irregular heartbeat, and diarrhea. This pharmaceutical is contraindicated in alcoholism, metabolic acidosis, hepatic disease, and heart failure, and increases the risk for lactic acidosis.

Sathyapalan et al. (2017) showed that, in animal studies, CB1 blockade reduces inflammation and neovascularization by decreasing vascular endothelial growth factor levels, associated with reduced inflammatory markers in obese women with PCOS.

Holistic treatments may include fertility treatments, lifestyle changes, and medications that can reduce symptoms and increase fertility rates. Weight management and exercise are recommended to decrease insulin resistance. Smoking cessation and limiting alcohol intake will help decrease the occurrence of adverse reactions with pharmaceutical management. A dietary consultation can help healthcare consumers make changes to their dietary intake. Nutraceuticals that may help manage PCOS symptoms include Resveratrol and Oleoylethanolamide (OEA). OEA reduces glycemic index, oxidative stress markers, and inflammation.

Early diagnosis and management of polycystic ovary syndrome (PCOS) can lead to successful management and a better quality of life while prevent complications. By identifying PCOS early, individuals can work with healthcare providers to address symptoms and reduce the risk of associated health issues, such as type 2 diabetes, cardiovascular disease, and fertility problems. Cannabinoid therapeutics may offer a novel treatment option to balance an individual's unique endocannabinoid system.

The phytocannabinoid THCV (delta-9-tetrahydrocannabivarin) has been shown to suppress appetite, promote weight loss, and restore insulin sensitivity in mice (Goldstein, 2020). This is a promising treatment option for diabetes and other metabolic disorders such as PCOS. THC and CBD may be used for pain management and inflammation. Product suggestions include tinctures, capsules, oral preparations, topicals, suppositories, and full-spectrum flower.

POST-COITAL PAIN

Post-coital pain, or pain after sexual intercourse, can be caused by a variety of factors and may affect both men and women. It is important to identify the underlying cause to address the condition appropriately. Common causes may include conditions such as vaginal dryness, pelvic inflammatory disease, endometriosis, uterine fibroids, interstitial cystitis, and infections such as urinary tract infections, yeast infections, or sexually transmitted infections. Per Hill & Taylor (2021), approximately 10% to 20% of women experience dyspareunia, which includes pain during or after intercourse. Post-coital pain is less commonly reported among men, and specific prevalence statistics are not as readily available.

Signs and symptoms in men can cause post-ejaculation discomfort. Women can experience pain in the vulvar region, vagina, uterus, or pelvis during vaginal penetration. Abdominal and or rectal pain may also be associated with anal penetration. Both sexes may experience skin inflammation or abrasions during penetration.

Traditional treatment may include pharmaceuticals such as Osphena. This medication is used to treat painful intercourse in post-menopausal women. Vaginal dilators can sometimes be used to reduce discomfort with penetration. Vaginal dilators work by gradually stretching and desensitizing the vaginal muscles, helping the person to become more comfortable with penetration over time. Typically, a set of dilators of increasing sizes is used, starting with a smaller size and gradually progressing to larger ones as comfort increases. This process is usually done in conjunction with pelvic floor physical therapy and under the guidance of a healthcare professional to ensure proper use and to address any underlying issues.

Cannabis may be considered as an option for managing post-coital pain due to its potential pain-relieving properties. Some people use cannabis to alleviate various types of pain and discomfort linked to sexual activity. It is believed that cannabis can help by reducing pain and inflammation, while also improving blood flow. It is thought that cannabis may help by reducing pain, inflammation, and improving blood flow, which can enhance relaxation and reduce anxiety.

Sexual intercourse has protective effects on sexual dysfunction (Belau et al., 2022). Lynn et al. (2020) showed in one survey of 373 women cannabis consumers, the 127 who used cannabis prior to sexual intercourse had a decrease in pain.

Topically, we know that CBD has anti-inflammatory properties and can reduce irritation sometimes caused by the first attempts at vaginal penetration (Barach et al., 2020). CBD is beginning to show promise as a pain blocker. Cannabigerol (CBG) can also block pain and inflammation. Tetrahydrocannabivarin (THCV) can reduce anxiety without altering moods. Products like topicals, infused lubricants, infused suppositories, infused bath products, tinctures, edibles, and full-spectrum flower can help reduce pain and inflammation associated with penetrative intercourse.

Discussing and assessing pain that occurs after intercourse can be challenging, primarily because the subject is personal and sexual health issues are often overlooked or not openly addressed. Many people may not seek medical assistance due to embarrassment or lack of awareness that their condition can be medically assessed and treated. To effectively address post-coital pain, it is important to identify and treat the underlying causes. Individuals who experience persistent or severe pain after intercourse should consult a healthcare professional to identify any serious health concerns and receive appropriate treatment. For those considering the use of cannabis for managing post-coital pain, it is crucial to seek medical advice, especially if they are taking other medications or have existing health conditions.

SEXUAL DIFFERENCES

According to Belau et al. (2022),there is limited research regarding women who frequently use cannabis, with at least one sexual dysfunction, who have a 4.7 times higher odds of developing depression than women who are abstinent and have no dysfunction. Women report sexual dysfunction more often than men.

ECS DIET AND HOLISTIC APPROACHES

A diet high in green beans, onions, mushrooms, berries, seeds, and omega-3 fatty acids (Konieczny, 2018). Green leafy vegetables, dairy fats, carrots, black pepper, maca, soybeans, fava beans, chickpeas, hot spices, and olive oil have also been identified in upregulating the endocannabinoid (Gertsch, 2017). Nutraceuticals such as DHA, EPA, and PEA can also regulate the endocannabinoid system.

Exercise offers numerous benefits for bone health, mental well-being, and emotional balance. Kegel exercises are particularly effective for strengthening the pelvic floor muscles, which can enhance core stability and support bladder control.

Additionally, weight-bearing exercises, aerobics, and strength training are highly recommended to help reduce the risk of osteoporosis by increasing bone density and maintaining muscle mass.

A holistic and multidisciplinary approach is crucial for comprehensive care. While cannabis may offer a novel approach to managing sexual wellness, it should not replace or overshadow other complementary aspects of treatment, such as psychotherapy, counseling, lifestyle modifications, and addressing underlying medical or psychological factors contributing to the disorder. Reducing substance use (tobacco, alcohol, etc.) can be a useful tool for decreasing sexual dysfunction.

Additional holistic approaches that may support the upregulation of the ECS are as follows:

- Cognitive behavioral therapy (CBT)
- Biofeedback
- Aromatherapy (bath products, diffusers, inhalers, and candles)
- Encourage talking about feelings
- Guided imagery
- Mindfulness
- Emotional freedom tapping
- Positive self-talk
- Earthing
- Support groups
- Progressive relaxation
- Meditation
- Calming music
- Art, painting, crafting, Drawing, gardening
- Pet therapy
- hobbies
- Stress management
- Yoga
- Deep breathing

ENVIRONMENT AND SETTINGS

When assessing a healthcare consumer's sexual activity, providers should have a welcoming environment that is respectful to all sexual identities. Providers should begin with open-ended questions. This communicates to the healthcare consumer that sexual activity is accepted and important, thus reducing the stigma surrounding sexual wellness. Some consumers may be comfortable discussing sexual topics, while others may experience anxiety. Be respectful of everyone's beliefs, sexual practices, and feelings. Environment and setting are also crucial for starting anything new, or for anything with a variety of possible outcomes. A controlled, safe environment is best when using cannabinoid therapeutics. This allows the cannabis consumer to control the severity of any unwanted side effects if needed. Overstimulation, lack of knowledge, and being underprepared can make any experience positive or negative. Cannabis consumers should be informed of what to do if unwanted side effects happen.

HEALTHCARE CONSUMER EDUCATION AND INFORMED CONSENT

Open and honest communication between healthcare providers and healthcare consumers is essential when considering the use of cannabis for FOD or any other medical condition. Healthcare providers should engage in thorough discussions with healthcare consumers regarding the potential risks, benefits, uncertainties, and alternatives of using cannabis as a treatment option. This process helps ensure that healthcare consumers understand what to expect and can make informed decisions about their healthcare.

Informed consent is a crucial aspect of this process, as it involves a healthcare consumer's understanding and agreement on the potential risks and benefits of using cannabinoid therapeutics for their condition.

Ongoing monitoring by healthcare providers is also essential to assess treatment effectiveness, monitor side effects, or changes in symptoms, and make necessary adjustments to the treatment plan. Consumers should be encouraged to keep a journal during this process. Journal entries should include a person's inventory, intentions, environment, product type, product content (cannabinoids and percentages), dosage, route of administration, and any wanted or unwanted side effects.

When beginning something new, it's important to start with a slow and gradual approach. Keep a journal to document the products you use, your goals, and any negative reactions. Remember that dosage, type of product, and method of consumption can greatly affect the results and significantly influence outcomes. To maximize benefits and reduce adverse events, please consult a cannabis nurse, healthcare provider, or pharmacist before adding any new treatments. It is essential for healthcare consumers considering cannabinoid therapeutics as a treatment option to work closely with healthcare professionals who can provide guidance on dosing, monitor any effects or changes, and help ensure a safe and effective approach.

ADVERSE EVENTS

Cannabis consumers should be aware that the use of cannabinoid therapeutics is not without risk and that the following list is not exhaustive of possible side effects or adverse reactions. Everyone has a unique endocannabinoid system, and what works for one person may not work for another. Each person's experience is unique and may not be replicable.

- Decreased appetite/increased appetite
- Drowsiness or lightheadedness
- Anxiety
- High-frequency users of THC may develop chronic anxiety and troublesome or worsening psychological disorders.
- Decrease in blood pressure or elevated heart rate.
- Increased fall risk
- Nausea and/or vomiting
- Impaired thinking
- Decreased motor functioning
- Dry mouth and dry eyes
- Coughing
- Blurred vision
- Paranoia or psychosis
- Cannabis hyperemesis syndrome/ cannabis use disorder

DRUG-TO-DRUG INTERACTIONS

Pharmaceuticals that use the CYP450 enzyme to metabolize, cannabis should be taken at least two hours after these pharmaceuticals. This includes, but is not limited to, antidepressants, antifungals, cardiac medications, and anticonvulsants (Parmelee et al., 2021). Drug interactions include the following medications: warfarin, steroids, calcium channel blockers, antihistamines, prokinetics, HIV antivirals, immune modulators, antiepileptics, beta-blockers, benzos, antiarrhythmics, antibiotics, anesthesia, antipsychotics, antidepressants, PPIs, and NSAIDs/COX inhibitors (Konieczny, 2018; Malka,2022). Adverse events are dose-, frequency-, and individual-chemistry-dependent. Cannabis can cause drug interactions. It can increase or decrease medication levels via CYP-mediated pathways (Malka, 2022).

PRODUCT DISCLAIMERS/ALLERGIES

The use of illicit drugs to treat or manage medical conditions in this chapter is not recommended without proper medical supervision. Cannabis consumers should be aware that some products may contain alcohol, MCT oil, coconut oil, corn syrup, and other genetically modified ingredients. Those with allergies should be aware of product ingredients and possible adverse reactions before use. Bath products such as infused Epsom salts, scrubs, and bath bombs should be used with caution. Consumers should be educated prior to using these products. Caution should be used to avoid falls.

UNDERSTANDING OVERCONSUMPTION

Overconsumption of cannabis, sometimes called "green out," occurs more frequently than many people realize and is often unintentional. It's crucial to keep in mind that low doses of cannabinoid therapeutics can enhance sexual response, whereas higher doses might impair or even suppress sexual function. The following safety guidelines can help if this happens. It's wise to prioritize safety in these situations. Cannabidiol (CBD) may be administered to mitigate adverse effects associated with excessive THC consumption. Incorporating CBD may help reduce undesirable side effects. Limonene, a terpene present in lemons, is recognized for its antistress and anti-anxiety effects. Black peppercorns contain beta-caryophyllene, which may help alleviate discomfort caused by overconsumption. Individuals may consider chewing a few peppercorns as a potential remedy. Other terpenes, such as those found in lavender and pine, may also enhance comfort. Stay hydrated when using cannabis to support one's well-being. Wearing sunglasses can limit overstimulation by shielding the eyes from harsh rays and relieving strain. Consider using earplugs, as loud noises might intensify discomfort during a challenging experience and, if need be, surround oneself with calming sounds. Overconsumption may persist for hours, so it's important to ensure you are in a safe environment.

TIPS AND TRICKS

Chemovars that include terpenes such as myrcene, limonene, beta-caryophyllene, and linalool are most effective in treating sexual dysfunction (Backes & Weil, 2017). It is imperative to remember that low doses of cannabinoid therapeutics may improve sexual response, while higher doses can impair and even suppress sexual function. Various factors, such as the specific type of cannabinoids (such as THC, CBD, etc.), the method of consumption (smoking, edibles, topical applications), dosage, and individual tolerance levels, can all influence how cannabis may affect individuals differently. Personalized and careful dosing is crucial not only to minimize potential side effects but also to optimize the potential therapeutic benefits of cannabis.

- Cannabinoid acids (those with an A at the end) should be kept in a cool, dark place to avoid activating psychoactive compounds.
- Eat with a fatty snack.
- Start low and go slow. One can always add more if needed. However, one cannot decrease the dose if you have overconsumed.
- Use whole-plant medicine rather than isolates to reduce adverse side effects.
- Use the mode of administration that promotes the least amount of harm (harms of smoking).
- When trying something new, always be in a safe, quiet environment to avoid overstimulation by outside distractions.
- Do not operate heavy machinery or drive until it is know how the plant will affect an individual.
- Always journal the product type and name, amount consumed, any wanted and unwanted side effects, time, and active ingredients.
- Use a cannabis clinician for the best results and assessments.
- Do not use products with high THC percentages. This can aggravate anxiety, depression, and PTSD symptoms.
- Chronic heavy use of THC-rich cannabis can cause a decrease in cannabinoid receptors that will lead to tolerance and eventually to a loss of effectiveness (Goldstein, 2020).
- Consumers should take a seven-day tolerance break to avoid overregulating the endocannabinoid system. Interchanging products, cannabinoids, and layering products can help prevent tolerance. Using other holistic modalities alongside diet and exercise is a healthy way to upregulate the endocannabinoid system and avoid the need for tolerance breaks.
- Cannabis use can increase avoidant behaviors. Be sure to monitor functional goals in addition to anxiety severity (Sulak, 2022).
- Limit caffeine, nicotine, and other central nervous system stimulants. Avoid use with alcohol (Gulanick & Myers, 2017).
- Do not use unregulated synthetic cannabinoids.
- Assess the effectiveness of the support system.
- Monitor sleep and activity patterns.
- Monitor prescriptive adherence.
- Assess Evaluate the Cannabinoid Use Disorder Identification Test (CUDIT-R) as outlined by Fratoni and Tutkus (2021). Research by Lo et al. (2022)

indicates that about 10% of regular cannabis users and 50% of chronic daily users may develop cannabis use disorder (CUD). It's important for consumers to undergo regular assessments. Treatment for CUD may involve pharmaceutical options such as antidepressants, gabapentin, and nabiximols, as well as holistic approaches like motivational enhancement, brief or psychosocial interventions, or cognitive-behavioral therapy.

CONCLUSION

In conclusion, while emerging research suggests that cannabis may hold promise as a treatment option for sexual wellness, further investigation and clinical evidence are needed to support its efficacy and safety. New evidence has shown that cannabidiol is very effective in menopausal symptoms, increasing sexual pleasure, and even for the relief of vulvodynia. Cannabinoid therapeutics can be used to enhance joy, connections, spirituality, and quality of life.

Healthcare providers and healthcare consumers should approach this topic with caution, sensitivity, and a collaborative decision-making process to ensure the best possible outcomes for individuals affected by sexual dysfunction. Human studies have not been able to precisely assess the appropriate dosing, timing, or methods of use. As our society works to eliminate the stigma surrounding sexual wellness and move away from shaming, clinicians should prioritize identifying underlying causes, respecting healthcare consumers' rights to choose their treatment options, and minimizing potential harm. Cannabinoid therapeutics is just a part of a holistic care plan and should never be considered a sole treatment option without other holistic modalities included. Care plans should be individualized, with education focused on the healthcare consumer's needs and learning abilities. Pertinent and age-appropriate information on the disease process, lifestyle modifications, and treatment options should be included.

- Use the route/cannabinoid with the least amount of harm.
- Use the route that provides the most relief.
- Start low and go slow.
- Only introduce one cannabinoid at a time.
- Take cannabinoids 1-2 hours after or prior to pharmaceuticals to avoid DDIs
- Always keep a record of the products used and the effects they provide.
- Always report adverse side effects.
- Do not use alcohol or other illicit substances.
- Lab work to follow liver profiles.
- A cannabis clinician should monitor clients to reduce harm.

Daily records should be sent to the provider weekly to monitor adverse reactions. Step down pharmaceuticals where appropriate.

ROUTES OF ADMINISTRATION

Inhalation: Onset 5-10 minutes, Duration 2-4 hours, Bioavailability 25-31% THC, 13-19% CBD.

Oral: Onset: 1-3 hours faster w/food. Duration: 5-8 hours Bioavailability: 6-20%. The unknown onset of edibles can increase the likelihood of overconsumption.

Sublingual: Onset: 15-45 minutes Duration: 6-8hours Bioavailability: 20-30%.

Topical: Onset: 30 minutes to 2 hours. Duration: 1-8 hours Bioavailability: varies.

Transdermal: Onset: 20 minutes. Duration: up to 48 hours. Bioavailability: CBD and CBN are approximately ten times more bioavailable than THC.

Suppository: Onset: 10-45 minutes. Duration: 2-8 hours. Bioavailability: 13-40%.

Cannabis is unique to everyone. Responses vary from consumer to consumer and product to product.

REFERENCES

American Sexual Health Association. (2018, October 22). *Female Orgasmic Disorder*. American Sexual Health Association. https://www.ashasexualhealth.org/orgasmic-disorder/

Anvari Aliabad, R., Hassanpour, K., & Norooznezhad, A. H. (2024). Cannabidiol as a possible treatment for endometriosis through suppression of inflammation and angiogenesis. *Immunity, Inflammation and Disease, 12*(8), e1370. DOI: 10.1002/iid3.1370 PMID: 39110084

Backes, M., & Weil, A. (2017). *Cannabis Pharmacy: The practical guide to medical marijuana*. Black Dog & Leventhal Publishers.

Barach, E., Slavin, M., & Earleywine, M. (2020). Cannabis and vulvodynia symptoms: A preliminary report. *Cannabis (Research Society on Marijuana), 3*(2), 139–147. DOI: 10.26828/cannabis.2020.02.001 PMID: 33426502

Belau, M. H., Wiessner, C., Becher, H., Von Rüden, U., & Briken, P. (2022). Frequent cannabis use moderates the relationship between sexual dysfunction and depression among female German adults. *Journal of Sexual Medicine, 19*(6), 940–949. DOI: 10.1016/j.jsxm.2022.03.610 PMID: 35431149

Blesching, U. (2025, January 18). *Erectile dysfunction (ED)*. Cannakeys. https://cannakeys.com/thc-cbd-for-erectile-dysfunction-ed/

Blesching, U. (2026, February 2). Menstrual Pain and Associated Conditions. *Cannakeys*. https://cannakeys.com/thc-cbd-for-menstrual-pain-and-associated-conditions/

Cannakeys. (2025). *Female Orgasmic Disorder*. Cannakeys.Com. https://cannakeys.com/thc-cbd-for-female-orgasmic-disorder-fod/

Carvalho, R. K., Souza, M. R., Santos, M. L., Guimarães, F. S., Pobbe, R. L. H., Andersen, M. L., & Mazaro-Costa, R. (2018). Chronic cannabidiol exposure promotes functional impairment in sexual behavior and fertility of male mice. *Reproductive Toxicology (Elmsford, N.Y.), 81*, 34–40. DOI: 10.1016/j.reprotox.2018.06.013 PMID: 29936126

Conjugated Estrogens Topical Side Effects: Common, Severe, Long Term. (2025, April 11). Drugs.Com. https://www.drugs.com/sfx/conjugated-estrogens-topical-side-effects.html

Crocq, M. A. (2020). History of cannabis and the endocannabinoid system. *Dialogues in Clinical Neuroscience, 22*(3), 223–228. DOI: 10.31887/DCNS.2020.22.3/mcrocq PMID: 33162765

Dahlgren, M. K., El-Abboud, C., Lambros, A. M., Sagar, K. A., Smith, R. T., & Gruber, S. A. (2022). A survey of medical cannabis use during perimenopause and postmenopause. *Menopause (New York, N.Y.), 29*(9), 1028–1036. DOI: 10.1097/GME.0000000000002018 PMID: 35917529

Dahlgren, M. K., Smith, R. T., Kosereisoglu, D., Sagar, K. A., Lambros, A. M., El-Abboud, C., & Gruber, S. A. (2024). A survey-based, quasi-experimental study assessing a high-cannabidiol suppository for menstrual-related pain and discomfort. *Npj Women's Health, 2*(1), 29. DOI: 10.1038/s44294-024-00032-0

Delvin, D., & Webber, C. (2014, September 24). *Lack of sex drive in women (lack of libido).* NetDoctor. https://web.archive.org/web/20151016134757/http://www.netdoctor.co.uk/sex_relationships/facts/lackingsexdrive.htm

Fratoni, M., & Tutkus, S. (2021). The Cannabis Care Nurse's Experience. In *Cannabis: A handbook for nurses* (pp. 402–445). Wolters Kluwer.

Gertsch, J. (2017). Cannabimimetic phytochemicals in the diet – an evolutionary link to food selection and metabolic stress adaptation? *British Journal of Pharmacology, 174*(11), 1464–1483. DOI: 10.1111/bph.13676 PMID: 27891602

Goldstein, B. (2020). *Cannabis is medicine: How medical cannabis and CBD are healing everything from anxiety to chronic pain* (1st ed.). Little Brown Spark.

Gulanick, M., & Myers, J. L. (Eds.). (2017). *Nursing care plans: Diagnoses, interventions, & outcomes* (9th ed.). Elsevier.

Hill, D. A., & Taylor, C. A. (2021). Dyspareunia in Women. *American Family Physician, 103*(10), 597–604. PMID: 33983001

Infertility. (2023, April 19). Cleveland Clinic. https://my.clevelandclinic.org/health/diseases/16083-infertility

Jarvis, C., Eckhardt, A., & Thomas, P. (2020). *Physical examination & health assessment* (Eighth). Elsevier.

Konick-McMahan, J. (2007). Endocrine Problems. In *Medical-surgical nursing: Assessment and management of clinical problems* (Seventh). Mosby Elsevier.

Konieczny, E. (2018). *Healing with CBD: How cannabidiol can transform your health without the high.* Ulysses Press.

Lane, D. (2022, September 4). 3 Penis Exercises That Improve Your Sex Life. *Black Doctor Org*. https://blackdoctor.org/penis-exercises-to-improve-sex-life/

Liang, A. L., Gingher, E. L., & Coleman, J. S. (2022). Medical cannabis for gynecologic pain conditions: A systematic review. *Obstetrics and Gynecology*, *139*(2), 287–296. DOI: 10.1097/AOG.0000000000004656 PMID: 35104069

Lilley, L. L., Collins, S. R., & Snyder, J. S. (Eds.). (2020). *Pharmacology and the nursing process* (9th ed.). Elsevier.

Lingegowda, H., Williams, B. J., Spiess, K. G., Sisnett, D. J., Lomax, A. E., Koti, M., & Tayade, C. (2022). Role of the endocannabinoid system in the pathophysiology of endometriosis and therapeutic implications. *Journal of Cannabis Research*, *4*(1), 54. DOI: 10.1186/s42238-022-00163-8 PMID: 36207747

Lo, J. O., Hedges, J. C., & Girardi, G. (2022). Impact of cannabinoids on pregnancy, reproductive health and offspring outcomes. *American Journal of Obstetrics and Gynecology*, *227*(4), 571–581. DOI: 10.1016/j.ajog.2022.05.056 PMID: 35662548

Lynn, B., Gee, A., Zhang, L., & Pfaus, J. G. (2020). Effects of Cannabinoids on Female Sexual Function. *Sexual Medicine Reviews*, *8*(1), 18–27. DOI: 10.1016/j.sxmr.2019.07.004 PMID: 31521567

Lynn, B. K., López, J. D., Miller, C., Thompson, J., & Campian, E. C. (2019). The Relationship between Marijuana Use Prior to Sex and Sexual Function in Women. *Sexual Medicine*, *7*(2), 192–197. DOI: 10.1016/j.esxm.2019.01.003 PMID: 30833225

Malka, D. (2022). *Medicinal cannabis: Pearls for clinical practice* (First edition). CRC Press, Taylor & Francis Group.

Mayo Clinic. (2024, February 29). *Anorgasmia in women—Symptoms and causes*. Mayo Clinic. https://www.mayoclinic.org/diseases-conditions/anorgasmia/symptoms-causes/syc-20369422

Moser, A., Ballard, S. M., Jensen, J., & Averett, P. (2023). The influence of cannabis on sexual functioning and satisfaction. *Journal of Cannabis Research*, *5*(1), 2. DOI: 10.1186/s42238-022-00169-2 PMID: 36658600

Mulvehill, S., & Tishler, J. (2024). Assessment of the effect of cannabis use before partnered sex on women with and without orgasm difficulty. *Sexual Medicine*, *12*(2), qfae023. Advance online publication. DOI: 10.1093/sexmed/qfae023 PMID: 38711949

Muthukumaran, D., Bin Jumah, J., Shanmugam, R., & Kamaraj, C. (2025). From Sunshine to Wellness: Understanding Vitamin D Impact on Menstrual Health. *Advances in Public Health, 2025*(1), 5296320. Advance online publication. DOI: 10.1155/adph/5296320

Parmelee, R., Sommers, D., & Clark, C. S. (2021). Cannabis pharmacology: From the whole plant to pharmaceutical applications. In C. S. Clark, *Cannabis: A handbook for nurses* (pp. 115–160). Wolters Kluwer.

Polycystic ovary syndrome. (2026, January 22). World Health Organization. https://www.who.int/news-room/fact-sheets/detail/polycystic-ovary-syndrome

Popescu-Spineni, D. M., Guja, L., Cristache, C. M., Pop-Tudose, M. E., & Munteanu, A. M. (2022). The influence of endocannabinoid system on women reproduction. *Acta Endocrinologica (Bucureşti), 18*(2), 209–215. DOI: 10.4183/aeb.2022.209 PMID: 36212249

Russo, E. B. (2016). Clinical Endocannabinoid Deficiency Reconsidered: Current Research Supports the Theory in Migraine, Fibromyalgia, Irritable Bowel, and Other Treatment-Resistant Syndromes. *Cannabis and Cannabinoid Research, 1*(1), 154–165. DOI: 10.1089/can.2016.0009 PMID: 28861491

Sathyapalan, T., Javed, Z., Kilpatrick, E. S., Coady, A.-M., & Atkin, S. L. (2017). Endocannabinoid receptor blockade increases vascular endothelial growth factor and inflammatory markers in obese women with polycystic ovary syndrome. *Horumon To Rinsho, 86*(3), 384–387. DOI: 10.1111/cen.13239 PMID: 27651218

Sulak, D. (2022). *Handbook of cannabis for clinicians: Principles and practice* (1st ed.). W.W. Norton & Company.

Sun, A. J., & Eisenberg, M. L. (2017). Association Between Marijuana Use and Sexual Frequency in the United States: A Population-Based Study. *Journal of Sexual Medicine, 14*(11), 1342–1347. DOI: 10.1016/j.jsxm.2017.09.005 PMID: 29110804

Tal, R., Seifer, D., & Arici, A. (2015). The Emerging Role of Angiogenic Factor Dysregulation in the Pathogenesis of Polycystic Ovarian Syndrome. *Seminars in Reproductive Medicine, 33*(3), 195–207. DOI: 10.1055/s-0035-1552582 PMID: 26036901

Zhu, L., Zhou, C., Li, X., Liu, Z., Tong, Y., & Yang, S. (2024). Global burden and trends in female premenstrual syndrome study during 1990-2019. *Archives of Women's Mental Health, 27*(3), 369–382. DOI: 10.1007/s00737-024-01426-4 PMID: 38280031

KEY TERMS AND DEFINITIONS

Conception: The process in which a sperm fertilizes an egg, initiating early pregnancy and influenced by hormonal, reproductive, and lifestyle factors.

Endocannabinoid System (ECS): A regulatory physiological system that supports balance in mood, pain, sleep, appetite, reproduction, and hormonal function through endogenous cannabinoids and receptor signaling.

Endometriosis: A chronic condition in which endometrial-like tissue grows outside the uterus, causing pelvic pain, inflammation, and fertility challenges.

Erectile Dysfunction (ED): The persistent difficulty achieving or maintaining an erection sufficient for sexual activity, often linked to vascular, neurologic, hormonal, or psychological factors.

Female Orgasmic Disorder: A sexual health condition characterized by delayed, infrequent, or absent orgasm despite adequate stimulation, often influenced by psychological, hormonal, or physiological factors.

Libido: An individual's desire for sexual activity, shaped by hormonal balance, emotional well-being, health status, and relationship factors.

Menopause: The natural end of menstrual cycles marked by declining ovarian hormone production, often accompanied by vasomotor, mood, sleep, and genitourinary symptoms.

Polycystic Ovarian Syndrome (PCOS): A hormonal and metabolic disorder characterized by irregular cycles, ovarian cysts, insulin resistance, and androgen excess.

Post-Coital Pain: Pain occurring after sexual intercourse, potentially related to pelvic floor dysfunction, infection, inflammation, or gynecologic conditions

Premenstrual Syndrome (PMS): A cluster of physical and emotional symptoms occurring before menstruation, related to hormonal fluctuations and individual sensitivity.

Chapter 8

Cannabis Care Nurses as Educational Leaders: Closing Knowledge Gaps in Military and Veteran Healthcare Systems

Mike Harvey
http://orcid.org/0009-0006-9572-1688
American Cannabis Nurses Association, USA

ABSTRACT

This chapter examines the essential role of Cannabis Care Nurses (CCNs) as educators addressing knowledge gaps about cannabis and cannabinoid therapies within military and Veterans healthcare. The Department of Defense (DoD) prohibits cannabis use among active-duty service members, imposing strict penalties for violations, but allows dependents limited access to FDA-approved cannabinoid medications through Tricare. Veterans face different access rules influenced by state laws and VA policies, which may permit broader use. The 2018 Farm Bill's legalization of hemp-derived products has further complicated compliance for service members. These regulations create ongoing challenges in understanding safe use, compliance, and stigma for military personnel, Veterans, dependents, and providers. CCNs are positioned to deliver evidence-based education and support informed decision-making, helping reduce stigma and ensuring all stakeholders can effectively navigate the evolving policies surrounding cannabis in healthcare.

DOI: 10.4018/979-8-2600-2035-7.ch008

INTRODUCTION: MILITARY OVERVIEW

The Department of Defense oversees healthcare services for around 1.3 million active-duty military personnel and about 1.5 million military dependents. Altogether, the Military Health System (MHS) provides care to nearly 9.5 million people, making it one of the largest healthcare systems in the United States, with over 700 facilities across the country, as well as hospitals located on military bases throughout the world and on the high seas.

Currently, the Department of Defense does not recognize the role of the Cannabis Care Nurse (CCN) or any role of the nurse in relation to cannabis or cannabinoids. This is mainly because the use of cannabinoid medicines is limited, and service members are strictly prohibited from using any cannabis or cannabinoid products.

However, DoD dependents can be prescribed FDA-approved cannabinoid treatments through the Tricare Pharmacy Program. Examples include Dronabinol (Marinol) for nausea and vomiting related to chemotherapy, and Epidiolex (Cannabidiol) for refractory seizure conditions like Dravet Syndrome, Lennox-Gastaut Syndrome, or Tuberous Sclerosis.

Active-duty service members are expressly prohibited from using any cannabis products, as this constitutes a violation of military law. Consumption of cannabis-derived substances may result in administrative separation pursuant to Article 112a of the Uniform Code of Military Justice (UCMJ), which addresses the wrongful use, possession, and related offenses concerning controlled substances. Significant drug violations can lead to a Dishonorable Discharge for enlisted personnel or Dismissal for officers, while lesser infractions may result in a Bad-Conduct Discharge.

Department of Defense Instruction 1010.04, Problematic Substance Use and Gambling Disorder, states that any illegal or improper use, possession, transfer, sale, or addiction involving controlled or psychoactive substances—including narcotics, cannabis, or other dangerous drugs—must be handled according to Executive Order 12968, DoD Manual 5200.02, and a memorandum from the Under Secretary of Defense for Intelligence dated August 30, 2006.

Greg Chadwick from the Air Force Materiel Command Health & Wellness Team wrote an article for Joint Base San Antonio's website titled "DOD prohibited substances: Marijuana, CBD and hemp" (Chadwick, 2022). In it, he notes that "the Department of Defense and each Service prohibit service members from consuming or using any hemp-derived products, including CBD, regardless of their THC content. This policy is in place to maintain military readiness and ensure the integrity of drug testing programs."

The rules regarding cannabis use apply equally to all military personnel, including those in reserve and National Guard units. The Department of Defense enforces these standards across every branch, so reservists and National Guard members must follow the same rules as active-duty members. This can create challenges for those living in states where cannabis is legal for medical or recreational use.

An additional concern relates to the increased availability of hemp-derived products permitted under the 2018 Farm Bill, which allows vendors to sell items with less than 0.3% THC by dry weight. Even with this legal change, service members who use hemp-based CBD products can violate Department of Defense policies and regulations. Some service members may not fully understand the risks and consequences of using hemp-derived products that are otherwise permitted by the 2018 Farm Bill, leaving them vulnerable to legal issues.

Given these strict policies and the evolving legal landscape, nurses and allied healthcare professionals play a vital role in reducing stigma and building trust around cannabinoid therapies for military families, while still complying with Department of Defense regulations. Nurses are especially well-positioned to provide education and support for service members and their families, helping them make informed decisions about the need for, use of, and risks associated with cannabis.

Due to the absence of standardized cannabis education, it is recommended that Department of Defense nurses and healthcare providers unfamiliar with cannabis utilize resources from the National Institute on Drug Abuse (2024), which presents current cannabis research to assist healthcare providers in making informed healthcare decisions. Furthermore, the National Council of State Boards of Nursing (2018) offers guidelines, including the Six Key Fundamentals of Essential Nursing Knowledge, aimed at improving both student and practitioner competency in the clinical application of cannabis. Staying current with legislative changes and scientific findings related to cannabis, as well as understanding its potential risks and benefits, enables nursing professionals to effectively educate military personnel and other beneficiaries about advancements in cannabis science and its prospective medical applications.

Given these rigorous policies and the changing legal context, nurses and allied health care professionals continue to hold a critical role in mitigating stigma and building trust around cannabinoid therapy for families, while remaining compliant with Department of Defense regulations. Nurses are uniquely positioned to educate service members and their beneficiaries by supporting the ability to make informed decisions concerning the justification, application, and potential risks associated with cannabis.

TRANSITIONING FROM UNIFORMED SERVICE: CANNABIS USE AND LEGAL CONSIDERATIONS

Navigating the intersection between military service and Veteran status reveals a complex and uncertain landscape for cannabis use. Individuals accessing VA healthcare may still hold active duty, reserve, or National Guard status, making them subject to Department of Defense regulations—including strict prohibitions under UCMJ Article 112a.

It is also essential to recognize that retired military personnel who use cannabis may encounter additional uncertainties. Existing case law establishes that retirees receiving military pay remain subject to UCMJ authority. Although such instances are rare, retired service members may be recalled to active duty, as was the case during Operation Desert Shield and Desert Storm. However, available records do not specify the number of retirees recalled or provide further details. Involuntary recalls have taken place during national emergencies; therefore, both retired service members and Cannabis Care Nurses should consider this possibility when deciding whether to use any cannabis or cannabinoids in the treatment of a health condition, or in recreational use.

The Department of Defense is highly unlikely to recall a former service member just to charge them with cannabis use. However, administrative recalls, medical evaluations, or records verification, and retiree musters do happen. These situations could potentially expose retired service members to legal risks regarding cannabis use during their civilian lives.

Cannabis Use Among Veterans

It is important to delineate the term "Veteran." As defined by the Merriam-Webster dictionary, a veteran refers to "a former member of the armed forces." However, for VA healthcare purposes, 38 U.S.C. § 101(2) specifies that a Veteran is "a person who served in the active military, naval, air, or space service, and who was discharged or released therefrom under conditions other than dishonorable." This clarification underscores a distinction: reservists and National Guard members typically do not qualify for VA health care unless they have been federally activated or have acquired a service-connected disability attributable to their service.

The Department of Veterans Affairs oversees 152 VA hospitals across the United States, along with more than 800 Community-Based Outpatient Clinics (CBOCs). Beyond the U.S. mainland, a VA Medical Center operates in San Juan, Puerto Rico, supported by additional CBOCs throughout the island. Facilities and services are also available in Guam, American Samoa, and the U.S. Virgin Islands. The Northern Mariana Islands have a limited VA presence, with care primarily provided through telehealth and referrals. Furthermore, the Manila VA Clinic in the Philippines serves veterans residing in this distinctive community.

It should be noted that all of the territories noted above have established cannabis legislation. Guam, the U.S. Virgin Islands, and the Northern Mariana Islands have each legalized both medical and recreational cannabis use. Puerto Rico permits medical cannabis but continues to prohibit recreational consumption. Only veterans residing in American Samoa or the Philippines lack access to either medical or recreational cannabis

As service members transition to Veteran status, they can now legally access cannabis through state-regulated dispensaries and products authorized under the 2018 Farm Bill. Cannabis is available both at retail establishments and via online platforms offering direct delivery services. The expanded accessibility of cannabis raises important concerns about Veterans potentially obtaining products that have not undergone third-party testing for cannabinoid content, heavy metals, pesticides, or other contaminants, thereby increasing the risk of exposure to unsafe or inadequately tested cannabis. Given the growing interest in medicinal cannabis by Veterans, comprehensive patient education is essential. A lack of communication between health care providers and Veterans on this topic may elevate risks associated with uninformed cannabis use, such as drug-drug interactions and increased risk for falls.

In 2019, 9.8% of Veterans reported cannabis use within the preceding year, while 11.9% indicated use during the previous six months. Among individuals aged 65-84 receiving care through the VA, 10.3% reported cannabis use within the past 30 days, which is nearly double the rate for civilian cannabis use. It should be noted that the proportion of Veterans who disclose cannabis use may differ from the actual number of users. Veterans who utilize cannabis as an adjunct to therapy, particularly those managing multiple health conditions, face an elevated risk of drug-drug interactions and additive pharmacological effects, potentially increasing the likelihood of harm or injury. Clear and impartial communication from the healthcare team plays a vital role in promoting patient safety, particularly as Veterans who are apprehensive about stigma may hesitate to disclose their cannabis use.

Now that we have a clearer picture of how many Veterans use cannabis, let's explore the possible reasons behind their choices. Out of 17.6 million Veterans, 1.3 million have service-connected Post-Traumatic Stress Disorder (PTSD). More than 180,000 are receiving treatment for Traumatic Brain Injury (TBI) (U.S. Department of Veterans Affairs, 2025), and the VA provides pain management services related to musculoskeletal problems for over 3 million Veterans. Many Veterans turn to cannabis to manage these conditions, along with other conditions, such as pain and issues with sleep.

According to VA News dated September 21, 2023, the Department of Veterans Affairs has substantially decreased the number of Veterans prescribed opioid medications from 874,897 in 2012 to 288,820 in 2023. This constitutes a 67% reduction as part of the Opioid Safety Initiative (OSI). Veterans now often receive non-opioid analgesics such as acetaminophen, nonsteroidal anti-inflammatory drugs (NSAIDs), selective serotonin reuptake inhibitors (SSRIs), tricyclic antidepressants (TCAs), anticonvulsants, topical agents, and muscle relaxants. Additionally, the VA has expanded its offerings in physical therapy, cognitive behavioral therapy, acupuncture, and chiropractic care, and introduced the Whole Health Program, which integrates conventional treatments with Complementary and Integrative Health (CIH) approaches.

The reduction in opioid prescriptions for chronic pain management, without an alternative pharmaceutical offering comparable efficacy, may be a contributing factor for Veterans in considering cannabis as a potential option for pain relief.

Changes in benzodiazepine prescribing practices have significantly impacted Veterans diagnosed with PTSD. In 2012, approximately 396,000 Veterans received new benzodiazepine prescriptions; however, this number was expected to decline to 336,000 by 2025, indicating a substantial reduction in the initiation of benzodiazepine therapy within this population. This trend reflects an estimated decrease of nearly 84.9% in new prescriptions. With close to 82,000 Veterans newly approved for PTSD in 2024, the decrease in benzodiazepine use suggests that alternative strategies for symptom management are being explored. Notably, there is growing interest in cannabis as a therapeutic option among veterans as an anxiolytic.

Veterans are aware of the research being conducted both within the US and from other developed nations, showing increased applications for cannabinoid pharmaceuticals for the treatment of a multitude of disease processes. Cannabinoid utilization for select seizure disorders, chemotherapy-induced nausea and vomiting, and anorexia in AIDS patients within the United States has been well established. Beyond the United States, cannabis as a pharmaceutical has achieved use in the treatment of chronic pain, multiple sclerosis, Parkinson's disease, Alzheimer's disease symptoms, PTSD, anxiety disorders, Crohn's/IBD.

There are currently no FDA-approved cannabinoid applications included within the VA formulary. The VA formulary indicates that the cannabinoid products are not on the VA national formulary and require a non-formulary drug request and prior approval to be dispensed. The cannabinoid options are listed as 'Undefined', which possibly suggests that there may be a potential pathway for a Veteran to access such products. However, it remains uncertain whether VA health care providers would be willing to submit an off-label request for a cannabinoid pharmaceutical, or if such a non-formulary drug request would encounter administrative barriers at initial review stages.

As with the Department of Defense, the Department of Veterans Affairs manages directives regarding cannabis utilization. In accordance with VHA Directive 1315

(Department of Veterans Affairs, 2023), the Department of Veterans Affairs does not withhold services from Veterans solely due to their participation in state-sanctioned cannabis programs. VA clinicians are directed to address cannabis use with patients utilizing harm reduction approaches. Maintaining transparent communication between health care providers and Veterans is essential, as Veterans may experience increased risks associated with cannabis use if potential harms are not discussed openly between health care providers and patients.

VHA Directive 1315 stipulates that VA clinicians are not permitted to recommend medical cannabis to Veterans, as cannabis is classified as a Schedule I substance under the Controlled Substances Act of 1970. Despite this restriction, providers have a primary responsibility to educate patients. The directive underscores the duty of health care teams to inform the Veteran about the potential risks of cannabis use but falls short of noting that providers should also document the potential medical benefits experienced from cannabis use by the Veteran. Ensuring open, transparent, and impartial communication between providers and patients is critical so that Veterans can make informed decisions regarding their use of cannabis.

Veterans encounter numerous barriers regarding both medicinal and recreational cannabis use. Foremost among these challenges is the stigma associated with cannabis consumption, accompanied by healthcare bias, potential implications of having negative annotations entered into their medical records, and insufficient education among healthcare professionals about cannabis-related issues.

The way in which a Veteran's cannabis use is perceived differs based on the state in which they live and receive medical care, as well as among individual healthcare professionals. Even in states where medical cannabis is permitted by law, there may be differing opinions within the same medical service, with some providers viewing cannabis use favorably while others may consider it potentially harmful. Generally, patients evaluated by general practitioners may encounter less bias regarding cannabis use compared to those seen by mental health professionals. Veterans who use cannabis are more likely to receive a diagnosis of Cannabis Use Disorder (CUD) during assessments conducted by mental health care providers.

CUD within the Veteran population has seen a steady increase since 2005, reflecting trends in both military and civilian groups. Specifically, CUD prevalence among veterans rose from 0.85% in 2005 to 1.92% by 2019 (Bonn-Miller et al., 2021). Variability in how CUD is diagnosed across medical specialties is a notable concern. This is evident in differing diagnostic practices between general practitioners and mental health professionals when evaluating Veterans who use cannabis daily or nearly daily, either as monotherapy or adjunct therapy.

In both VA and civilian healthcare settings, daily cannabis consumption—even when intended for therapeutic purposes—is frequently classified as misuse. Such diagnostic inconsistencies are particularly apparent in regions where Veterans have access to cannabis and choose it for issues like sleep disturbances or PTSD management, which often results in an automatic CUD diagnosis. There is also a tendency to diagnose CUD based on observed negative outcomes without adequately considering the therapeutic benefits experienced by individual Veterans using cannabis as part of their treatment regimen.

Legislation Pending

As of the writing of this chapter, federal legislation related to veterans' access to cannabis remains bogged down in various committees.

H.R. 966 – Veterans Cannabis Use for Safe Healing Act *(119th Congress, 2025–2026).*

- Ensure that the Department of Veterans Affairs (VA) does not impose any limitations on eligible Veterans seeking access to benefits related to participation in state-authorized medical cannabis programs.
- Talk to Veterans about cannabis use and modify the treatment plan as needed.
- Document this usage in the Veteran's medical records. Furthermore, the bill permits VA physicians and other healthcare providers to give recommendations or opinions to veterans residing in states with approved programs.

H.R. 2935-The PREPARE Act of 2025

- The purpose of this bill is to create a Commission on the Federal Regulation of Cannabis to prepare the market for a legally regulated market set in a post-prohibition era.
- This commission would comprise individuals from the Department of Justice (DOJ), Department of Health and Human Services (DHHS), US Department of Agriculture (USDA), Treasury Department, Federal Drug Administration (FDA), Drug Enforcement Agency (DEA), industry experts, researchers, and representatives from communities harmed by the 80 years of cannabis prohibition.
- While the PREPARE Act does not reschedule or decriminalize cannabis, it begins the framework for cannabis commerce.

H.R. 5060 – The MORE Act (Marijuana Opportunity Reinvestment and Expungement Act)

- Primary purpose is to decriminalize and reschedule cannabis
- Expungement of federal convictions

- Federal cannabis taxation
- Federal regulation through the permit process

PENDING RESEARCH OF INTEREST

Cannabis research in the United States faces challenges due to its Schedule I classification. Despite this barrier, studies are underway both nationally and internationally, including in Canada. Investigations into cannabis use among Veterans continue, although advancements are slow. The details below are based on data provided by clinicaltrials.gov.

- NCT06381180: Warrior CARE: Cannabis Behavioral Health is a randomized, controlled clinical trial sponsored by Wayne State University that aims to evaluate the therapeutic potential of cannabinoids—THC, CBD, and their combination—on PTSD symptoms and suicidal ideation in U.S. military Veterans. The trial plans to enroll 500 Veterans who meet DSM-5 criteria for PTSD and who currently use or have an interest in using cannabis. (ClinicalTrials.gov, 2025)

The Warrior CARE trial is designed to generate some of the first rigorous clinical evidence on whether smoked or vaporized cannabis (THC, CBD, or both) can reduce PTSD symptoms, suicidality, or improve behavioral health measures in Veterans. Its long-term goal is to inform future clinical guidelines and policy decisions regarding medical cannabis use in Veteran populations.

- NCT07224698: Title: *Inhaled Cannabis for Treatment of PTSD, is* sponsored by the Multidisciplinary Association for Psychedelic Studies (MAPS). Current status shows that they have not yet begun to recruit (ClinicalTrials.gov, 2025)

The study is scheduled to commence on February 1, 2026, with an anticipated completion date of June 30, 2027. The total projected enrollment is 320 participants. This Phase 2 multicenter, randomized, placebo-controlled, double-blind, parallel study will evaluate the safety and efficacy of inhaled cannabis in veterans diagnosed with posttraumatic stress disorder (PTSD). Eligibility criteria include individuals who are at least 18 years old, have been diagnosed as a Veteran with PTSD for more than six months, and meet the DSM-5 diagnostic criteria for PTSD. Although this is an FDA-approved clinical trial, it is not being conducted by the VA.

There has been other cannabis driven research conducted in which results are not available but may be of interest to the Veteran population. Each summary is as reported on the ClinicalTrials.gov website

- Enhancing Prolonged Exposure With Cannabidiol to Treat Posttraumatic Stress Disorder, NCT05132699. Sponsored by the University of Texas Health Science Center at San Antonio, with the primary goal of this pilot project to demonstrate the safety and feasibility of using Cannabidiol (CBD) in combination with standard of care prolonged exposure (PE) psychotherapy to reduce PTSD symptoms. Results posted Oct 2024 (ClinicalTrials.gov, 2024)
- Cannabidiol as a Treatment for PTSD and PTSD Comorbid With TBI. NCT04550377, sponsored by NYU Langone Health, is currently recruiting.

This will be a randomized, placebo-controlled study to test the efficacy of cannabidiol (CBD) as a treatment for symptoms of post-traumatic stress disorder (PTSD). Subjects, 120 in total, will be males and females with PTSD, half of whom will have comorbid mild traumatic brain injury (TBI). There will be three study arms, each with 40 subjects: 1) Oral CBD 400 mg daily; 2) Oral CBD 800 mg daily, and 3) Placebo daily. Treatment duration will be 8 weeks. The primary outcome will be a change in PTSD symptoms as measured by change in the Clinician-Administered PTSD Scale (CAPS-5) total score. ClinicalTrials.gov. (2025)

- Cannabidiol and Prolonged Exposure (CBD-PE). NCT03518801, sponsored by the VA Office of Research and Development. The trial will include a randomized control trial to evaluate the efficacy of using Cannabidiol (CBD), a non-intoxicating cannabinoid, as an adjunctive to Prolonged Exposure therapy (PE). The trial will compare PE + CBD to PE + placebo in a sample of 136 military Veterans with PTSD at the VA San Diego Medical Center. The study represents the logical and innovative next step for augmenting existing treatments and developing novel pharmacotherapy for PTSD. Findings from the proposed RCT will inform clinical practice and policy by investigating whether administration of CBD in the context of PE therapy will improve treatment outcomes for military Veterans with PTSD, ClinicalTrials.gov. (2025).

FACILITATING INFORMED CONVERSATIONS

Effective communication is essential to delivering high-quality patient care. Dialogue between healthcare providers and Veterans regarding cannabis use is often hampered by mutual apprehension. VA healthcare professionals may demonstrate hesitancy in addressing this topic due to limited knowledge. To facilitate informed conversations, the VA has released the VA Cannabis Provider Education Packet (Veterans Health Administration, 2020), available as a PDF. This comprehensive resource provides detailed information on the pharmacodynamics and pharmacokinetics of cannabis, as well as legal and ethical issues associated with its use.

Insufficient communication about cannabis between health care providers and Veterans may negatively affect interactions not only between providers and Veterans but also among providers themselves, especially when specialized care is necessary. Precise and impartial documentation of interactions with Veterans is vital for effective management of their care when cannabis is utilized. Health care professionals should systematically record the Veterans' perspectives regarding cannabis use and assess their understanding of cannabis as a potential therapeutic option, including awareness of possible adverse effects related to their health conditions.

Veterans frequently express concerns about the limited duration of face-to-face interactions with their healthcare providers, which restricts opportunities to address questions related to cannabis use. On a national level, the average patient visit lasts 18 minutes, with a range of 13 to 24 minutes. Comparable data for interaction times between VA providers and Veterans is not available, as the VA currently only monitors waiting times. If it is assumed that Veterans experience similar appointment durations, there may be insufficient time remaining after clinical assessment and review of medical history for meaningful discussion of additional questions, such as discussing cannabis.

In order to evaluate how accessible cannabis education is through Veterans Affairs (VA) providers, the author scheduled an appointment with their VA primary care provider. The author began this process using the 'My HealtheVet' application to email the provider. The email, titled "Education: Cannabis and health," was to request a discussion about cannabis use at the upcoming appointment. The aim was to better understand both the possible benefits and risks associated with cannabis use.

In response to the request, the VA health care provider initially recommended referring the subject to the mental health care team. The recommendation was based on observations indicating that cannabis use was primarily associated with mental health concerns, including depression, anxiety, and insomnia. In such cases, the involvement of a Cannabis Care Nurse may provide valuable support to Veterans seeking guidance on cannabis use, addressing their needs effectively while avoiding undue strain on the broader health care team.

POTENTIAL ROLE OF A CANNABIS CARE NURSE IN SUPPORTING VETERANS?

With the ongoing progress in endocannabinoid system (ECS) research, emerging therapeutic options are anticipated in the near future. Cannabis Care Nurses are equipped to take leadership roles across various healthcare fields, adapting to ongoing developments in cannabis science. The role of the Cannabis Care Nurse could closely mirror those of Anticoagulation Nurse Specialists (ACNS) and Diabetes Nurse Specialists (DNS). These nurses would collaborate with other healthcare professionals to assess, plan, deliver, and review patient care, both within the VA healthcare system and in independent clinics. (See Table 1)

Table 1.

Role	Anticoagulation Nurse	Diabetes Nurse Educator	Cannabis Care Nurse
Primary Focus	Anticoagulant therapy management	Diabetes self-management education	Medical cannabis therapy and patient advocacy
Key Responsibilities	Dose adjustment, INR monitoring, bleeding risk education	Glucose monitoring, insulin education, lifestyle counseling	Cannabis dosing guidance, ECS education, holistic care
Educational Background	RN license: BSN preferred; anticoagulation certification	RN license: BSN preferred; CDCES certification	RN license: BSN preferred; cannabis nursing education, pending cannabis certification
Specialized Knowledge	Coagulation pathways, drug-food interactions	Endocrinology, nutrition, and chronic disease management	Endocannabinoid system, cannabis pharmacology, legal frameworks

The Cannabis Care Nurse holds a key position in ensuring safe and evidence-based cannabis care for Veterans. This role encompasses facilitating effective communication, delivering thorough education, and promoting harm reduction initiatives. Through collaboration with VA healthcare providers, the Cannabis Care Nurse supports the customization of cannabinoid dosing regimens and the integration of cannabis use into care plans that comply with VA policies and federal regulations.

The Cannabis Care Nurse assists the Veteran by monitoring symptoms during cannabis therapy and advising on potential drug interactions. All actions are performed according to ethical standards and best practices to foster safety and comprehensive well-being. Additionally, the Cannabis Care Nurse operates within the defined scope and standards noted in the Cannabis Nursing Scope and Standards of Practice, as delineated by the American Nurses Association and the American Cannabis Nurses Association (2023).

The Cannabis Nursing Scope and Standards of Practice identifies the guidelines that the Cannabis Care Nurse must follow:

- Assessment – Collect comprehensive data on the patient's health and cannabis use.
- Diagnosis – Analyze assessment data to determine issues related to cannabis use.
- Outcomes Identification – Set measurable goals for safe cannabis integration.
- Planning – Develop individualized care plans incorporating cannabis considerations.
- Implementation – Execute interventions, including education and harm reduction.
- Coordination of Care – Collaborate with the health care team for integrated care.
- Health Teaching and Promotion – Educate patients on safe cannabis practices.
- Evaluation – Assess progress toward outcomes and adjust care plans.

Cannabis Care Nurses exhibit leadership within their field by offering support to nursing students, recent graduates, and seasoned professionals. They recognize their responsibility to ensure the nursing workforce possesses the comprehensive knowledge specified in the Six Principles of Essential Knowledge (S19-S21) established by the National Council of State Boards of Nursing (2018).

1. The nurse shall have a working knowledge of the current state of legalization of medical and recreational cannabis use.
2. The nurse shall have a working knowledge of the jurisdiction's MMP
3. The nurse shall have an understanding of the endocannabinoid system, cannabinoid receptors, cannabinoids, and the interactions between them.
4. The nurse shall have an understanding of cannabis pharmacology and the research associated with the medical use of cannabis.
5. The nurse shall be able to identify the safety considerations for patient use of cannabis.
6. The nurse shall approach the patient without judgment regarding the patient's choice of treatment or preferences in managing pain and other distressing symptoms.

CANADIAN VETERANS

In Canada, medical cannabis was legalized in 2001, followed by the legalization of adult-use cannabis in 2018. Canadian Veterans are eligible to apply for cannabis from external producers licensed by Health Canada, with reimbursement available for up to 3 grams per day, capped at $8.50 per gram. The approved cannabis products that the Veteran can purchase encompass oils, capsules, and dried flower.

Medical cannabis prescriptions are issued by physicians with expertise in cannabis dosing rather than by VAC physicians (Veterans Affairs Canada, 2019). Although VAC does not provide education on medical cannabis usage, there is a robust network of nurses across Canada specializing in cannabis as medicine who offer this training.

While national policy establishes a foundation for reimbursement and access, the quality of Veterans' day-to-day experiences and support is frequently determined by the expertise and commitment of individual community-based nurses. The relationship between policy and practical implementation is illustrated by professionals such as Kala Sanmartin, whose efforts demonstrate how specialized nursing roles effectively address the ongoing educational and care requirements of Veterans utilizing medical cannabis.

In an interview with Kala Sanmartin, BScN, CCHCNC, Managing Partner and Holistic Cannabis Nurse Coach at Vital Holistic Care, she outlines her responsibilities in delivering cannabis nursing services, with a focus on supporting Canadian Veterans diagnosed with pensioned health conditions. Eligible Veterans are entitled to reimbursement for up to 3 grams per day of medical cannabis, a benefit that has been available since the 2000s. Ms. Sanmartin assists her cannabis patients with cannabis education and guidance in response to a recognized need for these services. The significant demand has contributed to considerable expansion of the practice over the past two years.

Vital Holistic Care employs a holistic nursing approach to deliver comprehensive care and educate Veterans about their Endocannabinoid System and strategies for its maintenance. The organization curates and instructs on recommended cannabinoid care plans that encourage Veterans to participate in activities beyond cannabis use for ECS support—effectively promoting sustainable health practices. The primary focus is to use cannabinoids to establish foundational regulations of pain, sleep, and mood; from this foundation, coaching is provided to facilitate lifestyle changes using a holistic, non-judgmental methodology.

WHAT IS PENDING FOR THE FUTURE OF MEDICAL CANNABIS?

At the time of submission, cannabis is pending a review for potential rescheduling to Schedule III status. Should cannabis, as a plant-based medication, be reclassified as Schedule III, it may create expanded opportunities for Veterans to access FDA-approved, non-smokable cannabis products in the management of both service-related and non-service-related disabilities.

The Evolving Role of Compounding Pharmacies in Medical Cannabis Therapy

Medical cannabis treatments may move away from the traditional pharmacy model, where standard medications are given to broad groups of patients. Instead, compounding pharmacies are expected to play a key role in personalizing cannabinoid medications tailored to individual health conditions and specific delivery methods (such as oral or topical). This approach could also include titration or adjustable dosing to better address each patient's unique needs.

The implementation of individualized cannabinoid formulations represents a significant advancement over the conventional practice of dispensing dronabinol in standardized doses of 2.5, 5, and 10 mg. By utilizing compounding pharmacies, healthcare professionals can prepare cannabinoid medications with specialized formulations that allow for precise adjustments to THC and CBD ratios. This methodology enables clinicians to achieve targeted therapeutic outcomes more effectively and to accommodate patient preferences. The evaluation of therapeutic efficacy or dose failure is frequently informed by consultations, either in person or via telehealth, conducted by a Cannabis Care Nurse to assess the management of symptoms among Veterans.

The Cannabis Care Nurse customizes treatment plans for the Veteran, meeting the Veteran's needs. For example, a Veteran may receive a personalized prescription from the VA or other provider that includes a higher THC-to-CBD ratio with sleep-promoting terpenes for nighttime use. Conversely, a daytime formulation might feature a higher CBD-to-THC ratio and energizing terpenes to support daytime functioning. Each prescription is carefully crafted to match the Veteran's individual requirements, illustrating the flexibility and patient-centered nature of compounding in cannabis care.

Follow-up with the Veteran, who may be new to cannabis or is experiencing adverse effects, may be conducted through telehealth services or via a secure phone or computer application that enables the health care team to closely monitor the patient and provide recommendations regarding cannabinoid and terpene adjustments.

The Department of Veterans Affairs currently employs a telehealth program for patients suspected of hypertension, to help rule out the possibility that the Veteran's elevated blood pressure readings are not attributable to White Coat Syndrome. The Veteran may be referred for telehealth and followed by a nurse for blood pressure monitoring. The Veterans are provided with a tablet and a Bluetooth-enabled blood pressure monitor. This allows patients to regularly measure their blood pressure at home, while a telehealth nurse reviews the collected data to guide clinical decisions.

In addition to collecting data related to the Veteran's blood pressure monitoring, the Veteran responds to questions pertaining to falls, depression screening, and other relevant health concerns. Utilizing a platform such as the home telehealth blood pressure platform, the Cannabis Care Nurse could evaluate the Veteran on multiple levels, such as cannabis dosage, route, and outcome. Assess for falls, changes in sleep patterns, changes in appetite, increase in or decrease in physical activities, standardized mental health assessments, and quality-of-life questionnaires at specified intervals, and most importantly, the benefit over perceived risks of cannabis utilization

CONCLUSION

The Cannabis Care Nurse is equipped with the necessary educational qualifications to effectively support Veterans who incorporate cannabis into their medical treatment plans. It is essential that individuals who have served in the armed forces are provided with comprehensive options for managing their healthcare. As Florence Nightingale stated in her seminal work, "What nursing has to do in either case, is to put the patient in the best condition for nature to act upon him" (Nightingale, 1859).

The Cannabis Care Nurse is tasked with creating and maintaining optimal conditions to enhance the therapeutic benefits that Veterans may obtain from modern cannabis-based treatments, thereby supporting the patient's readiness for effective intervention.

REFERENCES

American Nurses Association, & American Cannabis Nurses Association. (2023). *Cannabis nursing: Scope and standards of practice* (1st ed.). American Nurses Association.

Bonn-Miller, M. O., Sisley, S., Riggs, P., Yazar-Klosinski, B., Wang, J. B., Loflin, M. J. E., Shechet, B., Hennigan, C., Matthews, R., Emerson, A., & Doblin, R. (2021). The short-term impact of three smoked cannabis preparations versus placebo on PTSD symptoms: A randomized cross-over clinical trial. *PLoS One*, *16*(3), e0246990. DOI: 10.1371/journal.pone.0246990 PMID: 33730032

Chadwick, G. (2022, September 12). *DOD prohibited substances: Marijuana, CBD and hemp*. Joint Base San Antonio. https://www.jbsa.mil/News/News/Article/3155658/dod-prohibited-substances-marijuana-cbd-and-hemp/

ClinicalTrials.gov. (2024). *Enhancing prolonged exposure with cannabidiol to treat posttraumatic stress disorder.* https://clinicaltrials.gov/study/NCT05132699

ClinicalTrials.gov. (2025). *Cannabidiol and prolonged exposure (CBD-PE) (NCT03518801).* https://clinicaltrials.gov/study/NCT03518801

ClinicalTrials.gov. (2025). *Cannabidiol as a treatment for PTSD and PTSD comorbid with TBI (NCT04550377).* https://clinicaltrials.gov/study/NCT04550377

ClinicalTrials.gov. (2025). *Inhaled cannabis for treatment of PTSD (NCT07224698).* https://clinicaltrials.gov/study/NCT07224698

ClinicalTrials.gov. (2025). *Warrior CARE: Cannabis Behavioral Health (NCT06381180).* https://clinicaltrials.gov/study/NCT06381180

Department of Veterans Affairs. (2023). *VHA Directive 1315: Access to VHA clinical programs for Veterans participating in state-approved marijuana programs.* Veterans Health Administration.

National Council of State Boards of Nursing. (2018). The NCSBN National Nursing Guidelines for Medical Marijuana: The Six Essential Areas of Nursing Knowledge. *Journal of Nursing Regulation*, *9*(2), S14–S21. https://www.journalofnursingregulation.com/article/S2155-8256(18)30131-1/fulltext

National Institute on Drug Abuse. (2024, September). *Cannabis (marijuana).* https://nida.nih.gov/research-topics/cannabis-marijuana

Nightingale, F. (1859). *Notes on nursing: What it is, and what it is not.* Harrison & Sons.

U.S. Department of Veterans Affairs. (2025). Traumatic brain injury and VA benefits. Retrieved from https://www.va.gov/health-care/traumatic-brain-injury/

U.S. Senate. Committee on Armed Services. (1991). *Status of certain retired members of the armed forces recalled to active duty in connection with Operation Desert Storm: Report to accompany S. 204*. U.S. Government Printing Office.

Veterans Affairs Canada. (2019). *Reimbursement policy for cannabis for medical purposes*. https://www.veterans.gc.ca/en/about-vac/reports-policies-and-legislation/policies/reimbursement-policy-cannabis-medical-purposes

Veterans Health Administration. (2020). *Cannabis provider education packet*. U.S. Department of Veterans Affairs.

Chapter 9

Therapeutic Cannabis and Older Adults:

Addressing Complex Health Needs Through Specialized Geriatric Nursing Care

Mohammed El Rhanbouri
http://orcid.org/0009-0006-9643-5181
Morpho-Science Research Laboratory, Faculty of Medicine and Pharmacy, Cadi Ayyad University, Marrakech, Morocco

Samia Boussaa
http://orcid.org/0000-0002-5599-1097
Higher Institute of Nursing Professions and Technical Health of Rabat, Morocco

Jamila Ouadaf
Polydisciplinary Faculty of Safi, Cadi Ayyad University, Safi, Morocco

Said Khaldouni
Morpho Science Research Laboratory, Faculty of Medicine and Pharmacy, Cadi Ayyad University, Marrakech, Morocco.

Reda Mzoura
http://orcid.org/0009-0000-1579-1499
Health Sciences, Education and Management Research Team. Health Care and Sustainable Development Laboratory. Higher Institute of Nursing Professions and Health Techniques (ISPITS), Casablanca, Morocco

Abdelati Oussous
http://orcid.org/0009-0002-9555-346X
Morpho-Science Research Laboratory, Faculty of Medicine and Pharmacy, Cadi Ayyad University, Marrakech, Morocco.

Mounia Amane
http://orcid.org/0000-0002-9273-4284
Higher Institute of Nursing Professions and Technical Health of Marrakech, Morocco

DOI: 10.4018/979-8-2600-2035-7.ch009

ABSTRACT

The use of medical cannabis in older adults represents a rapidly emerging clinical field characterized by unique challenges, including increased risk of falls, cognitive vulnerability, polypharmacy, and complex ethical considerations. Despite growing utilization, high-quality evidence remains limited, highlighting an urgent need for age-specific research. This chapter proposes a structured framework for nursing competencies in geriatric medical cannabis care, encompassing seven core domains: comprehensive geriatric assessment; therapeutic education; safe initiation and titration; continuous monitoring; management of drug interactions; and ethical, legal, and stigma-related considerations. Interprofessional collaboration, evidence-based practice, and patient-centered approaches are emphasized to ensure safety, efficacy, and adherence. Future research directions include randomized controlled trials in older adults, pharmacokinetic and pharmacodynamic studies, longitudinal safety evaluations, and optimization of THC/CBD ratios tailored to geriatric indications.

INTRODUCTION

The emergence of therapeutic cannabis as a legitimate treatment modality represents one of the most significant transformations in the contemporary healthcare landscape. After several decades of prohibition and profound stigmatization, medical cannabinoids are gradually securing their place within the modern therapeutic armamentarium, supported by a growing body of scientific evidence. Recent epidemiological data illustrate this remarkable shift: cannabis use among adults aged 65 years and older increased from less than 1.0% in 2005 to 4.2% in 2018 (Han et al., 2025) . This growth positions older adults as one of the demographic groups exhibiting the most rapid increases in cannabis use, far exceeding the rates observed in younger populations.

This pronounced trend reflects the convergence of several key determinants. Evolving legal frameworks across many jurisdictions have facilitated access to standardized, pharmaceutical-grade products. In the United States, medical cannabis is now authorized in 39 states and the District of Columbia (Rhee & Rosenheck, 2023), and several other countries have enacted comparable legislation. Concurrently, the gradual social acceptance of cannabis for legitimate medical purposes has helped reduce psychosocial barriers to its use, particularly among generations who have reached retirement age (Baumbusch & Sloan Yip, 2022).

Emerging clinical evidence strongly supports the increasing adoption of medical cannabis among older adults. Several prospective and observational studies have documented meaningful therapeutic benefits, including improvements in pain-related symptoms, sleep, and quality of life, along with a concomitant reduction in certain pharmacological treatments, such as opioids, which are particularly problematic in this population (Abuhasira et al., 2018; Hochberg et al., 2023; Pearson et al., 2024). These findings suggest substantial potential for medical cannabis to address the clinical needs of geriatric patients while mitigating risks associated with polypharmacy and adverse effects linked to conventional treatments.

Global demographic transition further underscores the urgency of developing specialized expertise in this emerging field. By 2070, the global population of individuals aged 65 years and older is projected to reach 2.1 billion according to the United Nations (United Nations, 2024), more than double current figures. In the United States, approximately 85% of adults aged 65 years and older have at least one chronic condition, while 60% live with two or more (Fong, 2019). This multimorbidity frequently leads to problematic polypharmacy: 35.8% of older adults concurrently use five or more medications, and 29% take five or more prescribed drugs (Qato et al., 2016). Opioids and benzodiazepines, commonly prescribed for pain and sleep disorders, respectively, are associated with substantial risks of dependence, falls, and cognitive impairment in this vulnerable population.

Within this complex clinical context, geriatric nurses occupy a central strategic position in the healthcare system. As professionals who spend the most time with patients and their families, they are uniquely positioned to provide comprehensive assessment, tailored therapeutic education, continuous monitoring, and sustained support required for the safe use of cannabinoids among older adults (American Nurses Association, 2020). The official recognition of the specialty of "Cannabis Nursing" validates the emergence of a distinct field of competencies and specialized knowledge (American Nurses Association, 2024). This recognition represents a decisive milestone in the professionalization of this emerging nursing practice.

Nevertheless, a substantial training deficit persists, creating a concerning dissonance between clinical needs and professional capacities. Data reported in the literature remain alarming: 76.47% of nurses report having received no training in therapeutic cannabis (King et al., 2023), and 90.9% explicitly express the need for additional education in this area (Paiva et al., 2024). This educational gap becomes particularly critical in geriatrics, where intrinsic pharmacological complexity and heightened patient vulnerability markedly amplify clinical challenges and the potential consequences of inappropriate care.

This chapter examines the critical interface between therapeutic cannabis and geriatric nursing care, a domain that remains largely underdocumented in the current scientific literature. In contrast to general cannabinoid guidelines that often adopt a uniform approach across populations, this analysis focuses exclusively on adults aged 60 years and older, explicitly integrating principles of comprehensive geriatric assessment and person-centered care. The specific objectives are as follows: (1) to present the physiological and pharmacological foundations of medical cannabis in the context of aging; (2) to identify and analyze clinical challenges specific to the geriatric population; (3) to propose practical solutions; and (4) to identify future directions for research and professional development. The chapter thus advances a framework of nursing competencies tailored to this population, clearly recognizing that standard approaches used in younger adults are insufficient—and potentially harmful—when applied without adaptation to older adults.

BACKGROUND

1. The Endocannabinoid System and Aging

The endocannabinoid system (ECS) represents a fundamental cellular signaling network that plays a central role in the regulation of physiological homeostasis. This complex system comprises three primary components: endogenously produced cannabinoids (primarily anandamide and 2-arachidonoylglycerol), cannabinoid receptors (CB1 and CB2), and the enzymes responsible for their synthesis and degradation. CB1 receptors are predominantly localized within the central nervous system, whereas CB2 receptors are primarily expressed in the immune system and peripheral tissues (Lu & Mackie, 2016; Pertwee, 2006; Vaughan & Christie, 2005). The ECS modulates numerous essential physiological functions, including pain perception, inflammation, sleep, mood, appetite, memory, and immune response.

Aging is associated with significant alterations in the ECS, with direct implications for the therapeutic use of cannabinoids. Research has documented reductions in CB1 receptor density in specific brain regions with advancing age, particularly in the hippocampus and prefrontal cortex. Concurrently, endogenous cannabinoid levels demonstrate tissue-specific and pathology-dependent variations. These age-related modifications may influence both therapeutic responses to exogenous cannabinoids and the profile of potential adverse effects. Some evidence suggests that the ECS may play a role in neurodegenerative and inflammatory processes associated with aging, offering potential therapeutic avenues for conditions such as Alzheimer's disease and Parkinson's disease. However, a comprehensive understanding of these mechanisms remains incomplete and constitutes an active area of research.

2. Geriatric Pharmacological Considerations

a. Pharmacokinetic Changes

Aging induces substantial pharmacokinetic changes that profoundly affect cannabinoid metabolism, with direct clinical implications for older adults.

Hepatic alterations — including a 20–40% reduction in liver volume, decreased hepatic blood flow, and diminished cytochrome P450 enzyme activity — significantly slow the phase I metabolism of both THC and CBD, prolonging their elimination half-life and increasing the risk of accumulation with repeated dosing (GRONICH, 2024). Critically, both cannabinoids inhibit multiple CYP450 isoenzymes, generating a clinically significant potential for drug–drug interactions that is particularly concerning in the context of geriatric polypharmacy (Doohan et al., 2021; Klotz, 2009).

Age-related changes in body composition — characterized by increased adipose tissue and reduced lean mass — further amplify this risk. As highly lipophilic molecules, cannabinoids accumulate preferentially in fat stores, prolonging terminal elimination and increasing exposure with chronic use (Mangoni & Jackson, 2004). Declining renal function may additionally impair the clearance of cannabinoid metabolites.

Taken together, these changes result in higher and more prolonged plasma concentrations in older adults compared to younger populations, underscoring the clinical imperative of the "start low, go slow" principle and close monitoring for adverse effects.

b. Pharmacodynamic Changes

Beyond pharmacokinetic alterations, aging is associated with pharmacodynamic changes that modify tissue responses to cannabinoids (Ginsburg & Hensler, 2022; Wu et al., 2023). Older adults exhibit increased sensitivity to the psychoactive effects of THC, even at doses considered moderate in younger adults (Velayudhan et al., 2021). This heightened sensitivity results from multiple factors, including changes in cannabinoid receptor density and function, alterations in blood–brain barrier permeability facilitating greater central nervous system penetration, and diminished homeostatic compensatory mechanisms.

These modifications create a distinct risk profile for this population. Cardiovascular effects warrant particular attention: THC may induce tachycardia and orthostatic hypotension, which can be especially dangerous in older adults with preexisting cardiovascular instability or those receiving antihypertensive therapy (Bouccin et al., 2016; Lapeyre-Mestre & Jouanjus, 2020; Storck et al., 2025). Psychomotor effects further increase the risk of falls, a major geriatric complication that can lead to fractures, hospitalization, and loss of autonomy (Workman et al., 2021).

Cognitive effects of THC—including impairments in short-term memory, attention, and executive functions—may be more pronounced and longer-lasting in older adults, particularly those with preexisting mild cognitive decline. Long-term cannabis use in older adults has been associated with reduced performance in executive function and processing speed (Stypulkowski & Thayer, 2022).

3. Therapeutic Indications in Geriatrics

The primary therapeutic indications for medical cannabis in geriatric populations correspond directly to the unmet health needs characteristic of this age group. According to the analysis by Pravosud et al. (2025), chronic pain accounts for 56.4% of cannabinoid use, followed by mood or mental health improvement (18.4%) and sleep enhancement (16.0%). These data reflect both the high prevalence of these conditions among older adults and the limitations of conventional therapeutic approaches.

Chronic pain represents a major burden for older adults, affecting up to 50% of community-dwelling individuals and as many as 80% of those residing in long-term care facilities (Cravello et al., 2019). Clinical evidence regarding the efficacy of cannabis for chronic pain in older adults is primarily derived from observational studies. Abuhasira et al. (2018) reported that 93.7% of geriatric patients experienced improvement after six months of cannabinoid therapy, with a substantial reduction in opioid use. More recent data from Pearson et al. (2024) confirmed significant improvements in both pain and quality of life among patients over 50 years old using medically supervised cannabis. However, Wolfe et al. (2023) noted in a systematic review that effects are inconsistent depending on specific conditions, and adverse associations sometimes outweigh benefits.

Sleep disorders constitute another major indication, affecting up to 50% of older adults (Tatineny et al., 2020). Chronic insomnia contributes to reduced quality of life, increased fall risk, and exacerbation of comorbid conditions. The endocannabinoid system plays an established role in circadian rhythm regulation, and exogenous cannabinoids exert measurable effects on human sleep architecture, which partly explains why sleep disorders are among the most frequently reported indications for medical cannabis use. Nevertheless, despite widespread use, high-quality clinical trial data remain limited (Minerbi et al., 2019). In a systematic review, Babson et al. (2017) suggested that CBD may have therapeutic potential for insomnia, possibly mediated via anxiolytic effects, as well as for REM sleep behavior disorders and excessive daytime sleepiness. Conversely, THC appears to exert bidirectional effects, combining short-term sedation with potential impairment of sleep quality during prolonged use.

Anxiety and depressive symptoms, common in geriatric populations, represent a more controversial indication. While some studies report improvements in these symptoms with medical cannabis use, Wolfe et al. (2023) highlighted associations between cannabis use and increased frequencies of depression and anxiety in older adults. This apparent dichotomy may reflect differences in formulations (THC:CBD ratios), dosages, and population characteristics.

Beyond these primary indications, preliminary data suggest potential benefits in several other geriatric conditions (Bilbao & Spanagel, 2022). In Parkinson's disease, some studies have reported improvements in rigidity, tremors, and sleep quality (Hafida et al., 2024), although the evidence remains limited. In contexts of cancer- or disease-related cachexia and anorexia, THC is approved for appetite stimulation, with potentially beneficial effects in older adults experiencing involuntary weight loss (Rogers & Pacanowski, 2023). In palliative care, medical cannabis is increasingly used for multisymptom management, including pain, nausea, anxiety, and insomnia, though data specific to older adults remain limited (Turcott et al., 2018). Despite its genuine therapeutic potential in specific indications, the use of cannabis or its derivatives cannot be considered entirely safe and must be strictly regulated due to its documented adverse effects (Solmi et al., 2023).

It is important to note that, despite these promising applications for multisymptom management, the overall level of evidence remains limited for several indications, particularly in older adults. Current data are largely derived from observational studies, case series, and small randomized controlled trials, often characterized by methodological limitations, including small sample sizes, short follow-up durations, and substantial heterogeneity in cannabis formulations (THC, CBD, varying ratios, and routes of administration).

Overall, the existing literature suggests potential symptomatic benefits; however, findings remain inconsistent and difficult to generalize to frail, multimorbid geriatric populations. The variability in study design and outcome measures further complicates the interpretation of results and limits the strength of clinical recommendations.

Consequently, although medical cannabis is increasingly incorporated into geriatric care for symptom management, its use should remain cautious and individualized. There is a critical need for large-scale, well-designed randomized controlled trials specifically targeting older adults, with particular attention to multimorbidity, polypharmacy, and age-related pharmacodynamic and pharmacokinetic changes. Future research should rigorously assess the benefit–risk balance, including drug–drug interactions, neuropsychiatric effects, and functional outcomes relevant to geriatric care.

MAIN FOCUS OF THE CHAPTER

Issues, Controversies, Problems

1. Geriatric-Specific Challenges

Older adults using medical cannabis face unique challenges that demand particular clinical attention. One of the most significant concerns is the increased risk of falls (Workman et al., 2021). Cannabinoids, particularly THC, may induce dizziness, ataxia, orthostatic hypotension, and impaired coordination (Bajtel et al., 2022), all of which substantially elevate fall risk. In older adults, falls can result in catastrophic outcomes, including hip fractures, traumatic brain injuries, prolonged hospitalizations, loss of autonomy, and increased mortality (Moreland et al., 2023).

Potential cognitive decline constitutes another major challenge. While some studies suggest that medically supervised cannabis use does not significantly impair cognitive function, other research has documented associations between cannabis use and cognitive deficits, particularly with THC-rich formulations. Stypulkowski & Thayer (2022) reported that long-term cannabis use in older adults is associated with reduced executive function and slower processing speed. Wolfe et al. (2023) identified cognitive decline as one of the frequently reported adverse associations of cannabis use in this population. For patients with preexisting mild cognitive impairment or early dementia, initiating medical cannabis requires baseline cognitive assessment and ongoing monitoring to detect any deterioration.

Polypharmacy and complex drug–drug interactions represent a particularly salient clinical challenge in geriatrics. In older adults taking an average of five to ten medications, the risk of clinically significant interactions increases exponentially. Notably concerning interactions have been documented with anticoagulants (warfarin), benzodiazepines, opioids, antihypertensives, antiepileptics, immunosuppressants, and numerous other medications metabolized via the CYP450 system (Caicedo et al., 2025).

Stigmatization constitutes a major psychosocial barrier. Current older adults experienced their youth and adulthood during the era of intensive cannabis prohibition, often internalizing negative attitudes and misconceptions about the substance (Dahlke et al., 2024; Krediet et al., 2020). This stigma may manifest in several ways: reluctance to discuss cannabis use openly with healthcare providers due to fear of judgment, anxiety, or guilt; familial or social opposition; and difficulty distinguishing legitimate medical use from recreational use (Bottorff et al., 2013). Evidence suggests that the separation between primary care and cannabis treatment, combined with perceived stigma, prevents many older adults from discussing this therapeutic option openly with their usual healthcare providers (Krediet et al., 2020).

2. Controversies and Areas of Uncertainty

The field of medical cannabis in geriatrics is characterized by numerous areas of scientific uncertainty and controversy that complicate clinical decision-making. The fundamental limitation is the lack of robust data from randomized controlled trials specific to older adults. The vast majority of available evidence derives from observational studies, uncontrolled cohort studies, or clinical trials conducted primarily in younger populations. Wolfe et al. (2023) emphasized that many studies were small, did not systematically evaluate adverse effects, and inadequately adjusted for confounding factors. This methodological limitation hinders the development of high-quality, evidence-based clinical recommendations.

The debate over optimal THC/CBD ratios for various geriatric indications remains unresolved. THC is the cannabinoid primarily responsible for analgesic and psychoactive effects, whereas CBD is reputed for its anxiolytic, anti-inflammatory, and potential neuroprotective properties (Hammell et al., 2016; Stella, 2023), and may mitigate certain THC-related side effects. However, recent data paradoxically suggest that CBD may inhibit the metabolism of THC and its active metabolite 11-OH-THC, potentially increasing adverse effects THC (Zamarripa et al., 2023). Balanced formulations (1:1 THC:CBD ratios) are often recommended for older beginners, but empirical support for this approach remains limited.

Ethical issues surrounding autonomy, informed consent, and decisional capacity raise complex clinical dilemmas. For older adults with mild to moderate cognitive decline, evaluating their capacity to understand potential risks and benefits of medical cannabis, weigh alternative therapies, and make an informed decision requires a nuanced approach (Appelbaum, 2007; Sacco et al., 2021). Principles of autonomy must be balanced with beneficence and non-maleficence. Shared decision-making frameworks involving the patient, family caregivers, and the healthcare team are recommended, yet practical implementation remains challenging.

Legal disparities between jurisdictions create significant clinical complications. In the United States, although medical cannabis is legalized at the state level, it remains a federally controlled substance, creating a paradoxical legal status. Regulations vary widely across states regarding qualifying conditions, certification processes, types of authorized products, possession limits, and employee protections. Internationally, regulatory frameworks range from full legalization in Canada and Uruguay to restrictive medical programs in some European countries, to strict prohibition in other jurisdictions (Cannabis Business Plan, 2025). This regulatory heterogeneity complicates patient mobility, access to care during travel, and consistency of clinical recommendations. For nurses practicing in diverse contexts, navigating these variable legal frameworks requires constant vigilance and regular knowledge updates.

SOLUTIONS AND RECOMMENDATIONS

1. Geriatric Medical Cannabis Nursing Competency Framework

In response to the challenges and controversies identified, the development of a nursing competency framework specifically adapted to geriatric populations is essential. This framework, structured around seven core domains, integrates the fundamental principles of geriatric nursing—including comprehensive assessment, person-centered care, preservation of autonomy, and prevention of iatrogenic complications—with specialized knowledge of the endocannabinoid system and therapeutic cannabinoids (Figure 1). Each domain encompasses specific competencies, requisite knowledge, and practical clinical skills that nurses must master to provide safe and effective care.

Figure 1. Geriatric Medical Cannabis Nursing Competency Framework

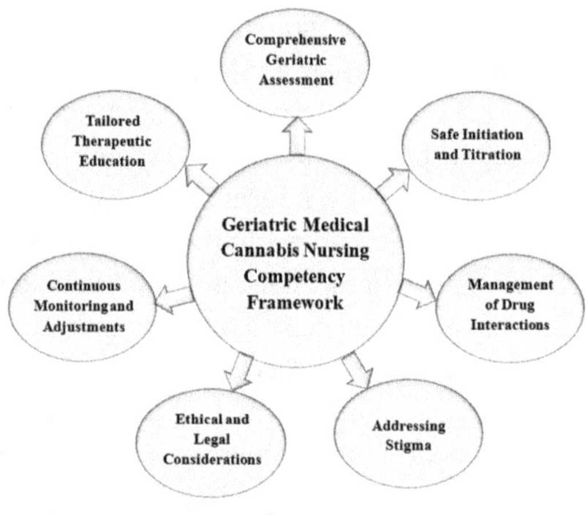

Comprehensive Geriatric Assessment
Tailored Therapeutic Education
Safe Initiation and Titration
Geriatric Medical Cannabis Nursing Competency Framework
Continuous Monitoring and Adjustments
Management of Drug Interactions
Ethical and Legal Considerations
Addressing Stigma

Domain 1: Comprehensive Geriatric Assessment

Comprehensive geriatric assessment (CGA) forms the foundation of all cannabinoid-related nursing care for older adults. This multidimensional evaluation extends beyond standard medical assessment to encompass functional, cognitive, affective, social, and environmental domains that influence health and well-being (Dimitriadou et al., 2025).

Functional assessment involves the use of standardized tools such as the Katz Activities of Daily Living (ADL) scale and the Lawton Instrumental Activities of

Daily Living (IADL) scale to evaluate autonomy (Katz, 1963; Lawton & Brody, 1969). Abuhasira et al. (2023) demonstrated that medical cannabis did not negatively affect functional abilities in 119 geriatric patients (mean age 79.3 years), with ADL and IADL scores remaining stable after six months of treatment.

Cognitive assessment is essential prior to initiating medical cannabis. Recommended tools include the Mini-Mental State Examination (MMSE) and the Montreal Cognitive Assessment (MoCA), the latter being more sensitive for detecting mild cognitive impairment (Folstein et al., 2014; Nasreddine et al., 2014). Baseline evaluation establishes a reference point and allows monitoring for potential changes over time. For patients with preexisting cognitive decline, more frequent monitoring is indicated, with regular reassessments to detect any changes.

Nutritional and appetite assessment is particularly important, as anorexia and cachexia are common in older adults, especially those with chronic illnesses. THC has well-documented orexigenic properties and is approved (as dronabinol) for the treatment of anorexia (Rogers & Pacanowski, 2023). Assessment should include recent dietary history, measurement of weight and body mass index, and screening for malnutrition using tools such as the Mini Nutritional Assessment (MNA) (Vellas et al., 1999).

Fall risk assessment is a critical safety measure. Standardized tools such as the Morse Fall Scale or Tinetti Performance-Oriented Mobility Assessment should be used systematically (Morse et al., 1989; Tinetti, 1986). Baseline evaluation identifies patients at high risk who will require enhanced preventive measures during cannabis initiation.

A thorough medication review is an essential component of the initial assessment. This review should include all prescribed medications, with particular attention to drugs metabolized by cytochrome P450 enzymes (CYP2C9, CYP2C19, CYP3A4, CYP2D6), as cannabinoids—particularly CBD—can inhibit these enzymes (Doohan et al., 2021).

Psychosocial assessment explores multiple dimensions: social isolation and available family support, attitudes and beliefs regarding cannabis, perceived or internalized stigma, financial situation and ability to afford medical cannabis not covered by insurance, access barriers (transportation, mobility), and anticipated adherence (Parker et al., 2018; Pomey et al., 2024). This holistic evaluation allows identification of potential obstacles to therapeutic success and the planning of appropriate supportive interventions.

Domain 2: Tailored Therapeutic Education

Therapeutic education is a central pillar of cannabinoid nursing care, particularly for geriatric populations who may have limited knowledge or misconceptions about medical cannabis. The educational approach should be adapted to the patient's cognitive and sensory capacities.

Explaining the differences between THC and CBD constitutes fundamental educational content. THC is the primary psychoactive cannabinoid responsible for the "high," with analgesic, orexigenic, antiemetic, and muscle-relaxant properties (Ng et al., 2025). However, it can also produce adverse effects including anxiety, tachycardia, orthostatic hypotension, sedation, short-term memory impairment, and psychomotor disturbances (Ng et al., 2025). CBD is non-psychoactive and exhibits anxiolytic, anti-inflammatory, anticonvulsant, and potentially neuroprotective properties. Importantly, CBD may modulate some THC effects, potentially mitigating anxiety and other psychoactive side effects (Luz-Veiga et al., 2023).

Education on different administration routes and their geriatric-specific considerations is essential for enabling patients to select the method best suited to their needs and capabilities. Sublingual oils provide a relatively rapid onset of action (15–45 minutes) with precise dosing via graduated droppers. Oral capsules are easy to use but have a slower onset (1–3 hours) due to first-pass hepatic metabolism, with longer duration of effect (6–8 hours). Topical formulations (creams, balms, lotions) allow localized application for joint or muscle pain without significant systemic effects but are limited to superficial structures. Vaporization offers very rapid onset (5–10 minutes) and precise titration but carries potential respiratory risks, particularly in older adults with preexisting pulmonary conditions, and requires specific equipment. Smoking is generally discouraged in geriatrics due to respiratory and cardiovascular risks (maccallum & Russo, 2018).

The principle "start low, go slow" must be explicitly taught and justified (maccallum & Russo, 2018). Due to age-related pharmacokinetic and pharmacodynamic changes, older adults typically require much lower starting doses than younger adults. A recommended approach is to initiate at very low doses and increase gradually based on tolerance and response. This gradual titration allows identification of the minimum effective dose while minimizing adverse effects. Patients must understand that, unlike many conventional medications, there is no "standard" dose of medical cannabis—the optimal dose is highly individualized and must be determined empirically.

Involving family caregivers in the educational process is strongly recommended, particularly for patients with cognitive deficits or requiring assistance with administration. However, patient autonomy must be respected, and consent should be obtained for caregiver involvement, balancing principles of confidentiality and family support.

Domain 3: Safe Initiation and Titration

Initiation protocols adapted to geriatric populations require a methodical and cautious approach. Recommended starting doses vary according to the administration route and product. For oral formulations (oils, capsules), a typical initial dose might be 1.25–2.5 mg THC once daily, preferably in the evening for early doses to minimize daytime fall risk. Similar doses are appropriate for sublingual formulations, with the advantage of faster onset allowing earlier evaluation of tolerance. For topicals, local application as needed generally does not require systemic titration, although a test application on a small area is recommended to exclude cutaneous reactions. Vaporization, if used, should begin with one or two inhalations of a low-THC product, with close monitoring during the first 30 minutes (maccallum & Russo, 2018).The progressive titration schedule should be conservative. A typical approach may include: maintaining the initial dose for at least 2 days to assess tolerance and initial effects; if well tolerated and benefit is insufficient, increase by 1.25–2.5 mg THC on days 3 and 4; repeat this process until achieving an acceptable therapeutic benefit or observing adverse effects, without exceeding 40 mg/day (Bhaskar et al., 2021; maccallum & Russo, 2018)..

Early adverse effect monitoring is essential for safety. Patients and caregivers should be instructed to observe and report: dizziness or lightheadedness, particularly with position changes; excessive sleepiness or fatigue; confusion, disorientation, or hallucinations; anxiety or agitation; nausea or gastrointestinal disturbances; tachycardia or palpitations; dry mouth or eyes; and any falls or near-falls ((Bajtel et al., 2022; Whiting et al., 2015).

Figure 2 presents an eight-step Clinical Decision Algorithm for Therapeutic Cannabis in Older Adults, synthesizing the core principles of this framework into a practical clinical reference. The algorithm guides nurses sequentially from indication assessment and CGA, through medication review, contraindication screening, and informed consent, to low-dose initiation applying the "start low, go slow" principle (THC: 1.25–2.5 mg/day; CBD: 5–10 mg/day), titration, monitoring, and final benefit-versus-risk evaluation. This structured tool is intended to support safe, individualized clinical decision-making in this vulnerable population.

Figure 2. Clinical decision algorithm for therapeutic cannabis in older adults

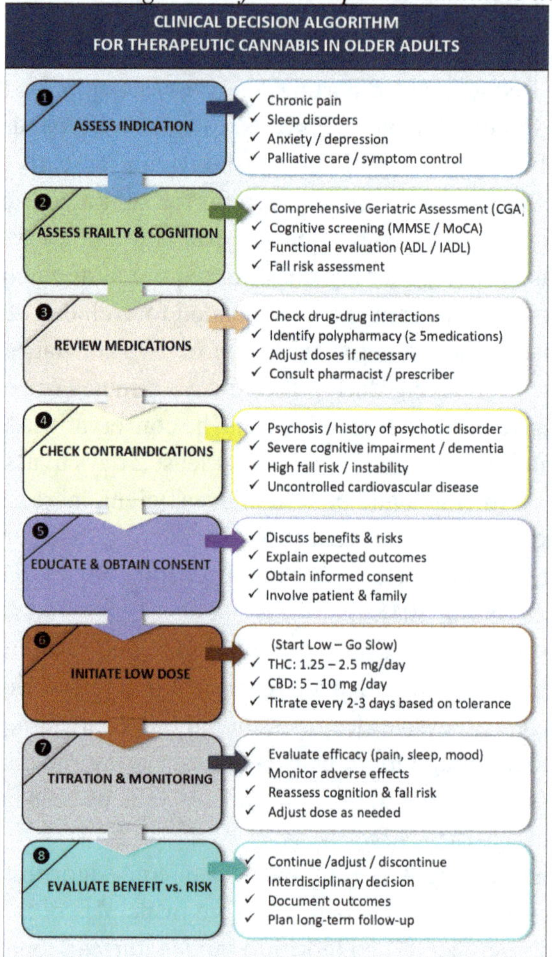

Domain 4: Continuous Monitoring and Adjustments

Ongoing monitoring is essential to optimize therapeutic benefits while minimizing risks. The frequency and content of nursing follow-ups should be adapted to the treatment phase and individual patient characteristics. During initiation and titration, frequent contacts are recommended: telephone follow-up 24–48 hours after the first dose, then after each dose increase; weekly in-person or telehealth visits during the first month; followed by biweekly visits during months 2–3. Once a stable and effective dose is established, monthly follow-ups are usually sufficient for most patients, although some may require closer monitoring (Abuhasira et al., 2019).

Symptom efficacy assessment should rely on validated scales tailored to the target symptoms (pain, sleep disturbances, anxiety/depression, appetite, and weight). This structured approach enables objective tracking of clinical evolution, facilitates interdisciplinary communication, and guides therapeutic adjustments.

Specific monitoring of cognitive function is particularly important in geriatrics (Scott et al., 2019). Caregivers and family members should be encouraged to report any changes in memory, attention, judgment, or executive function. If cognitive deterioration is observed, the risk–benefit ratio should be re-evaluated, potentially prompting a dose reduction or formulation change.

Balance and gait monitoring should be integrated into each consultation. Direct observation of walking, noting instability, shuffling, or difficulty initiating steps, is recommended. Systematic questioning about falls or near-falls since the last visit should be routine.

Cardiovascular monitoring includes regular measurement of blood pressure in both supine and standing positions to detect orthostatic hypotension, along with heart rate assessment. An increase in resting heart or the onset of palpitations warrants further evaluation and possible dose adjustment. For patients with cardiovascular history, periodic ECG monitoring may be indicated.

Mood and anxiety assessment should be systematic, as paradoxical effects may occur. Wolfe et al. (2023) identified associations between cannabis use and increased rates of anxiety and depression in older adults. Using standardized scales allows early detection of adverse effects requiring therapeutic adjustment.

Dose adjustment or cessation criteria should be clearly defined:

- **Increase dose:** insufficient therapeutic effect after an adequate trial, absence of significant side effects, and patient request with informed understanding.
- **Decrease dose:** mild but troubling adverse effects (dizziness, excessive somnolence), adequate therapeutic effect achieved at a lower dose, or emerging drug interactions.
- **Discontinue:** severe/intolerable side effects (injurious falls, severe confusion, hallucinations, significant cognitive decline), lack of therapeutic benefit after progressive titration, clinically significant drug interactions unmanageable by other means, or patient request.

Coordination with the multidisciplinary medical team is essential. Nurses should communicate regularly with the prescribing physician, clinical pharmacist (for drug interaction management), physical/occupational therapist (for mobility and fall risk evaluation), social worker (for access and cost issues), and any other professionals involved in the patient's care.

Domain 5: Management of Drug Interactions

Managing drug interactions is one of the most complex and critical aspects of cannabinoid nursing care in older adults. Many medications commonly prescribed in geriatrics have clinically significant interactions with cannabis, requiring heightened vigilance (table 1).

Table 1. Major drug–drug interactions between therapeutic cannabis and common medications in older adultS

Drug Class	Mechanism of Interaction	Clinical Consequence	Recommendation
Anticoagulants (warfarin)	CYP2C9 inhibition	↑ INR, increased bleeding risk	Close INR monitoring
Benzodiazepines	Additive CNS effects	Sedation, confusion, falls	Avoid or reduce doses
Opioids	Pharmacodynamic synergy	Respiratory depression, sedation	Close monitoring, respiratory rate surveillance, consider dose reduction
Antidepressants	CYP450 inhibition	Variability in drug concentrations	Clinical monitoring
Antiepileptics (clobazam)	↑ active metabolite levels	Excessive sedation	Dose adjustment
Antihypertensives	THC-induced vasodilation	Orthostatic hypotension, falls	Blood pressure monitoring, fall risk assessment

- **Anticoagulants:** Warfarin increases bleeding risk via elevated INR (Damkier et al., 2019; Smythe et al., 2023).
- **Benzodiazepines and other sedatives:** Enhanced sedation, cognitive impairment, and fall risk (Gaston et al., 2017; Ho et al., 2024).
- **Opioids:** Altered concentrations, with additive sedation and potential respiratory depression (Caicedo et al., 2025).
- **Antiepileptics:** CBD can lead to accumulation of norclobazam from clobazam, causing excessive sedation (Caicedo et al., 2025; Critchley et al., 2019).
- **Antihypertensives:** Cannabis, particularly THC, may induce vasodilation and reduce systemic vascular resistance, leading to orthostatic hypotension, dizziness, and increased fall risk in older adults, especially in those receiving antihypertensive therapy (Pacher et al., 2018). These effects may be poten-

tiated in frail patients or in the context of polypharmacy, warranting close blood pressure monitoring and cautious dose titration

- **Antidepressant:** Cannabinoids may interact with antidepressants through inhibition of cytochrome P450 enzymes, potentially altering plasma drug concentrations and increasing the risk of adverse effects such as sedation, dizziness, or serotonergic symptoms (Brown & Winterstein, 2019).

These interactions underscore the need for systematic medication review, targeted clinical and laboratory monitoring, and individualized dose adjustments when initiating or modifying therapeutic cannabis in older adults.

When medical cannabis provides clinical benefit (pain, sleep, anxiety), cautious deprescription of other medications may be considered. Deprescription should be gradual, structured, and individualized, prioritizing medications with an unfavorable risk–benefit profile, with careful monitoring for withdrawal or symptom recurrence to ensure patient safety.

Domain 6: Addressing Stigma

Stigma surrounding cannabis remains a major barrier to care and therapeutic success. Understanding its generational origins is key to effectively addressing it. Older adults were exposed for decades to intensive anti-drug messaging, criminalization, and negative media portrayals of cannabis (Bottorff et al., 2013)

Wang et al. (2023) identified stigma as a major barrier to medical cannabis access in older adults, manifesting as self-stigma, family and social stigma, and institutional stigma through restrictive policies in care facilities.

Empathic, nonjudgmental communication is essential to create a therapeutic environment. Nurses should provide a safe space for patients to express concerns, use neutral medical language, validate their worries, explore cultural representations of cannabis, and provide balanced, factual information on benefits and risks.

Explicitly distinguishing medical from recreational use legitimizes treatment: medical cannabis targets symptom relief and functional improvement, uses controlled doses, appropriate THC:CBD ratios, clinical supervision, and low-risk administration routes; recreational use is psychoactive-focused without medical oversight. This clarification promotes acceptance of cannabis as a therapeutic option (Krediet et al., 2020; Rowe et al., 2025).

Family involvement can reduce stigma: concerns should be addressed with clear information on legal framework, mechanisms of action, and documented benefits and risks, with participation in follow-up if the patient consents.

Anchoring medical cannabis in evidence-based practice (published clinical outcomes, scientific reports, pharmaceutical approvals) positions it as a legitimate component of the overall care plan, aligned with patient preferences and values.

Domain 7: Ethical and Legal Considerations

Ethical and legal issues in geriatric medical cannabis require particular nursing vigilance (American Nurses Association & American Cannabis Nurses Association, 2024). Informed consent, adapted to cognitive capacity, is central: it requires understanding of the treatment, appreciation of benefits and risks, reasoning ability, and expression of choice (Glickman & Sisti, 2020).

Information must be accessible and cover treatment nature, expected benefits, specific risks (falls, confusion, interactions), alternative therapies, voluntariness, and financial aspects, with rigorous documentation.

Respect for autonomy is fundamental: patient choices must be honored whether they accept, refuse, or discontinue treatment. When decision-making capacity is impaired, substitute decisions involving legal representatives or family are required, guided by the patient's presumed wishes (Glickman & Sisti, 2020).

Nurses must also master the regulatory framework in their jurisdiction (access conditions, authorized prescribers, products, institutional use) and maintain complete traceability: initial assessment, consent, care plan, follow-ups, adverse effects, adjustments, and interdisciplinary consultations. Practice must strictly adhere to the locally defined professional scope, with clear patient information on legal restrictions, including driving under influence..

2. Development of Training Programs

The integration of medical cannabis into the care of older adults highlights a specific training gap among nursing professionals (Paiva et al., 2024), particularly regarding age-related pharmacokinetic and pharmacodynamic changes, multimorbidity, polypharmacy, cognitive vulnerability, and ethical complexity. Contemporary reforms in health professional education emphasize competency-based learning as a central lever to address emerging clinical domains and to enhance care quality in complex populations (Frank et al., 2010).

In this context, the present chapter proposes a structured framework for continuing education, organized around seven core competency domains rather than a prescriptive syllabus. These domains can serve as the foundation for modular educational pathways, adaptable to institutional and regulatory contexts, in alignment with competency-based education principles.

The seven proposed domains are:

- Foundational knowledge, including the endocannabinoid system, cannabinoid pharmacology, and age-related pharmacokinetic and pharmacodynamic modifications;
- Comprehensive geriatric assessment adapted for medical cannabis use;
- Therapeutic education and communication with older adults and their caregivers;
- Safe initiation and cautious titration strategies;
- Ongoing monitoring and adverse effect management;
- Drug interactions in the context of geriatric polypharmacy;
- Ethical, legal, and anti-stigma considerations.

Structuring training by competency domains aligns directly with international competency-based education models, which prioritize the integration of knowledge, skills, and attitudes within authentic clinical situations (Frank et al., 2010; Ten Cate & Hennus, 2024).

Case-based learning constitutes a pedagogical cornerstone of this framework. Systematic reviews demonstrate that instruction grounded in clinical scenarios enhances clinical reasoning, knowledge integration, and learner engagement in health professional education (Thistlethwaite et al., 2012). In the geriatric context, proposed cases should reflect the real-world complexity of older patients, including multimorbidity, functional limitations, mild cognitive impairment, and polypharmacy patterns.

Simulation and role-playing approaches complement this framework by offering safe experiential learning for complex clinical and ethical situations. Health simulation has been associated with significant improvements in clinical skills, communication, and patient safety (Cook et al., 2011). Scenarios may include initial geriatric assessment consultations for medical cannabis, therapeutic education involving caregivers, management of family hesitancy, interprofessional coordination in the context of drug interactions, and evaluation of decision-making capacity.

This competency-based training model provides a structured, evidence-informed trajectory to prepare nurses for delivering safe, patient-centered care to older adults in the context of medical cannabis. By integrating geriatric assessment, pharmacological expertise, ethical reasoning, and interprofessional collaboration, the framework addresses the growing complexity of aging and supports the responsible integration of medical cannabis into geriatric practice.

3. Interprofessional Collaboration Models in Geriatric Cannabis Care

The increasing complexity of managing older adults using medical cannabis necessitates structured interprofessional care models capable of mobilizing complementary expertise to provide holistic, safe, and coordinated care (Reeves et al., 2017; Zwarenstein et al., 2009). Older adults frequently present with polypharmacy, multimorbidity, and heightened vulnerability to adverse effects, justifying the integration of specialized resources within a collaborative model.

Multidisciplinary clinics specialized in geriatric cannabis care could be established, comprising geriatric or family physicians, nurses trained in geriatric cannabinoid care, clinical pharmacists, physical or occupational therapists, social workers, and, as needed, geriatric psychologists or psychiatrists. These teams would provide comprehensive assessment, coordinated treatment planning, ongoing follow-up, and facilitated access to specialist consultations.

Regular case conferences promote communication and collaborative decision-making, with frequency adjusted to patient volume. Systematic documentation of these decisions within the medical record ensures continuity of care and enables longitudinal tracking.

Effective interprofessional collaboration relies on optimized communication systems, particularly electronic health records (EHRs), which allow structured, accessible sharing of clinical information among the team. Integrating medical cannabis follow-up data into the patient's primary record enhances coordination, reduces transmission errors, and supports safe clinical decision-making (Al-Ghamdi, 2023; Bates et al., 2001). EHRs also facilitate the detection of potential drug interactions, scheduling of follow-ups, and documentation of treatment modifications, all critical in a geriatric population frequently exposed to polypharmacy.

This interprofessional model minimizes polypharmacy-related risks, ensures continuous monitoring of adverse effects, and improves adherence and patient satisfaction (Al-Ghamdi, 2023; Bates et al., 2001). Structured coordination also supports patient and caregiver education, an essential aspect in older adults who are often vulnerable to medication-related complications and errors in cannabis management.

FUTURE RESEARCH DIRECTIONS

The field of medical cannabis in geriatrics remains characterized by substantial knowledge gaps, underscoring the need for rigorous, population-specific research. The majority of current evidence originates from uncontrolled observational studies or trials conducted in younger populations, limiting generalizability to older adults

(Beauchet, 2018). These limitations highlight the necessity of randomized controlled trials (RCTs) specifically targeting older patients to generate reliable, clinically applicable recommendations.

1. Randomized Controlled Trials in Older Adults

Well-designed RCTs should recruit exclusively or predominantly geriatric participants, stratify by age groups to assess age-dependent effects, and include patients with multimorbidity and polypharmacy to reflect real-world geriatric practice. Dosages and formulations must be tailored to the physiological characteristics of older adults. Furthermore, outcome measures should be relevant to geriatric care, such as physical function, quality of life, falls, and cognition, with a sufficient duration to capture medium- and long-term effects (Cesari et al., 2025). Such methodological rigor ensures that trial results are directly translatable to clinical practice.

2. Pharmacokinetic and Pharmacodynamic Studies

Precise characterization of cannabinoid pharmacokinetics (PK) and pharmacodynamics (PD) in older adults is essential for dose optimization and risk minimization (Wu et al., 2023). These studies should compare PK parameters between younger and older adults, assess the impact of age-related alterations (hepatic and renal function, body composition), and examine PK/PD relationships to understand how plasma concentrations translate into therapeutic and adverse effects. Investigating interindividual variability, predictive factors of response, and the effects of chronic use—including potential accumulation—would support evidence-based dosing recommendations specifically for older adults.

3. Optimization of THC/CBD Ratios

Research on optimal THC/CBD ratios for specific geriatric indications is needed to clarify the most appropriate formulations. Comparative studies should evaluate different ratios for common conditions such as chronic pain, insomnia, anxiety, anorexia, and Parkinsonian symptoms. Understanding pharmacological interactions between CBD and THC, particularly the potential for CBD to inhibit THC metabolism (Zamarripa et al., 2023), requires both mechanistic and clinical investigation.

4. Longitudinal Studies and Long-Term Follow-Up

Prospective cohorts of older adults using medical cannabis should be followed over several years to assess long-term safety and effectiveness. Periodic assessments should include cognitive function, physical function, independence, frequency of falls and fractures, progression of comorbidities, polypharmacy, cardiovascular events, and all-cause mortality. These studies would provide critical data on long-term benefit–risk profiles, which are difficult to capture in short-duration RCTs (Newman, 2010).

5. Development and Validation of Specific Assessment Tools

The creation of standardized, reproducible instruments would enable consistent evaluation of cannabis efficacy on geriatric symptoms, side effect burden, fall risk, quality of life, and patient satisfaction. Validated tools would facilitate cross-study comparisons, support accumulation of coherent evidence, and guide clinical practice (Kimberlin & Winterstein, 2008).

6. Comparative Research with Standard Treatments

To position medical cannabis within the geriatric therapeutic algorithm, comparative studies are required. These should evaluate cannabis relative to conventional first-line treatments—opioids for chronic pain, hypnotics for insomnia, anxiolytics for anxiety, pharmacologic appetite stimulants—and as adjunctive therapy to standard care. Such studies would inform clinical decision-making and potentially influence reimbursement policies.

7. Nursing Education and Implementation Research

Evaluation of nursing education programs represents another research priority. It is essential to assess the impact of educational interventions on nurses' knowledge, skills, and confidence, as well as on clinical practice changes and patient outcomes (satisfaction, safety, effectiveness). Comparing different training modalities (in-person vs. online, simulation vs. case-based learning, short vs. extensive courses) would help identify the most effective approaches for specialized geriatric cannabis education (King et al., 2023; Paiva et al., 2024).

CONCLUSION

The emergence of medical cannabis in older adults represents both a promising clinical opportunity and a complex challenge requiring specialized expertise. The rapid increase in its use, combined with global population aging, underscores the urgency of developing nursing competencies adapted to this emerging reality.

This chapter has proposed a competency framework for geriatric medical cannabis nursing, integrating the physiological, pharmacological, and psychosocial particularities of older adults. The framework acknowledges that standard approaches applied to younger adults are insufficient—and may even be hazardous—when applied without adaptation to a population characterized by complex polypharmacy, increased fall risk, and heightened pharmacological sensitivity to cannabinoids.

Nurses occupy a uniquely strategic role in this context. As professionals in constant contact with patients and families, they are ideally positioned to perform comprehensive assessments, provide tailored therapeutic education, conduct ongoing monitoring, and ensure safe cannabinoid use. Yet, existing training programs rarely provide content specifically adapted to geriatric considerations, making the development of specialized curricula an urgent priority.

The call to action spans multiple levels: educational, through development of adapted curricula; research, through geriatric-specific clinical trials; and institutional, through the creation of standardized guidelines and clinical tools.

In conclusion, developing specialized nursing competencies in geriatric medical cannabis is not optional—it is imperative. The proposed framework offers a practical roadmap grounded in the best available scientific evidence, positioning nurses as autonomous, expert professionals—not merely executors of prescriptions—playing a central role in navigating this complex and emerging therapeutic domain. Investment in training, research, and the establishment of practice standards today will directly determine the quality and safety of care provided to the millions of older adults who may benefit from medical cannabis in the decades ahead.

REFERENCES

Abuhasira, R., Ron, A., Sikorin, I., & Novack, V. (2019). Medical Cannabis for Older Patients-Treatment Protocol and Initial Results. *Journal of Clinical Medicine*, *8*(11), 1819. DOI: 10.3390/jcm8111819 PMID: 31683817

Abuhasira, R., Schleider, L. B.-L., Mechoulam, R., & Novack, V. (2018). Epidemiological characteristics, safety and efficacy of medical cannabis in the elderly. *European Journal of Internal Medicine*, *49*, 44–50. DOI: 10.1016/j.ejim.2018.01.019 PMID: 29398248

Abuhasira, R., Schwartz, L., & Novack, V. (2023). Medical Cannabis Is Not Associated with a Decrease in Activities of Daily Living in Older Adults. *Biomedicines*, *11*(10), 2697. DOI: 10.3390/biomedicines11102697 PMID: 37893071

Al-Ghamdi, S. (2023). Implementation of Electronic Health Records (EHR) In an Interprofessional Collaboration Model of Care to Improve Patient Outcomes : A Systematic Literature Review. *Journal of Financial Accounting and Managerial Studies*, *10*(1), 32–60.

American Nurses Association. (2020). *Gerontological nursing scope and standards of practice* (2nd ed.). American Nurses Association.

American Nurses Association (Ed.). (2024). *Cannabis nursing : Scope and standards of practice* (1st ed.). American Nurses Association.

Appelbaum, P. S. (2007). Assessment of Patients' Competence to Consent to Treatment. *The New England Journal of Medicine*, *357*(18), 1834–1840. DOI: 10.1056/NEJMcp074045 PMID: 17978292

Babson, K. A., Sottile, J., & Morabito, D. (2017). Cannabis, Cannabinoids, and Sleep : A Review of the Literature. *Current Psychiatry Reports*, *19*(4), 23. DOI: 10.1007/s11920-017-0775-9 PMID: 28349316

Bajtel, Á., Kiss, T., Tóth, B., Kiss, S., Hegyi, P., Vörhendi, N., Csupor-Löffler, B., Gede, N., Hohmann, J., & Csupor, D. (2022). The Safety of Dronabinol and Nabilone : A Systematic Review and Meta-Analysis of Clinical Trials. *Pharmaceuticals (Basel, Switzerland)*, *15*(1), 100. DOI: 10.3390/ph15010100 PMID: 35056154

Bates, D. W., Cohen, M., Leape, L. L., Overhage, J. M., Shabot, M. M., & Sheridan, T. (2001). Reducing the Frequency of Errors in Medicine Using Information Technology. *Journal of the American Medical Informatics Association : JAMIA*, *8*(4), 299–308. DOI: 10.1136/jamia.2001.0080299 PMID: 11418536

Baumbusch, J., & Sloan Yip, I. (2022). Older adults experiences of using recreational cannabis for medicinal purposes following legalization. *The International Journal on Drug Policy*, *108*, 103812. DOI: 10.1016/j.drugpo.2022.103812 PMID: 35930902

Beauchet, O. (2018). Medical cannabis use in older patients : Update on medical knowledge. *Maturitas*, *118*, 56–59. DOI: 10.1016/j.maturitas.2018.10.010 PMID: 30415756

Bhaskar, A., Bell, A., Boivin, M., Briques, W., Brown, M., Clarke, H., Cyr, C., Eisenberg, E., de Oliveira Silva, R. F., Frohlich, E., Georgius, P., Hogg, M., Horsted, T. I., MacCallum, C. A., Müller-Vahl, K. R., O'Connell, C., Sealey, R., Seibolt, M., Sihota, A., & Moulin, D. E. (2021). Consensus recommendations on dosing and administration of medical cannabis to treat chronic pain : Results of a modified Delphi process. *Journal of Cannabis Research*, *3*(1), 22. DOI: 10.1186/s42238-021-00073-1 PMID: 34215346

Bilbao, A., & Spanagel, R. (2022). Medical cannabinoids : A pharmacology-based systematic review and meta-analysis for all relevant medical indications. *BMC Medicine*, *20*(1), 259. DOI: 10.1186/s12916-022-02459-1 PMID: 35982439

Bottorff, J. L., Bissell, L. J. L., Balneaves, L. G., Oliffe, J. L., Capler, N. R., & Buxton, J. (2013). Perceptions of cannabis as a stigmatized medicine : A qualitative descriptive study. *Harm Reduction Journal*, *10*(1), 2. DOI: 10.1186/1477-7517-10-2 PMID: 23414118

Bouccin, E., Eloye, H., & Hantson, P. (2016). Complications vasculaires périphériques, cardiaques et cérébrales associées à l'utilisation du cannabis. *Toxicologie Analytique et Clinique*, *28*(2), 115–128. DOI: 10.1016/j.toxac.2016.01.002

Brown, J., & Winterstein, A. (2019). Potential Adverse Drug Events and Drug–Drug Interactions with Medical and Consumer Cannabidiol (CBD) Use. *Journal of Clinical Medicine*, *8*(7), 989. DOI: 10.3390/jcm8070989 PMID: 31288397

Caicedo, D. A., Pérez-Mañá, C., Farré, M., & Papaseit, E. (2025). An Overview of the Potential for Pharmacokinetic Interactions Between Drugs and Cannabis Products in Humans. *Pharmaceutics*, *17*(3), 319. DOI: 10.3390/pharmaceutics17030319 PMID: 40142983

Cannabis Business Plan. (2025). Cannabis Legalization World Map : October 2025 Updated. *Cannabis Business Plan*. https://cannabusinessplans.com/cannabis-legalization-map/

Cesari, M., Canevelli, M., Zhang, W., Thiyagarajan, J. A., Azzolino, D., Cherubini, A., Chhetri, J. K., Dias, A., Ferriolli, E., Gentili, S., Gregson, C. L., Jang, H., Kalula, S., Lloyd-Sherlock, P., Matijevic, R., Quarata, F., Sadana, R., Banerjee, A., & Moorthy, V. (2025). Enhancing the methodology of clinical trials in older people : A scoping review with global perspective. *The Journal of Nutrition, Health & Aging*, *29*(6), 100582. DOI: 10.1016/j.jnha.2025.100582 PMID: 40373493

Cook, D. A., Hatala, R., Brydges, R., Zendejas, B., Szostek, J. H., Wang, A. T., Erwin, P. J., & Hamstra, S. J. (2011). Technology-Enhanced Simulation for Health Professions Education : A Systematic Review and Meta-analysis. *Journal of the American Medical Association*, *306*(9). Advance online publication. DOI: 10.1001/jama.2011.1234 PMID: 21900138

Cravello, L., Di Santo, S., Varrassi, G., Benincasa, D., Marchettini, P., de Tommaso, M., Shofany, J., Assogna, F., Perotta, D., Palmer, K., Paladini, A., di Iulio, F., & Caltagirone, C. (2019). Chronic Pain in the Elderly with Cognitive Decline : A Narrative Review. *Pain and Therapy*, *8*(1), 53–65. DOI: 10.1007/s40122-019-0111-7 PMID: 30666612

Critchley, D., Szaflarski, J., Patsalos, P., Gidal, B., VanLandingham, K., & Morrison, G. (2019). Drug-drug Interaction Studies with Coadministration of Cannabidiol (CBD) and Clobazam, Valproate, Stiripentol or Midazolam in Healthy Volunteers and Adults with Epilepsy. *Epilepsy & Behavior*, *101*, 106735. DOI: 10.1016/j.yebeh.2019.08.010

Dahlke, S., Butler, J. I., Hunter, K. F., Toubiana, M., Kalogirou, M. R., Shrestha, S., Devkota, R., Law, J., & Scheuerman, M. (2024). The Effects of Stigma : Older Persons and Medicinal Cannabis. *Qualitative Health Research*, *34*(8-9), 717–731. DOI: 10.1177/10497323241227419 PMID: 38305270

Damkier, P., Lassen, D., Christensen, M. M. H., Madsen, K. G., Hellfritzsch, M., & Pottegård, A. (2019). Interaction between warfarin and cannabis. *Basic & Clinical Pharmacology & Toxicology*, *124*(1), 28–31. DOI: 10.1111/bcpt.13152 PMID: 30326170

Dimitriadou, I., Toska, A., Eloranta, S., Mört, S., Korsström, N., Lundberg, A., Häger, M., Melbarde-Kelmere, A., Circenis, K., Šteinmiller, J., Skuladottir, S. S., Hjaltadóttir, I., & Fradelos, E. C. (2025). Comprehensive Geriatric Assessment : Addressing Unmet Healthcare Needs in Older Adults. *Health Care*, *13*(21), 2715. DOI: 10.3390/healthcare13212715 PMID: 41228082

Doohan, P. T., Oldfield, L. D., Arnold, J. C., & Anderson, L. L. (2021). Cannabinoid Interactions with Cytochrome P450 Drug Metabolism : A Full-Spectrum Characterization. *The AAPS Journal*, *23*(4), 91. DOI: 10.1208/s12248-021-00616-7 PMID: 34181150

Folstein, M. F., Folstein, S. E., & McHugh, P. R. (2014). *Mini-Mental State Examination* [Jeu de données]. DOI: 10.1037/t07757-000

Fong, J. H. (2019). Disability incidence and functional decline among older adults with major chronic diseases. *BMC Geriatrics*, *19*(1), 323. DOI: 10.1186/s12877-019-1348-z PMID: 31752701

Frank, J. R., Snell, L. S., Cate, O. T., Holmboe, E. S., Carraccio, C., Swing, S. R., Harris, P., Glasgow, N. J., Campbell, C., Dath, D., Harden, R. M., Iobst, W., Long, D. M., Mungroo, R., Richardson, D. L., Sherbino, J., Silver, I., Taber, S., Talbot, M., & Harris, K. A. (2010). Competency-based medical education : Theory to practice. *Medical Teacher*, *32*(8), 638–645. DOI: 10.3109/0142159X.2010.501190 PMID: 20662574

Gaston, T. E., Bebin, E. M., Cutter, G. R., Liu, Y., & Szaflarski, J. P.UAB CBD Program. (2017). Interactions between cannabidiol and commonly used antiepileptic drugs. *Epilepsia*, *58*(9), 1586–1592. DOI: 10.1111/epi.13852 PMID: 28782097

Ginsburg, B. C., & Hensler, J. G. (2022). Age-related changes in CB1 receptor expression and function and the behavioral effects of cannabinoid receptor ligands. *Pharmacology, Biochemistry, and Behavior*, *213*, 173339. DOI: 10.1016/j.pbb.2022.173339 PMID: 35077729

Glickman, A., & Sisti, D. (2020). Prescribing medical cannabis : Ethical considerations for primary care providers. *Journal of Medical Ethics*, *46*(4), 227–230. DOI: 10.1136/medethics-2019-105759 PMID: 31852743

Gronich, N. (2024). Central Nervous System Medications : Pharmacokinetic and Pharmacodynamic Considerations for Older Adults. *Drugs & Aging*, *41*(6), 507–519. DOI: 10.1007/s40266-024-01117-w PMID: 38814377

Hafida, E. G., Rachid, S., Halima, G., & Najib, K. (2024). CBD's potential impact on Parkinson's disease : An updated overview. *Open Medicine : a Peer-Reviewed, Independent, Open-Access Journal*, *19*(1), 20241075. DOI: 10.1515/med-2024-1075 PMID: 39479465

Hammell, D. C., Zhang, L. P., Ma, F., Abshire, S. M., McIlwrath, S. L., Stinchcomb, A. L., & Westlund, K. N. (2016). Transdermal cannabidiol reduces inflammation and pain-related behaviours in a rat model of arthritis. *European Journal of Pain (London, England)*, *20*(6), 936–948. DOI: 10.1002/ejp.818 PMID: 26517407

Han, B. H., Yang, K. H., Cleland, C. M., & Palamar, J. J. (2025). Trends in Past-Month Cannabis Use Among Older Adults. *JAMA Internal Medicine*, *185*(7), 881. DOI: 10.1001/jamainternmed.2025.1156 PMID: 40455425

Ho, J. J. Y., Goh, C., Leong, C. S. A., Ng, K. Y., & Bakhtiar, A. (2024). Evaluation of potential drug-drug interactions with medical cannabis. *Clinical and Translational Science*, *17*(5), e13812. DOI: 10.1111/cts.13812 PMID: 38720531

Hochberg, U., Ingelmo, P., Solé, E., Miró, J., Rivera, G., & Perez, J. (2023). Early Interventional Treatments for Patients with Cancer Pain : A Narrative Review. *Journal of Pain Research*, *16*, 1663–1671. DOI: 10.2147/JPR.S405808 PMID: 37223437

Katz, S. (1963). Studies of Illness in the Aged : The Index of ADL: A Standardized Measure of Biological and Psychosocial Function. *Journal of the American Medical Association*, *185*(12), 914. DOI: 10.1001/jama.1963.03060120024016 PMID: 14044222

Kimberlin, C. L., & Winterstein, A. G. (2008). Validity and reliability of measurement instruments used in research. *American Journal of Health-System Pharmacy*, *65*(23), 2276–2284. DOI: 10.2146/ajhp070364 PMID: 19020196

King, D. D., DeCarlo, M., Mylott, L., & Yarossi, M. (2023). Cannabis knowledge gaps in nursing education : Pilot testing cannabis curriculum. *Teaching and Learning in Nursing*, *18*(4), 474–479. DOI: 10.1016/j.teln.2023.06.012

Klotz, U. (2009). Pharmacokinetics and drug metabolism in the elderly. *Drug Metabolism Reviews*, *41*(2), 67–76. DOI: 10.1080/03602530902722679 PMID: 19514965

Krediet, E., Janssen, D. G., Heerdink, E. R., Egberts, T. C., & Vermetten, E. (2020). Experiences with medical cannabis in the treatment of veterans with PTSD : Results from a focus group discussion. *European Neuropsychopharmacology*, *36*, 244–254. DOI: 10.1016/j.euroneuro.2020.04.009 PMID: 32576481

Lapeyre-Mestre, M., & Jouanjus, E. (2020). Cannabis et pathologies cardiovasculaires. *La Presse Médicale Formation*, *1*(4), 355–363. DOI: 10.1016/j.lpmfor.2020.08.009

Lawton, M. P., & Brody, E. M. (1969). Assessment of Older People : Self-Maintaining and Instrumental Activities of Daily Living. *The Gerontologist*, *9*(3 Part 1), 179–186. DOI: 10.1093/geront/9.3_Part_1.179 PMID: 5349366

Lu, H.-C., & Mackie, K. (2016). An Introduction to the Endogenous Cannabinoid System. *Biological Psychiatry*, *79*(7), 516–525. DOI: 10.1016/j.biopsych.2015.07.028 PMID: 26698193

Luz-Veiga, M., Azevedo-Silva, J., & Fernandes, J. C. (2023). Beyond Pain Relief : A Review on Cannabidiol Potential in Medical Therapies. *Pharmaceuticals (Basel, Switzerland)*, *16*(2), 155. DOI: 10.3390/ph16020155 PMID: 37259306

MacCallum, C. A., & Russo, E. B. (2018). Practical considerations in medical cannabis administration and dosing. *European Journal of Internal Medicine*, *49*, 12–19. DOI: 10.1016/j.ejim.2018.01.004 PMID: 29307505

Mangoni, A. A., & Jackson, S. H. D. (2004). Age-related changes in pharmacokinetics and pharmacodynamics : Basic principles and practical applications. *British Journal of Clinical Pharmacology*, *57*(1), 6–14. DOI: 10.1046/j.1365-2125.2003.02007.x PMID: 14678335

Minerbi, A., Häuser, W., & Fitzcharles, M.-A. (2019). Medical Cannabis for Older Patients. *Drugs & Aging*, *36*(1), 39–51. DOI: 10.1007/s40266-018-0616-5 PMID: 30488174

Moreland, B. L., Legha, J. K., Thomas, K. E., & Burns, E. R. (2023). Hip Fracture-Related Emergency Department Visits, Hospitalizations and Deaths by Mechanism of Injury among Adults Aged 65 and Older, United States 2019. *Journal of Aging and Health*, *35*(5-6), 345–355. DOI: 10.1177/08982643221132450 PMID: 36210739

Morse, J. M., Morse, R. M., & Tylko, S. J. (1989). Development of a Scale to Identify the Fall-Prone Patient. *Canadian Journal on Aging*, *8*(4), 366–377. DOI: 10.1017/S0714980800008576

Nasreddine, Z. S., Phillips, N. A., Bédirian, V., Charbonneau, S., Whitehead, V., Collin, I., Cummings, J. L., & Chertkow, H. (2014). *Montreal Cognitive Assessment* [Jeu de données]. DOI: 10.1037/t27279-000

Newman, A. B. (2010). An Overview of the Design, Implementation, and Analyses of Longitudinal Studies on Aging. *Journal of the American Geriatrics Society*, *58*(s2). Advance online publication. DOI: 10.1111/j.1532-5415.2010.02916.x PMID: 21029055

Ng, T., Gupta, V., & Keshock, M. C. (2025). Tetrahydrocannabinol (THC). In *StatPearls*. StatPearls Publishing., https://www.ncbi.nlm.nih.gov/books/NBK563174/

Pacher, P., Steffens, S., Haskó, G., Schindler, T. H., & Kunos, G. (2018). Cardiovascular effects of marijuana and synthetic cannabinoids : The good, the bad, and the ugly. *Nature Reviews. Cardiology, 15*(3), 151–166. DOI: 10.1038/nrcardio.2017.130 PMID: 28905873

Paiva, C., Santos, T., Cunha-Oliveira, A., Rosendo, I., & Pita, J.-R. (2024). Knowledge, opinions and experiences of nurses and nursing students in Portugal regarding the use of medical Cannabis. *BMC Nursing, 23*(1), 788. DOI: 10.1186/s12912-024-02443-5 PMID: 39468501

Parker, S. G., McCue, P., Phelps, K., McCleod, A., Arora, S., Nockels, K., Kennedy, S., Roberts, H., & Conroy, S. (2018). What is Comprehensive Geriatric Assessment (CGA)? An umbrella review. *Age and Ageing, 47*(1), 149–155. DOI: 10.1093/ageing/afx166 PMID: 29206906

Pearson, B., Walker, M., Tempero, J., Ong, K., & Lucas, P. (2024). Medical Cannabis for Patients Over Age 50 : A Multi-site, Prospective Study of Patterns of Use and Health Outcomes. *Cannabis (Research Society on Marijuana)*. Advance online publication. DOI: 10.26828/cannabis/2024/000239 PMID: 39968489

Pertwee, R. G. (2006). Cannabinoid pharmacology : The first 66 years. *British Journal of Pharmacology, 147 Suppl 1*(Suppl 1), S163-171. DOI: 10.1038/sj.bjp.0706406

Pomey, M.-P., Jutras-Aswad, D., Paquette, J., Saadi, K., Taguemout, M., Ikene, D.-L., Arbour, N., Zertal, A., Fréjeau, N., Morin, D., Ouellette, J.-S., Alami Marrouni, K., & Duquette, P. (2024). Perceptions and engagement of patients with chronic conditions on the use of medical cannabis : A scoping review. *European Journal of Medical Research, 29*(1), 211. DOI: 10.1186/s40001-024-01803-w PMID: 38561859

Pravosud, V., Lum, E., Vali, M., Cohen, B. E., Hoggatt, K. J., Byers, A. L., Austin, P. C., Walter, L. C., Hasin, D., Zaman, T., & Keyhani, S. (2025). Cannabis Use Among Older Adults. *JAMA Network Open, 8*(5), e2510173. DOI: 10.1001/jamanetworkopen.2025.10173 PMID: 40366653

Qato, D. M., Wilder, J., Schumm, L. P., Gillet, V., & Alexander, G. C. (2016). Changes in Prescription and Over-the-Counter Medication and Dietary Supplement Use Among Older Adults in the United States, 2005 vs 2011. *JAMA Internal Medicine, 176*(4), 473–482. DOI: 10.1001/jamainternmed.2015.8581 PMID: 26998708

Reeves, S., Pelone, F., Harrison, R., Goldman, J., & Zwarenstein, M. (2017). Interprofessional collaboration to improve professional practice and healthcare outcomes. *Cochrane Database of Systematic Reviews, 2018*(8). Advance online publication. DOI: 10.1002/14651858.CD000072.pub3 PMID: 28639262

Rhee, T. G., & Rosenheck, R. A. (2023). Increasing Use of Cannabis for Medical Purposes Among U.S. Residents, 2013-2020. *American Journal of Preventive Medicine*, *65*(3), 528–533. DOI: 10.1016/j.amepre.2023.03.005 PMID: 36918131

Rogers, C. I., & Pacanowski, C. R. (2023). The relationship between cannabis and anorexia nervosa : A scoping review. *Journal of Eating Disorders*, *11*(1), 186. DOI: 10.1186/s40337-023-00887-9 PMID: 37858278

Rowe, E. C., Coles, A. R. L., Harris-Lane, L. M., Harris, N., Bishop, L., Howells, R., & Donnan, J. (2025). Exploring cannabis consumption stigma in Canada with consideration of age and gender differences. *Addictive Behaviors Reports*, *21*, 100608. DOI: 10.1016/j.abrep.2025.100608 PMID: 40438612

Sacco, G., Noublanche, F., Blazek, F., Hue, C., Carballido, L., Asfar, M., Allain, P., & Annweiler, C. (2021). How to deal with the consent of adults with cognitive impairment involved in European geriatric living labs? *Philosophy, Ethics, and Humanities in Medicine; PEHM*, *16*(1), 3. DOI: 10.1186/s13010-021-00101-1 PMID: 34130730

Scott, E. P., Brennan, E., & Benitez, A. (2019). A Systematic Review of the Neurocognitive Effects of Cannabis Use in Older Adults. *Current Addiction Reports*, *6*(4), 443–455. DOI: 10.1007/s40429-019-00285-9 PMID: 32477850

Smythe, M. A., Wu, W., & Garwood, C. L. (2023). Anticoagulant drug–drug interactions with cannabinoids : A systematic review. *Pharmacotherapy*, *43*(12), 1327–1338. DOI: 10.1002/phar.2881 PMID: 37740600

Solmi, M., De Toffol, M., Kim, J. Y., Choi, M. J., Stubbs, B., Thompson, T., Firth, J., Miola, A., Croatto, G., Baggio, F., Michelon, S., Ballan, L., Gerdle, B., Monaco, F., Simonato, P., Scocco, P., Ricca, V., Castellini, G., Fornaro, M., & Dragioti, E. (2023). Balancing risks and benefits of cannabis use : Umbrella review of meta-analyses of randomised controlled trials and observational studies. *BMJ (Clinical Research Ed.)*, *382*, e072348. DOI: 10.1136/bmj-2022-072348 PMID: 37648266

Stella, N. (2023). THC and CBD : Similarities and differences between siblings. *Neuron*, *111*(3), 302–327. DOI: 10.1016/j.neuron.2022.12.022 PMID: 36638804

Storck, W., Elbaz, M., Vindis, C., Déguilhem, A., Lapeyre-Mestre, M., & Jouanjus, E. (2025). Cardiovascular risk associated with the use of cannabis and cannabinoids : A systematic review and meta-analysis. *Heart (British Cardiac Society)*, *111*(22), 1047–1056. DOI: 10.1136/heartjnl 2024 325429 PMID: 40527600

Stypulkowski, K., & Thayer, R. E. (2022). Long-Term Recreational Cannabis Use Is Associated With Lower Executive Function and Processing Speed in a Pilot Sample of Older Adults. *Journal of Geriatric Psychiatry and Neurology*, *35*(5), 740–746. DOI: 10.1177/08919887211049130 PMID: 34583547

Tatineny, P., Shafi, F., Gohar, A., & Bhat, A. (2020). Sleep in the Elderly. *Missouri Medicine*, *117*(5), 490–495. PMID: 33311760

Ten Cate, O., & Hennus, M. P. (2024). Entrustable professional activities and entrustment decision-making for competency-based education in the health professions : An introduction. In Ten Cate, O., Burch, V. C., Chen, H. C., Chou, F. C., & Hennus, M. P. (Eds.), *Entrustable Professional Activities and Entrustment Decision-Making in Health Professions Education* (pp. 3–14). Ubiquity Press., DOI: 10.5334/bdc.a

Thistlethwaite, J. E., Davies, D., Ekeocha, S., Kidd, J. M., MacDougall, C., Matthews, P., Purkis, J., & Clay, D. (2012). The effectiveness of case-based learning in health professional education. A BEME systematic review : BEME Guide No. 23. *Medical Teacher*, *34*(6), e421–e444. DOI: 10.3109/0142159X.2012.680939 PMID: 22578051

Tinetti, M. E. (1986). Performance-Oriented Assessment of Mobility Problems in Elderly Patients. *Journal of the American Geriatrics Society*, *34*(2), 119–126. DOI: 10.1111/j.1532-5415.1986.tb05480.x PMID: 3944402

Turcott, J. G., Del Rocío Guillen Núñez, M., Flores-Estrada, D., Oñate-Ocaña, L. F., Zatarain-Barrón, Z. L., Barrón, F., & Arrieta, O. (2018). The effect of nabilone on appetite, nutritional status, and quality of life in lung cancer patients : A randomized, double-blind clinical trial. *Supportive Care in Cancer*, *26*(9), 3029–3038. DOI: 10.1007/s00520-018-4154-9 PMID: 29550881

United Nations. (2024). *World Population Prospects 2024 : Summary of Results* [PDF]. United Nations. https://population.un.org/wpp/assets/Files/WPP2024_Summary-of-Results.pdf

Vaughan, C. W., & Christie, M. J. (2005). Retrograde Signalling by Endocannabinoids. In Pertwee, R. G. (Ed.), *Cannabinoids* (Vol. 168, pp. 367–383). Springer-Verlag., DOI: 10.1007/3-540-26573-2_12

Velayudhan, L., McGoohan, K., & Bhattacharyya, S. (2021). Safety and tolerability of natural and synthetic cannabinoids in adults aged over 50 years : A systematic review and meta-analysis. *PLoS Medicine*, *18*(3), e1003524. DOI: 10.1371/journal.pmed.1003524 PMID: 33780450

Vellas, B., Guigoz, Y., Garry, P. J., Nourhashemi, F., Bennahum, D., Lauque, S., & Albarede, J.-L. (1999). The mini nutritional assessment (MNA) and its use in grading the nutritional state of elderly patients. *Nutrition (Burbank, Los Angeles County, Calif.)*, *15*(2), 116–122. DOI: 10.1016/S0899-9007(98)00171-3 PMID: 9990575

Wang, Y., Robinson, K. R., Fechtel, H., & Hartog, A. (2023). Medical Cannabis Use and Its Impact on Health Among Older Adults : Recent Research Findings and Future Directions. *Current Addiction Reports*, *10*(4), 837–843. DOI: 10.1007/s40429-023-00519-x PMID: 38586531

Whiting, P. F., Wolff, R. F., Deshpande, S., Di Nisio, M., Duffy, S., Hernandez, A. V., Keurentjes, J. C., Lang, S., Misso, K., Ryder, S., Schmidlkofer, S., Westwood, M., & Kleijnen, J. (2015). Cannabinoids for Medical Use : A Systematic Review and Meta-analysis. *Journal of the American Medical Association*, *313*(24), 2456. DOI: 10.1001/jama.2015.6358 PMID: 26103030

Wolfe, D., Corace, K., Butler, C., Rice, D., Skidmore, B., Patel, Y., Thayaparan, P., Michaud, A., Hamel, C., Smith, A., Garber, G., Porath, A., Conn, D., Willows, M., Abramovici, H., Thavorn, K., Kanji, S., & Hutton, B. (2023). Impacts of medical and non-medical cannabis on the health of older adults : Findings from a scoping review of the literature. *PLoS One*, *18*(2), e0281826. DOI: 10.1371/journal.pone.0281826 PMID: 36800328

Workman, C. D., Fietsam, A. C., Sosnoff, J., & Rudroff, T. (2021). Increased Likelihood of Falling in Older Cannabis Users vs. Non-Users. *Brain Sciences*, *11*(2), 134. DOI: 10.3390/brainsci11020134 PMID: 33494171

Wu, X., Sia, J. E. V., Hai, M., Lai, X., Li, H., Cui, C., & Liu, D. (2023). Physiologically Based Pharmacokinetic Model for Older Adults and Its Application in Geriatric Drug Research. *Current Drug Metabolism*, *24*(3), 211–222. DOI: 10.2174/1389200224666230509104404 PMID: 37165496

Zamarripa, C. A., Spindle, T. R., Surujunarain, R., Weerts, E. M., Bansal, S., Unadkat, J. D., Paine, M. F., & Vandrey, R. (2023). Assessment of Orally Administered Δ9-Tetrahydrocannabinol When Coadministered With Cannabidiol on Δ9-Tetrahydrocannabinol Pharmacokinetics and Pharmacodynamics in Healthy Adults : A Randomized Clinical Trial. *JAMA Network Open*, *6*(2), e2254752. DOI: 10.1001/jamanetworkopen.2022.54752 PMID: 36780161

Zwarenstein, M., Goldman, J., & Reeves, S. (2009). Interprofessional collaboration : Effects of practice-based interventions on professional practice and healthcare outcomes. In The Cochrane Collaboration (Éd.), *Cochrane Database of Systematic Reviews* (p. CD000072.pub2). John Wiley & Sons, Ltd. DOI: 10.1002/14651858.CD000072.pub2

KEY TERMS AND DEFINITIONS

Cannabidiol (CBD): Major non-psychoactive cannabinoid of cannabis with anxiolytic, anti-inflammatory, anticonvulsant, and potential neuroprotective properties, primarily metabolized by the hepatic enzymes CYP2C19, CYP2C9, and CYP3A4.

Comprehensive Geriatric Assessment (CGA): Multidimensional process aimed at evaluating an older adult's functional (ADL/IADL), cognitive (MMSE, MoCA), psychosocial, nutritional status, and fall risk to optimize individualized care plans.

Cytochrome P450 (CYP450): Hepatic enzyme system responsible for oxidative phase I metabolism of approximately 60–80% of medications. Isoenzymes CYP2C9, CYP2C19, CYP2D6, and CYP3A4 are frequently inhibited by cannabinoids, creating a potential for drug–drug interactions.

Endocannabinoid System (ECS): Fundamental cellular signaling system discovered in the 1990s, consisting of endocannabinoids, cannabinoid receptors (CB1, CB2), and synthesizing/degrading enzymes, regulating homeostasis and multiple physiological functions.

Geriatric Pharmacokinetics: Study of age-related changes affecting drug absorption, distribution, metabolism, and elimination in older adults, including a 35–40% reduction in hepatic blood flow, decreased renal function, and increased adipose tissue.

Medical Cannabinoids: Compounds derived from cannabis or synthetically produced for therapeutic purposes, including tetrahydrocannabinol (THC) and cannabidiol (CBD), prescribed or recommended under professional supervision for various medical conditions.

Polypharmacy: Concurrent use of multiple medications, typically defined as five or more drugs, affecting approximately 39% of older adults and exponentially increasing the risk of drug interactions and adverse effects.

'Start Low, Go Slow' Principle: Fundamental geriatric therapeutic approach involving initiation at very low doses with gradual titration to identify the minimum effective dose while minimizing adverse effects.

Tetrahydrocannabinol (THC): Principal psychoactive cannabinoid of cannabis responsible for the "high," possessing analgesic, orexigenic, antiemetic, and muscle-relaxant properties, but potentially causing anxiety, tachycardia, orthostatic hypotension, and cognitive impairment, particularly in older adults.

Chapter 10
Gerontological Nursing: Riding the Green Tsunami

Alexandria Scoggins
http://orcid.org/0000-0003-3747-8473
Cannability Consulting, USA

ABSTRACT

The intersection of gerontology and cannabinoid therapeutics represents one of the most critical frontiers in modern nursing. As the global population ages, often referred to as the "Silver Tsunami," healthcare providers are likewise witnessing a "Green Wave" of increased cannabis utilization among older adults who are challenged with aging and chronic disease and looking for harm-reduction tools for polypharmacy. The mission of this chapter is to equip the nursing workforce and other allied professionals with the essential knowledge for the assessment, implementation, and evaluation of cannabis use in an older adult's plan of care, grounded in the competencies of the Cannabis Nursing Scope and Standards of Practice and Gerontological Nursing Scope and Standards of Practice. (American Cannabis Nurses Association [ACNA] & American Nurses Association [ANA], 2024; American Nurses Association [ANA], 2019).

INTRODUCTION

The intersection of gerontology and cannabinoid therapeutics represents one of the most critical frontiers in modern nursing. Gerontological nursing has historically focused on maximizing quality of life and function while minimizing the burden of chronic disease. Cannabis provides a transformative modality to support these goals, particularly in challenging behavioral and psychological symptoms of dementia (BPSD), pain management, and improving sleep. However, the introduc-

DOI: 10.4018/979-8-2600-2035-7.ch010

tion of cannabinoids into an older adult's plan of care is not without risk. A highly specialized nursing approach is essential for this patient population. This approach must address altered pharmacokinetics and pharmacodynamics, the challenges posed by polypharmacy, potential cognitive vulnerabilities or difficulties with activities of daily living, and the specific regulatory framework governing inpatient care settings that older adults may encounter on an acute or long-term basis.

This chapter seeks to provide the nursing workforce and other allied professionals with the knowledge needed to understand the population-specific differences that older adults face when considering cannabis as a therapeutic intervention. It aims to legitimize the use of cannabis as a harm-reduction tool for polypharmacy and a method for optimizing the endocannabinoid system for a population where many are challenged with aging and chronic disease. Chapter objectives include:

- Recognize the historical impact of cannabis prohibition on beliefs and attitudes of the gerontological population.
- Evaluate the potential impacts of the endocannabinoid system on challenges largely unique to older adults.
- Determine the implications of population specific differences in pharmacokinetics, pharmacodynamics, and pharmaceutical use.
- Characterize the role of the cannabis nurse in advocating for professional standards, quality of life, and residents' rights, especially the right to self-determination, in federally regulated facilities.
- Investigate the legal status of cannabis in federally regulated facilities, laws that aim to facilitate access in these settings, and setting-specific differences that can impact cannabis care.
- Articulate the necessary competencies for safe, effective gerontologic cannabis care.
- Outline future considerations for the gerontologic cannabis nurse.

CANNABIS: AN OVERVIEW

The consistently shifting but ever-expanding federal and state regulatory landscape surrounding medical cannabis, recreational cannabis, and hemp-derived cannabis necessitates that the gerontological cannabis nurse possesses a thorough understanding of each regulatory context and its potential applicability to their patients. This knowledge is vital for providing safe, effective, and legally compliant care.

Medical Cannabis

As of November 2025, 40 states, three territories, and the District of Columbia allow the medical use of cannabis for qualified patients (National Council of State Legislatures, 2025). However, millions of Americans who rely on federal programs for support, housing, and healthcare face a challenging predicament: using cannabis lawfully under their state's medical cannabis program defies federal prohibition and is considered "unlawful drug use." The disparity between federal and state cannabis laws negatively affects several older adult populations, including veterans, Medicare beneficiaries, those in federally subsidized housing, and individuals receiving care in inpatient healthcare settings.

An Executive Order was signed by President Donald Trump on December 18th, 2025, to expedite the rescheduling of cannabis to the Schedule III classification. Schedule III drugs are classified as having less potential for abuse, a currently accepted medical use in the United States, and a potential for moderate or low physical dependence or high psychological dependence in the event of drug abuse (Exec. Order No. 14,370, 2025). At the time of this writing, medical marijuana products regulated by a state medical marijuana license and FDA-approved products containing marijuana were moved to be Schedule III controlled substances within the Controlled Substances Act. Further hearings are needed to fully remove marijuana from Schedule I (Office of Public Affairs, 2026).

Regardless of schedule, the placement of cannabis within the Controlled Substances Act presents unique and major challenges to the implementation and coordination of care for the older adult. This is especially true within the stringent regulatory framework of federally regulated healthcare settings, such long-term care, home care, and hospice agencies, which are overseen by the Centers for Medicare and Medicaid Services (CMS), and discussed later in this chapter.

Hemp-Derived Cannabis

The rise of hemp-derived cannabis products provides an often overlooked, but imperative avenue for integrating cannabinoid therapeutics into the care of older adults. Governed by the 2018 Farm Bill, hemp-derived products containing less than 0.3% Delta-9 tetrahydrocannabinol (THC) by dry weight are, at the time of this writing, federally legal, effectively bypassing many of the federal-state conflicts that make medical cannabis programs impractical for many. For the gerontological cannabis nurse, hemp derived cannabis represents a low barrier, high impact therapeutic tool that directly addresses common geriatric issues while sidestepping many of the institutional and legal barriers associated with traditional medical marijuana.

Cannabidiol (CBD) is the most abundant phytocannabinoid in industrial hemp (Clark, 2021). CBD has been widely studied for its anti-inflammatory and analgesic potential. Given the high prevalence of chronic conditions like osteoarthritis and anxiety in older adults, CBD can be a powerful tool to combat chronic inflammation and oxidative stress. Additionally, full-spectrum hemp-derived cannabis often contains a combination of minor, non-intoxicating cannabinoids such as cannabigerol (CBG), cannabinol (CBN), and cannabichromene (CBC) (Clark, 2021). For older adults, this means better access to a holistic product that can address multiple symptoms simultaneously, a benefit often lacking in medical cannabis programs that focus heavily on THC concentration.

Another benefit to hemp-derived cannabis that is sometimes absent from medical cannabis programs is the ability to consistently reorder the same product, which decreases the risk of adverse events associated with product variability. However, the variability of state-based regulatory oversight of the hemp-derived cannabis industry in terms of product development, packaging, labeling, testing, and distribution poses additional challenges that cannot be dismissed. Over or underlabeling product contents, product quality, and contamination are valid concerns due to a lack of standardization. The gerontological cannabis nurse must ensure the older adult and their caregivers understand how to evaluate the quality, safety, and transparency of the hemp-derived products they are considering. This includes validating that the product has a batch number and the certificate of analysis associated with the product matches this number (MacCallum et al., 2023).

A further sign of shifting perspectives at the federal level is the Substance Access Beneficiary Engagement Initiative (BEI). This BEI is optional for Accountable Care Organization (ACO) REACH, Enhancing Oncology, and Long-Term Enhance ACO Design (LEAD) model participants. The Substance Access BEI allows model participants to consult with eligible beneficiaries and provide up to $500 of eligible hemp products per year for symptom control. Eligible products must be federally legal, compliant with state and local laws, contain no more than 0.3% delta-9 THC, contain no more than 3mg of tetrohydrocannabinols per serving, and be tested by a third party for potency, contaminants, and microbial hazards. Inhalable products and products containing synthetic cannabinoids are excluded. A physician must determine appropriate use and document, at minimum, a discussion of potential benefits and risks, goals and preferences, and a medication review for potential interactions. The shared decision making process must also include follow-up planning. Should the legal limits for hemp-derived cannabis products change, CMS will adjust safeguards to this program accordingly (Centers for Medicare & Medicaid Services, 2026).

THE UNIQUE NEEDS OF THE OLDER ADULT

The older adult demographic is rapidly expanding, and so is the demographic of older adults utilizing cannabis for therapeutic purposes. By 2030, all members of the baby boom generation will be 65 or older. The United States population of individuals 65 and older is projected to grow to 82 million by 2050 (Alzheimer's Association, 2024). A deepened understanding of the unique physiological, psychological, and social needs inherent to the gerontologic cannabis patient is vital to providing competent, informed care to this rapidly growing population. This section will introduce some of the needs discussed in the chapter and discuss the potential implications of ECS modulation for aging and the challenges chronically faced by older adults.

Beliefs and Attitudes Towards Cannabis

Integrating cannabinoid therapeutics into gerontological care cannot be successful without bringing awareness to the deep-seated stigma and various attitudes towards cannabis commonly held by older adults. These views are often not uniform but can be linked generationally to the political and media messaging towards cannabis during each group's formative years. Table 1 illustrates these views for each older adult generation. For the gerontological cannabis nurse, understanding this historical context is essential for effective communication, assessment, and patient education.

Stigmas surrounding cannabis use are a direct legacy of sharp prohibitionist campaigns, most notably the "Reefer Madness" era. The Silent and Greatest generations largely came of age during a time when cannabis was portrayed as a gateway drug leading to insanity, a life of crime, and moral failure. These unconscious, fear-based beliefs may persist despite the mounting scientific and clinical evidence illustrating the therapeutic potential of cannabis. The shift in societal perception- the "Green Wave" of legalization and acceptance- has accelerated rapidly over recent years. However, some generational differences in understanding and approval still exist.

Table 1. Generational, historical, and media influences towards cannabis

Generation	Born	Formative Years	Historical and Media Influences
Silent and Greatest	Before 1946	Pre-1945 to 1960's	• *Reefer Madness* (1936) • Marijuana Tax Act (1937) outlawed cannabis in the United States • Cannabis was removed from the United States Pharmacopeia and National Formulary (1941)
Baby Boom	1946-1964	1960s to 1980s	• Counter-culture experimentation (late 1960s,1970s) • Controlled Substances Act passed, placing marijuana as a Schedule I substance (1970) • "War on Drugs" began (1971)
Generation X	1965-1980	1980s to 2000s	• Reagan's "Just Say No" campaign (1982) • Gateway Drug theory

Source: (Clark, 2021; Santos et al., 2019)

While historical memories can lend to skepticism, recent statistics reveal a growing overlap between the aging population and cannabis use. As of 2024, of U.S. adults aged 50 and older, one in ten reported using cannabis within the past year. Furthermore, among these older adults who used cannabis, a third used it at least four times weekly (Fernandez et al., 2024). This disparity between historical belief and current use necessitates a specialized nursing approach. By acknowledging the major influence of the past on individual attitudes, the gerontological cannabis nurse can facilitate open dialogue to safely integrate cannabis into the older adult's plan of care. Table 2 outlines competencies the gerontological cannabis nurse can utilize to bridge the gap and ultimately overcome the barrier of stigma.

Table 2. ACNA and ANA standards and competencies that address potential barriers to cannabis care

Standard of Practice	Gerontological Cannabis Nurse Competency
Assessment	Identify the patient's values, preferences, needs (expressed and unexpressed), culture, state of health, and current knowledge regarding their health situation and cannabis
Diagnosis	Recognize actual/potential risks or barriers to health or safety (e.g., environmental, interpersonal, cultural, spiritual, or systematic)
Outcomes Identification	Facilitate identification of expected outcomes that consider culture, health and cannabis related values, and ethical concerns
Planning	Create a plan in conjunction with the patient and all relevant stakeholders that considers beliefs, choices, values, preferences, and age
Implementation	Assist in the educational and informational needs of the patient and their caregivers

continued on following page

Table 2. Continued

Standard of Practice	Gerontological Cannabis Nurse Competency
Coordination of Care	Collaborate with the interprofessional team, community-based resources, and the patient to provide safe transitions and manage cannabis care based on mutually agreed outcomes
Health Teaching and Health Promotion	Provide education tailored to their learning needs, values, and beliefs; engage consumer advocacy groups in health teaching activities
Evaluation	Share evaluation data with the patient and other stakeholders to promote transparency in outcomes

Source: (ACNA & ANA, 2024; ANA, 2019)

Dementia

The most critical and unique need of the older adult that this chapter must address is dementia, mainly because of its high prevalence and distinct clinical considerations that apply almost exclusively to this age demographic. It is estimated that, as of 2024, 6.9 million Americans aged 65 and older have Alzheimer's dementia, meaning that approximately 1 in 9 people are affected (Alzheimer's Association, 2024). The number of Americans with Alzheimer's disease is expected to increase to 13.85 million in 2060 (Rajan et al., 2021). Addressing dementia is essential for understanding the specific challenges involved in utilizing cannabis-based therapies in this vulnerable population.

Dementia is a general term for symptoms that affect a person's ability to complete everyday tasks, including difficulty with thinking skills, memory, problem-solving, and language. Alzheimer's disease is the most common cause of dementia. Other common causes include cerebrovascular disease, frontotemporal degeneration, Lewy body disease, hippocampal sclerosis, and Parkinson's disease. More than one brain change that contributes to the cause of dementia can be present, and that is called mixed dementia (Alzheimer's Association, 2024).

Regardless of the cause, a person living with dementia often needs caregivers to assist with activities of daily living (ADL), instrumental activities of daily living (IADL), provide supervision, assist with medication management, manage behavioral symptoms, coordinate care, and maintain their home. Unpaid caregiving by a family member or friend was performed by more than 11 million Americans and accounted for $350 billion dollars in 2023 (Alzheimer's Association, 2024). Caregiver burnout, lack of caregiver support, or increased care needs often lead to transfers to a regulated long-term care setting. Mitchell et al. (2005) estimated that 66.9% of dementia related deaths occur in a nursing home. This fact, combined with accelerated population growth since its discovery, and the therapeutic potential of cannabis in symptom management for persons living with dementia, becomes particularly relevant in the discussion of nursing home care later in this chapter.

To date, there is no cure for dementia, and there are just eight FDA-approved medications for its treatment. Five medications (donepezil, rivastigmine, galantamine, memantine, and memantine combined with donepezil) aim to improve symptoms in the early stages of the disease. Aducanumab and Iecanemab have the potential to slow disease progression, but Aducanumab was discontinued on November 1, 2024. Refractory agitation, aggression, and insomnia can be distressing for the resident, caregivers, and long-term care clinicians and often result in the off-label use of antipsychotics, benzodiazepines, and other psychotropic or black-box label medications (Alzheimer's Association, 2024). The eighth medication is an atypical antipsychotic, brexpiprazole, FDA-approved in May 2023, for dementia-related agitation but maintains its Boxed Warning for an increased risk of stroke and death in older adults with dementia-related psychosis. It is not to be used on an as-needed basis, and non-pharmacological interventions should be attempted first (Otsuka America Pharmaceutical, 2025).

As of this writing, nineteen of the thirty-eight states (50%) with medical cannabis programs list Alzheimer's disease as a qualifying condition (Bonair et al., 2025). It is important to note that not all states require practitioners to specify a qualifying medical condition. Instead, some states may only require the practitioner to confirm that the patient has a chronic condition that could potentially be alleviated by cannabis use (Certification For Use of Cannabis for Treatment, 2021/2023). A variety of treatments and clinical trials aiming to treat the pathologies of Alzheimer's disease are underway. Mechanisms include tau accumulation, plaque deposition, neuroinflammation, glutamate excitotoxicity, gut-brain axis dysfunction, and oxidative stress (Xing et al., 2025). It's important to note that many functions of the endocannabinoid system (ECS) can impact those mechanisms, and ECS dysregulation is implicated in the pathophysiology of neurological disorders like Alzheimer's and Parkinson's disease (Ferreira et al., 2023)

Coordination of Care

Coordination of care is an essential pillar of any specialty, but is particularly important within gerontology due to the often complex care network of an aging patient. The typical gerontological patient has a large, diverse healthcare team that may include primary care providers, multiple specialists, pharmacies, rehabilitation therapists, home health services, and more. For the gerontological cannabis nurse, coordination is not merely scheduling; it is the deliberate act of identifying the older adult's personal goals for quality of life and ensuring these goals are shared and internalized by all stakeholders involved in the patient's care. Especially if the older adult is unable to articulate their goals due to cognitive or language challenges, engaging formal and informal caregivers to discern what one's highest practical level of wellbeing is imperative. The introduction of cannabinoid therapeutics requires frequent, transparent communication to the older adult's care network about the dosing, rationale, and response to cannabis use. This comprehensive approach to information sharing is mandatory for advocating dignified and holistic care, competencies directly mirrored in both the *Cannabis Nursing Scope and Standards for Practice* and the *Gerontological Nursing Scope and Standards of Practice* (ACNA & ANA, 2024; ANA, 2019).

Endocannabinoid System Modulation

Aging can result in a chronic state of inflammation that is nonspecific to a particular area and can contribute to chronic illness onset and progression. The endocannabinoid system (ECS) is a complex network of receptors, cannabinoids, and signaling molecules that are key for maintaining homeostasis by regulating key physiological processes such as pain, mood, sleep, appetite, and immune response (Clark, 2021). Cannabinoids have potential in age-related neurodegenerative diseases like Alzheimer's Disease and Parkinson's disease, bone changes, osteoarthritis, and cardiovascular aging (Tudorancea et al., 2022). The neuroregulatory functions of the ECS are crucial to our body's ability to reduce inflammation, counter oxidative stress, and promote homeostasis. Studies on animals, tissues, and cells have revealed various ways in which the ECS can protect the nervous system from trauma, excitotoxicity, ischemia, and inflammation associated conditions such as seizures, stroke, and traumatic brain injury (Duncan et al., 2024).

PHARMACOLOGY FOR THE OLDER ADULT

Per the National Council of State Boards of Nursing [NCSBN] (2018), a key principle of a nurse's knowledge surrounds an understanding of cannabis pharmacology, including how one's condition and current medications influence safe cannabis use. The pharmacological management of the older adult population presents unique challenges that profoundly impact how conventional pharmaceuticals and cannabinoid therapeutics are utilized. Due to the high prevalence of chronic illness in older adults, they frequently experience polypharmacy. Detailed medication discussions are vital to combat polypharmacy and increased drug-drug interaction risks in older adults (Varghese et al., 2025; WHO, 2019). This section will explore the critical differences in pharmacokinetics and pharmacodynamics in older adults, analyze the risk posed by polypharmacy and potentially inappropriate medications, and provide a framework for assessing potential drug-cannabis interactions.

Polypharmacy

Polypharmacy is defined as "the regular use of five or more medications at the same time." As the United States has one of the highest medication rates globally, polypharmacy presents a challenge to healthcare providers (Varghese et al., 2025). Despite the numerical definition, the World Health Organization (WHO, 2019) emphasizes that providers should aim to reduce inappropriate polypharmacy. A medication contributes to inappropriate polypharmacy when it lacks an evidence-based indication, the indication is no longer valid, the dose is too high, it is not achieving its intended objective, the patient cannot or will not take it as intended, or it contributes to the potential for an adverse drug event (WHO, 2019).

Older adults often experience polypharmacy because they see several specialists for their chronic conditions, may have medications filled at multiple pharmacies, or manage symptoms with over-the-counter medications and supplements. This can lead to more than one medication being prescribed in the same medication class, major medication interactions, or duplicative therapy. Additionally, polypharmacy often causes prescribing cascades, where a symptom that is potentially a side effect of a medication appears and is treated with another medication (Meiner & Yeager, 2019). Methods to prevent polypharmacy and improve medication safety include (Meiner & Yeager, 2019; Varghese et al., 2025; WHO, 2019):

- Maintain an accurate medication list that includes all medications, including prescription, OTC, supplements, and herbal preparations. Update it as needed.
- Review medications during any care transition. Use a collaborative approach, incorporating caregivers, pharmacists, and other health professionals when possible.
- Incorporate evidence-based tools such as the American Geriatrics Society Beers Criteria, STOPP (Screening Tool of Older Person's Prescriptions), and START (Screening Tool to Alert to Right Treatment) to facilitate deprescribing and evaluate appropriate prescribing.
- Attempt to associate each medication with a confirmed diagnosis while scanning for drug-drug and drug-disease interactions.
- Use the minimal amount of medication, at the smallest dose, with the simplest possible regimen.
- If potential side effects of other medicines appear, try to avoid starting medications to combat them.

- Provide any changes in writing, whenever possible, and review with patients and, when applicable, their caregivers.

Potentially Inappropriate Medications

The American Geriatrics Society (AGS) Beers Criteria for Potentially Inappropriate Medications (PIM) Use in Older Adults is an evidence-based tool designed to support shared clinical decision-making in prescribing PIMS to adults aged 65 and older. The report serves as an educational resource for clinicians, patients, their families, regulators, policymakers, and researchers. Special consideration is given to specific diseases or syndromes, altered renal function, and specific drug combinations. The AGS emphasizes that while medications within the criteria are potentially inappropriate, they are not definitely inappropriate. The criteria are simply a starting point for a comprehensive medication review that ideally involves the patient and their family. An understanding of the rationale, recommendations, and caveats associated with the medication is needed to assess its potential, when possible, and offer safer alternatives or non-pharmacologic interventions (American Geriatrics Society [AGS] 2023 Update Expert Panel, 2023).

In 2018, Medicare Part D enrollees received 7.3 billion potentially inappropriate doses, as defined by the American Geriatrics Society's Beers Criteria. The most commonly prescribed medication classifications were proton pump inhibitors (45%), benzodiazepines (31%), and tricyclic antidepressants (9%) (Fralick et al., 2020). It is of note that the AGS 2023 Update Expert Panel (2023) considers benzodiazepines potentially inappropriate for delirium, dementia, cognitive impairment, and a history of falls or fractures (see Table 3). Yet, benzodiazepines were the second most commonly prescribed medication classification in the study conducted by Fralick et al. (2020).

Table 3. An excerpt of AGS Beers Criteria for common conditions affecting older adults

Disease or Syndrome	Drugs	Rationale
Delirium	• Anticholinergics • Antipsychotics • Benzodiazepines • Corticosteroids • H2-receptor Antagonists • Cimetidine • Famotidine • Nizatidine • Nonbenzodiazepine benzodiazepine receptor agonists hypnotics ("Z-drugs") • Esozopiclone • Zaleplon • Zolpidem • Opioids	Potential to induce or worsen delirium - avoid in older adults with or at high risk for delirium. Antipsychotics: Avoid for BPSD or delirium unless non-pharmacological interventions are contraindicated or failed and there is substantial threat to harm self or others. Periodic assessment and gradual dose reduction necessary. May be necessary if concurrent schizophrenia, bipolar, or other mental health conditions are present. Corticosteroids: Monitor for delirium if they must be used. Use the lowest dose for the shortest duration. Opioids: Emerging data links opioid administration and delirium. Use a balanced, multimodal approach and validated pain assessment tools to minimize use.
Dementia or Cognitive Impairment	• Anticholinergics • Antipsychotics, chronic or persistent as needed use • Benzodiazepines • Nonbenzodiazepine benzodiazepine receptor agonist hypnotics ("Z-drugs") • Esozopiclone • Zaleplon • Zolpidem	Avoid due to adverse effects on the central nervous system. Antipsychotics: Increased risk of cognitive decline and mortality with a dementia diagnosis, also increases risk for stroke. Avoid for BPSD or delirium unless non-pharmacological interventions are contraindicated or failed and there is substantial threat to harm self or others. Periodic assessment and gradual dose reduction necessary. May be necessary if concurrent schizophrenia, bipolar, or other mental health conditions are present.
History of Falls or Fractures	• Anticholinergics • Antidepressants (SNRIs, SSRIs, tricyclic antidepressants) • Antiepileptics • Antipsychotics • Benzodiazepines • Nonbenzodiazepine benzodiazepine receptor agonists hypnotics ("Z-drugs") • Esozopiclone • Zaleplon • Zolpidem • Opioids	May cause impaired gait or psychomotor function, syncope, or additional falls. Avoid unless safer alternatives are not available. If one medication must be used, consider reducing other central nervous system medications that also increase risk of falls or fractures and implement additional fall prevention strategies. Benzodiazepines: Shorter acting is not more safe than long acting.

Source: (AGS 2023 Beers Criteria® Update Expert Panel, 2023)

Pharmacokinetics and Pharmacodynamics

Cannabinoid therapeutics have the potential to interrupt prescribing cascades, aid in the reduction of polypharmacy, and avoid potentially inappropriate medications by substituting multiple drugs with a single option. However, careful consideration of pharmacokinetics, pharmacodynamics, and potential medication interactions is necessary for a safe and effective experience.

In addition to alterations as a result of chronic disease, there are many normal age-related changes that can impact how an older individual may process cannabis or prescription medications. The four stages of pharmacokinetics: absorption, distribution, metabolism, and elimination outline how the body processes a substance from ingestion to excretion (Meiner & Yeager, 2019). Absorption changes are minimal in the older adult population, meaning dosage adjustments based solely on age are typically not needed. However, a strong propensity for delayed or reduced gastric emptying can affect the release of enteric-coated medications and the absorption of calcium carbonate (Ngcobo, 2025). The normal distribution is affected by increased body fat and decreased total body water. Lipophilic substances may take longer to distribute, leading to prolonged action and increased effects (Ngcobo, 2025). THC is lipid soluble and CBD is lipophilic (Chayasirisobhon, 2020). Topical drug absorption is affected by reduced subcutaneous fat, which is a normal age-related change (Meiner & Yeager, 2019). The kidneys are primarily responsible for excretion, and kidney function generally declines with age (Ngcobo, 2025). Metabolism will be discussed in the following section.

Altered pharmacokinetics and pharmacodynamics of the older adult underscore the standard call for all cannabis patients to "start low, go slow" in their dose titration to minimize the chance of undesired effects, as outlined in professional practice references for cannabis nursing (ACNA & ANA, 2024; NCSBN, 2018). Additionally, full-spectrum products that are CBD dominant can further reduce the occurrence of undesired effects (MacCallum & Russo, 2018). This effect and the mechanisms of action of CBD contribute to why CBD dominant or CBD only products are often preferred by the older adult population (Choi et al., 2025; Yang et al., 2021).

Cannabis-Drug Interactions

Cytochrome P-450 (CYP-450) isoenzymes in the liver are responsible for metabolizing cannabis. First pass metabolism and CYP enzyme activity decrease with age, primarily due to reduced hepatic blood flow and liver mass. Drug clearance may be reduced by 30-40% due to decreased hepatic CYP-450 mediated metabolism and decreased in first-pass metabolism (Chayasirisobhon, 2020; Meiner & Yeager, 2019). This is especially significant in the context of cannabinoid therapeutics since most cannabis-drug interactions are related to the CYP-450 enzymes that metabolize cannabis (Clark, 2021). It is important to note that the relevance of cell or animal findings to humans regarding CYP interactions has not yet been well established. However, if a patient is taking medications that induce or inhibit CYP enzymes, altered serum cannabinoid levels can cause cannabis-drug interactions (MacCallum et al., 2021).

The CYP2C19 enzyme oxidizes phytocannabinoids THC and metabolizes cannabidiol (CBD) and is of particular importance for the gerontologic cannabis patient (Just et al., 2024; MacCallum et al., 2021). Low liver CYP2C19 expression can lead to enzyme saturation, thereby impacting the metabolism of CYP2C19 substrates. This is notably concerning with polypharmacy or medications with a narrow therapeutic range, as it may specifically increase the risk of falls. Therefore, a crucial preventative measure is to carefully personalize the dosage and duration of treatment for known CYP2C19 substrates, which include many antidepressants, opioids, antiparkinsonian drugs, and sedatives. Additionally, other CYP2C19 substrates, such as proton pump inhibitors, should be used with caution (Just et al., 2024).

Although more studies are needed, it is believed that, generally, cannabis can be safely used with most medications. While formal cannabis-drug interactions are limited, one class of particular relevance for heightened caution is central nervous system (CNS) depressants such as benzodiazepines, tricyclic antidepressants, antipsychotics, antiepileptics, opioids, and alcohol. Concurrent use of CNS depressants and cannabis can contribute to cognitive impairment and increased likelihood of sedation (MacCallum et al., 2021). As previously mentioned, several CNS depressants are known to be potentially inappropriate for older adults on their own and are commonly prescribed (AGS 2023 Update Expert Panel, 2023; Fralick et al., 2020). Approaches for managing potential cannabis-drug interactions and adverse events include (MacCallum et al., 2021):

- Be aware of and inform the patient of potential cannabis-drug interactions.
- Initiate cannabis at a low dose.
    - Consider dosing based on the milligrams of THC, rather than product percentage concentration.
    - Consider CBD-dominant products for daytime use, especially for medically fragile populations.
- Slowly titrate upward, only as needed, to achieve the intended effect.
- Establish a monitoring plan based on medical status, comorbidities, ability to adhere to the plan, and previous cannabis experience.
    - Include an evaluation of new, altered dose or frequency, or discontinued medications.
- If an interaction or adverse effect presents itself:

- Modify either THC or CBD dose.
- Switch chemovars or chemotypes.
- Switch the route of administration.
- Consider discontinuing cannabis use.

INPATIENT HEALTH CARE FOR THE OLDER ADULT

A significant number of older adults ultimately require inpatient assistance in a nursing center, assisted living, or hospice. The decision to transition to inpatient care is typically driven by the patient's escalating medical, functional, or supervisory needs. The challenges and complexity of care—including managing multiple medications, safely transferring a non-ambulatory patient, or providing consistent supervision for an individual with severe cognitive impairment—frequently exceed the physical, emotional, or financial capacity of the patient's existing support systems. Some older adults may lack caregiver support and can benefit from the community and the supervision that comes along with it.

As you read further, it is essential to critically visualize the distinct challenges these older adults face in independently managing their own therapeutic cannabis use. Consider the potential profound limitations in the abilities of a terminally ill patient or nursing home resident to independently obtain, safely store, and correctly administer their own cannabis products, as often required, whether for pain management, appetite stimulation, or other medical conditions. Their dependence on facility staff for basic ADLs and medication administration highlights a critical area of concern for integrating cannabis into the comprehensive care models of these regulated environments.

CMS Certified Nursing Homes

Centers for Medicare and Medicaid Services (CMS) generally requires compliance with federal, state, and local laws. Their regulations do not explicitly address the use of medical cannabis or hemp in healthcare settings. This fact is highlighted by personal communications with CMS shared by Wilbert and Adinoff (2023):

> *Medicare or Medicaid regulations do not address the use of medical marijuana or CBD oil. Surveyors do look at topics such as medication storage, appropriate self- administration of medications, and safe smoking policies, fire safety, etc. – but there is nothing explicitly in the Medicare/Medicaid survey and certification process related to the use of marijuana or CBD oil. CMS regulations generally require compliance with federal, state, and local laws. CMS would not cite this unless that other body (the authority having jurisdiction-in this case the DOJ)*

has made an adverse finding. We are not aware of a provider that has specifically lost funding or been penalized for permitting the use of marijuana or CBD oil; however, there have been citations cited when there has been non-compliance related to the other areas above (fire safety issues in smoking marijuana in a resident/patient room, safe storage, etc.). (p. 2)

Yet, concern persists within healthcare facilities that the federal prohibition of cannabis can lead to the cessation of federal research funds or Medicare and Medicaid reimbursement for care and services provided (Wilbert and Adinoff, 2023). The gerontological cannabis nurse can exercise Ethics and Advocacy competencies within the *Cannabis Nursing Scope and Standards of Practice* and *Gerontological Nursing Scope and Standards of Practice* to help shift this (ACNA & ANA, 2024; ANA, 2019). To effectively champion the voice of the gerontological cannabis patient, an understanding of key aspects of federal regulations that govern CMS nursing homes is necessary. It is important to note that the regulations are nursing home-specific, but the intent is similarly found in state-regulated ALFs and in the federal hospice code.

Quality of life is a fundamental principle that applies to all care and services provided to facility residents. Each resident must receive and the facility must provide the necessary care and services to attain or maintain the highest practicable physical, mental, and psychosocial well-being, consistent with the resident's comprehensive assessment and plan of care. (Quality of Life, 2016)

To promote quality of life, it is expected that nursing home staff provide person-centered care that fosters the resident's ability to make independent choices and exercise control (Quality of Life, 2016). This includes honoring the residents' rights to (Resident Rights, 2024):

- Be informed of and participate in the planning and implementation of their plan of care.
- Choose health care and providers and services that align with their interests and preferences.
- Be informed by a physician, other practitioner, or other healthcare professionals of the risks and benefits and alternative treatments to the proposed plan of care.
- Choose their preferred alternative or option, pending the physician's deeming that treatment is appropriate for their medical condition.
- Refuse, discontinue, or request treatment or participation in experimental research.

It is required that all services provided and outlined in one's comprehensive care plan meet professional standards of quality (Comprehensive Person-Centered Care

Planning, 2016). The State Operations Manual Appendix PP Guidance to Surveyors for Long Term Care Facilities (CMS, 2025, Section F658) states that:

> *"Professional standards of quality" means that care and all services are provided according to accepted standards of clinical practice. Standards may apply to care provided by a particular clinical discipline or in a specific clinical situation or setting. Standards regarding quality care practices may be published by a professional organization, licensing board, accreditation body or other regulatory agency. Recommended practices to achieve desired resident outcomes may also be found in clinical literature. Possible reference sources for standards of practice include:*

- *Current manuals or textbooks on nursing, social work, physical therapy, etc.*
- *Standards published by professional organizations such as the American Dietetic Association, American Medical Association, American Medical Directors Association, American Nurses Association, National Association of Activity Professionals, National Association of Social Work, etc.*
- *Current professional journal articles.*

Long Term Care

CMS-certified and regulated nursing facilities totaled 14,742 as of July 2025 (Chidambaram & Burns, 2025). According to the Medicare Payment Advisory Commission (MedPAC, 2025), approximately 1.2 million Medicare beneficiaries live in nursing homes due to cognitive or functional limitations that impede their ability to live independently in the community. In the almost 15,000 nursing homes nationwide, residents receive 24-hour care to meet their medical needs and assistance with activities of daily living. Most individuals, 64% of the nursing home population, stay on average for 25 days to receive post-acute care following a hospital stay. The typical goal of a short stay is to regain as much functional independence as possible and return home as safely as possible, given the limitations of their condition. (American Health Care Association National Center for Assisted Living [AHCA-NCAL], 2026b).

Chronic medical conditions are prevalent among nursing home residents. Specifically, 62% of residents have hypertension, 37% have diabetes, 34% have depression, 31% have non-ischemic heart disease, 23% have dementia, and 19% have ischemic heart disease (AHCA-NCAL, 2026b). The state of the endocannabinoid system—whether balanced or imbalanced—may considerably impact the progression of both illness and wellness across all these conditions. Fortunately, nursing home residents benefit from close healthcare provider oversight, which can support the call for close monitoring of special populations outlined by MacCallum and colleagues (2021) and the NCSBN (2018). A physician, nurse practitioner, physician's assistant, or clinical nurse specialist must visit long-stay residents within 30 days of admission, every 30 days until they've resided in the community for 90 days, and then every 60 days thereafter (MedPAC, 2025).

The high prevalence of needing assistance with activities of daily living (ADLs)—including bathing (87%), using the restroom (79%), dressing (72%), transfers (70%), bed mobility (60%), hygiene (47%), and ambulation (47%)—is a critical consideration (AHCA-NCAL, 2026b). This necessity for assistance becomes distinctly imperative when reviewing compassionate care law requirements regarding a patient's ability to obtain, store, and administer their medical cannabis, which will be discussed later in this chapter.

Assisted Living

An assisted living facility (ALF) provides residential care that bridges the gap between independent living and skilled nursing facilities for more than one million older adults nationwide. This care can be delivered through large communities, residential care centers, personal care homes, and other similar terms. ALFs typically offer 24-hour supervision and less-intensive activities of daily living assistance, housekeeping, maintenance, dining services, medication management, personal care services, and transportation assistance. While ALFs do not directly provide therapy, pharmacy, podiatry, hospice, dental, skilled nursing, and mental health services, they work with other providers to ensure the residents' needs are met (ACHA-NCAL, 2026a).

More than half (58%) of all ALF residents have hypertension, 44% have a diagnosis of Alzheimer's Disease or dementia, a third (33%) experience heart disease, and 26% are diagnosed with depression. Specialized dementia care services, either in a designated area or the entire community, are provided in 29% of the approximately 32,231 ALFs nationwide. ALF residents require supervision or hands-on assistance from a caregiver for at least one activity of daily living. Common needs include assistance with bathing (75%), walking (71%), dressing (60%), bed transfer (57%), and toileting (51%) (ACHA-NCAL, 2026a). Similar to nursing home residents, the functional limitations of ALF residents can restrict their ability to obtain, self-administer, and safely store medical cannabis.

Medicare does not cover assisted living services. and although Medicaid does not cover the cost of room and board, on a state-by-state basis, some residents receive Medicaid assistance with daily services (AHCA-NCAL, 2026a). Licensing and certification requirements and regulations governing service operations are enforced at the state level. The diverse philosophies underpinning ALF models of care encourage innovation and flexibility in designing care models that meet consumer demands in each state. Consequently, the scope of care, service limitations, and requirements related to quality, education, staffing models, and medication management can vary significantly (AHCA-NCAL, 2025). Therefore, it is imperative for the gerontological cannabis nurse to thoroughly understand the specific constraints and permissions regarding cannabis care within the ALFs of their respective state.

Hospice Care

Hospice is a Medicare-covered resource for patients with terminal conditions to receive medical care, pain management, and psychosocial support. Hospice benefits include medication and medical equipment, caregiver education, grief support and counseling, volunteer support, and case management. While hospice is often provided at home with a family member acting as the patient's primary caregiver, hospice is also provided in ALFs, nursing homes, hospitals, and free-standing hospice facilities. Of all Medicare beneficiaries who passed away in 2022, 49.1% were enrolled in hospice at the time of their passing and received at least one day of hospice care. The average length of hospice care received was 109 days in a nursing home and 165 days in an ALF (National Hospice and Palliative Care Organization [NHCPO], 2024).

The principal diagnosis assigned to each patient, which is the diagnosis that most contributes to their terminal prognosis, shows a strong concentration in a few key areas. In 2022, Alzheimer's disease, other nervous system disorders, and organic psychosis collectively represent 25% of all principal diagnoses. The two next most common categories are cancer and circulatory diseases. Notably, Parkinson's disease is the fifth most frequent principal diagnosis overall, and the most common principal cancers listed are those of the lung, prostate, pancreas, and colon (NHCPO, 2024).

While a goal of hospice care is to promote comfort, it is often not without tradeoffs in adverse effects of the medications utilized to manage distressing symptoms. Opioid pain medications are often used for pain management, and psychotropic medications are often prescribed to manage anxiety and terminal restlessness, at times causing undesired effects of sedation or confusion.

The Institutional Challenge: Reconciling Patient Needs with Regulatory Barriers

Functional challenges and complex medical needs of older adults in long-term care settings such as nursing homes, ALFs, and hospice facilities present substantial operational and ethical challenges for the gerontological cannabis nurse. The data previously presented illustrates a fundamental issue: the population who can benefit from cannabis the most is also the population least able to self-manage this treatment (see Table 4).

Table 4. Key challenges to cannabis use in long-term care settings

Care Setting	Data Summary	Implications for Cannabis Use
Nursing Homes	• High prevalence of chronic conditions (e.g. 62% hypertension, 37% diabetes, 34% depression, 23% dementia) • High prevalence of critical activities of daily living assistance (e.g. 87% bathing, 70% transfers, 60% bed mobility)	• Patients likely require staff assistance with aspects of cannabis care such as procurement, storage, and administration. • Cognitive impairment adds complexity to potential barriers.
Assisted Living Facilities	• High prevalence of chronic conditions (e.g., 58% hypertension, 44% Alzheimer's disease or dementia, 33% heart disease, 26% depression) • High need for ADL assistance (e.g., 75% bathing, 71% walking). • Scope of care is highly variable by state/facility.	• Functional limitations (walking, transfers) restrict the ability to obtain and store products independently. • Cognitive impairment adds complexity to potential barriers. • State-level regulatory differences create a patchwork of policies that the nurse must navigate to ensure compliance.
Hospice Care	• Primary focus on aggressive symptom management at end-of-life. • Common diagnoses: Alzheimer's/nervous system disorders (25%), cancer, and circulatory diseases.	• The dying process can lessen one's functional and cognitive abilities to procure, store, and self-administer cannabis.

Source: (AHCA-NCAL, 2025; AHCA-NCAL, 2026a; AHCA-NCAL, 2026b; NHCPO, 2024)

The necessity for hands-on assistance—from bathing and transfers to medication management—makes the concept of "self-administration" of medical cannabis, as often required by state laws and implicitly demanded by federal regulations, practically impossible for a significant majority of residents. This functional dependency directly translates into an institutional dependency, one that organizations will not meet due to fear of perceived consequences. This operational conflict is where institutional regulation intersects with personal stigma, creating a profound barrier to comprehensive, person-centered care. The nurse's ability to uphold professional practice standards and promote the patient's right to self-determination—core principles enshrined in the State Operations Manual Appendix PP (2025) and professional nursing standards—is severely compromised by this regulatory ambiguity and lingering historical stigma.

RYAN'S LAW: A NATIONAL LANDMARK PROGRESS

Receiving inpatient care in an acute care hospital or residing in a long-term care facility tends to preclude a qualifying patient from using their lawful cannabis medicine. The need to change this unfortunate gap in palliative and end-of-life care was highlighted by the story of Ryan Bartell, a 41-year-old diagnosed with Stage 4 pancreatic cancer. Bartell found he could remain lucid and pain-free through the use of cannabis, which was prohibited by the hospital. This prohibition left him with the sole alternative of overly-sedating Fentanyl to manage his pain until his family could find another hospital that would permit cannabis use. His father made it his personal mission to ensure families would not have to endure a similar challenge and waste precious time trying to find a place that would accept cannabis use as therapeutic (Americans for Safe Access, 2025).

What is Ryan's Law?

SB 311, also known as "Ryan's Law" or the "Compassionate Access to Medical Cannabis Act," was signed by California Governor Gavin Newsom on September 28th, 2021 with the intent to support safe medical cannabis use for terminally ill patients within specified health care facilities. Health care facilities covered by this law include general acute care hospitals, skilled nursing facilities, special hospitals, congregate living health facilities, and hospice facilities. Chemical dependency recovery hospitals and state hospitals are explicitly excluded from this law, and the law does not apply during emergency services and care. Terminally ill means the patient has "a medical condition resulting in a prognosis of life of one year or less, if the disease follows its natural course." Upon the passage of the bill, California health care facilities are now required to (Compassionate Access to Medical Cannabis Act or Ryan's Law, 2021/2022/2023):

1. Prohibit smoking and vaping as methods of using medical cannabis.
2. Document the use of medical cannabis within patient records.
3. Require the patient to provide a copy of their valid identification card or their written documentation.
4. Reasonably restrict storage and delivery methods, including requiring medical cannabis to be stored in a locked container.
5. Develop and implement written guidelines for medical cannabis use at the healthcare facility.

In 2022, SB 988 further clarified health care facility staff requirements to include the prohibition of health care professionals, health care facility staff, and home health staff from administering medical cannabis or retrieving medical cannabis from storage. This includes, but is not limited to, physicians, nurses, and pharmacists. The passage of this bill also required a patient or their primary caregiver to be solely responsible for acquiring, retrieving, administering, and removing medical cannabis (Compassionate Access to Medical Cannabis Act or Ryan's Law, 2021/2022/2023).

In 2023, the Law's provisions were expanded to include home health agencies and update the definition of a patient. Under SB 302, patients, in addition to being terminally ill, could also be over 65 years old with a chronic disease that has been assessed by a physician to be a "serious medical condition" and for which medical cannabis use is appropriate. A serious medical condition, in the state of California, is defined as (California Medical Marijuana Program, 2003/2023):

1. Acquired immune deficiency syndrome (AIDS).
2. Anorexia.
3. Arthritis.
4. Cachexia.
5. Cancer.
6. Chronic pain.
7. Glaucoma.
8. Migraine.
9. Persistent muscle spasms, including, but not limited to, spasms associated with multiple sclerosis.
10. Seizures, including, but not limited to, seizures associated with epilepsy.
11. Severe nausea.
12. Any other chronic or persistent medical symptom that either:
    a. Substantially limits the ability of the person to conduct one or more major life activities as defined in the federal Americans with Disabilities Act of 1990 (Public Law 101-336).
    b. If not alleviated, may cause serious harm to the patient's safety or physical or mental health.

While there are still gaps for California citizens and the law has not been widely implemented elsewhere, it shines a signal of hope for the continued advancement of compassionate cannabis care. The passage of Ryan's Law was a catalyst for legislative recognition of cannabis therapeutics as a legitimate and necessary intervention for palliative and end-of-life care. Its framework has served as a model and reference point for policymakers who are advocating for medical cannabis patients, especially in long-term care or hospice, to begin or retain their access to their treatment. The landmark legislation of Ryan's Law has become a catalyst for proposed, considered, and enacted compassionate use bills in other states.

Pitfalls and Opportunities: A Vignette

Although Ryan's Law was groundbreaking, its implementation has highlighted several gaps that require refinement to ensure practical use for all terminally ill patients or patients with a serious medical condition, irrespective of their functional status or support system. Specific pitfalls that impede the compassionate use of cannabis, along with potential advocacy strategies for the gerontological nurse, are detailed in the vignette below and in Table 5.

Mary is an 85-year-old female living in a CMS-certified nursing home receiving hospice care for a terminal diagnosis of protein-calorie malnutrition. She has severe dementia and routinely experiences behavioral and psychological symptoms of dementia (BPSD), including anxiety, agitation, aggression, and sleep disturbances. While staff are trained in person-centered dementia care and attempt many non-pharmacological interventions to minimize the frequency and intensity of these symptoms, she is very easily triggered and can be difficult to redirect.

For example, she was recently observed pacing and wringing her hands near the front exit. A Certified Nursing Assistant (CNA) gently approached her and asked, "Mary, I see you're looking for something. Can I help you?" Mary immediately became aggressive, shouting, "I have to go home! My children need me!" When the CNA let her know her children were safe at school and attempted a redirection by offering a puzzle—a favored activity for Mary in the past—Mary slapped the puzzle pieces off the table, hitting the CNA's arm, and retreated to her room, where she continued to yell and bang on the wall for over an hour. This aggressive episode required two staff members to monitor her until she eventually calmed down, significantly disrupting care delivery on the unit.

Outbursts such as these have become chronic and persistent, despite frequent evaluation and updating of her person-centered care plan. Mary has been prescribed several pharmaceutical medications to help manage her BPSD. She currently takes buspirone, an antidepressant, and memantine routinely and sometimes requires as-needed lorazepam when she cannot be redirected. Other medications have been previously tried and were completely ineffective or caused sedation. Mary's practitioner is considering prescribing an antipsychotic as a last resort due to the high number of previously unsuccessful interventions.

Her daughter, who is her Healthcare Power of Attorney, is aware of the potential risks associated with antipsychotic medications and has requested that cannabis be considered as an option. Fortunately, her attending provider feels that the benefits could outweigh the risks. Mary lives in a state that has a compassionate cannabis law essentially identical to Ryan's Law, and she qualifies both as a terminally ill patient and a patient with a serious medical condition. Unfortunately, Mary's long-term care facility does not have a policy that supports compassionate access to medical cannabis. Additionally, she does not have a local friend or caregiver who can serve as her primary caregiver.

Table 5. Pitfalls/challenges in compassionate cannabis legislation

Area	Pitfalls/Challenges
Policy Development	• Organizational hesitancy to develop written guidelines for medical cannabis use • Lack of awareness on how to create a policy that meets compassionate use requirements and federal requirements • Unclear federal protection on implementing state based policies
Acquiring Medical Cannabis	• Patients with terminally ill or serious medical conditions may be unable to procure medical cannabis due to inability to navigate ordering technology, inability to drive, or cognitive impairment • If the ability to acquire cannabis is present, this may change due to the progressive nature of the illness • Not all patients have access to someone who can act as their cannabis caregiver
Administering and Storing Medical Cannabis	• Patients with terminally ill or serious medical conditions may not have the functional or cognitive abilities to administer or store their own medicine • If the ability to store or administer is present, this may change due to the progressive nature of the illness • Not all patients have access to someone who can act as their cannabis caregiver

THE FUTURE OF GERONTOLOGICAL CANNABIS CARE

The therapeutic potential of the cannabis plant can be transformative. For instance, it can enable a patient struggling with the challenging behavioral and psychological symptoms of dementia (BPSD) to experience a significant reduction in agitation, often allowing them to decrease or even discontinue conventional psychoactive medications, which frequently carry "black box" warnings and undesirable side effects. A patient suffering from debilitating chronic pain due to conditions such as severe arthritis may regain the ability to participate in social activities, such as playing croquet with friends, thereby restoring connections and physical function. Similarly, for a patient with Parkinson's disease experiencing tremor, a carefully managed cannabinoid regimen might improve motor control enough to allow them to hold a spoon steady and feed themselves with independence, a small act that profoundly restores dignity.

The core professional responsibility of the gerontological cannabis nurse is to serve as the critical bridge, connecting the rapidly evolving science of the endocannabinoid system—the body's intrinsic regulatory mechanism—with the compassionate, highly-skilled, and patient-centered practice of gerontological nursing. This calling necessitates the embodiment of the professional standards and competencies set forth by our professional organizations (ACNA & ANA, 2024; ANA, 2019). As we ride the "green wave," nurses must take on multiple critical roles (ACNA & ANA, 2024):

Dedicated Advocates: Stand as unwavering advocates, championing essential policy change to ensure responsible access and equitable availability of cannabinoid therapies, addressing foundational barriers that disproportionately affect older adults (p. 74).

Stewards of Quality: Use creativity and innovation to enhance care and ensure therapeutic, holistic cannabis care is efficient, equitable, person-centered, safe, and timely (p. 85).

Compassionate Educators: Act as compassionate and informed educators for a generation that was historically subjected to decades of anti-cannabis propaganda. Our role is to build trust, dispel long-held fears, and reestablish confidence in the therapeutic utility of a plant many were once profoundly influenced to fear and avoid (p. 54).

Dignified Role Models: Serve as role models to the interprofessional health care team by defining clear roles, practicing effective communication, tracking measurable outcomes, and creating efficient processes that meet the needs of our patients (p. 79).

ACKNOWLEDGMENT

The author is grateful for the support of Westminster Canterbury on Chesapeake Bay, The Westminster Canterbury Foundation, and the American Cannabis Nurses Association. The development of this chapter received no specific grant from any funding agency in the public, commercial, or not-for-profit sectors.

REFERENCES

Act, C. S. 21 U.S.C. §§ 801 et seq. (1970 & rev. 2025). https://www.govinfo.gov/app/details/COMPS-10355

Alzheimer's Association. (2024, April 30). 2024 Alzheimer's disease facts and figures. *Alzheimer's & Dementia, 20*(5), 3708–3821. DOI: 10.1002/alz.13809 PMID: 38689398

American Cannabis Nurses Association & American Nurses Association. (2024). *Cannabis nursing: Scope and standards of practice*. ANA.

American Geriatrics Society 2023 Beers Criteria® Update Expert Panel (2023). American Geriatrics Society 2023 updated AGS Beers Criteria® for potentially inappropriate medication use in older adults. *Journal of the American Geriatrics Society,* 71(7), 2052–2081. https://doi.org/DOI: 10.1111/jgs.18372

American Health Care Association National Center for Assisted Living. (2025). *Assisted Living State Regulatory Review.* https://www.ahcancal.org/Assisted-Living/Policy/Documents/2025_RegReview_Overview%20and%20Executive%20Summary.pdf

American Health Care Association National Center for Assisted Living. (2026a). *Assisted Living Facts and Figures.* Retrieved January 17th, 2026 from https://publish.ahcancal.org/Assisted-Living/Facts-and-Figures/Pages/default.aspx

American Health Care Association National Center for Assisted Living. (2026b). *Fast Facts.* Retrieved January 21st, 2026 from https://www.ahcancal.org/Data-and-Research/facts/Pages/default.aspx

American Nurses Association. (2019). *Gerontological nursing: Scope and standards of practice* (2nd ed.). ANA.

Americans For Safe Access. (2025). *California Health Care Facility Implementation Guide - Compassionate Access to Medical Cannabis Act.* Retrieved January 11th, 2026 from https://assets.nationbuilder.com/americansforsafeaccess/pages/17098/attachments/original/1763572308/Ryan's_Law_Health_Care_Facility_Guide_2025.pdf?1763572308

California Medical Marijuana Program. Ca. Code § 11362.7 (2003, rev. 2022) https://leginfo.legislature.ca.gov/faces/codes_displaySection.xhtml?lawCode=HSC&sectionNum=11362.7

Centers for Medicare & Medicaid Services. (2026). Substance Access Beneficiary Engagement Incentive. Retrieved May 1, 2026 from https://www.cms.gov/priorities/innovation/substance-access-beneficiary-engagement-incentive

Certification For Use of Cannabis for Treatment. Va. Code § 4.1-1601 (2021, rev. 2023). https://law.lis.virginia.gov/vacodefull/title4.1/chapter16/

Chayasirisobhon, S. (2020). Mechanisms of action and pharmacokinetics of cannabis. *The Permanente Journal*, *25*(1), 1–3. DOI: 10.7812/TPP/19.200 PMID: 33635755

Chidambaram, P., & Burns, A. (2025). *A look at nursing facility characteristics in 2025.* Retrieved February 8, 2026, from https://www.kff.org/medicaid/a-look-at-nursing-facility-characteristics/

Choi, N. G., Marti, C. N., & Choi, B. Y. (2025). Cannabidiol use among older adults: Associations with cannabis use, physical and mental health, and other substance use. *Clinical Gerontologist*, *48*(5), 1255–1267. DOI: 10.1080/07317115.2024.2429595 PMID: 39575982

Clark, T. M. (2021). Scoping review and meta-analysis suggests that cannabis use may reduce cancer risk in the United States. *Cannabis and Cannabinoid Research*, *6*(5), 413–434. DOI: 10.1089/can.2019.0095 PMID: 33998861

Compassionate Access to Medical Cannabis Act or Ryan's Law. CA Health & Safety Code § 1250 (2021 & rev. 2023).

Comprehensive Person-Centered Care Planning. 42 C.F.R. § 483.21. (2016). https://www.ecfr.gov/current/title-42/chapter-IV/subchapter-G/part-483/subpart-B/section-483.21

Duncan, R. S., Riordan, S. M., Gernon, M. C., & Koulen, P. (2024). Cannabinoids and endocannabinoids as therapeutics for nervous system disorders: Preclinical models and clinical studies. *Neural Regeneration Research*, *19*(4), 788–799. DOI: 10.4103/1673-5374.382220 PMID: 37843213

Executive Order No 14,370, 3 C.F.R. 60541 (2025). https://www.federalregister.gov/documents/2025/12/23/2025-23846/increasing-medical-marijuana-and-cannabidiol-research

Fernandez, A. C., Coughlin, L., Solway, E. S., Singer, D. C., Kullgren, J. T., Kirch, M., & Malani, P. N. (2024). Prevalence and frequency of cannabis use among adults ages 50-80 in the United States. *Cannabis and Cannabinoid Research*, *9*(1), 59–64. DOI: 10.1089/can.2023.0056 PMID: 38010715

Ferreira, P. C. L., Bellaver, B., Povala, G., Brum, W. S., Tissot, C., Badji, A., Sloan, M. E., Benedet, A. L., Rosa-Neto, P., Ashton, N. J., Pascoal, T. A., Leuzy, A., & Zimmer, E. R. (2023). Endocannabinoid system biomarkers in Alzheimer's disease. *Cannabis and Cannabinoid Research*, *8*(1), 77–91. DOI: 10.1089/can.2022.0151 PMID: 36394442

Fralick, M., Bartsch, E., Ritchie, C. S., & Sacks, C. A. (2020). Estimating the use of potentially inappropriate medications among older adults in the United States. *Journal of the American Geriatrics Society*, *68*(12), 2927–2930. DOI: 10.1111/jgs.16779 PMID: 32841366

Just, K. S., Pott, L. M., Sommer, J., Scholl, C., Steffens, M., Denkinger, M. D., Rothenbacher, D., Dallmeier, D., & Stingl, J. C. (2024). Association of polymorphic cytochrome p450 enzyme pathways with falls in multimedicated older adults. *Journal of the American Medical Directors Association*, *25*(11), 105235. DOI: 10.1016/j.jamda.2024.105235 PMID: 39236770

MacCallum, C. A., Lo, L. A., & Boivin, M. (2021). "Is medical cannabis safe for my patients?" A practical review of cannabis safety considerations. *European Journal of Internal Medicine*, *89*, 10–18. DOI: 10.1016/j.ejim.2021.05.002 PMID: 34083092

MacCallum, C. A., Lo, L. A., Pistawka, C. A., & Boivin, M. (2023). A clinical framework for evaluating cannabis product quality and safety. *Cannabis and Cannabinoid Research*, *8*(3), 567–574. DOI: 10.1089/can.2021.0137 PMID: 35049330

MacCallum, C. A., & Russo, E. B. (2018). Practical considerations in medical cannabis administration and dosing. *European Journal of Internal Medicine*, *49*, 12–19. DOI: 10.1016/j.ejim.2018.01.004 PMID: 29307505

Medicare Payment Advisory Commission. (2025). *Medicare and the health care delivery system*. https://www.medpac.gov/wp-content/uploads/2025/06/Jun25_MedPAC_Report_To_Congress_SEC.pdf

Meiner, S. E., & Yeager, J. J. (2019). *Gerontologic Nursing* (6th ed.). Elsevier.

Mitchell, S. L., Teno, J. M., Miller, S. C., & Mor, V. (2005). A national study of the location of death for older persons with dementia. *Journal of the American Geriatrics Society, 53*(2), 299–305. DOI: 10.1111/j.1532-5415.2005.53118.x PMID: 15673356

National Council of State Legislatures. (2025). *State Medical Cannabis Laws*. Retrieved January 11th, 2025 from https://www.ncsl.org/health/state-medical-cannabis-laws

National Hospice and Palliative Care Organization. (2024). *NHPCO Facts and Figures 2024 Edition*. https://allianceforcareathome.org/wp-content/uploads/2024/09/Facts-Figures-2024_FINAL.pdf

Ngcobo, N. N. (2025). Influence of ageing on the pharmacodynamics and pharmacokinetics of chronically administered medicines in geriatric patients: A review. *Clinical Pharmacokinetics, 64*(3), 335–367. DOI: 10.1007/s40262-025-01494-4 PMID: 39798015

Office of Public Affairs. (2026, April 23). *Justice Department Places FDA- Approved Marijuana Products and Products Containing Marijuana Subject to a Qualifying State-issued License in Schedule III, Strengthening Medical Research While Maintaining Strict Federal Controls* [Press Release]. https://www.justice.gov/opa/pr/justice-department-places-fda-approved-marijuana-products-and-products-containing-marijuana

Otsuka America Pharmaceutical. (2025). Rexulti [package insert]. Retrieved February 4th, 2026, from https://www.rexulti.com/ https://www.otsuka-us.com/media/static/Rexulti-PI.pdf

Quality of Life. 42 C.F.R. § 483.24. (2016). https://www.ecfr.gov/current/title-42/chapter-IV/subchapter-G/part-483/subpart-B/section 483.24

Rajan, K. B., Weuve, J., Barnes, L. L., McAninch, E. A., Wilson, R. S., & Evans, D. A. (2021). Population estimate of people with clinical Alzheimer's disease and mild cognitive impairment in the United States (2020-2060). *Alzheimer's & Dementia, 17*(12), 1966–1975. DOI: 10.1002/alz.12362 PMID: 34043283

Rights, R. 42 C.F.R. § 483.10. (2024). https://www.ecfr.gov/current/title-42/chapter-IV/subchapter-G/part-483/subpart-B/section-483.10

Santos, A. F., Meier, E. M., Board, T. E., Scanlan, L. N., Wynn, T. H., Bowler, M. C., Francia, P. L., & Braithwaite, A. (2019). *Let's be blunt: Public opinion on the legalization of marijuana in the United States*. Eastern Carolina University Center for Research. https://news.ecu.edu/wp-content/pv-uploads/sites/80/2019/12/CSR-Marijuana-Report-FINAL-12.17.19.pdf

The National Council of State Boards of Nursing. (2018). The NCSBN National Nursing Guidelines for Medical Marijuana [July 2018 Supplement]. *Journal of Nursing Regulation*, *9*(2), S1–S58. DOI: 10.1016/S2155-8256(18)30082-6

Tudorancea, I. M., Ciorpac, M., Stanciu, G. D., Carata u, C., Săcărescu, A., Ignat, B., Burlui, A., Rezu , E., Creangă, I., Alexa-Stratulat, T., Tudorancea, I., & Tamba, B. I. (2022). The therapeutic potential of the endocannabinoid system in age-related diseases. *Biomedicines*, *10*(10), 2492. DOI: 10.3390/biomedicines10102492 PMID: 36289755

Wilbert, E., & Adinoff, B. (2023). *Legislative and administrative guidelines for regulating cannabis use in healthcare facilities: A DFCR white paper.* Doctors for Cannabis Regulation. https://vngoc.org/wp-content/uploads/2023/03/Legislating-Cannabis-Use-in-Healthcare-Facilities-reduced.pdf

World Health Organization. (2019). *Medication Safety in Polypharmacy: Technical Report (WHO/UHC/SDS/2019.11).* https://iris.who.int/server/api/core/bitstreams/be139493-0474-49cd-9767-b72069bf42d6/content

Varghese, D., Ishida, C., Patel, P., Haseer Koya, H. (2025). *Polypharmacy.* In StatPearls [Internet]. StatPearls Publishing.

Xing, H., Yue, S., Qin, R., Du, X., Wu, Y., Zhangsun, D., & Luo, S. (2025). Recent advances in drug development for Alzheimer's disease: A comprehensive review. *International Journal of Molecular Sciences*, 26(8), 3905. https://doi.org/10.3390/ijms26083905

Yang, K. H., Kaufmann, C. N., Nafsu, R., Lifset, E. T., Nguyen, K., Sexton, M., Han, B. H., Kim, A., & Moore, A. A. (2021). Cannabis: An emerging treatment for common symptoms in older adults. *Journal of the American Geriatrics Society*, 69(1), 91–97. https://doi.org/10.1111/jgs.16833

KEY TERMS AND DEFINITIONS

Cannabinoid Therapeutics: The medicinal use of cannabis-derived compounds, including phytocannabinoids such as THC and CBD, to treat various health conditions by modulating the endocannabinoid system to achieve therapeutic outcomes.

Gerontological Cannabis Nurse: A registered nurse with specialized knowledge in both gerontological nursing and cannabinoid therapeutics who provides evidence-based care, education, and advocacy for older adults using or considering medical cannabis, while navigating the unique pharmacological, regulatory, and ethical considerations of this patient population.

Gerontological Nursing: An evidence-based nursing specialty focused on the comprehensive care of older adults that emphasizes maximizing quality of life, maintaining functional independence, preventing illness and injury, managing chronic disease, and addressing the unique physiological, psychological, and advocacy needs of the aging population.

Older Adult: An individual typically aged 65 years or older.

Polypharmacy: The concurrent use of five or more medications by a single patient, which increases the risk of adverse drug interactions, medication errors, and potentially inappropriate prescribing, particularly prevalent among older adults with multiple chronic conditions.

Potentially Inappropriate Medications (PIM): Medications identified by evidence-based tools such as the American Geriatrics Society Beers Criteria that pose greater risks than benefits for older adults due to factors including lack of indication, adverse effects, drug interactions, or availability of safer alternatives.

Start Low, Go Slow: A fundamental dosing principle in cannabis therapeutics and geriatric pharmacology that emphasizes initiating treatment with minimal doses and gradually titrating upward to achieve therapeutic benefit while minimizing adverse effects and drug interactions.

Chapter 11
Medical Use of Cannabis: Patient Education and the Role of Oncology Nurses

Divya Aroodi Puttaraju
Sri Sathya Sai University for Human Excellence, India

Ramya Raghavan
http://orcid.org/0000-0002-9953-543X
Sri Sathya Sai University for Human Excellence, India

ABSTRACT

Medical cannabis is a transformative, multidisciplinary modality in symptom management. A growing pharmaceutical market is driving the evolution of clinical and public health frameworks. There is a need for a socially responsive curriculum to enhance nursing students' knowledge and understanding of their role in cannabis-related practice. Cannabis nursing has implications for nursing educators in countries where cannabis is legal or is being legalized. Rapid expansion of medical cannabis uses in oncology place expectations on oncology nurses to provide accurate, evidence-based guidance. However, gaps in knowledge, clinical preparedness, and institutional support challenge cannabis nursing. In future oncology nurses training will reflect in patient education within a fragmented regulatory environment. The therapeutic potential of cannabis will be realized through continued research, harmonized guidelines, and comprehensive healthcare provider education.

INTRODUCTION

Cancer is a leading cause of death globally, and conventional chemotherapy has limitations and the development of drug resistance, impacting patients' quality of

DOI: 10.4018/979-8-2600-2035-7.ch011

life. There is a growing trend among patients to use phyto cannabinoids for symptom relief with standard chemotherapy. (Nahler, 2024) Cannabis and its derivatives have undergone a remarkable transformation from stigmatized substances to promising therapeutic agents. Cannabis has a long history of use for medicinal purposes. The therapeutic application of cannabis originated in Central Asia and subsequently spread to India, North Africa, and Europe. In India, cannabis was employed for a variety of health-related purposes, including relaxation and anxiety reduction. Ancient text discusses cannabis for seizure management, pain relief, and appetite stimulation. By the nineteenth century, medical interest in cannabis increased in the United Kingdom, following reports from physicians in India. Inclusion in the British and American Pharmacopoeias added Cannabis treatment for convulsive disorders and as a hypnotic agent. However, cannabis was removed from these official medical texts in the mid-twentieth century (1932 in the UK and 1941 in the US).

In palliative care settings, medical cannabis can serve as an adjunct therapy that enhances quality of life when conventional treatments provide limited relief. Nursing professionals must conduct comprehensive assessments of symptom burden and integrate cannabis therapy into individualized care plans under the supervision of qualified clinicians. This includes monitoring for efficacy, side effects, and changes in symptom trajectories while maintaining detailed documentation to support ongoing evaluation. Emphasis should be placed on interdisciplinary communication to ensure that physicians, pharmacists, and caregivers share a unified approach to patient-centered care.

Education and ongoing professional development are critical for nurses navigating this evolving field. Structured training programs should encompass pharmacology, legal considerations, ethical implications, and communication strategies. Nurses must also develop cultural competence, recognizing diverse patient attitudes toward cannabis use that may be influenced by social, religious, or generational perspectives. Through a combination of evidence-based knowledge, empathy, and advocacy, oncology and palliative care nurses can cultivate trust and ensure that cannabis is used judiciously and compassionately to enhance symptom management and dignity in care.

The effective medical use of cannabis in oncology and palliative care ultimately depends on a balanced integration of scientific understanding, ethical sensitivity, and patient empowerment. Nurses, as frontline practitioners, have a unique opportunity to bridge the gap between emerging cannabinoid research and bedside practice. By embracing their roles as educators, advocates, and caregivers, they help ensure that medical cannabis contributes meaningfully to the holistic well-being of patients facing the challenges of cancer and end-of-life care. The present chapter aims to delineate the role of the registered nurse in assisting patients with the legal, clinical, and educational complexities associated with medicinal cannabis. Registered nurses play a critical role in patient care; however, many report feeling unprepared to discuss medicinal cannabis and express a need for further education. It is essential that registered nurses are equipped to engage in informed conversations with patients regarding medicinal cannabis. Nurse leaders express support for the legalization of medical cannabis to better meet patients' needs. Yet, there is a significant concern among nurse leaders about the stereotype of cannabis, highlighting the need for education and awareness. (Kurtzman et al., 2022) Our paper argues that oncology nurses are central, though often under-recognized, agents in making medical cannabis use safer and more clinically meaningful for patients with cancer. Drawing on evidence from nursing education, integrative oncology, and supportive care literature, it examines how nurse-led patient education can move beyond surface-level reassurance toward structured, safety-focused guidance.

Figure 1. Medical Use of Cannabis: Need for Patient Education and the Challenging Roles of Oncology Nurses. Oncologists feel uncomfortable advising on cannabis due to a lack of formal training and evidence-based guidelines. It positions specialized cannabis nursing as the solution to bridge these deficits, providing the clinical expertise and protocols necessary for the healthcare system

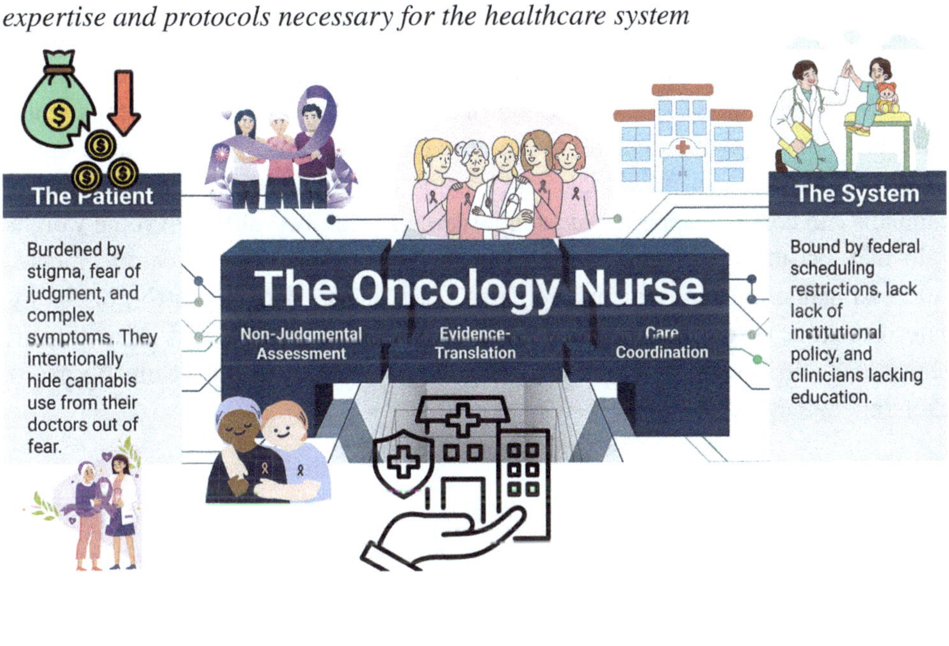
The Patient
Burdened by stigma, fear of judgment, and complex symptoms. They intentionally hide cannabis use from their doctors out of fear.
The Oncology Nurse
Non-Judgmental Assessment
Evidence-Translation
Care Coordination
The System
Bound by federal scheduling restrictions, lack lack of institutional policy, and clinicians lacking education.

CANNABINOID RECEPTORS AND *CANNABIS SPP.* EFFECTS ON HUMAN HEALTH

The human body has a complex signaling system called the endocannabinoid system, which includes specific sites called cannabinoid receptors. These receptors are primarily classified into two types:

- CB1 Receptors: These receptors are predominantly located in the nervous system, including the cortex, cerebellum, basal ganglia, limbic system, hypothalamus, and hippocampus. Activation of CB1 receptors is responsible for the psychoactive effects associated with cannabis use.
- CB2 Receptors: These receptors are primarily found outside the central nervous system, including in the immune system, bone marrow, lungs, pancreas, and smooth muscle.

The discovery of cannabinoid receptors, such as CB1 and CB2, in the human body, along with the identification of compounds like THC and CBD, has spurred scientific interest in the use of cannabis for symptom relief in cancer patients, The management of chemotherapy-induced nausea, chronic pain, and wasting syndrome has coincided with a notable increase in "cannabis-seeking" behaviors among cancer patients. Anorexia and cachexia are significant challenges for many cancer patients. Pure THC and its synthetic analogs are utilized to stimulate appetite and promote weight maintenance, in individuals with wasting syndromes. Research indicates that cannabis can enhance appetite and support weight stability, although some weight gain may be attributable to fluid retention rather than increased caloric intake. Addressing anorexia and cachexia remains a critical aspect of supportive oncology care. Cannabis medication issues with unpredictable shelf-life and variability in plant composition were overcome by the development of more stable cannabis based chemotherapeutic drugs and opiates.

Table 1. Mechanisms of action in cancer (Bellas et al., 2025) (Correa & Tucci, 2026)

Mechanism	Receptor Involvement	Notes
Inhibition of proliferation	CB1, CB2, others	Cell cycle arrest in various cancers
Induction of apoptosis	CB1, CB2, others	Programmed cell death in tumor cells
Anti-angiogenesis	CB1, CB2	Inhibits new blood vessel formation
Inhibition of metastasis	CB1, CB2	Reduces invasion and spread
Immune modulation	CB2	Alters the tumor microenvironment
Palliative symptom management	CB1, CB2	Pain, nausea, appetite

The body produces its own cannabinoids, known as endogenous cannabinoids or endocannabinoids, such as anandamide and 2-arachidonoylglycerol. These lipid-based molecules bind to cannabinoid receptors throughout the body, playing a crucial role in regulating physiological processes and maintaining homeostasis. Exogenous cannabinoids, also known as phytocannabinoids, are complex compounds derived from the *Cannabis sativa* plant. The plant contains over 100 distinct phytocannabinoids, each with unique properties and potential therapeutic effects. The route of cannabis administration influences the onset, intensity, and duration of its effects.

THC (delta-9-tetrahydrocannabinol): THC is the primary psychoactive component of cannabis. It exerts its effects by binding to CB1 receptors in the brain, mimicking the action of endogenous cannabinoids. This interaction produces euphoria, relaxation, and analgesia.

CBD (cannabidiol): CBD is not psychoactive because it does not bind to the CB1 receptor. However, it has other pharmacological properties, including being a promising anticonvulsant.

PHARMACOTHERAPY SAFETY ISSUES

Cancer patients are already using cannabis, whether clinicians like it or not. A significant proportion of cancer survivors report cannabis use, often alongside opioids. The primary reasons are painfully predictable: pain, nausea, anxiety, sleep issues, and appetite loss. Many patients report perceived symptom relief, sometimes substantial.

The body produces its own cannabinoids, known as endogenous cannabinoids or endocannabinoids, such as anandamide and 2-arachidonoylglycerol. These lipid-based molecules bind to cannabinoid receptors throughout the body, playing a crucial role in regulating physiological processes and maintaining homeostasis. Exogenous cannabinoids, also known as phytocannabinoids, are complex compounds derived from the *Cannabis sativa* plant. The plant contains over 100 distinct phytocannabinoids, each with unique properties and potential therapeutic effects. The route of cannabis administration influences the onset, intensity, and duration of its effects.

THC (delta-9-tetrahydrocannabinol): THC is the primary psychoactive component of cannabis. It exerts its effects by binding to CB1 receptors in the brain, mimicking the action of endogenous cannabinoids. This interaction produces euphoria, relaxation, and analgesia.

CBD (cannabidiol): CBD is not psychoactive because it does not bind to the CB1 receptor. However, it has other pharmacological properties, including being a promising anticonvulsant. Some even believe cannabis has anticancer effects, despite weak clinical evidence. At the same time, patients are not exactly experts in pharmacology. Awareness of risks and side effects is low, including drug interactions and psychiatric effects. Use is often self-directed, based on informal advice rather than medical guidance. In complex pharmacotherapy, for older adults with chronic conditions, AI and graph neural networks are revolutionizing the detection of drug-drug interactions (DDIs). Unlike traditional methods that rely on retrospective reporting, AI-driven clinical decision support systems can proactively predict rare or population-specific interactions, enhancing safety and accuracy in medication management. Estimates on the prevalence of cigarette-cannabis co-use among adult cancer survivors found that 3.28% reported co-use, with 12.00% currently using cigarettes and 10.36% using cannabis in the past 30 days.

The research identified individual-level factors associated with higher odds of cigarette-cannabis co-use. (Raziani et al., 2025) AI-based conversational agents (chatbots) are increasingly used to support clinical decision-making, mental health, and the promotion of healthy lifestyles. While promising, in areas like smoking cessation and substance use, the overall effectiveness of these tools varies, highlighting a need for standardization in their development.

Figure 2. Receptor topography determines clinical and psychoactive effects

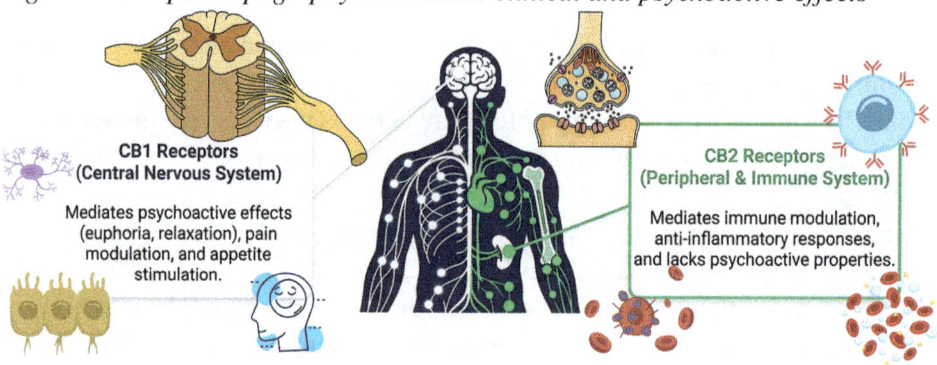

Dosing Protocols

Cannabinoids exhibit dose-dependent effects, a phenomenon known as a biphasic response. The therapeutic window can be narrow and varies between individuals. Evidence indicates that dosage influences both efficacy and safety. Low Doses usually make people feel happy and calm. Inaccurate or high doses can lead to unhappy, anxious, panic attacks, or hallucinations. In some cases, it can even cause psychosis from THC effects. The interaction of cannabinoids with the endocannabinoid system in regulating mood and sleep emphasizes that optimal dosing, cannabinoid ratios, and administration routes are not well established. There are potential risks associated with cannabis use, dependency, cognitive impairment, and adverse interactions with cancer treatments. (Reddy et al., 2026) Nursing students and professionals have identified significant knowledge gaps regarding dosing best practices, effectiveness, and regulations, highlighting the need for socially responsive curricula to prepare nurses for this role. (Hudspeth, 2024) Because many patients rely on unregulated internet sources for medical cannabis information, nurses play a critical role in providing evidence-based guidance to support informed decision-making. (Camp et al., 2025) CBD-predominant protocols start with 5 mg CBD twice daily, titrated as needed. Chronic pain may need THC if required; titrate slowly. The balanced THC: CBD ratio protocols start with 2.5–5 mg each, titrate every 2–3 days up to 40 mg/day THC. Oral preparations are commonly preferred, as oils and capsules are safer than inhaled forms. Participants identified challenges related to cost, availability of physicians, restrictive guidelines, and stigma, which hinder their access to prescribed cannabis. The literature emphasizes that cannabis use in oncology involves multiple safety risks. The uncertainty in dosing and standardization can lead to potential adverse effects and drug interactions. There is a risk of misuse or co-use with tobacco or other substances, especially among ill populations (pediatric, palliative, or comorbid patients). Further research is required to determine the effects of varying cannabinoid dosages on patients. Establishing evidence-based dosing guidelines is essential to ensure the safe and effective clinical use . For example, monitoring the use of substances such as cannabis alongside opioids and other treatments is recommended to improve patient safety and outcomes.

Table 2. Delivery methods of medicinal cannabis

Method	Onset	Duration	Pros	Risks
Smoking	Minutes	1–3 hours	Fast relief	Lung irritation, carcinogens
Vaping	Minutes	1–3 hours	Fast relief, less smoke	Lung risks, device safety Use with caution, not first-line
Edibles	30–120 min	4–8 hours	Long-lasting, discreet	Delayed onset, risk of overconsumption Good for chronic symptoms, careful dosing
Tinctures	15–45 min	2–4 hours	Rapid, titratable, and avoids inhalation	Taste, mouthfeel Highly appropriate, especially for rapid relief
Topicals	Minutes–1 h	Varies	Localized, non-psychoactive	No systemic relief Good for localized pain/ inflammation
Trans dermal	30–60 min	Hours	Sustained, systemic, or local	Limited availability Promising for sustained relief

NEED FOR PATIENT EDUCATION: SYSTEMIC GAP IN ONCOLOGY CARE

Oncology patients increasingly turn to medical cannabis to manage cancer-related symptoms such as pain, nausea, anxiety, and sleep disturbances. Yet, despite its growing use, a critical gap persists: patients are not receiving structured, evidence-based education about safe and effective cannabis use. This gap is not merely incidental but is strongly linked to insufficient education and preparedness among oncology nurses and healthcare providers. Evidence suggests that a substantial proportion of cancer survivors actively use cannabis for symptom management, often without adequate clinical guidance. For instance, cannabis use among cancer patients is driven primarily by symptom relief needs, including pain, stress, nausea, and sleep disturbances, with many patients perceiving significant benefit . However, this use frequently occurs in the absence of professional consultation, creating risks related to dosing, drug interactions, and adverse effects. Compounding this issue is the reluctance or inability of healthcare professionals to engage in meaningful discussions about cannabis. Nurses and physicians often report insufficient knowledge and discomfort in addressing cannabis-related questions, resulting in missed opportunities for patient education and harm reduction . Thus, the problem is twofold: high patient demand and low provider readiness.

Figure 3. Healthcare professionals face variability in regulations, formulations, routes of administration, and clinical evidence. Cannabis nursing overcomes the uncertain patients care navigating cannabis use alongside conventional oncology treatments. Oncology nurses occupy a pivotal role in patient education, safety monitoring, and clinical advocacy

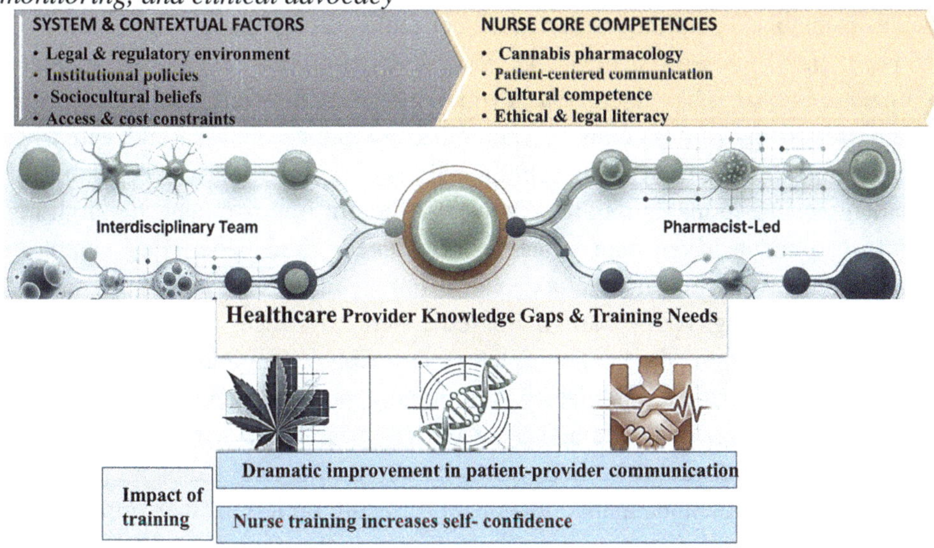

Table 3. Barriers, risks, and oncology nursing roles in cannabis care

Barriers Identified	Associated Risks	Core Oncology Nursing Roles
Lack of formal cannabis training; absence of standardized curricula	Inaccurate counseling, unsafe dosing, and misinformation	Educator, evidence translator, patient counselor
Limited evidence for some oncology indications; unclear dosing	Adverse effects, drug–drug interactions, misuse	Clinical assessor, symptom monitor, safety advocate
Complex legal frameworks; inconsistent institutional policies	Delayed access, inequitable care	Navigator, policy interpreter, patient advocate
High cost of products; lack of reimbursement	Financial toxicity, discontinuation of therapy	Supporter, referral coordinator
Stigma, patient nondisclosure, and clinician discomfort	Hidden use, unmanaged risks	Trusted communicator, rapport builder
Anxiety, distress, and comorbid substance use	Co-use with tobacco or alcohol, impaired outcomes	Holistic assessor, mental health screener
Poor storage practices; limited anticipatory guidance	Accidental pediatric exposure	Family educator, risk-mitigation leader
Fragmented interdisciplinary coordination	Inconsistent care and monitoring	Care coordinator, documentation leader

UNMET PALLIATIVE CARE AND ONCOLOGY PATIENT NEEDS AND EDUCATIONAL DEFICITS

The literature consistently demonstrates that oncology patients experience significant unmet palliative care needs, which drive the use of complementary therapies such as cannabis. Symptom burden in cancer populations remains high, including persistent pain, nausea, cachexia, anxiety, and depression, even with standard treatments. Cannabis has emerged as a widely used adjunct therapy in this context. Patients report using it to manage chemotherapy-induced nausea and vomiting, chronic pain, appetite loss, and psychological distress. Importantly, more than half of patients using cannabis report perceived symptom improvement, highlighting its role in patient-driven care strategies. Evidence-based benefits of symptom management in cancer care include pain relief, reduced chemotherapy-induced nausea and vomiting (CINV), and increased appetite in cancer patients. Approved and emerging cannabis medications such as Dronabinol, nabilone (for CINV and appetite), target CB1/CB2 modulators. Additionally, suppositories are noted for their relatively rapid onset of action and bioavailability compared with oral ingestion. A successful collaboration between investigators and a state cannabis program, suggesting that medical cannabis may be a promising option for managing severe symptoms in cancer patients, warrants further investigation. A qualitative study involving pediatric oncology providers revealed three main themes: perceptions of pain management, available pharmacological and nonpharmacological treatment options, and the challenges associated with opioid pain management. There are barriers to effective pain management for youth in oncology settings, and providers are encouraged to refer patients to pain specialists when possible, as a better understanding of cancer-related pain can help identify those at risk for chronic pain and inform tailored interventions. (Reddy et al., 2026) (Rogers et al., 2026)

The increasing legalization and accessibility of cannabis has led to its widespread use among cancer patients for managing psychological symptoms, anxiety, depression, and sleep disturbances. While many patients report moderate to high levels of symptom relief from cannabis use, the clinical evidence supporting its efficacy is mixed. Cannabis may be considered for refractory pain, nausea, appetite loss, and sleep disturbances when standard therapies fail. Patient education is essential to discuss risks, benefits, legal status, and realistic expectations. (Reddy et al., 2026) Improved communication between patients and physicians to enhance equitable access to medicinal cannabis. Cannabis improves overall symptom burden and patient-reported Quality of Life outcomes. Sativex (nabiximols, for Multiple Sclerosis and off-label cancer pain), Epidiolex (CBD, for epilepsy, cancer research), preclinical data suggest phytochemicals, fungi have anti-tumor properties. (Nanjundeshwara et al., 2025)

However, awareness of risks remains alarmingly low. Many patients lack knowledge about potential adverse effects such as psychiatric symptoms, drug interactions, or paradoxical nausea syndromes. Cannabis or mushroom knowledge gap underscores the need for clinician involvement to understand the cardiovascular effect. (Lakshmaiah & Raghavan, 2026) At the same time, provider-side barriers are well documented in education and legal matters. Nurses identify lack of knowledge, social stigma, and absence of institutional guidance as primary obstacles to discussing cannabis use with patients . Similarly, broader clinical literature highlights inconsistent guidelines, regulatory challenges, and limited high-quality evidence as systemic barriers to integrating cannabis into oncology care. The result is a paradox: patients want guidance, providers are expected to provide it, but neither side is adequately supported.

Figure 4. Healthcare providers lack evidence-informed information on potential side effects, such as cognitive alterations, dizziness, or fatigue, as well as possible drug interactions with chemotherapy agents, analgesics, or sedatives. Ultimately, targeted training has been shown to dramatically improve patient-provider communication and bolster nursing staff's professional confidence

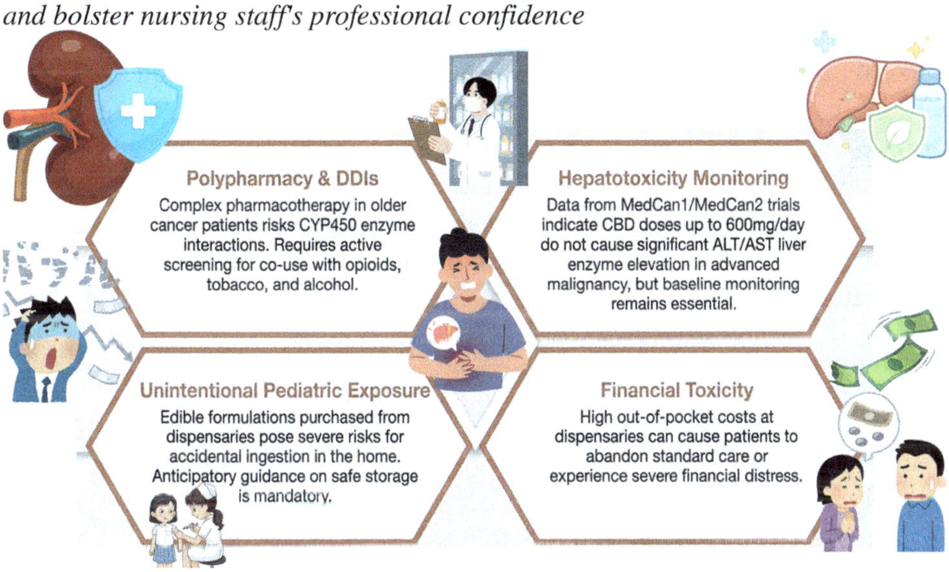

CHALLENGING ROLES OF THE NURSES WORKING WITH MEDICAL CANNABIS PATIENTS

Cannabis (CBD) as a medical modality is at the nexus of biomedical innovation, evolving clinical practice, pharmaceutical industry growth, and public health policy. Preliminary data indicate that combining phytocannabinoids with conventional chemotherapy may enhance anti-cancer effects, reduce resistance, and improve survival rates. The management of chemotherapy-induced nausea, chronic pain, and wasting syndrome has coincided with a notable increase in "cannabis-seeking" behaviors among cancer patients. Cancer survivors frequently initiate discussions about its use when conventional treatments, such as opioids, are insufficient. Patients experiencing psychosocial distress frequently use cannabis to manage symptoms such as anxiety, depression, and insomnia. For example, approximately 70% of breast cancer patients report using cannabis to aid sleep, and over 50% use it to alleviate anxiety and stress. Many patients perceive cannabis as improving their quality of life during treatment. Research indicates that up to 93% of clinical conversations regarding medicinal cannabis are initiated by patients or their caregivers rather than healthcare providers. Additionally, due to complex legal access pathways and high financial costs, many patients request cannabis during inpatient hospital care. Patient education and therapeutic guidance by nurses are instrumental in bridging the gap between patients' interest in cannabis and the lack of standardized clinical advice. Oncology veteran patients often feel their physical conditions are underestimated. Nurses are uniquely positioned to provide specialist advice from diagnosis through treatment. Veteran nursing services include educating patients on pharmacological and non-pharmacological approaches, including medical cannabis. (Joseph & Taylor, 2025)

Table 4. Literature review on cannabis use in oncology nursing

Theme	Key Findings from Literature	Implications for Oncology Nursing Practice
Knowledge gaps in cannabis care	Nurses and nursing students report limited knowledge of cannabis regulations, dosing, pharmacology, and evidence of effectiveness.	Necessitates structured pre- and in-service education and competency-based training
Patient reliance on non-clinical sources	The majority of oncology patients obtain cannabis information from the internet rather than healthcare teams.	Increases risk of misinformation, unsafe use, and unrealistic expectations
Patient education as a safety intervention	Education improves symptom self-management, reduces polypharmacy, and supports informed decision-making.	Positions nurses as frontline educators and safety gatekeepers

continued on following page

Table 4. Continued

Theme	Key Findings from Literature	Implications for Oncology Nursing Practice
Vulnerable populations	Pediatric, palliative, and comorbid oncology patients face higher safety risks.	Requires tailored education, screening, and monitoring strategies
Regulatory and access complexity	Legal, cost, and product availability barriers limit equitable access	Nurses must support navigation of systems and advocate for patients
Communication gaps	Cannabis use is often undisclosed due to stigma or clinician discomfort	Highlights the need for nonjudgmental, routine cannabis discussions
Interdisciplinary fragmentation	Limited coordination between oncology teams regarding cannabis	Reinforces the need for nurse-led coordination and documentation
Ethical and cultural considerations	Attitudes toward cannabis vary by culture and belief systems	Calls for culturally sensitive, patient-centered communication

PATIENT EDUCATION AND THE ROLE OF ONCOLOGY NURSES

The clinical application of medicinal cannabis in oncology is primarily focused on palliative care and symptom management rather than direct tumor treatment. Many healthcare providers emphasize that evidence is most robust for managing the side effects of conventional treatments. Nurses and clinicians collaborate on dosing, administration, and monitoring. Patients with controlled or uncontrolled pain are in shared decision-making regarding the use of cannabis. The role of nurses in patient education and intervention is to advocate for evidence-based, nonjudgmental care. In oncology, the primary use of medicinal cannabis is to improve patient comfort and manage symptoms, rather than to treat the cancer itself. Healthcare providers emphasize its value in alleviating the adverse effects of conventional cancer treatments.

Chemotherapy-induced nausea and vomiting (CINV) is a common and distressing side effect for many cancer patients. When standard antiemetic medications are ineffective, medicinal cannabis or THC has demonstrated efficacy in reducing both anticipatory and refractory nausea. There is substantial evidence supporting the use of cannabis for CINV, and many clinicians endorse its use based on its mechanism of action within the nervous system to reduce the frequency and severity of nausea. Thus, an interprofessional team approach for effective palliative care delivery, treatment status, pain levels, and cannabis use. Comprehensive risk-benefit education requires ongoing education about side effects, drug interactions, and legal status. (P. et al., 2025) At the beginning of the 21st century, nurses felt unprepared to engage in these discussions, citing social stigma, lack of knowledge, and insufficient workplace guidance as major barriers. Additionally, a significant number of participants expressed a need for continuing education and written resources on the topic. (Shim et al., 2023) Cannabis effects in symptom management for cancer and chronic conditions show strong evidence for pain, nausea, and appetite stimulation. While preclinical data suggest direct anticancer effects, clinical translation remains limited and is an area of active research. Communication barriers exists on cannabis use between young cancer patients and their healthcare highlighting the influence of age and treatment stage on these discussions. Over half (50.4%) of the surveyed cancer patients did not disclose their cannabis use to their cancer doctor or care team, with younger patients (aged 20–39 years) being more likely to be non-disclosers compared to older patients. Patients report that cannabis plays a critical role in addressing cancer-related pain through its opioid-sparing effects; by enhancing pain relief, it allows patients to reduce their opioid intake, thereby lowering the risk of dependency and side effects. Logistic regression analysis indicated that newly diagnosed patients and younger patients had lower odds of discussing cannabis use with their healthcare providers. (Baral et al., 2025) The legalization of medical cannabis is increasing globally, leading to heightened interest in its potential benefits for cancer patients and caregivers. The psychosocial moderation hypothesis posits that psychosocial factors can influence the effectiveness of pharmacological analgesics by either enhancing or diminishing their pain-relieving effects. (Rogers et al., 2026)

The biopsychosocial model of pain in relation to pharmacological treatments promotes a more comprehensive approach that considers patients' psychosocial context. There is a significant knowledge gap among oncologists regarding the use of cannabis in patient care, which causes frustration for patients seeking guidance. Oncology nurses serve as primary educators, advocates, and safety monitors; they require ongoing training and institutional support. (Valente et al., 2024) The pharmaceutical industry is rapidly innovating, with new products and delivery systems expanding therapeutic options. However, challenges in regulation, standardization, and evidence generation persist. There is a significant lack of research on long-term risks, dosage standardization, and treatment benefits of cannabinoids. Public health efforts must focus on equitable access, robust education, and ongoing research to ensure safe and effective integration of cannabis into modern medicine.(McIntosh et al., 2024) Regulatory Hurdles for Cannabis remain a Schedule I substance in many jurisdictions. Standardization is complicating research and access. Variability in strains, formulations, and dosing requires more high-quality randomized controlled trials.

Global regulatory practices for medical cannabis are heterogeneous, based on three main models (conservative medical, balanced procedural, and liberal). The importance of context-sensitive research, given the heterogeneity in study designs and policy contexts, is crucial for informing future drug policy decisions, thereby complicating the establishment of unified clinical guidelines and posing barriers for patients. (Korrapati et al., 2026)

Figure 5. Effective nurse education and interdisciplinary approach can support informed decision-making. Oncology nurses can normalize disclosure, integrate cannabis discussions into routine symptom assessments, and coordinate care with physicians, pharmacists, and palliative care teams

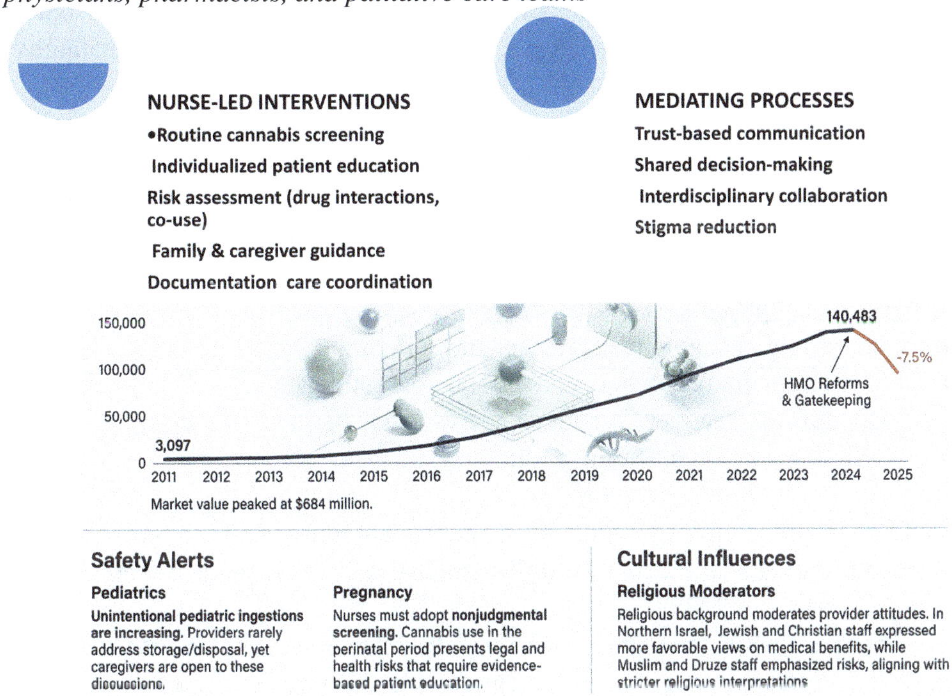

DEFINING THE NEW ROLE OF THE ONCOLOGY NURSE IN MEDICAL CANNABIS CARE

Today's oncology care still fails to control symptoms. Patients continue to experience chemotherapy-induced nausea, pain, fatigue, and psychological distress, even with standard treatments. Palliative needs in both adult and adolescent cancer populations remain high and inadequately addressed. This unmet need is a major driver behind cannabis use and other complementary therapies. There is emerging interest in anti-tumor effects, but evidence is weak and largely preclinical. Clinical trials face regulatory, logistical, and methodological challenges, which limit the availability of high-quality data.(Wolff et al., 2026)

The effectiveness of nurses in this role depends on addressing the current educational deficit. Studies consistently show that healthcare professionals lack sufficient knowledge about medical cannabis, including its indications, dosing, and safety profile. To prepare nurses adequately, several strategies must be implemented:

Curriculum Integration: Cannabis pharmacology and clinical applications should be incorporated into undergraduate and graduate nursing education.

Continuing Education Programs: Targeted training programs have demonstrated effectiveness in improving knowledge, confidence, and clinical practice in palliative care settings.

Clinical Guidelines Development: Standardized protocols for cannabis use in oncology care are needed to reduce uncertainty and variability in practice.

Simulation and Case-Based Learning: Real-world scenarios can enhance clinical decision-making and communication skills related to cannabis use.

- Educating patients on safe cannabis use
- Supporting symptom management and self-care
- Assisting with treatment decisions and goal setting
- Monitoring effectiveness and adverse effects
- Facilitating communication within the care team

There is also evidence that nurse-led educational interventions improve patient outcomes and clinical practice, and that funding and implementing them is warranted.(Baral et al., 2025)

Emerging inpatient cannabis programs and palliative care models further demonstrate that structured, nurse-led interventions can improve symptom management and patient satisfaction. These models highlight the feasibility and necessity of integrating cannabis education into routine oncology nursing practice. The oromucosal sprays (Nabiximols) documented route in oncology patient experiences are currently limited to a few cases. Phytocannabinoids, especially cannabidiol, may help alleviate chemotherapy-related side effects such as nausea, vomiting, loss of appetite, peripheral neuropathic pain, and anxiety, while also potentially protecting organs from chemotherapy-induced toxicity. (Nahler, 2024)

Case Vignette: Oncology Nurse-Led Cannabis Education in Advanced Cancer

Mrs. A, a 68-year-old woman with metastatic breast cancer, reports moderate to severe bone pain and poor sleep despite optimal opioid analgesia and adjuvant agents. She asks her oncology nurse whether "medical marijuana" might help her pain and appetite. The nurse begins by reviewing her current medications, cognitive status, and fall risk, and confirms that she has no history of psychosis or substance-use disorder.

The nurse explains that medical cannabis may modestly improve pain and sleep in some patients but is not a substitute for her current pain regimen. Together, they establish a clear goal: a 1–2 point reduction in worst pain intensity over 24 hours and improved restfulness, with a firm limit on sedation or dizziness. The prescriber then selects a low-dose, THC-dominant oromucosal spray, starting at 2 mg per dose, and the nurse documents the plan, including dose, timing, and criteria for follow-up.

Over the next two weeks, the nurse telephones Mrs. A weekly to review pain scores, any dizziness or confusion, and her ability to perform daily activities. At the second call, Mrs. A reports mild sedation and improved sleep but no meaningful change in pain. The nurse discusses these findings with the prescriber, and the team decides to slightly increase the dose while reinforcing non-pharmacologic strategies such as sleep hygiene and physical therapy. The nurse also documents the shared decision, Mrs. A's preferences, and ongoing safety monitoring, illustrating how oncology nurses can operationalize evidence-based, nurse-led cannabis care within a structured guideline framework.

Figure 6. From a systems perspective, oncology nurse engagement in medical cannabis education contributes to standardized, equitable care. The future of nursing competencies in cannabis science relies on legal frameworks and ethical considerations

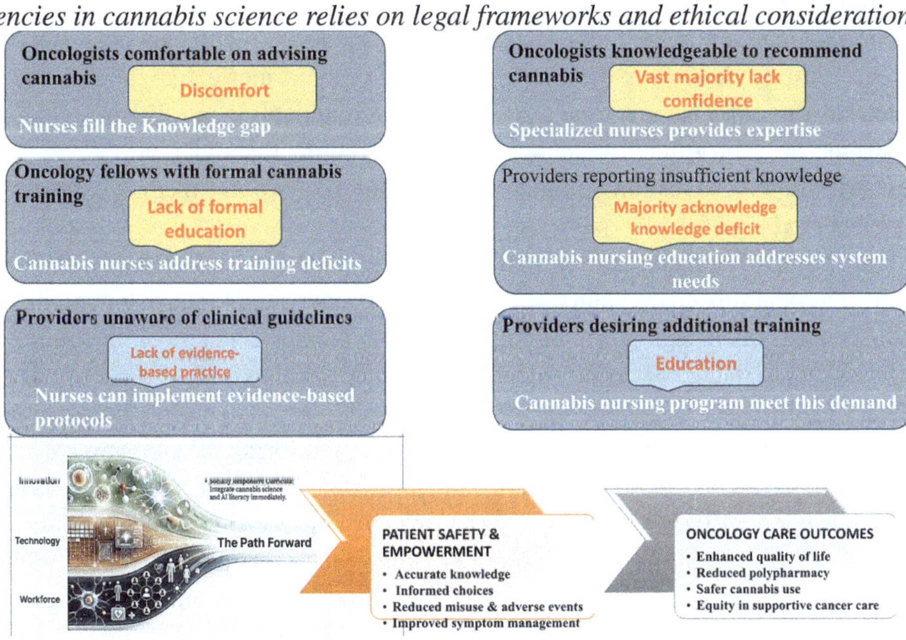

ONCOLOGY AND PAIN MANAGEMENT

In oncology settings, nurses should assess mental health, social support, and sleep quality before initiating analgesic therapies. Monitoring for substance use, including cannabis, is part of ensuring patient safety and adherence, when managing complex pharmacotherapy or potential opioid misuse. (Rogers et al., 2026) Nurses act as gatekeepers for safety, screening for risks, and managing comorbidities across various patient populations.

Nurses are responsible for patient education, screening, and intervention strategies regarding cannabis use. The role requires providing evidence-based, nonjudgmental care to optimize outcomes while navigating the legal landscape. The clinicians must also provide anticipatory guidance to patients regarding the risks of unintentional cannabis ingestion. Counseling caregivers on proper storage and disposal techniques to mitigate safety risks in the home. (Valente et al., 2024)

ADDRESSING STIGMA AND CULTURAL FACTORS

The cultural and religious background can influence a nurse's attitude toward medical cannabis. For instance, research in Northern Israel showed that religious affiliation moderated the evaluation of cannabis's therapeutic potential versus its risks, underscoring the need for culturally tailored education to facilitate clinical integration. (Correa & Tucci, 2026)

Nurses are essential in addressing the stigma associated with cannabis use, for patients with gender issues who may have faced years of ineffective therapies and societal dismissal. (Kcomt et al., 2026) Medical cannabis clinics also highlight disparities based on ethnicity, gender, and income, noting that older individuals and those with higher education and income are more likely to use medical cannabis. (Ataiants et al., 2025)

Perceptions of cannabis have shifted in recent years. Previously regarded primarily as a recreational substance, cannabis is now being investigated for its potential therapeutic benefits in managing challenging symptoms. Cannabis nursing is becoming a specialty due to rising cancer prevalence, regulatory changes, and advances in drug delivery. (Shim et al., 2023) Pipeline Innovations in delivery systems (nanoemulsions, transdermal patches), and combination therapies are exploring the cannabis effects. GW Pharmaceuticals/Jazz, Cara Therapeutics, and Cannabics Pharmaceuticals are expanding Clinical Trials to focus on symptom management and potential antitumor effects. Legalization and policy reform are expanding access, but require robust public health frameworks to ensure safe, evidence-based use. The endocannabinoid system CB1/CB2 receptors, endocannabinoids influences immune infiltration, tumor-stroma crosstalk, making spatial profiling ideal for studying cannabinoid effects. (M et al., 2026) Cannabis nursing has to form a specialized role focused on patient education and biomedical research innovations. Oncology nurses face the divide between patient expectations of nursing expertise and the current lack of evidence-based resources provided to clinicians, as well as the integration of cannabis therapeutics into holistic care plans. Nurses are increasingly viewed as the "best professionals" to guide patients through medical cannabis treatment due to their position at the intersection of clinical care, patient advocacy, and symptom management. (Joseph & Taylor, 2025) Nurse leaders express overwhelming support for the legalization of medical cannabis to better meet patients' needs. There is a significant concern among nurse leaders about the stereotype of cannabis, highlighting the need for education and awareness. (Kurtzman et al., 2022) Future needs to delineate the role of the registered nurse in assisting patients with the legal, clinical, and educational complexities associated with medicinal cannabis. Registered nurses play a critical role in patient care; however, many report feeling unprepared to discuss medicinal cannabis and express a need for further education. It is essential that registered nurses are equipped to engage in informed conversations with patients regarding medicinal cannabis. (Correa & Tucci, 2026)

Table 5. Machine learning (ML) and artificial intelligence (AI) enhance personalization in cannabis dosing and symptom prediction for oncology/palliative patients

Technology	Application in Cannabis Care	Benefits for Oncology	Examples
Machine Learning	Predictive analytics for dosing; symptom trajectory forecasting (pain, nausea)	Reduces trial-and-error; minimizes side effects like dizziness	LSTM/CNN models predict chemo symptom escalation (accuracy >85%); challenge: data privacy
Deep Learning	Analyze cannabinoid interactions; patient response modeling	Tailors THC/CBD for cancer pain/sleep; opioid sparing	CNNs process imaging/ genomics for personalized regimens; needs large datasets
Artificial Intelligence	Clinical decision support; chatbots for patient education	Improves adherence in palliative symptom management	AI recommends strains/doses based on history; ethical issues in bias
Neuromorphic Computing	Spiking neural networks mimicking brain synapses	Real-time symptom monitoring (pain response to CBD); low-power edge devices for wearables	Energy-efficient for remote palliative monitoring; limited cannabis-specific studies
Quantum Computing	Superposition/entanglement for complex simulations	Cannabinoid-receptor binding prediction; personalized dosing via quantum ML	VQE simulates THC-CB1 interactions 100x faster; scales to multiomics for cancer cachexia
Quantum ML (Hybrid)	Quantum enhanced neural networks	Cancer drug matching (cannabinoids + chemo); trajectory prediction	QDRL for radiotherapy decisions (+10% accuracy); early-stage, qubit limitations

FUTURE DIRECTIONS

Looking ahead, several emerging tools and policy developments are likely to shape the nurse's role in medical cannabis. Digital health applications, including symptom-tracking apps and cannabis-diary platforms, can support the self-titration process by providing structured templates for dose logging, side-effect reports, and patient-reported outcomes that nurses can review remotely. Artificial intelligence–assisted clinical decision-support tools and virtual-reality-based training scenarios may further enhance nurses' ability to simulate complex cannabis-related conversations, assess risk, and practice interprofessional coordination in a safe, low-stakes environment.(Ilie et al., 2026)

Artificial Intelligence and Predictive Analytics

Artificial Intelligence (AI) and machine learning are transforming clinical practice from reactive responses to proactive, personalized interventions. a digital educational intervention aimed at enhancing oncology nurses' professional practice to support safe cannabis use among young adults (aged 18-39) diagnosed with cancer, addressing a gap in existing educational resources. (Lakshmaiah et al., 2025)

The results indicated strong feasibility, with 89% of the intervention group completing the whole program, and a significant increase in intention to support safe cannabis use among intervention participants compared with controls ($P = .016$). The findings suggest that tailored, theory-informed educational strategies can effectively enhance oncology nursing practices and indicate potential for further research and larger trials to scale the intervention. (Vinette et al., 2022) Emerging healthcare technologies and digital tools are fundamentally reshaping patient-centered clinical practice by enabling proactive risk management, expanding therapeutic modalities through virtual environments, and altering how patients access and utilize medical information. These advancements allow for more personalized, accessible, and interdisciplinary care models, in oncology, pain management, and mental health. AI is being integrated into supportive oncology to personalize interventions and improve patient-reported outcomes. AI tools facilitate symptom monitoring and predictive analytics for adverse events, allowing clinicians to provide timely symptom relief and optimized care recommendations. (Ilie et al., 2026) However, implementing AI requires addressing challenges related to data privacy, algorithmic bias, and rigorous validation.

Virtual Reality (VR) is emerging as a powerful modality for pain management and behavioral skill-building. The offering of immersive environments complements traditional care between fatalistic cancer beliefs and risky health behaviors. (Zaidi et al., 2024) Cannabis use with tobacco smoking, electronic cigarette use, and heavy alcohol drinking, among adults with a history of cancer, is reported. The findings indicate that higher levels of cancer fatalism are associated with a 30% increase in the odds of engaging in these risky behaviors. (Hudspeth, 2024)

Youth in the questioning and transgender classes exhibited higher levels of curiosity and intention to use substances (alcohol, nicotine/tobacco, and cannabis) compared to cisgender youth, with adjusted odds ratios indicating significant associations. Members of the naïve class were less likely to report curiosity, intention, or actual use of substances compared to cisgender youth, suggesting a lower risk profile for substance use. (Zaidi et al., 2024) Diversity-based study findings highlight the importance of understanding gender diversity among preadolescent youth to inform the development of targeted early prevention services for substance use, during critical developmental periods. (Kcomt et al., 2026) Understanding this relationship can help tailor digital cancer prevention outreach programs to meet the needs of individuals and communities better. VR is being explored as a pain management and therapy method. It offers distraction from pain and the clinical environment, or conversely, helps youth with cancer focus, providing a sense of comfort. In the broader field of pain management, research trends are shifting toward virtual reality and e-health as key emerging technologies. (Correa & Tucci, 2026)

Table 6. Technology applications in cannabis oncology

Tech nology	Application in Cannabis Care	Benefits for Oncology
Machine Learning	Predictive analytics for dosing; symptom trajectory forecasting	Reduces trial-and-error; minimizes side effects LSTM/CNN models predict chemo symptom escalation (accuracy >85%); challenge: data privacy
Deep Learning	Analyze cannabinoid interactions; patient response modeling	Tailors THC/CBD for cancer pain/sleep; opioid-sparing CNNs process imaging/genomics for personalized regimens; needs large datasets
Artificial Intelligence	Clinical decision support; chatbots for patient education	Improves adherence in palliative symptom management AI recommends strains/doses based on history; ethical issues in bias
Neuromorphic Computing	Spiking neural networks mimicking brain synapses	Real-time symptom monitoring; low-power edge devices Energy-efficient for remote palliative monitoring; limited cannabis-specific studies
Quantum Computing	Superposition/entanglement for complex simulations	Cannabinoid-receptor binding prediction; personalized dosing VQE simulates THC-CB1 interactions 100x faster, scales to multiomics for cancer cachexia
Quantum ML Hybrid	Quantum-enhanced neural networks	Cancer drug matching; trajectory prediction QDRL for radiotherapy decisions (+10% accuracy); early-stage, qubit limitations

Mental Health Interventions

The development of the intervention involves collaboration with patient partners (young adults with cancer) and health professionals (nurses and doctors) using the VR in adolescent suicide prevention. The "Practice Experiences for School Reintegration" (PrESR) intervention uses VR to allow hospitalized adolescents to practice therapeutic skills (affect regulation, problem-solving) in simulated stressful school settings before discharge. This approach has proven feasible and acceptable, bridging the gap between inpatient care and real-world stressors. (Correa & Tucci, 2026) Patients at medical cannabis clinics were less likely to seek treatment for chronic pain but more likely for mental health conditions. However, participants reported lower satisfaction with various aspects of care, including consultation duration and information on potential harms and benefits. (Lintzeris et al., 2025) The use of Digital Monitoring treatment approaches and the associated treatment costs suggest higher consumer satisfaction. Smartphone-based self-report instruments are enabling the longitudinal monitoring of mental health in the general population. These digital tools predominantly measure deficit-based constructs (like depression and anxiety) but have the potential to support holistic self-monitoring if evolved to include strength-based measures. (Kcomt et al., 2026) Digital tools are also helping bridge gaps in access to specialized care. For example, in the context of medical cannabis patients often rely on unregulated internet sources. There is a critical need for digitally integrated education to support informed decision-making. Furthermore, bibliometric analyses indicate that future research in pain management is increasingly focused on telemedicine and digital health to personalize treatment approaches. (Brittain et al., 2025)

Figure 7. AI is being integrated into oncology to personalize patient interventions and improve patient-reported outcomes. AI tools facilitate symptom monitoring and provide predictive analytics on adverse events, enabling clinicians to deliver timely symptom relief and optimize care recommendations

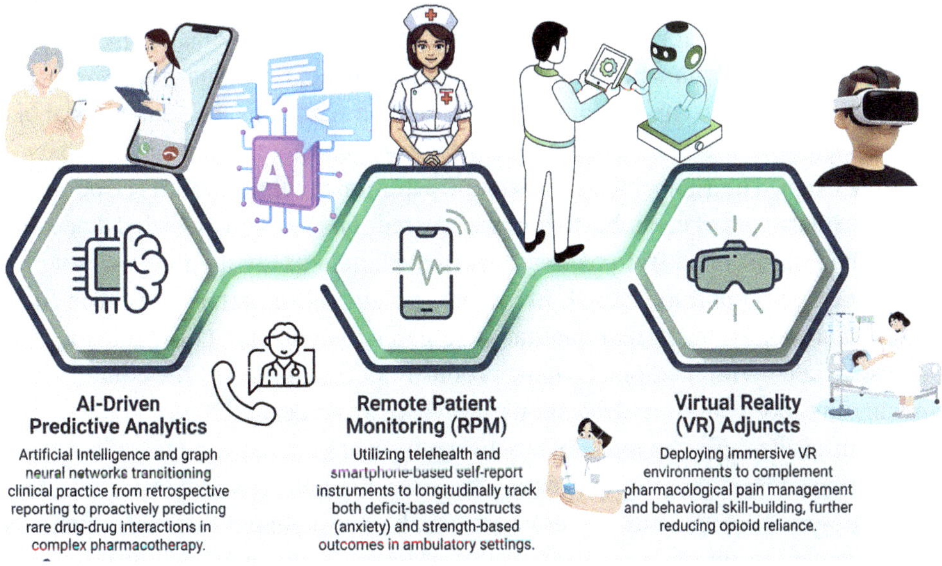

Telehealth and Remote Care Models

Digital tools extend clinicians' reach, enabling ambulatory and interdisciplinary Remote Pain Management. Telehealth supports the clinical capabilities necessary to address concerns about prescribing unapproved treatments. Cannabis remote care nursing debunks negative perceptions within the medical community and the clinical utility of medicinal cannabis. (Dobson et al., 2024) Telehealth interventions can effectively deliver interdisciplinary cancer pain management. For example, a single-session telehealth intervention combining medical education and behavioral pain treatment was found acceptable and resulted in reduced pain intensity, interference, and depression. By collaborating with patient partners and health professionals, the intervention will be tested for feasibility and acceptability among nurses to improve their ability to guide patients effectively. Digital monitoring and educational tools facilitate risk-stratified ambulatory care for conditions such as malignant bowel obstruction. By using proactive nursing phone calls and interdisciplinary team guidance, patients can often be managed as outpatients with high rates of symptom resolution, reducing hospital stays. Nurses report key barriers in the time and involvement required for the cannabis clinic program. Cannabis facilitators include a positive perception of the program's design and the home setting for therapeutic education sessions.

The proliferation of digital platforms has transformed patients into active information seekers, requiring clinicians to navigate a landscape of online health information and crowdsourced support. It finds that individuals with chronic pain are more likely to use cannabis for medical or dual purposes. Medical cannabis users report access to medicinal cannabis through telehealth consultations, and single-purpose dispensaries are welcome. Despite high satisfaction with cannabis, concerns about stigma, legal issues, and lack of medical disclosure highlight significant challenges faced by users. The financial barriers and frustrations with initial prescriptions of cannabis oil instead of cannabis flower were noted. The research revealed that some individuals transitioned from recreational to medicinal use, with dual-use motives (both recreational and medicinal) being present among the informants. The findings indicate a need for further qualitative research to understand the behaviors and risks associated with medicinal cannabis consumption, in light of the complexities surrounding motivations and access pathways. (Dawson et al., 2025)

A central theme is the mismatch between patient demand for cannabis-related information and healthcare professionals' readiness to deliver it. For instance, many healthcare practitioners and trainees report feeling unprepared to counsel patients about cannabis despite its increasing clinical relevance. Patients frequently turn to the internet for medical information. For instance, breast cancer patients increasingly use YouTube for treatment information; while credible sources exist, the quality varies, necessitating that clinicians guide patients toward reliable content. Similarly, analysis of Google Trends and Wikipedia indicates a sustained public interest in online information regarding schizophrenia diagnosis and management. A major challenge identified is patients' reliance on non-clinical sources for cannabis information. Among head and neck cancer patients, 70% relied on the internet for information, while only 20% consulted their cancer care team. (Raghavan et al., 2025)

Medical Crowdfunding Platforms like GoFundMe have become tools for families to manage the financial toxicity of serious illnesses like pediatric cancer. These campaigns allow families to share illness narratives and garner financial and emotional support, although they also expose the burden of deductibles and employment disruptions. The "digital-intelligent age" presents challenges in assessing the credibility of information. Medical students and professionals must develop the capability to discern reliable health information amidst the complexity of generative AI and big data to advise patients effectively. (Baral et al., 2025)

Public Health: Policy, Access, and Education

Oncology nurses are positioned as key mediators between scientific evidence and patient understanding. Their responsibilities include explaining the risks, benefits, and limitations of cannabis use. Cannabis nursing addresses misconceptions and unrealistic expectations by tailoring education to vulnerable populations. Upcoming innovations integrate cannabis discussions into holistic symptom management. Product choice and dosing require a cautious, individualized approach. CRISPR could engineer ECS modulation (CB1/CB2 receptors) for anti-tumor effects or synthetic cannabinoid production, complementing cannabis's role in pain/nausea relief. (Pallavi et al., 2026) Whenever possible, teams should use regulated, standardized products with known THC and CBD concentrations, favoring oral or oromucosal preparations over inhaled routes to reduce pulmonary risk and improve dose titration. A "start low, go slow" strategy should be used, beginning with low doses, gradually titrating based on symptom response and tolerability, and clearly documenting dose changes, timing, and formulations in the medical record. Oncology nurses can reinforce adherence to titration plans by reviewing patient-reported symptom relief and adverse effects at each contact. (Ananthakumar et al., 2025)

However, the literature repeatedly stresses that nurses require advanced training and institutional support to fulfil these roles effectively. A national strategy for the circulation of medical cannabis due to the increasing number of patients with chronic pain and post-traumatic stress disorders. There is a global variation in the regulatory and policy landscape. Legal status and access to medical cannabis vary widely, affecting clinical practice and patient access. Ongoing efforts to standardize recommendations and ensure patient safety. Patient access and equity barriers are legal restrictions, cost, and a lack of standardized. Public and professional education is essential to dispel myths, reduce stigma, and promote informed decision-making. (Valente et al., 2024) The role of nurses and clinicians as frontline educators can bridge knowledge gaps and support patient autonomy. Nurses expressed a desire for meaningful discussions with patients about medicinal cannabis but reported feeling underprepared and lacking confidence in their ability to support these patients effectively. (McIntosh et al., 2024) The importance of evidence-based education for nurses and their involvement in policy development will enhance patient care related to medicinal cannabis. Psychosocial factors are categorized into three groups: dispositional psychological factors, situational cognitive or affective factors, and contextual and social factors, highlighting the complexity of pain management. A significant majority (75%) of cancer patients reported using at least one psychotropic medicinal plant in oncology settings. The study identified neuroactive plants, including Valeriana officinalis, Lavandula angustifolia, Hypericum perforatum, and Urtica, which are commonly known and used by patients. (Nahler, 2024) The main ethical concerns in psychedelic research and practice: standards of practice, equity, integrity, cultural appropriation, and epistemic justice. There were notable differences in plant usage between genders, with women using more psychotropic plants than men, and higher usage rates were found in patients with breast cancer and head and neck cancer. The absence of consensus among stakeholders (researchers, clinicians, patients, and regulators) on managing ethical challenges in psychedelic research and therapy. (Brittain et al., 2025) The research emphasizes the need for structured preoperative assessments of herbal use due to potential interactions with anesthetic and analgesic medications, which is crucial for enhancing perioperative safety. (Wolff et al., 2026) Future recommendations include developing clear competency frameworks, engaging with Indigenous and priority populations, establishing guidelines for Indigenous recognition, managing post-trial care, and ensuring proper governance of psychedelic prescribing practices. (Bellas et al., 2025)

Figure 8. Oncology nurses are ideally positioned as primary educators, advocates, and safety monitors in cannabis-integrated oncology and palliative settings. Cannabis Nursing responsibilities extend beyond education to encompass surveillance for adverse reactions, documentation of clinical outcomes, and reporting of any regulatory or ethical concerns (P. et al., 2025)

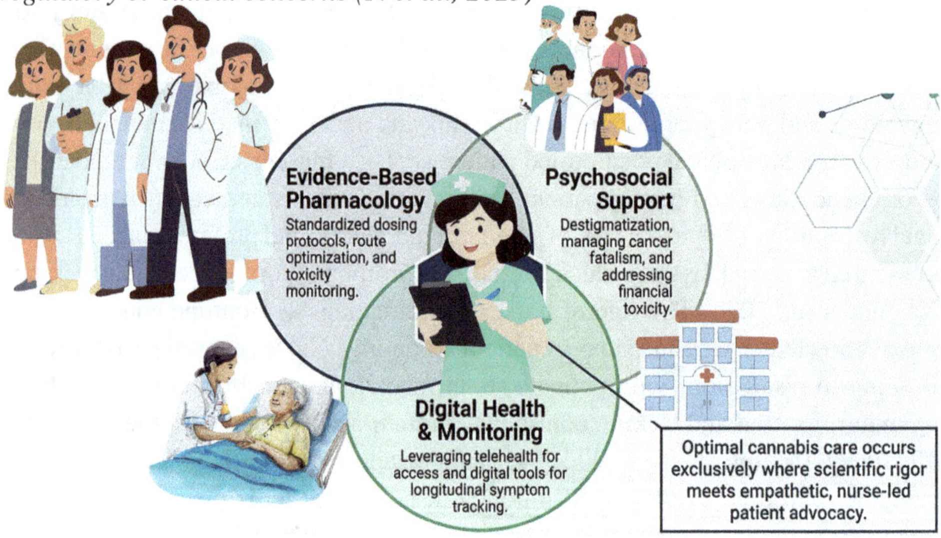

Recommendations

Nursing must evolve from passive information providers to proactive educators and safety advocates. Integration of cannabis education into nursing curricula and continuing professional development. The objective is to empower nurses to transition from uncertainty to active advocacy, ensuring that medicinal cannabis is integrated safely and holistically into patient treatment plans.(Dawson et al., 2025)

- Development of standardized patient education frameworks.
- Institutional policies supporting open, stigma-free communication.
- Interdisciplinary collaboration to ensure safe and evidence-based cannabis use.
- Risk screening (mental health, substance co-use, vulnerability)
- Education on safe storage, dosing variability, and formulation risks

Importantly, educational interventions must go beyond knowledge acquisition to include communication skills, ethical reasoning, and interprofessional collaboration. Despite these barriers, the role of the oncology nurse in supporting patients using medical cannabis is both well-defined in principle and underutilized in practice. Frameworks such as those from NCSBN (2018), ANA, and ACNA emphasize the nurse's responsibility in patient education, symptom management, and interprofessional collaboration. When applied to medical cannabis, this role expands into several critical domains. (Brittain et al., 2025)

- First, nurses must develop foundational knowledge of the endocannabinoid system (ECS) and cannabinoid pharmacology. Understanding how cannabinoids interact with ECS receptors to modulate pain, inflammation, and mood is essential for informed patient guidance.
- Second, nurses play a key role in goal setting and care planning. Patients often approach cannabis use with vague or unrealistic expectations, including curative intent. Nurses must help align cannabis use with realistic palliative goals such as symptom relief and quality-of-life improvement.
- Third, interprofessional coordination is crucial. Cannabis may interact with chemotherapy agents, immunotherapies, or supportive medications. Nurses must collaborate with physicians and pharmacists to evaluate safety within the patient's treatment regimen.
- Fourth, nurses guide product selection and administration routes. Evidence indicates that cannabis is administered through multiple routes, including oils, edibles, and inhalation, each with different pharmacokinetics and risk profiles. Nurses must help patients choose appropriate formulations and understand onset times and duration of effects.
- Fifth, patient education on self-titration and monitoring is essential. Safe cannabis use requires gradual dose escalation, symptom tracking, and adjustment based on therapeutic response and side effects.

- Sixth, nurses must address safety, adverse effects, and risk mitigation. Cannabis use carries risks including cognitive impairment, psychiatric effects, and potential interactions with other medications. Nurses are responsible for educating patients on recognizing and managing these risks.
- The legal and ethical considerations must be incorporated into care. Regulatory variability and institutional policies influence access to and use of care, requiring nurses to remain informed and to advocate for patient-centered care within legal frameworks.

Interprofessional collaboration and ongoing education strengthen quality and safety. Oncology nurses, physicians, pharmacists, and palliative care specialists should coordinate care plans, share updates on evolving evidence, and clarify roles in assessment, prescribing, education, and follow-up. (Vinette et al., 2022) Because evidence and regulations around medical cannabis continue to evolve, institutions should provide continuing education in cannabinoid pharmacology, symptom assessment, shared decision-making, and documentation, explicitly incorporating the oncology nurse's role as educator, advocate, and safety monitor. Embedding these clinical guidelines into routine workflows allows oncology nurses to support safe, consistent, and patient-centered integration of medical cannabis into cancer and palliative care. (Shim et al., 2023)

ETHICAL CONSIDERATIONS

Nursing must evolve from passive information providers to proactive educators and safety advocates. Safety monitoring is a core responsibility, and nurses are central to this process. Oncology nurses should systematically assess for common adverse effects such as sedation, dizziness, orthostatic symptoms, cognitive changes, and mood alterations, with particular vigilance in frail, older, or polypharmacy patients. They should also actively screen for drug–drug interactions between cannabis and opioids, sedatives, antidepressants, and select chemotherapeutic agents, and promptly communicate concerns to prescribers. Regular reassessment using standardized tools for pain, nausea, sleep, and function, combined with clear documentation, supports timely dose adjustments or discontinuation when risks outweigh benefits. Vulnerable populations, older adults, patients with cognitive impairment, those with psychiatric comorbidities, or those with substance-use histories, warrant particular attention. Nurses must adjust education and monitoring strategies for these groups, including more conservative titration, closer follow-up, and explicit caregiver involvement to ensure safety and adherence. Inpatient cannabis programs that have successfully integrated nurse-led education, self-report tracking tools, and interprofessional review meetings provide useful models for structured, safe cannabis use in hospital and palliative-care settings.

Integration of cannabis education into nursing curricula and continuing professional development. The objective is to empower nurses to transition from uncertainty to active advocacy, ensuring that medicinal cannabis is integrated safely and holistically into patient treatment plans. (Wolff et al., 2026)

- Development of standardized patient education frameworks.
- Institutional policies supporting open, stigma-free communication.
- Interdisciplinary collaboration to ensure safe and evidence-based cannabis use.
- Risk screening (mental health, substance co-use, vulnerability)
- Education on safe storage, dosing variability, and formulation risks

The main ethical concerns in psychedelic research and standards of practice are equity, integrity, cultural appropriation, and epistemic justice. There were notable differences in usage between genders, with women using more psychotropic plants than men, and higher usage rates were found in patients with breast cancer and head and neck cancer. The absence of consensus among stakeholders (researchers, clinicians, patients, and regulators) on managing ethical challenges in psychedelic research and therapy. (Brittain et al., 2025) Institutional policies and legal frameworks must guide cannabis-related practice. Oncology services should adopt written protocols covering eligibility criteria, consent, prescribing processes, documentation standards, and nurse responsibilities for patients authorized to use medical cannabis. Nurses must remain informed about local regulations governing medical cannabis authorization, possession, and administration, and should carefully document patient-reported use even when cannabis is obtained outside formal medical channels. Ethical practice requires balancing respect for patient autonomy with adherence to professional standards and legal boundaries, while maintaining nonjudgmental communication even when patients use non-prescribed cannabis products. The research emphasizes the need for structured preoperative assessments of herbal use due to potential interactions with anesthetic and analgesic medications, which is crucial for enhancing perioperative safety. (Wolff et al., 2026) Future recommendations include developing clear competency frameworks, engaging with Indigenous and priority populations, establishing guidelines for Indigenous recognition, managing post trial care, and ensuring proper governance of psychedelic prescribing practices. (Rogers et al., 2026)

CONCLUSION

Oncology nurses are central agents in patient education, safety regulation, and therapeutic communication in the context of cannabis use. Cannabis use in oncology is increasing, but clinical governance, education systems, and nursing training infrastructures have not evolved in parallel. Without formal integration into oncology nursing practice frameworks, cannabis remains a parallel therapy system rather than a clinically governed supportive-care modality. Nurse-led dialogues, which emphasize nonjudgmental, structured, and proactive communication, can normalize disclosure and reduce stigma. Addressing this gap requires structured nurse-led education systems, formal safety frameworks, and institutional policy alignment, transforming cannabis from an informal coping strategy into a clinically accountable component of supportive oncology care.

REFERENCES

Ananthakumar, B., Nagaraja, B. G., Umesh, S. M., & Raghavan, R. (2025). Predictive Medicine: A New Era of Pain Management for Assistive Augmentative Rehabilitation Systems. *Predictive Algorithms for Rehabilitation and Assistive Systems*, 291–314. DOI: 10.4018/979-8-3373-0194-5.ch011

Ataiants, J., Fedorova, E. V., Cocchiaro, B., Kleber, L., Sayyid, A., Ardeleanu, K., & Lankenau, S. E. (2025). Assessing anxiety longitudinally among medical cannabis patients in Pennsylvania. *The American Journal of Drug and Alcohol Abuse*, *51*(6), 750–760. DOI: 10.1080/00952990.2025.2588273 PMID: 41368882

Baral, A., Diggs, B.-N. A., Aka, A., Williams, R., Ortega, N. H., Fellah, R. M. E., Islam, J. Y., Camacho-Rivera, M., Penedo, F. J., & Vidot, D. C. (2025). Experiences and Comfort of Young Cancer Patients Discussing Cannabis with Their Providers: Insights from a Survey at an NCI-Designated Cancer Center. *Journal of Cancer Education*, *40*(2), 256–265. DOI: 10.1007/s13187-024-02507-9 PMID: 39294413

Bellas, O. M., Cao, K., Bowen, J., Smid, S., Shakib, S., Crawford, G. B., Zannettino, A., Yeung, D. T., Kichenadasse, G., Boublik, J., Louise, J., Marker, J., Cambareri, B., Price, T., & Wardill, H. R. (2025). Medicinal CANnabis (CBD/THC) to prevent the symptoms and side effects of chemotherapy in people with advanced CANcer (CANCAN): Protocol for a phase II, randomised, double-blind, placebo-controlled trial. *BMJ Open*, *15*(3), e089336. DOI: 10.1136/bmjopen-2024-089336 PMID: 40032389

Brittain, N., Higgins, N., Barber, M., Choi, W., Carter, A., & Gardner, J. (2025). Ethical Issues and Recommendations in Psychedelic Research and Practice: A Scoping Review. *Journal of Bioethical Inquiry*. Advance online publication. DOI: 10.1007/s11673-025-10454-3 PMID: 40773130

Camp, L., Babicheva, V., Conahan, C., Hayes, S., & Sherburne Hawkins, S. (2025). Cannabis Use and Disclosure in the Oncology Setting: A Cross-Sectional Survey Exploring Information Needs Among Cancer Survivors. *Clinical Journal of Oncology Nursing*, *29*(2), 157–164. DOI: 10.1188/25.CJON.157-164 PMID: 40096564

Correa, L. G., & Tucci, A. M. (2026). Impact of Medical Cannabis on the Quality of Life of Cancer Patients: A Critical Review. *Journal of Integrative and Complementary Medicine*, *32*(1), 18–26. DOI: 10.1177/27683605251377417 PMID: 40932699

Dawson, D., Stjepanović, D., McClure-Thomas, C., Lorenzetti, V., Hall, W., Sun, T., & Leung, J. (2025). Motivations and Pathways: A Thematic Analysis of Interviews with Medicinal Cannabis Consumers in Australia. *Substance Use & Misuse*, *0*(0), 1–5. DOI: 10.1080/10826084.2025.2560074 PMID: 40970421

Dobson, O., Barber, M., Graham, M., Carter, A., & Savic, M. (2024). 'The wild west of medicine': A qualitative investigation of the factors influencing Australian health-care practitioners' delivery of medicinal cannabis. *Drug and Alcohol Review*, *43*(5), 1280–1293. DOI: 10.1111/dar.13847 PMID: 38630896

Hudspeth, R. S. (2024). Outcomes From a Decade of Risk Evaluation Mitigation Strategies and Safe Opioid Prescribing Education. *The Journal for Nurse Practitioners*, *20*(1), 104830. DOI: 10.1016/j.nurpra.2023.104830

Ilie, G., Murphy, S., MacDonald, C., & Rutledge, R. D. H. (2026). Digital delivery of a 6-month home-based empowerment program improves mental health in rural adults with chronic conditions: A single-arm prospective interventional trial. *Digital Health*, *12*, 20552076251413351. DOI: 10.1177/20552076251413351 PMID: 41585304

Joseph, L. M., & Taylor, L. (2025). Veterans' Health: Insights for Nurse Practitioner Practice. *The Journal for Nurse Practitioners*, *21*(2), 105301. DOI: 10.1016/j.nurpra.2024.105301

Kcomt, L., Veliz, P. T., Jardine, J., Evans-Polce, R. J., Clift, J., McCabe, S. E., & Arslanian-Engoren, C. (2026). Gender Diversity, Substance Cognitions, and Alcohol, Nicotine/Tobacco, and Cannabis Use Among Youth. *LGBT Health*, *13*(1), 1–10. DOI: 10.1177/23258292251385564 PMID: 41060835

Korrapati, C., Chowdareddy, S., Suresh, C., & Raghavan, R. (2026). Cancer Cell Membrane-Coated Nanoparticles: Therapeutic Advancements and Hybrid Systems. *Applications of Nanomaterials for Oncology*, 131–160. DOI: 10.4018/979-8-3373-3765-4.ch005

Kurtzman, E. T., Greene, J., Begley, R., & Drenkard, K. N. (2022). "We want what's best for patients." nurse leaders' attitudes about medical cannabis: A qualitative study. *International Journal of Nursing Studies Advances*, *4*, 100065. DOI: 10.1016/j.ijnsa.2022.100065 PMID: 38745605

Lakshmaiah, A., Korrapati, C., Suresh, C., & Raghavan, R. (2025). Synthetic Biology and AI. *Spatially Variable Genes in Cancer*, 265–290. DOI: 10.4018/979-8-3693-7728-4.ch010

Lakshmaiah, A., & Raghavan, R. (2026). Cardiovascular Protector Activity of Medicinal Mushrooms. *Medicinal Mushrooms: Conservation and Bioprospecting*, 209–218. DOI: 10.1007/978-1-0716-4993-0_28

Lintzeris, N., Arnold, J. C., McGregor, I. S., & Mills, L. (2025). Consumer perspectives of accessing medicinal cannabis treatment from cannabis clinics versus generalist health settings in Australia. *Journal of Cannabis Research*, *7*(1), 83. DOI: 10.1186/s42238-025-00338-z PMID: 41146248

McIntosh, N., Wilson, N. J., Povalej, P., Hunt, L., & Lewis, P. (2024). An Exploration of Registered Nurses' Experiences Caring for Patients Taking Medicinal Cannabis. *Nursing Open*, *11*(10), e70063. DOI: 10.1002/nop2.70063 PMID: 39455290

Nahler, G. (2024). Phytocannabinoids as Chemotherapy Adjuncts—A Review for Users. *Onco*, *4*(4), 287–321. DOI: 10.3390/onco4040021

Nanjundeshwara, N., Lakshmaiah, A., & Raghavan, R. (2025). Aflatoxigenic Fungi. *Aflatoxigenic Fungi*, 225–239. DOI: 10.1201/9781003487043-29

Pallavi, V. N., Chowdareddy, S., Byalahunasishetter, B. I., & Raghavan, R. (2026). CRISPR-Cas9 Technology for Precision Cancer Medicine: Target Discovery, Disease Modeling, and Therapeutics. *CRISPR-Cas9 Technology for Precision Medicine*, 35–72. DOI: 10.4018/979-8-3373-4857-5.ch002

Raghavan, R., Moger, S. S., Umesh, S., & Bhuvana, G. N. (2025). Revolutionizing Pain Management. *Unveiling Technological Advancements and Interdisciplinary Solutions for Pain Care*, 129–164. DOI: 10.4018/979-8-3693-9501-1.ch005

Raziani, Y., Sarkar, S., Zaidi, M., & Poghosyan, H. (2025). Prevalence and determinants of cigarette-cannabis co-use among US cancer survivors. *Journal of Cancer Survivorship: Research and Practice*. Advance online publication. DOI: 10.1007/s11764-025-01789-2 PMID: 40156654

Reddy, A. C., Wilson, P., Shah, J., Schmitz, N., & Chewning, B. (2026). Use of cannabis in psychological symptom management among patients with cancer: A narrative review. *Journal of the American Pharmacists Association*, *66*(1), 102954. Advance online publication. DOI: 10.1016/j.japh.2025.102954

Rogers, A. H., Pester, B. D., Fligelman, S. J., Pielech, M., Groenewald, C. B., Ketterl, T. G., Vest, B. M., & Palermo, T. M. (2026). Pediatric Oncology Providers' Perceptions on Pain Management and Opioid Use for Adolescents and Young Adults With Cancer: A Qualitative Study. *Pediatric Blood & Cancer, n/a*(n/a), e70131. DOI: 10.1002/1545-5017.70131

Shim, M., Nguyen, H., & Grootendorst, P. (2023). Lessons from 20 years of medical cannabis use in Canada. *PLoS One, 18*(3), e0271079. DOI: 10.1371/journal.pone.0271079 PMID: 36952564

Valente, A. C., Lopes, L. P. N., & Matheus, M. E. (2024). Medical cannabis use in oncology and associated outcomes: A scoping review. *Journal of Oncology Pharmacy Practice, 30*(4), 737–751. DOI: 10.1177/10781552241239006 PMID: 38477532

Vinette, B., Côté, J., & Bilodeau, K. (2022, December 17). (2022). Evaluation of a Digital Educational Intervention to Enhance Oncology Nurse Professional Practice to Support Safe Cannabis Use: A Pilot Study. *The Journal of Continuing Education in the Health Professions*. Advance online publication. DOI: 10.1097/CEH.0000000000000631 PMID: 41427816

Wolff, A., Hübner, J., Büntzel, J., & Büntzel, J. (2026). Psychotropic Medicinal Plant Use in Oncology: A Dual-Cohort Analysis and Its Implications for Anesthesia and Perioperative Care. *Applied Sciences (Basel, Switzerland), 16*(1), 481. DOI: 10.3390/app16010481

Zaidi, M., Sarkar, S., Arakelyan, S., & Poghosyan, H. (2024). Relationship Between Fatalistic Cancer Beliefs and Risky Health Behaviors. *Western Journal of Nursing Research, 46*(10), 757–765. DOI: 10.1177/01939459241273388 PMID: 39161288

KEY TERMS AND DEFINITIONS

Artificial Intelligence (AI): Broad field using data-driven algorithms (including ML and deep learning) to support clinical decisions, automate symptom monitoring, and personalize cannabis-based oncology care.

Cancer Cachexia: A syndrome of severe weight loss and muscle wasting in cancer patients; computational models and multiomics approaches help identify optimal cannabis-based interventions to alleviate symptoms.

Cannabinoid Interactions: Modeling how different cannabinoids (THC, CBD) interact with each other and patient-specific factors, using AI to optimize combinations for cancer symptom management.

Cannabinoid-Receptor Binding Prediction: Computational modeling (using AI or quantum algorithms) to predict how cannabinoids interact with specific receptors, informing selection and dosing of cannabis-based treatments for cancer patients.

Chatbots for Patient Education: Conversational AI systems delivering tailored information and guidance to cancer patients about cannabis use, improving engagement and adherence.

Clinical Decision Support: AI-powered tools that provide evidence-based recommendations (cannabis dosing, symptom management) to clinicians, enhancing oncology care.

CNN (Convolutional Neural Network): Deep learning models that extract features from structured data (medical images, genomics) to personalize cannabis regimens and assess risk of side effects.

Deep Learning Advanced ML: using multi-layered neural networks to analyze complex data (genomics, patient histories), helping discover optimal cannabis formulations and predict individual responses.

Edge Devices / Wearables for Palliative Monitoring: Sensor-equipped technologies worn by patients to continuously monitor physiological and behavioral data, supporting real-time, personalized interventions and remote management of cannabis-based therapies in oncology.

LSTM (Long Short-Term Memory): A neural network type designed for sequential data (daily symptom logs), enabling accurate prediction of symptom escalation or relief with cannabis therapies.

Machine Learning (ML): Algorithms that learn from patient data (symptoms, genomics) to support personalized cannabis dosing and predict symptom changes, reducing trial-and-error in oncology care.

Multiomics: Integration of diverse biological data types (genomics, proteomics, metabolomics) to provide a comprehensive view of patient biology, supporting personalized cannabis therapies and biomarker identification for cancer symptom management.

Neuromorphic Computing: Brain-inspired hardware and algorithms that mimic neural processing, enabling ultra-low-power, real-time analysis of biomedical data for remote symptom monitoring and adaptive cannabis dosing in oncology.

Opioid-Sparing: AI-driven analytics to identify cannabis regimens that reduce opioid use in cancer pain management, minimizing opioid-related risks and side effects.

Patient Response Modeling: AI/ML techniques that predict how individual cancer patients will respond to cannabis therapies, integrating clinical and genomic data for tailored interventions.

Predictive Analytics for Dosing: ML models that analyze individual patient data to forecast optimal cannabis dosing, aiming to maximize benefits and minimize side effects in cancer treatment.

QDRL (Quantum Deep Reinforcement Learning): Integrates quantum computing with deep reinforcement learning to optimize sequential decision-making, potentially improving adaptive dosing and treatment planning in cannabis-based oncology care.

Quantum Computing: Uses quantum bits (qubits) and phenomena like superposition and entanglement for massively parallel computations, enabling simulation of complex molecular interactions (cannabinoid-receptor binding) and accelerating drug discovery.

Quantum ML (Hybrid/Quantum-Enhanced Neural Networks): Combines quantum computing with classical neural networks to enhance pattern recognition and prediction, such as matching cannabinoids to patient-specific cancer profiles or forecasting symptom trajectories.

Qubit Limitations: Challenges in quantum hardware (limited qubit numbers, short coherence times, error rates) that currently constrain the scalability and practical application of quantum algorithms in drug discovery and personalized oncology.

Spiking Neural Networks (SNNs): Neural networks that process information via discrete spikes, emulating biological neurons effective for analyzing temporal biomedical signals (pain) in wearables for personalized palliative care and cannabis response prediction.

Superposition and Entanglement: Quantum properties allowing qubits to exist in multiple states and be interdependent, enabling efficient simulation of molecular systems and optimization of cannabis compound effects in cancer care.

Symptom Trajectory Forecasting: Use of ML/deep learning to predict how symptoms like pain or nausea will evolve, enabling proactive cannabis-based interventions for cancer patients.

VQE (Variational Quantum Eigensolver): A hybrid quantum-classical algorithm for finding lowest energy states of molecules, valuable for simulating cannabinoid-receptor interactions and optimizing drug candidates for oncology.

Chapter 12
Bridging Comfort and Care:
The Role of the Cannabis Nurse in Palliative and End-of-Life Care

Lesley Anne Affeldt
http://orcid.org/0009-0004-3204-7839
Integrative Holistics Nursing Corp, USA

ABSTRACT

Cannabis nurses play a transformative role in palliative and end-of-life care through integrating cannabis-based therapies to enhance comfort, dignity, and emotional well-being for patients with life-limiting conditions. Cannabis nursing uniquely bridges conventional palliative care and evolving therapeutic options, positioning cannabis nurses as key advocates, educators, and caregivers. This chapter reviews the specialty of palliative care, explores the advocacy and holistic management roles of cannabis nurses, and discusses the therapeutic benefits and challenges of cannabis in symptom management. By combining professional knowledge with compassionate care, cannabis nurses are reshaping palliative medicine and calling for greater recognition of their contributions amongst healthcare organizations, policymakers, and educators.

INTRODUCTION

The specialties of Palliative, Hospice, and Cannabis nursing combine perfectly to address the multimodal needs of patients and their families. The aim of this chapter is to offer insight into palliative and hospice care and how cannabis nursing benefits patients with chronic life-limiting or terminal illnesses. As you read, you will learn

DOI: 10.4018/979-8-2600-2035-7.ch012

about the philosophies of palliative and hospice care focusing on symptom relief and stress reduction to improve the quality of life for patients and their families. Ethical principles guide all nurses. Cannabis nurses embody advocacy, justice, autonomy, and nonmaleficence by supporting patient access to cannabis-based treatments. This chapter addresses the therapeutic use of cannabis-based therapies in palliative and end-of-life care to manage symptoms and improve comfort, dignity, and emotional well-being. The author will outline challenges and barriers in cannabis nursing for this vulnerable population. Practice application will demonstrate how cannabis-based therapies fit within our nursing practice. In closing, this chapter will address future directions for cannabis nursing in palliative and end-of-life care, and part with a call to action.

A BRIEF HISTORY OF PALLIATIVE AND HOSPICE CARE

Palliative care emerged from the modern Hospice movement of the 1960s. Dr. Cicely Saunders, a nurse, social worker, and physician, founded St. Christopher's Hospice in 1967, London. Her work focused on whole-person care encompassing physical, psychological, social, and spiritual suffering in those with terminal diseases. In 1969, Elizabeth Kubler-Ross's book, "On Death and Dying" further changed attitudes about end-of-life care. In 1971, Dr. Florence Wald, Yale Dean of Nursing, launched the American Hospice movement by opening Connecticut Hospice. She later developed a Hospice Education Program for nurses at Yale University School of Nursing (Hospice and Palliative Nurses Association & American Nurses Association, 2025). Palliative care grew from the hospice model, which was first focused cancer patients with short prognoses. Advances in cancer and chronic disease treatments now allow palliative care to last longer, providing support during both periods of decline and stabilization along the disease journey.

Palliative care is a medical sub-specialty for those facing serious, chronic, or life-limiting illnesses gaining official recognition within the United States in 2006. It addresses physical, emotional, social, and spiritual suffering with an interdisciplinary approach, helping patients and families navigate care decisions as well as manage transitions in care. The interdisciplinary team, including palliative physicians, nurses, social workers, and chaplains, supports patients by ensuring continuity of care, facilitating care planning, and promoting comfort and dignity throughout their disease trajectory. Palliative care can be provided at any age or stage of serious illness and may occur alongside curative treatment. Individuals may benefit from palliative care for years, depending on their diagnosis and disease course (National Coalition for Hospice and Palliative Care, 2018).

National Coalition For Hospice And Palliative Care (2018).*Clinical practice guidelines for quality palliative care*. National Coalition For Hospice And Palliative Care defines palliative care as:

> *Palliative care focuses on expert assessment and management of pain and other symptoms, support for caregiver needs, and coordination of care. Palliative care attends to the physical, functional, psychological, practical, and spiritual consequences of a serious illness. It is a person– and family-centered approach to care, providing people living with serious illness relief from the symptoms and stress of their illness. Early integration into the care plan for seriously ill patients improves the quality of life for both the patient and the family.*

National Coalition For Hospice And Palliative Care (2018). *Clinical practice guidelines for quality palliative care* further outline eight core care domains, setting the framework for providing high- quality, patient-and family-centered palliative care as follows:

- Structure and Processes of Care – Focuses on organizational and care-delivery structures.
- Physical Care – Pain and symptom management.
- Psychological and Psychiatric Care – Attending to emotional and mental health.
- Spiritual, Religious, and Existential Care – Address spiritual needs and beliefs.
- Social Aspects – Navigating the social determinants of patients and families.
- Cultural Sensitivity – Honoring diverse values and traditions.
- End-of-Life care – Provides compassionate, patient-focused end-of-life care.
- Ethical and Legal Aspects of Care – Upholding autonomy and informed decision-making pertaining to palliative needs.

Aside from Palliative Care as its own specialty, it is important to know the terms primary palliative care or generalist palliative care. This is palliative care provided by non-specialists. Examples include primary care providers, disease-oriented specialists (e.g., oncologists and nephrologists), as well as nurses, social workers, pharmacists, or chaplains who are not certified in palliative care. Nursing always seeks to relieve suffering and advocate for patients, their families, and their communities. This embodies all principles of palliative nursing.

Hospice

Hospice-focused care is a philosophy of care for patients with end-stage, life-limiting diseases. It applies when disease-modifying treatments have failed or patients no longer seek treatment. Hospice requires specific criteria for enrollment. Medicare requires a prognosis of six months or less, physician certification, and agreement with a comfort-focused care plan. Many private and commercial insurance plans also offer hospice benefits with similar requirements. Regular patient evaluation ensures they continue to meet hospice criteria.

When comfort and quality become the main goals, hospice offers crucial support for patients and families through an interdisciplinary team. This period can be incredibly stressful, so a hospice team provides reassurance and comfort. Hospice also gives bereavement support to families for 13 months after their loved one's death. Palliative care can start at diagnosis and continue without a time limit. Hospice care is for the advanced or terminal phase of illness and requires specific eligibility. All end-of-life care involves those in the imminent death phase, regardless of hospice status. Not all palliative care is hospice or end-of-life care, but all hospice and end-of-life care is palliative.

Palliative Care is a unique specialty. It centers on patient-focused, whole-person care that honors each patient and their family's personal goals. Care aims to meet people where they are, relieve suffering in every domain, clarify care goals, and improve quality of life as patients define it. Palliative and hospice specialists are expert educators. They give information, support, and guidance about the disease, manage side effects, and help with informed decisions. Patients and families are active in care planning to align care with their goals.

Palliative, Hospice, and the Cannabis Nurse

Now that the specialties of palliative and hospice care have been addressed, let us explore the perfect adjunctive specialty of cannabis nursing. Much of what palliative and hospice specialists do is expertly manage disease symptoms, medication, and treatment side effects. Cannabis has many clinically approved indications, as well as patient and caregiver anecdotal support confirming that cannabis medicine provides critical relief and improves quality of life for those suffering (Doppen et al., 2022). Having nurses who can competently assist patients and caregivers navigate cannabis as a valuable medicine is a growing necessity. In 2023, the American Nursing Association (ANA, 2023) recognized Cannabis Nursing as a nursing specialty. Patients utilizing cannabis-based medicines are increasing at a staggering rate now that most states offer either medical use, adult use, or both. However, they are most often left to navigate products and dosing on their own through self-research, family and friends, or budtender recommendations. Physicians and medical professionals are grossly undereducated when it comes to the endocannabinoid system, medical cannabis indications, leaving them unable to offer basic education, administration, and dosage guidance to assist their patients. The intention here is not to blame medical professionals for this shortcoming, as it is a complicated issue that includes systemic bias, a lack of medical institutional buy-in, local and national bureaucracy, and politics, among other factors.

Incorporating the knowledge of cannabis-based medicine within the specialties of palliative and hospice care offers patients and families the benefit of highly skilled counsel. This guidance provides patients access to cannabis-medicines that provide symptom relief and, in many cases, improve the effectiveness of other medications, resulting in dosage reductions or discontinuation of other pharmaceuticals. This is often a welcome benefit as most patients and families desire deprescribing and simplifying medication regimens whenever possible.

ETHICAL PRINCIPLES

Nursing is guided by core ethical principles that should be practiced and applied in every patient experience and professional nursing encounter. The ANA, in partnership with ACNA, published the *Cannabis Nursing Scope and Standards of Practice* (2024), *Cannabis: A Handbook for Nurses* by Carey S. Clark (2021) as well as the HPNA *Scope, Standards, and Competencies for the Hospice and Palliative RN and APRN* (2025) offers clear and succinct guidance that this author will be referencing throughout this section.

The profession of nursing, regardless of the specialty, is guided by core principles of ethics, including autonomy, justice, beneficence, and nonmaleficence. Within the specialty of palliative and hospice care these principles expand to include advocating for informed decision making, interdisciplinary and multidisciplinary collaboration, legal and ethical counseling when appropriate. Nurses must embody a devotion to the advancement of the specialty of palliative care through responsible research, promotes health equity through cultural competence and championing social justice, and uphold a professional and viable healthcare environment practicing fiduciary competence (Hospice And Palliative Nurses Association & American Nurses Association, 2025, p. 23). In addition to what has been previously mentioned, the specialty of cannabis nursing requires nurses to act with high fidelity to the principles of totality and integrity, as well as knowledge of local and federal cannabis laws. "Cannabis care nurses are called to be caring, compassionate, social justice warriors to ensure that all patients in need have the opportunity to access cannabis therapeutics along their palliative and healing journeys" (Clark, 2021, p. 271).

Autonomy

Autonomy is respecting patients' beliefs and health care wishes, even when they differ from your own, and recognizing patients' right to make their own decisions as they navigate their disease process. We do this as "advocates for the rights of cannabis health care consumers and populations regarding informed decision-making and self-determination in relation to cannabis as a medicine" (American Nurses Association & American Cannabis Nurses Association, 2024, p. 71). Providing appropriate education and support is key to helping patients make well-informed care decisions. Once a decision is made, the nurse must have the confidence to fully support the patient with ongoing education and treatment coaching. Let us consider some possible situations you may come across when supporting a patient's autonomy.

- The patient would like to utilize cannabis as medicine, and their provider is non-supportive and/or dismissive.
- Perhaps the patient's family or support system is not supportive and discourages the use of cannabis medicine.

How would you apply your critical thinking skills to support the patient's autonomy while being responsive to fellow colleagues/peers and family members' concerns?

Justice

When nurses advocate for Justice, we consider the geographical, societal, cultural, political, and economic determinants of the health care disparities our patients may be experiencing. "Practice cannabis nursing from a framework of caring ethics and social justice with a non-discriminatory, caring and compassionate approach" (American Nurses Association & American Cannabis Nurses Association, 2024, p.73) is a great way to ensure we maintain a big-picture perspective when caring for our patients. Whether cannabis is being utilized as medicine or recreationally, it still carries with it continued discrimination, bias, stigma, and fear associated with its utilization. Unfortunately, access to cannabis medicine is still not equal. A patient's geographic location greatly affects one's access. People of color, those living in lower-income communities, have been and continue to be disproportionately targeted with increased legal consequences compared to someone from a wealthier white community. Many who were prosecuted and incarcerated for cannabis infractions prior to cannabis laws changing in their state still have not been exonerated and remain incarcerated, though the law and public views have changed. Confronting social justice issues is an active, ongoing topic that nurses are perfectly positioned to tackle. As nurses, we do this by remaining curious, continually expanding our knowledge, and applying best practices. Embracing the role of educator, taking every opportunity to share our knowledge with peers, patients, and our communities. It is imperative to stay current with local and federal laws to properly advise our patients and care facilities. As nurses we must never stop advocating and moving the needle of progress forward for our patients, improving the overall health of our communities.

Beneficence

Beneficence, in its simplest definition, is the art of doing good. Nurses have an ethical duty to do nothing that would promote harm, always weighing risks versus benefits. This means our patients are well informed about treatment options, allowing them to make the best decision that is consistent with their care goals. Cannabis has many indications in the treatment of many palliative diseases process. The nurse provides education about using cannabis medicine as it is a viable treatment option for many indications throughout a patient's entire palliative journey. Carey Clark, in her book, *Cannabis: A Handbook for Nurses*, gives a great example outlining a learning opportunity of cannabis care at the end of life, focusing on the ethical practice of beneficence:

> *When we consider the principle of beneficence, it becomes clear that we want patients to experience 'more good than harm' in their end-of-life care. If cannabis can help support quality of life at the end of life, despite the lack of phase II/III clinical trials, shouldn't the hospice team or physician be ethically obligated to suggest the use of cannabis for palliation at the end of life? Carey Clark further challenges nurses: if you were working in a legal cannabis state, where hospice patients can access medical cannabis at the end of life, how might you use the ethical principle of beneficence, in combination with your knowledge of cannabinoid therapeutics, to guide your conversation with health care providers, the hospice team, patients, and caregivers? (p. 375)*

Nonmaleficence

Nonmaleficence, at its core, is avoiding harm, or the intent to do the least amount of harm in some cases. Let us consider a plausible scenario that Carey Clark proposes as a case study in her book, *Cannabis: A Handbook for Nurses*:

> *In brief, a 72-year-old female with a diagnosis of stage II uterine cancer just started her chemotherapy treatment. She reported that she had lost all her hair after her first round of chemo. She shares that she is having abdominal pain that radiates to her back. The patient is using a mixture of opioids and low-dose whole plant cannabis 5 mg THC TID. However, the patient continues to have frequent nausea, fatigue, anxiety, and depression. She shares that the chemotherapy is*

ruining her life, and she wants to speak with her oncologist about stopping her current chemotherapy treatment and using full-spectrum cannabis oil (FECO) to cure her cancer. The patient has asked her palliative nurse with cannabis care education to assist her with this conversation. The patient reports that she wants to feel better so she can enjoy being with her grandchildren. (p. 377)

- How would you apply the ethical decision-making process, considering the principle of nonmaleficence?
- What further information might you need to gather from the patient and other sources?
- How would you best use motivational interviewing?
- Does the decision-making process change if this were a minor or a person deemed vulnerable?
- Do ethical issues change if the diagnosis, staging, and/or prognosis change?

What are your thoughts? How would you best support this patient from a nonmaleficence perspective? Are there other ethical principles that should also guide your counseling?

Fidelity, Totality, and Integrity

The ethical principles of fidelity, totality, and integrity provide the foundation for our nursing compasses. Fidelity upholds patient/community trust, safety, and the integrity of the nursing practice. Totality is an ethical approach a nurse takes, guaranteeing that all decisions consider the well-being of the whole person. Weighing the benefits versus the adverse effects, does the *greater good* outweigh the *bad*? When patients use cannabis medicine, they may experience side effects (This can usually be remedied with a dose or chemovar modification). We must evaluate whether this side effect is interfering with the overall benefit the patient is receiving. The nursing profession, regardless of specialty, is foundationally driven by our code of ethics. With nursing entering its 23rd consecutive year as the most honest and ethical profession, we are tasked with continuing this legacy for those who came before us and those who will come after.

APPLYING CANNABIS-BASED THERAPIES IN PALLIATIVE CARE

Therapeutic application of cannabis-based therapies in palliative and end-of-life care has proven to be clinically significant in managing many symptoms, providing enhanced comfort, dignity, and emotional well-being for patients facing life-limiting illnesses. This is not a new or novel idea. Cannabis medicine has been utilized palliatively since the earliest civilizations and throughout history. Dr. William O'Shaugnessy in 1838, utilized cannabis in the treatment of epilepsy, rheumatic pains and fatal tetanus with "remarkable success" (Russo, 2018). Though cannabis-based medicine has been in use for thousands of years, we are still lacking high-quality human studies to support palliative cannabis use. Most data to date is composed of meta-analysis, observational, expert and anecdotal data that support palliative patients utilizing cannabis-based medicine. "The results for the improvement of symptoms and the quality of life of palliative patients are excellent, with an improvement in adverse effects, anxiolytic, antitumor, antiemetic, and analgesic with synergism with opioid actions and increased appetite, improved sleep, and significant reduction of the drug load of these patients" (da Costa & de Carvalho, 2022). Dr. Beckes points out, "WAMM, the respected Santa Cruz medical cannabis collective, has specialized in cannabis palliative care with a range of terminal illnesses and reported remarkable success for over two decades" (Beckes, 2017, p. 250). This is not to say that we do not have quality phase II/III RCTs data supporting medicinal cannabis use in supporting palliative symptom management, as we do. We need more!

Providing education on best-practice titration strategies remains essential to assisting patients minimize adverse effects and gradually develop tolerance to the psychoactive effects of THC. It is important to remember that therapeutic benefit does not require experiencing psychoactive or intoxicating effects. Medicinal cannabis users typically prefer CBD-dominant chemovars with small amounts of THC, in contrast to recreational consumers. For patients with chronic conditions and complicated symptomology, long-acting oral and transdermal formulations should serve as the foundation of therapy, with vaporized (inhaled) products reserved for prn (as needed) use to manage breakthrough or exacerbated symptoms. Incorporating CBD can assist in tempering unwanted THC-related psychoactivity if taken 60-90 minutes prior, particularly during daytime use or when activities require preserved cognitive function.

It is important to remember that nurses can provide coaching regarding patients and their cannabis use. This would include providing information and education on the ECS, different cannabinoids, administration methods, titration, Certification of Analysis (COA), safety, storage, adverse effects, drug interactions, and contraindications. Nurses cannot procure, handle, or administer cannabis-based medicine in many locations. It is imperative that nurses stay up to date with their local, state, and federal cannabis laws. Providing education on the procurement of cannabis- based medicine, reading cannabis product labels, and requesting Certificate of Analysis (COA) is important to ensure that patients are consuming safe, quality products. In addition to a comprehensive medical review and assessment, motivational interviewing is a beneficial tool for understanding the desire/need for medicinal cannabis. A key principle within the palliative care model is goals of care planning. Understanding what the patient values and desires from their care should drive their individualized treatment plan. With all cannabis use, it would be beneficial to have the patient keep a medication diary to log each dose, frequency, and chemovar/terpene profile along with insightful details of its effects to determine if the medication is addressing the desired need as well as any adverse side effects experienced.

The Endocannabinoid System (ECS)

Why does the cannabis plant offer such wonderful therapeutic benefits? Dr. Ethan Russo explains it well in his paper, Beyond Cannabis: Plants and the Endocannabinoid System. *Trends in Pharmacological Sciences*, "There is hardly any physiological process that is not affected by it to some degree: pain, movement, emotion, digestion, skin, and even bone health. It is surprising then to realize that the ESC was unknown prior to three decades ago." It is concerning to say that most physicians and clinical professionals continue to be undereducated regarding the ECS and, along with it, the benefits of cannabis-based medicines. The ECS is an important system that utilizes endogenous cannabinoids, regulated by regulatory enzymes and receptors, to monitor and maintain homeostasis. When the ECS is in a deficit or excess for prolonged periods, many believe this initiates disease processes and leads to an unfortunate progression. The body can be prompted to optimize the ECS using holistic practices such as diet, exercise, sleep, and activities that promote joy (music, art, dance, meditation, yoga, etc.). Cannabis-based medicine can be a good supplement to a holistic, mindful practice to promote balance within the ECS. "The endocannabinoid system is a recently discovered regulatory physiologic system that holds great promise for improvements in human quality of life. To date, it has not received the attention that it deserves in physician and patient education, nor in research expenditures. Should these shortcomings be rectified, it stands to reason that the public health would benefit enormously" (Russo, 2016).

Chemovar

Let us now explore the different chemovar types and their benefits. First, it is not appropriate to refer to cannabis types as "Strains". The cannabis plant is not a bacteria nor virus. As medical professionals, we are professionally tasked with ensuring we use the most appropriate terminology. This will translate to properly educated peers, patients, and the community. The Cannabis plant (Chemovar) has dominant cannabinoids that identify its Chemovar type. THC (Tetrahydrocannabinol) and CBD (Cannabidiol) are the most common cannabinoids found in cannabis;

there are over 100 that have been identified with many holistic benefits of their own. Below is a table outlining the Chemovar type and its content description.

Table 1. Chemovar types based on information from Your Cannabis CBD:THC Ratio, Uwe Blesching, Ph.D., pp 13-14. 2020

Chemovar Type	**Dominate Cannabinoid Content**	**Description**
I	THC	Dominate THC content
II	THC/CBD	Balanced THC:CBD ratio
III	CBD	Dominate CBD content
IV	CBG	Dominate CBG content
V	No/Minimal Cannabinoid	No/Minimal cannabinoid content
VI	THCV	Dominate THCV content

Terpenoids

Once we identify the appropriate chemovar type, we need to identify the terpenoid profile that would be most beneficial. "Terpenes are the aromatic compounds in fruits, vegetables, trees, a few insects, and flowering plants, with over 50,000 terpenes found in nature and over 100 different terpenes identified in cannabis" (Clark, 2021, p. 123). Terpenes give cannabis its fragrances and flavors and provide the plant with natural protection from insects, animals, fungi, bacteria, and other environmental stressors.

The most prevalent terpenoids are referred to as major terpenoids, and the less prominent, minor terpenoids. As terpenes have their own notable medicinal benefits when paired with the appropriate Chemovar Type, this leads to the most ideal therapeutic outcome for the patient. The table below, "Common Major and Minor Terpenes," is provided for your review.

Table 2. Major & minor terpenoids and their primary effects based on information from Clark, 2021, pp.125-128

Major Terpenes	**Effects**
Myrcene	Analgesic, anti-inflammatory, antibacterial, antifungal, antioxidant, neuroprotective, sedating and relaxing effects
Limonene	Antioxidant, anxiolytic, antibacterial, mood elevator, antifungal, antiacid, stress reducer

continued on following page

Table 2. Continued

Pinene	Anti-inflammatory, bronchodilator, expectorant, antibiotic, analgesic, anticonvulsant
Caryophyllene (Terpene & Cannabinoid)	Anti-inflammatory, antianxiety, mood elevator, anticancer, antibacterial, analgesic effect
Humulene	Anorectic, anti-inflammatory, antibacterial, antineoplastic, analgesic effect
Linalool	Anti-inflammatory, antianxiety, antidepressant, antileptic, boost immunity, calming, sedating effect
Terpinolene	Antianxiety, anticancer, sedation, cognitive clarity
Camphene	Cholesterol and triglyceride reducer
Terpineol	Antibacterial, antioxidant, calming, sedative
Minor Terpenes	**Effects**
a-bisabolol	Antibacterial and analgesic
Borneol	Insect repellent, anticancer
Carene	Analgesic, improves memory
Eucalyptol	Analgesic, antibacterial, antifungal
Geraniol	Neuroprotectant, antioxidant
Ocimene	Anti-inflammatory, antiviral, antifungal
Nerolidol	Antifungal, antioxidant, antimicrobial, anti-inflammatory
Phellandrene	Antifungal

Routes of Administration

The route of administration will have a direct effect on how the cannabis medicine is absorbed and processed. It would be beneficial to investigate in detail the pharmacokinetics and pharmacodynamics of cannabis to fully understand this process. Below is a table outlining the different routes of administration, the onset and duration of effects, and the pros and cons of each route.

Table 3. Routes of administration based on information from MacCallum & Russo, 2018; Clark, 2021, p. 139; Goldstein, 2020, pp. 121-126

Route	Onset (min.)	Duration (hr.)	Pro's	Con's
Inhalation Smoking / Vaporization	5-10	2-4	Good for acute, episodic symptoms (Nausea, Breakthrough Pain). Avoid first- pass metabolism for a faster onset and more potent effect. Vaporization is considerably less harmful than smoking.	Multi step process requires good dexterity. Vaporizers can be expensive. Portability is an issue. Noxious odor associated with use. Smoking is not recommended for medicinal patients due to pulmonary irritation and harmful biproducts.
Oral ingestion	60-180	6-8	More discrete, convenient, no noxious odor associated with use. Better for longer symptom control.	Delayed onset can make titration a bit more challenging. Higher risk for over medicating.
Oromucosal - Nabiximol (Sativex)	15-45	6-8	Pharmaceutical preparation (Nabiximols) has a documented safety and efficacy use profile for many clinical indications. Avoid first-pass metabolism for a faster onset.	Unfortunately, it does not have FDA approval in the USA. (Currently approved in 30 countries). It is an expensive preparation.
Topical	10-30	3-6	Good for local applications, less systemic effect.	Only affects local area. Generally, it has a superficial benefit.
Suppository PR	15-30	4-8	May address local, GI disorders and pelvic symptoms. Avoids first-pass metabolism.	Absorption is variable, making it a challenge to treat symptoms systemically. Titration is challenging
Suppository PV	15-30	4-12	May address many gynecological symptoms. The female reproductive tract has many endocannabinoid receptors. Avoids first-pass metabolism.	Oil-based suppositories can compromise the integrity of latex condoms. Use oil-resistant products, such as nitrile or polyurethane, if appropriate.

When initiating cannabis-based medicine, the recommendation is always to start low and slow. The treatment dose is the lowest dose that addresses the symptom with little to no side effects. It will take time to fine-tune the dose. Everyone is unique and dosing needs to be patient-specific. Most medical cannabis patients will utilize between 1 and 3 g of herbal cannabis per day. To help visualize this, a standard paperclip weighs 1 g.

Table 4. Inhalation titration method THC & CBD based on information from Clark, 2021, p. 144

Inhalation	Time (min.)	Instructions
1	15	Start with 1 inhalation, then wait at least 15min.
1	15-30	May increase by 1 inhalation every 15-30 min. until the desired symptom is controlled. A higher THC content should yield to a lower amount needed to achieve symptom control.

The recommendation for oral dosing is to start THC-dominant cannabis medicine at bedtime (HS) to help the patient adjust and develop some tolerance to the THC while limiting adverse effects. When starting a THC-dominant cannabis medicine during the day, think about a more stimulating chemovar unless sedation is the desired effect. Following the same principle as at bedtime (HS), continue increasing by 1.5-2.5 mg every 2 days up to 15 mg, divided BID or TID. It is not common for patients to require more than 20-30 mg/day. This puts patients at increased risk of adverse events and induced tolerance, without the benefits of efficacy. When initiating CBD remember, Cannabidiol is biphasic, meaning it is energizing and uplifting at lower doses and sedating at higher doses. It may take several weeks of medication adjustments for the patient to reach the desired therapeutic benefit. When utilizing a chemovar with both CBD and THC, the THC component is what you would use to guide your dosing and titration recommendations. Epidiolex is the only FDA-approved CBD that is 98% pure CBD isolate medication. The table below is provided as a reference for oral cannabis-based medicine initiation and titration.

Table 5. Oral titration method of THC & CBD based on information from Clark, 2021, p. 144

Days	Dose	Instruction THC Dominate Bedtime Initiation & Titration
1-2	2.5 mg	Start at bedtime (HS), may start at lower dose 1.25 mg for young, elderly, or other concerns.
3-4	1.25-2.5 mg	Increase if previous dose was well tolerated at bedtime (HS).
5-6	1.25-2.5 mg	Continue to increase at HS every 2 days if well tolerated until the patients desires effect is achieved. If adverse effects are noted, reduce back to last well tolerated dose.
Days	**Dose**	**Instructions THC Dominate Daytime Initiation & Titration**
1-2	2.5 mg	Start with administration once per day.
3-4	2.5 mg	May increase to twice per day BID.
Days	**Dose**	**Instructions CBD Dominate Initiation & Titration**

continued on following page

Table 5. Continued

1-3	5-10 mg	Starting dose, prefer during the day as lower doses can have an energizing benefit.
3-6	5-10 mg	Increase every 3-4 days until the patient feels their symptoms have improved. May divide dosing to BID or TID if indicated. If a dose is required at bedtime, a reduced or half-dose may be wise, as at lower doses, CBD can interfere with sleep and be alerting to some.

Disease Processes / Symptomology

When we think about all the potential palliative and terminal disease processes that cannabis medicine could be utilized for, it can feel overwhelming. This section will outline specific symptoms, as many disease processes share similar symptomology. The table below is a good representation of many of the conditions with associated symptoms that can be addressed with cannabis medicine; it is certainly not all-inclusive.

Table 6. Symptomology for which cannabis-based treatments have been utilized based on information from MacCallum & Russo, 2018; Russo, 2018, p.5; Clark, 2021, p.220, NASEM Report; Goldstein, 2020, pp. 290-301; Blesching, 2020, pp.195-207.

Symptomology	Suggested Cannabinoid / Terpene Profile	Level of Evidence
Agitation / Aggression	THC, CBD, linalool, myrcene, borneol, nerolidol, terpinolene	Limited, Observational, Anecdotal
Anorexia/Cachexia	THC, CBD, CBG	Limited
Anxiety	CBD, THC (low dose), THCA, CBDA, linalool, limonene, myrcene	Limited
Cancers (including Glioma)	THC, THCA, CBD, CBG	Insufficient
Chronic Pain	THC, CBD, CBDA, nabiximol, beta-myrcene, beta-caryophyllene	Conclusive / Substantial
CINV (Chemo Induced Nausea & Vomiting)	THC, THCA, CBD, CBDA, nabiximol	Conclusive / Substantial
Depression	THC, CBD, CBG, CBC, limonene, linalool, myrcene	Limited
Epilepsy (Dravet and Lennox-Gastaut Syndrome)	Cannabidiol (Epidiolex), CBD, THC (low dose), linalool	Conclusive / Substantial
EOL Symptomology- anxiety, pain, terminal agitation, restlessness, SOD, depression	THC, CBD, linalool, myrcene, caryophyllene, alpha-pinene, limonene	Limited, Insufficient, Anecdotal
Glaucoma- intraocular pressure	THC, CBD	Moderate

continued on following page

Table 6. Continued

Symptomology	Suggested Cannabinoid / Terpene Profile	Level of Evidence
IBS symptoms	THC, CBD, THCA, CBDA, limonene, alpha-pinene, beta-caryophyllene, terpinolene	Insufficient, Observational, Anecdotal
Inflammation	THC, THCA, THCV, CBD, CBDA, CBC, CBD, CBDA, CBG, alpha-bisabolol, beta-caryophyllene, alpha-pinene, geraniol, limonene, linalool, myrcene	Moderate
Insomnia / Restlessness	THC, CBN, linalool, myrcene, nerolidol	Moderate
Lower urinary tract symptoms (LUTS) MS	THC, CBD, nabiximol	Moderate
Memory	THC, THCA, THCV, CBD, CBG, alpha-bisabolol, alpha-pinene, geraniol	Insufficient
Migraines	THC, CBD, CBG	Limited
Movement issues – bradykinesia, dyskinesia, dystonia, rigidity, spasticity, tremor	THC, CBD, THCA, CBDA, THCV, nabiximol, myrcene	Spasticity - Conclusive / Substantial Limited, Insufficient, Anecdotal
Post-Traumatic Stress Disorder (PTSD)	THC (low dose), CBD, THCV	Limited
Psychosis	CBD, THCA	Insufficient
Schizophrenia (Positive and Negative symptoms)	CBD	Limited
Spiritual Distress- sadness, despair, feeling of abandonment, loss of hope, questioning life's meaning	THC, CBD, linalool, myrcene, limonene	Limited, Insufficient, Anecdotal
Traumatic Brain Injury (TBI) / Intercranial Hemorrhage – (CTE) Chronic Traumatic Encephalopathy symptoms	THC, CBD, THCA, CBDA	Limited

End-of-Life (EOL) Considerations

When a patient has progressed to the terminal phase of their disease, the primary goal is to stress comfort and enhance quality of life. Cannabis-based medicine is a great option offering symptom relief with minimal burden, relieving common end-of-life symptoms such as chronic pain, anxiety, appetite, nausea/vomiting, restlessness, and spiritual distress. It is important to note that cannabis-based medicine level of evidence is limited, observational and anecdotal for EOL indications. It is imperative that compassionate, timely education be provided to prepare patients and families for the dying process and the symptoms that accompany it. In many cases, cannabis-based medicine can work adjunctively with traditional end-of-life medications to minimize unwanted side effects while synergistically improving medication efficacy. Let's take a closer look at specific EOL symptoms and how cannabis-based medicine can help.

Pain: Cannabis can provide effective pain control, especially for chronic or neuropathic pain types, without the unwanted side effect of respiratory depression, constipation and nausea, which are common side effect of opioid use. In referencing one study, "patients undergoing cancer treatment who used 10 mg THC experienced pain reduction proportional to 60 mg codeine" (da Costa & de Carvalho, 2022). When used adjectively with opioids, cannabis has a synergistic benefit, often causing decreased opioid dosing needed to achieve pain relief as well as decreased opioid-associated constipation. Available in tincture form, as a transdermal patch for longer-acting relief, or as a vaporizer for inhalation, can also be helpful for many when PRN dosing is needed.

Anxiety/Spiritual Distress/Fear: At the end-of-life, anxiety can be due to multiple reasons, such as uncontrolled symptoms, fear, spiritual distress, or, unfortunately, a result of the progressing disease process. Cannabis-based medicine may induce relaxation, improve mood, and elevate overall emotional well-being for patients. "Israeli research has shown that 80% of patients believe that cannabis relieved physical and psychological stress, improving the way they deal with the situation" (da Costa & de Carvalho, 2022). Utilizing chemovars that are higher in CBD content would be the recommendation in addition to appropriate religious / spiritual support persons for a multimodal approach.

Appetite: For patients who still have a desire to eat, but do not have an appetite, a cannabis-based medicine that is higher in THC can stimulate one's appetite. This can particularly be helpful in disease processes that experience anorexia or cachexia.

Nausea/Vomiting: Cannabis-based medicine has conclusive support for this particular indication. Utilizing cannabis-based medicine for CINV is well studied and known to be very beneficial. "Cannabinoids have been shown to be more effective than various antiemetics, such as prochlorperazine, metoclopramide, chlorpromazine, trimethylpyridine, domperidone, and alizapride" (da Costa & de Carvalho, 2022).

Restlessness/Agitation: Unfortunately, this is a common symptom observed in the weeks to days before death to varying degrees. Traditionally managed with benzodiazepines or antipsychotics, utilizing cannabis-based medicine offers calming effects that can be used as a primary treatment or adjunctively with traditional medications to address this challenging symptom.

Cannabis-based medicine is a great option for patients and families as a tool to enhance quality of life, addressing comfort, dignity, and connection. It often allows patients to feel less sedated, more alert and engaged, able to create meaningful connections and lasting memories for themselves and their families during their final days. It can lead to decreased medication needs, addressing the "Pill Burden" that patients and families often feel when managing so many symptoms. However, due to the lack of quality studies to understand its entire MOA and the known interactions cannabinoids have with numerous medications used by this patient population, the administration of cannabis-based medicine must be done with care (da Costa & de Carvalho, 2022). Cannabis-based medicine is consistent with the hospice philosophy by respecting our patients and their families' particular preferences for their end-of-life care.

Adverse Effects

The adverse effects experienced with cannabis use are often chemovar, dose, or administration related. Once this is adjusted and education provided, patients tolerate the cannabis medication well. Just like any other medication, there will be those who do not tolerate cannabis, and other treatment options will need to be explored. As the dose of THC-dominant chemovars increases, patients are at an increased risk of experiencing adverse side effects. As stated before, medication efficacy is not determined by psychoactive/intoxicating side effects. This is not necessary to achieve therapeutic benefit, and most patients should not require more than 20-30mg of THC/day. It is important to educate patients and families about what a potential THC drug overdose could look/feel like and how to manage prior to the initiation of cannabis-medication use. If a patient experiences an overdose of THC, it is important to be reassured that there is no danger of respiratory arrest or death. Patients can experience tachycardia, paranoia, anxiety, delusions, increased sedation, and a sense of doom. It is very important to stay calm and reassure the patient and those with them that this will pass. Distractions can be helpful, along with a calm and supportive environment. Table 7 below outlines adverse events associated with cannabis use.

Table 7. Adverse events associated with cannabis-based medicines, based/updated information from MacCallum & Russo, 2018.

Adverse effect	Most common	Common	Rare
Drowsiness/fatigue	X		
Dizziness	X		
Dry Mouth	X		
Cough, phlegm, bronchitis (smoking only)	X		

continued on following page

Table 7. Continued

Adverse effect	Most common	Common	Rare
Anxiety	X		
Nausea	X		
Cognitive effect	X		
Euphoria		X	
Blurred vision		X	
Headache		X	
Orthostatic hypotension			X
Toxic psychosis/paranoia			X
Depression			X
Ataxia/ dyscoordination			X
Tachycardia (post titration)			X
Cannabinoid Hyperemesis Syndrome			X
Diarrhea			X

The adverse effects of CBD are dose-dependent and follow the same dosing recommendation as THC patients, with starting low and slow to find one's ideal dose. CBD is extremely beneficial for patients, and often medicinal cannabis use is CBD-dominant chemovars with low-dose THC. Some conditions and disease processes benefit from high-dose CBD. Once dosing exceeds 750 mg, adverse events are reported. This can usually be modified with dose adjustments and support. CBD has a very safe medication profile, even at very high dosing. With some disease processes like Epilepsy (Dravet and Lennox-Gastaut Syndrome), CBD has been studied with conclusive supportive evidence. It is a misconception that CBD does not have any psychoactive effects. CBD does have psychoactive effects / benefits as it can have positive effects on anxiety and mood. The correct way to explain this is, CBD does not have intoxicating effects. Table 8 describes possible CBD adverse events.

Table 8. CBD adverse effects based on information from Clark, 2021, pp. 197-198

Adverse Event	Common	Rare
Dizziness	X	
Lightheadedness	X	
Tachycardia	X	
Jitteriness	X	
Drowsiness	X	

continued on following page

Table 8. Continued

Adverse Event	Common	Rare
Diarrhea	X	
Headache	X	
Irritability		X
Decreased appetite		X
Palpitations		X
Increased Seizures		X

Drug to Drug Interactions

Providing education in relation to cannabis and potential drug interactions is a must as a clinical provider. The *CMAJ* article "Drug Interactions with Cannabinoids" offers essential considerations summarized below that you should incorporate into your practice.

- Common medications that CYP450, CYP3A4 & CYP2C9 metabolize can increase THC & CBD concentrations, causing increased psychoactive effects and elevated transaminase.
- Cannabinoids can also affect the therapeutic levels of other medications. For example, CBD inhibits CYP2C19, increasing the active metabolite of clobazam by 3x. Cannabis is known to increase the serum levels of Warfarin, increasing bleeding risk, and must be monitored.
- When inhaling cannabis regularly, medication metabolized by CYP1A2 can increase clearance of theophylline by 40%. Olanzapine would also be affected. Occasional inhalation does not seem to have this effect.
- Cannabis can also potentiate other medications' side effect profiles. When combined with central nervous system depressants (Alcohol, Opioids and Benzodiazepines), there could be an increase in drowsiness or ataxia. When taken with anticholinergics (Atropine or Hyoscyamine), one may experience increased tachycardia and confusion (Antoniou et al., 2020).

Patients should always inform their clinical provider or pharmacist if they are utilizing cannabis. Most drug interactions can be mitigated by staggering medication administration and cannabis medication by 1-2 hours. Patients should consider their cannabis medicine as they would any other prescribed medication. If a new cannabis medication is being initiated, it is recommended that the patient be home or in a safe and comfortable location for the first few hours to ensure they are tolerating the medication well. Patients should not drive while taking THC or combine it with alcohol consumption. This could lead to increased adverse effects, including excessive impairment, poor judgment, and injury.

Contraindications

Cannabis-based medicines are well tolerated when implemented for a medical indication and under the guidance of a clinical professional. Clinicians must understand physiologic decline / dying process and adjust cannabis- base medications based on pharmacokinetic and pharmacodynamic tolerance. Data has established some conditions under which cannabis-based medicine should be used with caution or abstained from altogether. Particularly patients with cardiovascular disease, pulmonary conditions, pregnancy/breastfeeding, and a concern for the pediatric population due to their developing brains. Let's keep in mind the risks of driving while actively under the influence, and unfortunately, if a patient has been diagnosed with Cannabinoid Hyperemesis Syndrome, the only treatment is to abstain from cannabis completely. These concerns are with THC-dominant chemovars, and patients should be well counseled on the risks vs. benefits. CBD-dominant chemovars have a very safe medication profile; however, they can have notable pharmacokinetic effects that were briefly addressed in the section discussing drug-to-drug interactions. It must also be mentioned that a patient would rarely receive a recommendation to smoke cannabis from a medical professional. If inhalation would be of benefit, vaporization would be the recommended mode. If a patient choose smoking cannabis-based medicine as their preferred delivery method, they must be properly counseled to the associated risks.

Safety Considerations

With the States legalizing medical and adult use of cannabis, the accidental ingestion has drastically increased. In most cases, pets and children are unintentional victims of accidental ingestion. Though cannabis has a high safety profile, a cannabis overdose can be very scary. Cannabis-based medicine needs to be cared for and stored as you would other medications in child-proof containers, up out of reach and in a secure location would be the recommendation. As a nurse, it is within or scope and responsibility to provide ample education on the importance and methods for ensuring safe storage. If accidental ingestion occurs, advise the patient and family to call the American Association of Poison Control Centers at 1-800-222-1222 (*American Association of Poison Control Centers*, n.d.).

Tolerance/Sensation Protocol

If tolerance is suspected, a therapeutic break can reset the ECS. Dr. Sulak has developed an ideal protocol for this very need, outlined below.

Table 9. Sulak cannabis sensation protocol based on information from Carey Clark, 2021, Table 3.14, p.147, Sulak Cannabis Sensation Protocol

Day	Instruction
0	The day prior to initiation of the protocol, track cannabis use and review cannabis diary.
1	Cannabis use as usual, then store away all product and associated administration tools. Be sure to note your 48hr cannabis fasting start time.
2	Supplement your ECS with endocannabinoid-enhancing foods, rest, movement that brings enjoyment, and plenty of water.
3	On day 3, the intention is to use as little cannabis product to reach therapeutic effect. This takes a good mindful practice, taking inventory of how your body, mind, mood are feeling before and after cannabis use. For Inhalation: Take 1 inhalation, then wait 5min., while staying connected to your body, mind, and mood for any changes or enhancements. If no change at all is noted, take 1 more inhalation. For Tinture: Take about ½ of your usual administration dose. Wait 30min., taking an inventory of body, mind, and mood for any subtle change or enhancements. If no change is noted, take another dose after the initial 30min. has passed. Repeat up to 3x /day. Continue to nurture your ECS with plenty of water, rest, enjoyable activities, and ECS supportive diet.
4-5	Continue with day 3 protocol. Staying mindful and taking an inventory prior and post cannabis use. Keep your findings noted in your cannabis diary. Continue with max use of 3x / day. Upregulate your ECS with plenty of water, rest, enjoyable activities, and ECS supportive diet.
6	Finding the optimal dose. It is essential to continue to keep a mindful approach, taking inventory of your body, mind, and mood, and documenting in your cannabis diary. Continue to supplement your ECS with healthy eating/hydration, joyful movement, and rest. Now you should be fine-tuning the dose to meet where symptoms are relieved. Once the optimal dose has been established, cannabis use can be used as needed without the mindful waiting period between doses.

APPLIED CANNABIS MEDICINE

Cancer

This author could select from a catalogue of cancer patients with beneficial cannabis experiences encountered in clinical practice; however, none is as meaningful as the experience of an immediate family member. She was diagnosed with stage IV melanoma shortly after her 29th birthday. Prior to diagnosis, there were no indications of severe illness, and the cancer was discovered incidentally. Her medical team was unable to identify an external primary lesion. Treatment was initiated immediately, consisting of an oral immunotherapy combination regimen along with radiation therapy to multiple metastatic sites, and she was given an estimated life expectancy of five years.

Her disease course rapidly became complicated by intractable pain related to multiple pathological fractures, compounded by the emotional and psychological distress of being a young mother facing terminal cancer. From the outset, treatment was physically demanding, with significant pain and numerous adverse effects. Cannabis was briefly suggested by her oncologist; however, little additional guidance was provided, leaving the patient and her family, like many others, to navigate cannabis-based care independently.

Cannabis-based medicine became an essential part of her symptom management. At the time, she was receiving extremely high doses of both long- and short-acting opioids, as well as antidepressant medications that caused significant sedation and limited her ability to interact meaningfully with her young daughter. The introduction of cannabis allowed for a reduction in opioid dosing, enabling greater alertness and presence with her daughter. She utilized oral cannabis formulations, including tinctures and gummies, which were especially helpful for mood stabilization and relief from persistent nausea, while also reducing anticipatory anxiety and distress related to disease progression.

Despite multiple interruptions throughout treatment and periods of disease-related complications, cannabis remained a consistent and sustaining therapy. Ultimately, her five-year prognosis became a survival trajectory of 378 days. Her cancer journey was defined by repeated challenges; however, cannabis-based medicine served as a lifeline, supporting improved comfort, preserved connection, and enhanced quality of life throughout the course of her illness.

Multiple Sclerosis

Judy is a 70-year-old Caucasian female diagnosed with secondary progressive multiple sclerosis (SPMS) in her early thirties. At the time of assessment, she had just enrolled in a home hospice program and was bedbound, with physical findings notable for frailty, muscle atrophy, and limited range of motion. Despite these physical limitations, she remained cognitively intact and able to perform many activities of daily living with intermittent assistance. She maintained full decisional capacity and independently directed her healthcare.

A review of her medication regimen revealed long-term utilization of cannabis-based medicine for symptom management. While her early cannabis use was recreational, this shifted to therapeutic use following disease progression. Her primary indication for cannabis was the management of painful muscle spasms. She utilized a balanced THC:CBD chemovar, dosed at 5 mg orally at bedtime and 2.5 mg in the morning, administered as a gummy formulation. This regimen had remained stable for approximately 15 years. She did not require opioid analgesics and used baclofen and acetaminophen on an as-needed basis. Judy's symptoms were so well controlled, and her clinical status remained stable, which ultimately resulted in discharge from hospice services due to an extended prognosis.

Alzheimer's

John is an 88-year-old Japanese American male with a 12-year history of Alzheimer's disease. His daughter serves as his primary caregiver and seeks guidance regarding the reinitiation of cannabis-based therapy. John had previously utilized cannabis edibles approximately seven years prior for a duration of one year, with unclear benefit and undocumented reasons for discontinuation.

At the time of reassessment, John was functioning at a Functional Assessment Staging Tool (FAST) score of 6a, with nightly episodes of sundowning characterized by agitation and behavioral issues. These episodes were managed with lorazepam, administered two to three times per week. John's daughter expressed interest in a more consistent, non-sedating approach to symptom management to improve nighttime agitation and total sleep quality.

A Type I chemovar was recommended, initiated at bedtime at a dose of 2.5 mg THC, delivered via tincture and administered approximately 45 minutes prior to sleep. The chemovar was selected for its terpenoid profile, including myrcene and terpineol, which support sedative and anxiolytic effects. Within two weeks of implementation, the caregiver reported a significant reduction in agitation, with lorazepam use decreasing to two total doses during that period. Overall, sleep quality improved, and the patient consistently awoke calmer and more positive.

Based on the results, upward titration to 5 mg at bedtime was discussed to optimize symptom control. At follow-up, John's daughter reported complete resolution of sundowning symptoms. In conjunction with cannabis-based therapy, environmental modifications were implemented to reduce evening stimulation and reinforce consistent sleep hygiene. John has maintained this cannabis dosing regimen for just over one year, with sustained symptom management and decreased dependence on benzodiazepine therapy.

CHALLENGES AND BARRIERS FACING CANNABIS-BASED MEDICINE

As this chapter is being written, the national landscape regarding cannabis is very active. Some information provided will certainly have changed by the time this book is published. With that said, nurses must stay apprised of the changing cannabis landscape to properly guide patients and colleagues in the course of these changes.

Late October (2025). H.R. 5371 added statutory definitions for hemp products that were omitted by the 2018 Farm Bill, intended to close the "hemp loophole" that has allowed unregulated intoxicating hemp-derived products to take hold nationwide. These provisions take effect on November 11, 2026, amending section 297A. Americans for Safe Access has a great outline of the proposed changes that you can review below:

HEMP PROVISIONS IN FY2026 AG BILL (H.R. 5371: SEC 781)

Amends Section 297A of the Agricultural Marketing Act of 1946 (7 U.S.C. § 1639o); provisions do not expire with FY2026.

Effective Date: November 11, 2026

- Establishes new definitions for Industrial hemp, intermediate hemp-derived cannabinoid products, and hemp-derived cannabinoid products.
- Explicitly excludes cannabinoid products from the definition of industrial hemp.
- Revises the THC threshold to include "total THC" (<0.3%), capturing all detectable tetrahydrocannabinol compounds, including THCA, on a dry-weight basis.
- Prohibits all synthetic cannabinoids.
- Prohibits products containing more than 0.4 mg THC per container.
- Prohibits seeds capable of producing cannabis varieties exceeding 0.3% THC.

(*2025 Federal Medical Cannabis Policy: What Changed & What 2026 Will Mean for Patient Access*, 2025)

This will affect millions of patients, especially patients who live in states without a functional medical cannabis program that have been able to purchase full-spectrum hemp to manage complicated chronic health issues. "Without intervention, patients who already live at the margins of the healthcare system risk losing one of the few therapeutic options available to them (*Safe Access 4 All*, 2024)".

President Trump signed an Executive Order, *"Increased Medical Marijuana and Cannabidiol Research,"* on December 18, 2025. The order directs many federal agencies to actively research and propose policies related to medical cannabis and cannabinoid products. Below is an outline of the tasks that different federal agencies are charged with completing, provided by ASA:

- **The Attorney General** is to expedite completion of the ongoing process to reschedule marijuana to Schedule III of the Controlled Substances Act (CSA).

- **The White House Deputy Chief of Staff for Legislative, Political, and Public Affairs** will work with Congress to allow Americans to benefit from access to appropriate full-spectrum CBD products, while restricting products that pose serious health risks.
- **The Department of Health and Human Services (HHS)** is to develop research methods and models utilizing real-world evidence to improve access to hemp-derived cannabinoid products in accordance with federal law and to inform standards of care.

(*2025 Federal Medical Cannabis Policy: What Changed & What 2026 Will Mean for Patient Access*, 2025)

It is vital to understand the Executive Order did not reschedule Cannabis. It remains a Schedule I drug. In October of 2022, President Biden initiated the rescheduling process, and the DEA is responsible for the formal rescheduling process, which has reached the final stages of an Administrative Law Judge hearing. However, the process has been stalled by an interlocutory appeal. Rescheduling Cannabis to a Schedule III class provides recognition that cannabis has medical value, but it does not:

- Legalize medical cannabis.
- Improve state medical cannabis programs.
- Restore federal rights for patients.
- Protect patients from discrimination.
- Ensure nationwide access.
- Integrate cannabis into federal healthcare systems (ASA).

(*2025 Federal Medical Cannabis Policy: What Changed & What 2026 Will Mean for Patient Access*, 2025)

As a Schedule III medication, Cannabis remains federally illegal and under tightly regulated federal oversight. Patients remain vulnerable to the potential loss of employment, VA benefits, parental rights, housing, and other serious consequences by utilizing cannabis-based medicines. States are currently protected through the annual renewal of the CJS medical cannabis amendment, which only applies to medical cannabis programs, not adult use.

The 2026 year is packed with a very active timeline for legislation that will alter the future of cannabis in our country. Advocacy for access and patients' rights has never been more important.

State-Based Considerations / MMP (Medical Marijuana Program)

In researching the most current information at the time of writing, 40 states and 3 territories, as well as the District of Columbia, permit medical use of cannabis and are considered to have a comprehensive Medical Cannabis Program. 24 states, 3 territories, and the District of Columbia regulate cannabis for non-medical/ recreational use by adults. 8 states permit CBD-dominant, low-THC in limited situations for medical reasons. The NCSL (National Conference of State Legislatures) does not consider high-CBD, low-THC states as having a comprehensive medical use program. "NCSL uses criteria similar to other organizations tracking this issue to determine if a program is 'comprehensive'", outlined below:

- Protection from criminal penalties for using cannabis for a medical purpose.
- Access to cannabis through home cultivation, dispensaries, or some other system is likely to be implemented.
- It allows a variety of strains or products, including those with more than "low THC."
- It allows either smoking or vaporization of some kind of cannabis products, plant material, or extract.
- It is not a limited trial program.

(National Conference of State Legislatures, 2024)(CDC, 2024)

Nurses must be well informed about the process of obtaining an MMP card in their counties and state, and guide patients and caregivers through the process. In states where recreational and medicinal cannabis use is accepted, patients may not feel a need to seek out an MMP card; however, there could be benefits. Patients would be protected as the MMP verifies medical needs. In addition, many dispensaries offer medicinal discounts, donating products, or assistance with tax costs for patients who have an MMP. As of March 2020, the state of California permits terminally ill patients to receive cannabis donations tax-exempt without the need for an MMP card (*Americans for Safe Access Urges California Governor Gavin Newsom to Sign SB 34*, 2024). Caregiver is defined as well as cannabis possession and growing of cannabis plants.

Care Locations / Access / Cost & Product Variability

Patients face many obstacles in relation to access to cannabis-based medicine, restrictions due to care locations, as well as cost and product variability. Physical access can be an issue due to individual state laws and the patient's geographical location. More rural locations lack access to dispensaries and require patients/caregivers to travel long distances, sometimes crossing state lines and incurring increased legal risk, or relying on limited access to what can be provided through online ordering/shipping. Marginalized communities continue to be disproportionately underrepresented regarding equitable access.

Patient care locations often dictate whether cannabis-based medicine can be utilized. Once a patient is receiving care within a care facility, their cannabis use is subject to strict facility guidelines and, in most instances, prohibited in any form. This is a combination of a lack of a comprehensive Medical Cannabis program, but mostly due to a lack of facilities creating cannabis-based medicine policies. Cannabis is still federally illegal, with many facilities stating they are concerned with reimbursement and all the logistics that go with managing a Schedule I drug. Most palliative and certainly EOL patients qualify under most states' Compassionate Use Acts and have a legal right to initiate or continue to utilize the cannabis-based medicines that provide symptomatic relief, provided that they do not smoke/vape while on facility property. ASA has wonderful resources that provide facilities and providers with the direction needed for facility compliance. An impatient Medical Oncology Unit based in Southern California implemented Ryan's Law (SB311) from May 2022 to June 2024. Findings reported better patient experiences and positive nursing satisfaction. The article outlines the steps facilities should follow to comply with SB311 and its health and safety provisions, as well as the Donabedian model for implementation (Implementing Ryan’s Law on an Inpatient Medical Oncology Unit, 2025).

Once a patient enrolls in a Hospice program, it also continues to be an issue with cannabis-based medicine access. Many Hospices are still not prepared to support patients and their caregivers. Hospice agencies share that their primary concern is related to Medicare reimbursement, as cannabis is federally illegal. A national survey was conducted and sent to 500 hospice organizations, with 310 respondents across 40 states. Results sites 91% reported support for cannabis-based medicine, yet physicians share that they rarely write orders to certify patients for Cannabis-based medicines, further share that they feel uneducated to make recommendations, and do not discuss unless asked. Most of the hospices surveyed stated that they do not have any policies regarding cannabis-based medicines. As cannabis remains federally illegal, hospices do not administer, procure, dispose of, or cover the cost of cannabis-based medicine. Clearly, hospices see the benefit of cannabis-based medicine as a safe, effective modality for patients facing the end of their lives; however, lack of education, federal legal status, equitable access, and policy formation remain barriers to formal implementation (Salvador, 2024).

Quality Studies for Palliative & Hospice Patients

As mentioned previously, cannabis has a history of medical application likely exceeding that of the written word (MacCallum & Russo, 2018). Cannabis Prohibition and the global grip it had and continues to have has had lasting consequences regarding research. Many countries have stepped out of the prohibition era, leading the way in cannabis research. Conducting quality studies, utilizing Phase III RCTs within the United States is nearly impossible due to the Schedule I status. However, many countries are conducting high-quality research and publishing daily. We have ample information, including high-quality research studies using both quantitative and qualitative methods, as well as extensive expert and anecdotal evidence. With the cannabis landscape continuing to shift, it opens the door for high-quality studies that specifically address palliative and hospice populations.

Bias & Stigma

Cannabis prohibition was fueled by a racist and anti-immigration agenda, focusing on Mexican and Black communities, creating racialized policies. Harry Anslinger was the first head of the Federal Bureau of Narcotics from 1930 to 1962. Anslinger was the primary catalyst in molding drug policy through criminalizing cannabis, exaggerated claims regarding its danger, and promoting racial profiling and rhetoric. This widened system-wide inequalities and resulted in mass incarcerations. A highly recommended read, *Chasing the Scream* by Johann Hari, takes us back to the start of Anslinger's grasp and beyond, giving valuable insight into the beginning of America's War on Drugs.

It is imperative that nurses recognize and understand their personal biases. It is through acknowledgement that we can address and or move aside bias to best serve our patients. This is an invitation to explore your biases regarding cannabis-based medicine. Explicit bias is a conscious belief (s) or attitude (s) that individuals openly express about certain groups, commonly leading to discriminatory behavior. This type of bias is generally easier to identify, address, and rectify. Implicit bias or prejudice is more challenging because it operates unconsciously and is not outwardly recognized. This is more challenging to snuff out, so here are a few questions you could ask yourself to help identify any implicit bias: Have you experienced any negative outcomes from cannabis use? How do you approach decisions regarding cannabis? Cannabis has risks and benefits. What is your perception? Do you typically approach unknown or new information about cannabis with curiosity or wariness? These questions can help identify implicit bias, enabling us to better serve our patients and their personal cannabis journey.

Many patients conceal their medical cannabis use from clinicians and even family due to the fear of stigma (a mark of disgrace associated with a particular circumstance, quality, or person), bias, legal consequences, and general fear. This is a serious concern/barrier to properly caring for patients. Nurses must be asking and properly assessing patients for cannabis use. Incorporating it into your standard assessment and treating cannabis questions as you would any other assessment question will help patients normalize this information.

Lack of Clinical & Public Education

It is truly unfortunate that cannabis was criminalized starting in the 1910s and 20s, stemming from moral panic rather than evidence-based knowledge or public health data. To further discredit cannabis and its medicinal uses, cannabis was removed from the US Pharmacopeia in 1942, despite the American Medical Association arguing for cannabis's substantial value and benefits. Clinicians have spent decades without this valuable knowledge and have been prohibited from researching cannabis. "In a national survey of US medical school curriculum deans, 66.7% reported that their graduates were not at all prepared to prescribe medical cannabis. Despite growing educational needs, medical cannabis was mentioned in only 9% of medical school curricula in the 2015-2016 academic year" (Zolotov et al., 2025). When clinicians are surveyed directly, they echo the same concern about being underprepared to confidently advise patients on use and on risks vs. benefits.

In 1996, medical cannabis was first legalized in California under the Compassion Use Act, setting the ball in motion, directly challenging federal prohibition via the pathway of medical access. As of February 2024, 3 states (ID, KS, NE, and American Samoa) do not yet have a legal cannabis program (CDC, 2024). Yet almost 3 decades later, formal cannabis education has still lagged. A JAMA Network Open Article, *Developing Medical Cannabis Competencies* was published, outlining 6 medical cannabis competencies for medical education, summarized below:

- Understanding the basics of the ECS.
- Explain the main components of the cannabis plant and their biological effects.
- Review the legal and regulatory landscape of cannabis in the U.S.
- Describe the evidence base for health conditions that are commonly managed with cannabis.
- Understand the potential risks of medical cannabis use.
- Understand basic clinical management with medical cannabis. (Zolotov et al., 2025)

For nursing, cannabis education is slowly being incorporated into the curricula, but it is not yet included within the NCLEX. The NCSBN has formalized guidelines that address the nursing care for patients utilizing cannabis-based medicine. In addition, the ANA, in partnership with the ACNA, published *Cannabis Nursing: Scope and Standards of Practice* 2024, which coincided with the ANA's September 2023 announcement that Cannabis Nursing was a recognized nursing specialty. A national certification exam is being developed and will further cement cannabis nursing specialty in a profound way.

Educating the public will be challenging. Years of stigma, bias, racial profiling, and the plethora of misinformation must be addressed. We do this by properly educating our clinical professionals, supporting the legalization of cannabis, having clinical professionals within dispensaries, guaranteeing equitable access, standardized cannabis product testing, and educating the public regarding credible cannabis information versus identifying misinformation. Nurses must take every opportunity to provide appropriate cannabis education when the occasion arises.

Patients face many barriers to accessing equitable cannabis-based medicine. Public perception, bias, stigma, lack of clinical education, access disparities, and years of prohibition have led us to where we are. Cannabis crusaders continue to fight for equitable access for all, with the ultimate goal of descheduling cannabis and implementing a comprehensive national cannabis program.

FUTURE DIRECTION AND CALL TO ACTION

The future of cannabis-based medicine is hopeful. As its medicinal indications grow, the country and the world are gradually recognizing its inherent benefits. Broadening quality clinical research will provide support and evidence-based confirmation for its indications, limitations, interactions, and any associated harms. Providing standard, structured education for clinicians will further validate the medicinal benefits. The true victory will be when cannabis is descheduled and has a dedicated oversight committee. As we progress through this key year within the U.S., each legislative step will have a direct impact on the steps to follow.

Call to Action

With 2026 being such a pivotal year, have you thought about your personal call to action? What way will you support legislative momentum and patient access? Perhaps you will join a national organization like ACNA, CNN, ASA, NORML, SCC, etc. Provide donations to support the monumental costs this mission entails. Organize informational meetings within your organization to ensure that they are well-informed and up to date with their state's Compassion Use Acts, upholding patients' rights. Introduce yourself and your support for cannabis-based medicine to your local and state representatives. Maybe you will find yourself in Washington, DC, on Capitol Hill, providing in-person support at a monumental legislative hearing. The messaging here is that you take the initial step to become better informed and let that lead you to advocate in a way that speaks to you.

CONCLUSION

As this chapter concludes, the hope is that you feel informed, as well as inspired to seek more knowledge to grow your palliative cannabis-based medicine nursing practice. Palliative patients and patients facing the end of their lives require care that is holistic, addressing mind, body, spirit, and their emotional needs. Palliative clinicians must be knowledgeable in cannabis-based medicine to maximize treatment and symptom relief while limiting adverse effects, promoting the best quality of life for our patients. The key lies in remaining curious and open-minded in your interactions with patients and colleagues. Take every opportunity to advocate and support patients' rights. Become an activist for medical cannabis, and as Clark stated, "nurses are social justice warriors." Join professional nursing organizations and volunteer groups, becoming a steward of change. That you honor and care for your own ECS, leading by example as you care for others.

In closing, may this work honor those who inspired it and strengthen our shared mission to promote compassionate, evidence-informed care. May the curiosity and advocacy at the heart of our nursing practice continue to light the way forward.

"We will only survive and advance the field if we speak in a collective voice as united disciplines" (Ferrell, 2007).

ACKNOWLEDGMENT

The depth of my gratitude and appreciation is truly vast. To my colleagues, mentors, and professional affiliations, whose encouragement, guidance, and shared expertise have profoundly shaped who I am as a nurse, educator, and mentor—thank you. Your influence continues to guide my growth with purpose and integrity.

A heartfelt expression of thanks goes to Llewellen Dawn Smith for her belief in me, her steady encouragement, and her thoughtful, constructive feedback through this process as a first-time writer. I am also deeply grateful to the American Cannabis Nurses Association (ACNA) for providing a platform and voice for the specialty of Cannabis Nursing, helping shape its future and illuminating the path forward. In addition, I recognize the Hospice and Palliative Nurses Association (HPNA) for their outstanding guidance and professional resources, which enrich my daily practice in Palliative and Hospice care.

My personal gratitude extends to my sister Robynne, whose journey ignited my passion for these nursing specialties and introduced me to the meaningful intersection of Palliative, Hospice, and Cannabis-based medicine. Her influence is at the heart of the work I do.

To my husband Bruce, thank you for your constant love, support, and steadiness—your consistency has sustained me through every personal, professional, and academic endeavor. And to my daughter, Grace, my true North and greatest joy, thank you for choosing me as your mom and for inspiring me every day.

REFERENCES

American Association of Poison Control Centers. (n.d.). Poisoncenters.org. https://poisoncenters.org/

American Nurses Association. (2024). *American Nurses Association*. ANA. https://www.nursingworld.org/ana/

American Nurses Association. (2024). *American Cannabis Nurses Association*. Cannabis Nursing Scope and Standards of Practice.

Americans for Safe Access. https://www.safeaccessnow.org/americans_for_safe_access_urges_california_governor_gavin_newsom_to_sign_sb_34#gsc.tab=0

Americans for Safe Access Urges California Governor Gavin Newsom to Sign SB 34. (2024).

ANA. (2023, September 27). *ANA Officially Recognizes Cannabis Nursing as a Specialty Nursing Practice*. ANA. https://www.nursingworld.org/news/news-releases/2023/ana-officially-recognizes-cannabis-nursing-as-a-specialty-nursing-practice/

Antoniou, T., Bodkin, J., & Ho, J. M.-W. (2020). Drug interactions with cannabinoids. *Canadian Medical Association Journal*, *192*(9), E206–E206. DOI: 10.1503/cmaj.191097 PMID: 32122975

Blesching, U. (2020). *Your Cannabis CBD:THC Ratio*. Ed Rosenthal.

CDC. (2024). *State Medical Cannabis Laws*. Cannabis and Public Health. https://www.cdc.gov/cannabis/about/state-medical-cannabis-laws.html

Clark, C. S. (2021). *CANNABIS: a handbook for nurses*. Wolters Kluwer Medical.

da Costa, V. F. D. D., & de Carvalho, W. S. R. (2022). Use of Medicinal Cannabis for Palliative Care Patients: A Systematic Review. *Journal of Biosciences and Medicines*, *10*(09), 242–252. DOI: 10.4236/jbm.2022.109017

Doppen, D., Kung, S., Maijers, I., John, M., Dunphy, H., Townsley, H., Eathorne, A., Semprini, A., & Braithwaite, I. (2022, November). M., Kung, Dr. S., Maijers, Dr. I., John, Dr. M., Dunphy, Dr. H., Townsley, Dr. H., Eathorne, M. A., Semprini, P. A., & Braithwaite, P. I. (2022). Cannabis in palliative care: A systematic review of current evidence. *Journal of Pain and Symptom Management*, *64*(5), e260–e284. Advance online publication. DOI: 10.1016/j.jpainsymman.2022.06.002 PMID: 35705116

2025 Federal Medical Cannabis Policy. What Changed & What 2026 Will Mean for Patient *Access*. (2025). Americans for Safe Access. https://www.safeaccessnow.org/2025_federal_cannabis_policy#gsc.tab=0

Ferrell, B. (2007). On Finding a Balance. *Journal of Palliative Medicine*, *10*(2), 309–312. DOI: 10.1089/jpm.2006.9981 PMID: 17472501

Goldstein, B. (2020). *Cannabis Is Medicine*. Little, Brown Spark. Implementing Ryan's Law on an Inpatient Medical Oncology Unit. (2025). *Clinical Journal of Oncology Nursing*. Advance online publication. DOI: 10.1188/25.CJON.86-90

MacCallum, C. A., & Russo, E. B. (2018). Practical considerations in medical cannabis administration and dosing. *European Journal of Internal Medicine*, *49*(49), 12–19. DOI: 10.1016/j.ejim.2018.01.004 PMID: 29307505

National Coalition For Hospice And Palliative Care. (2018). *Clinical practice guidelines for quality palliative care*. National Coalition For Hospice And Palliative Care.

National Conference of State Legislatures. (2024, July 12). *State Medical Cannabis Laws*. Www.ncsl.org. https://www.ncsl.org/health/state-medical-cannabis-laws

Russo, E. B. (2016). Beyond Cannabis: Plants and the Endocannabinoid System. *Trends in Pharmacological Sciences*, *37*(7), 594–605. DOI: 10.1016/j.tips.2016.04.005 PMID: 27179600

Russo, E. B. (2018). Cannabis Therapeutics and the Future of Neurology. *Frontiers in Integrative Neuroscience*, *12*, 51. DOI: 10.3389/fnint.2018.00051 PMID: 30405366

Salvador, (2024). Salvadore, E. (2024). A Survey of hospice professionals regarding medical cannabis practice Review of *A Survey of hospice professionals regarding medical cannabis practice*, by Costantino. *Journal of Palliative Medicine,22*(10),1208–1212

ADDITIONAL READING

American Nurses Association. (2024). *American.* Cannabis Nursing Scope and Standards of Practice.

Backes, M., Weil, A., & McCue, J. D. (2017). *Cannabis pharmacy: the practical guide to medical marijuana*. Black Dog & Leventhal Publishers.

Blesching, U. (2020). *Your Cannabis CBD:THC Ratio*. Ed Rosenthal.

Blesching, U. (2021). The Cannabis Health Index. *Logos.*

Clark, C. S. (2021). *CANNABIS: a handbook for nurses*. Wolters Kluwer Medical.

Ferrell, B., Paice, J., & Coyle, N. (2019). *Oxford textbook of palliative nursing* (5th ed.). Oxford University Press. DOI: 10.1093/med/9780190862374.001.0001

Guide: Cannabis 6-day Dosage Protocol. (n.d.). Healer. https://healer.com/programs/sensitization-protocol/

Hari, J. (2015). *Chasing the scream: The first and last days of the war on drugs*. Bloomsbury.

Hospice And Palliative Nurses Association, & American Nurses Association. (2025). *Hospice and palliative nursing: scope and standards of practice*. American Nurses Association.

Konieczny, E., & Wilson, L. (2018). *Healing with CBD: How cannabidiol can transform your health without the high*. Ulysses Press.

MacCallum, C. A., & Russo, E. B. (2018). Practical considerations in medical cannabis administration and dosing. *European Journal of Internal Medicine*, *49*(49), 12–19. DOI: 10.1016/j.ejim.2018.01.004 PMID: 29307505

National Conference of State Legislatures. (2024, July 12). *State Medical Cannabis Laws*. Www.ncsl.org. https://www.ncsl.org/health/state-medical-cannabis-laws

National Council of State Boards of Nursing. (2018). NCSBN National Nursing Guidelines for Medical Marijuana. *Journal of Nursing Regulation*, *9*(2), S1–S40. https://www.ncsbn.org/nursing-regulation/practice/marijuana-guidelines.page

NORML. (2015). *National Organization for the Reform of Marijuana Laws - NORML – Working to Reform Marijuana Laws*. Norml.org. https://norml.org/

Patient's Guide to Ryan's Law. (2024). Americans for Safe Access. https://www.safeaccessnow.org/ryanslaw_patientresources#gsc.tab=0

Physician's Guide to Ryan's Law. (2024). Americans for Safe Access. https://www.safeaccessnow.org/ryanslaw_physicianresources#gsc.tab=0

Russo, E. B. (2016). Beyond cannabis: Plants and the endocannabinoid system. *Trends in Pharmacological Sciences*, *37*(7), 594–605. DOI: 10.1016/j.tips.2016.04.005 PMID: 27179600

Russo, E. B. (2018). Cannabis therapeutics and the future of neurology. *Frontiers in Integrative Neuroscience*, *12*, 51. DOI: 10.3389/fnint.2018.00051 PMID: 30405366

KEY TERMS AND DEFINITIONS

ACNA: American Cannabis Nurses Association, established in 2015.

Advanced Care Planning: a process that supports patients of any age or health stage in understanding and sharing their personal values, life goals, and preferences for future medical care. It involves discussions about values, goals, and treatment preferences in the context of serious illness or end-of-life.

Advocacy: means promoting the desired goal of a person or group. Advocacy may also include participation in policy and legislative development.

ANA: American Nursing Association, established in 1911.

ASA: Americans for Safe Access, established in 2002.

Autonomy: the capacity of an individual to independently make well-informed choices regarding their own healthcare, in the absence of undue influence or persuasion.

Beneficence: defined as the obligation of health care providers to act in their patients' best interests, actively motivating practitioners to help others and promote their well-being.

Comfort Kit: a pre-packaged supply of prescription medications kept in a hospice patient's home/ location of care. The kit's purpose is to allow for rapid symptom management and provide immediate relief for sudden, acute symptoms like severe pain, anxiety, nausea, constipation, or breathlessness. This ensures patients have access to medication when needed.

Eight Domains of Palliative Care: Based on the NCP guidelines, 8 domains of palliative care have been established: 1- The Structure and Processes of Care, 2- Physical Aspects of Care, 3- Psychological and Psychiatric Aspects, 4- Social Aspects of Care, 5- Spiritual, Religious and Existential Aspects of Care, 6- Cultural Aspects of Care, 7- Care of the Actively Dying Patient, 8- Ethical and Legal Aspects of Care.

HPNA: Hospice and Palliative Nursing Association, established in 1988.

Interdisciplinary: a multidisciplinary approach in healthcare in which professionals from various disciplines collaborate to provide integrated patient care, assuring that all aspects of a patient's health are addressed.

Justice: the fair allocation of healthcare resources, access, and outcomes across all populations, regardless of socioeconomic status, race, gender, or geographic location.

Nonmaleficence: the term originates in Latin and translates to "first, do no harm," emphasizing the paramount importance of avoiding harm to patients in all aspects of care.

Schedule I: *Drugs* are substances/chemicals defined as drugs with no currently accepted medical use and a high potential for abuse. Examples of Schedule I drugs are: heroin, lysergic acid diethylamide (LSD), marijuana (cannabis), methaqualone, and peyote.

Schedule III: *Drugs* are substances/chemicals defined as drugs with a moderate to low potential for physical and psychological dependence. The abuse potential of Schedule III drugs is less than that of Schedule I and Schedule II drugs but more than Schedule IV.

Chapter 13
Oncology Nurses and Medical Cannabis:
Integrating Evidence-Based Therapeutics Into Cancer Care

Said Khaldouni
Morphoscience Laboratory, Faculty of Medicine and Pharmacy of Marrakech, Morocco

Mohammed El Rhanbouri
http://orcid.org/0009-0006-9643-5181
Faculty of Medicine and Pharmacy of Marrakech, Morocco

Fatiha Laghouasli
http://orcid.org/0009-0008-6716-812X
Morphoscience Laboratory, Faculty of Medicine and Pharmacy of Marrakech, Morocco

Zaoui Khalifa
http://orcid.org/0009-0004-6938-5372
Faculty of Medicine and Pharmacy of Marrakech, Morocco

Mouna Khouchani
Morphoscience Laboratory, Faculty of Medicine and Pharmacy of Marrakech, Morocco

ABSTRACT

The growing use of medical cannabis in oncology has generated significant clinical, ethical, and professional challenges for healthcare providers, particularly oncology nurses. This chapter explores the role of medical cannabis as a complementary

DOI: 10.4018/979-8-2600-2035-7.ch013

intervention in cancer care, focusing on its pharmacological foundations, clinical indications, safety profile, and potential drug–drug interactions relevant to oncology practice. Emphasis is placed on the endocannabinoid system and the therapeutic properties of tetrahydrocannabinol (THC) and cannabidiol (CBD) in the management of cancer-related symptoms. The chapter further highlights the pivotal role of oncology nurses in patient assessment, education, monitoring, and interdisciplinary collaboration. By synthesizing current evidence, this chapter aims to support evidence-based nursing practice and promote safe, patient-centered integration of medical cannabis in oncology and palliative care settings

I. INTRODUCTION

Over the past decade, cannabis has shifted from a peripheral and highly stigmatized substance to an increasingly debated component of cancer care, driven by legal reforms, expanding social acceptance, and strong patient demand.

Observational studies and national surveys consistently demonstrate that a substantial proportion of cancer patients report current or recent cannabis use, with prevalence estimates in the United States ranging from 5% to 26%, and reaching up to 40% in certain contemporary cohorts (Amin et al., 2024; McClure et al., 2023; Nugent et al., 2020; Tehranchi et al., 2025). Patients most commonly seek cannabis for cancer-related pain, chemotherapy-induced nausea and vomiting (CINV), sleep disturbance, anxiety, and appetite loss, often reporting perceived symptom relief (Abu-Amna et al., 2021; Amin et al., 2024; Braun et al., 2021, 2024; Nugent et al., 2020). However, this patient-reported benefit frequently exceeds the strength of available high-quality randomized evidence, underscoring the need for critical appraisal within oncology practice.

This chapter distinguishes non-medical, unregulated cannabis use from medical cannabis and pharmaceutical cannabinoids (dronabinol, nabilone, nabiximols). While pharmaceutical options have been evaluated in randomized trials, other forms include standardized herbal or oil preparations within regulated programs. These categories differ in cannabinoid composition and evidentiary support, yet their clinical boundaries often overlap, complicating patient counseling (Braun et al., 2021; Turgeman & Bar-Sela, 2019; Woerdenbag et al., 2023). Although cancer is a leading qualifying condition for medical cannabis, oncology teams often feel insufficiently informed regarding therapeutic benefits, drug–drug interactions, and legal considerations (Patel et al., 2024; Tehranchi et al., 2025; Worster et al., 2022). Evidence for cannabis as an antitumor therapy remains unconvincing, while its support for symptom management beyond refractory CINV remains tentative (Abrams, 2022; Abu-Amna et al., 2021; Braun et al., 2024).

This chapter examines cannabis and cannabinoids in oncology: use patterns, global legislation, pharmacology, clinical evidence for symptom management (pain, CINV, cachexia, quality of life), drug interactions with anticancer and immunotherapies, and clinical implementation (indication, product selection, dosing, monitoring, shared decision-making). It emphasizes oncology nurses' evolving role and addresses ethical, legal, and cultural dimensions of palliative use, outlining future research and policy directions.

II. CANNABIS USE BY CANCER PATIENTS OUTSIDE A FORMEL MEDICAL CONTEXT

Many people with cancer use cannabis on their own initiative, for both symptom relief and recreational reasons, often without medical supervision or prescriptions.

1. Prevalence and Patterns of Non-Medical Use

Cannabis use among cancer patients is far more prevalent and complex than often assumed. Across major surveys in the United States and Europe, approximately 25–33% of cancer patients report using cannabis after their diagnosis, with a significant portion describing recreational or mixed use rather than purely medical purposes.(Amin et al., 2024; Azizoddin et al., 2023; Donovan et al., 2023; Ellison et al., 2024, 2024; McIntosh et al., 2024; Pergam et al., 2017; Rashid et al., 2025; Salz et al., 2023).

Among cancer survivors who use cannabis, over half do so for nonmedical reasons, with heavy alcohol use and male sex emerging as predictive factors(Rashid et al., 2025). Young adults navigating cancer particularly stand out, frequently using cannabis weekly or more often, driven by recreational motivations alongside medical needs such as pain, anxiety, nausea, and sleep disturbances(Donovan et al., 2023; Schubel et al., 2025). Notably, even in regions without legal access, roughly one-quarter of patients report cannabis use, often obtained informally through friends and family or via illicit markets (McClure et al., 2023; Nielsen et al., 2022).

2. Reasons for Use and Patient Perceptions

Cancer patients use cannabis for symptom relief (pain, insomnia, mood, appetite) and coping (relaxation, social connection, emotional processing), blending medical and recreational motivations (Amin et al., 2024; Donovan et al., 2023; McClure et al., 2023; Nielsen et al., 2022; Salz et al., 2023; Vinette et al., 2022). Most users hold notably positive perceptions of cannabis safety and efficacy, with 70–90% reporting perceived symptom improvement and relatively few experiencing worsening symptoms, though these remain subjective assessments rather than findings from controlled clinical trials(Amin et al., 2024; Ellison et al., 2024; McClure et al., 2023; Nielsen et al., 2022; Salz et al., 2023). A concerning gap emerges in information-seeking: many cannabis users rely primarily on the internet, media, and peer networks for guidance, while conversations with oncologists remain sparse, and 30–45% of users do not disclose their cannabis use to their healthcare providers(Cousins et al., 2023; Donovan et al., 2023; Ellison et al., 2024; Pergam et al., 2017; Salz et al., 2023) .

3. Risks, Disparities, and Knowledge Gaps

Use is notably more prevalent in younger patients, males, those with concurrent tobacco or alcohol use, and individuals from socioeconomically disadvantaged backgrounds, revealing important disparities that warrant clinical attention(Amin et al., 2024; Azizoddin et al., 2023; Cousins et al., 2023; Ellison et al., 2024; Gonzalez et al., 2024; Rashid et al., 2025). Beyond these epidemiological patterns lie substantive clinical concerns: recreational or unsupervised cannabis use raises legitimate questions about potential drug interactions, neurocognitive impairment, impaired driving ability, and the risk that cannabis consumption might substitute for or delay evidence-based cancer treatments (Azizoddin et al., 2023; Cousins et al., 2023; Ellison et al., 2024; Gonzalez et al., 2024; McClure et al., 2023; Rashid et al., 2025). A critical knowledge gap persists: most research fails to distinguish between strictly medical and recreational cannabis use, leaving the long-term health impacts of non-medical cannabis consumption in cancer populations poorly understood (Amin et al., 2024; Gonzalez et al., 2024; Helzlsouer et al., 2024; McClure et al., 2023; Schubel et al., 2025; Vinette et al., 2022).

4. Clinical Implications for Oncology Practice

Cannabis derivatives (nabilone, dronabinol, nabiximols) are used for cancer pain, chemotherapy-induced nausea and vomiting, sleep disturbance, appetite loss, and mood symptoms. Evidence is strongest for pain and CINV, moderate for sleep disturbance, and weaker for appetite stimulation and anxiety relief (Damsky Dell, Msn, Aprn, Aocn, Lnc & P. Stein, Md, 2021; Worster et al., 2022). Many patients self-experiment with cannabis beyond symptom palliation, sometimes viewing it as a potential anti-cancer therapy despite absent clinical evidence supporting such use (Patel et al., 2024; Shalata et al., 2024; Vinette et al., 2022; Worster et al., 2022). Cannabis use during active cancer treatment proves surprisingly common, with recent surveys indicating that 15–25% of patients report ongoing use while undergoing therapy(Nugent et al., 2020; Vinette et al., 2022; Zhou et al., 2022) This prevalence underscores the pressing need for evidence-based guidance and clinical integration of cannabis discussions within oncology practice.

III. MEDICAL CANNABIS LEGISLATION AND SOCIAL ACCEPTANCE

1. Global Legislative Landscape

Global regulation balances standardized pharmaceutical approval with compassionate access, distinguishing licensed cannabinoid medicines (nabiximols, synthetic THC) from herbal cannabis. Europe and North America have approved cannabinoid pharmaceuticals, but few jurisdictions authorize herbal cannabis exceptions include Canada, Germany, Israel, and select US states (Abuhasira et al., 2018; Baratta et al., 2022; De Souza et al., 2022a; Jardim & Delgado-Charro, 2025). By the early 2020s, at least 36 countries had established formal medical cannabis frameworks, differing in permitted product types, quality standards, and access routes ranging from standard authorization to compassionate use schemes(Aguilar et al., 2018; Baratta et al., 2022; De Souza et al., 2022a; Ruheel et al., 2021). Some nations including Brazil, Australia, and the UK employ less-regulated "cannabis product" categories with minimal pre-marketing safety data, typically accessed through special authorization pathways prioritizing patient access while potentially compromising evidence standards(Baratta et al., 2022; De Souza et al., 2022b; Jardim & Delgado-Charro, 2025; Ravindra B. Malabadi et al., 2024).

2. Facilitators and Barriers to Regulation

Successful implementation of medical cannabis regulation requires navigating both enabling factors and substantial obstacles. Key facilitators include alignment between state and federal regulatory frameworks, transparent administrative procedures, and meaningful engagement of patients, clinicians, and industry stakeholders in policy development (Ruheel et al., 2021). Significant barriers persist: ideological opposition, social stigma surrounding cannabis use, fragmented evidence bases, and labyrinthine bureaucratic processes that paradoxically delay patient access even after legal authorization (Aguilar et al., 2018; De Souza et al., 2022b; Ravindra B. Malabadi et al., 2024; Ruheel et al., 2021). Effective regulation demands coordinated governance, evidence-informed policy, and sustained commitment to dismantling institutional and cultural barriers to equitable access.

3. Public and Professional Acceptance

Public acceptance of medical cannabis has underged dramatic expansion in high-income countries, with overwhelming majorities now supporting legalization exemplified by 81% of Americans favoring medical legalization in a 2016 poll (Ruheel et al., 2021). International surveys reveal that users widely characterize cannabis as a "natural, safe medicine," frequently exceeding what empirical evidence supports(Castle et al., 2025; Cohen et al., 2023; Eldering et al., 2025; Hossain & Chae, 2024; Khademi et al., 2023; Taylor et al., 2025).

Among healthcare professionals, approximately half support medical cannabis legalization according to a systematic review of 40 studies, with support growing over time. (Weisman & Rodríguez, 2021). The global TASMAN oncology survey found most oncologists and palliative care providers recognize a potential role for cannabis in symptom management, yet over 90% remain unaware of clinical guidelines and few prescribe it routinely, citing legal uncertainty and insufficient evidence(Trapani et al., 2025).

Cancer patients themselves express high interest and perceive substantial benefits, yet harbor significant misconceptions about efficacy and safety, obtaining information predominantly from media and social networks rather than clinical discussions(Cohen et al., 2023; Eldering et al., 2025; Nayak et al., 2023; Nugent et al., 2020; Taylor et al., 2025). Persistent stigma particularly within medical environments discourages disclosure, with many survivors concealing their cannabis use from their healthcare teams(Hossain & Chae, 2024; Nayak et al., 2023; Nugent et al., 2020).

4. Implications for Oncology and Nursing Practice

Nurses are pivotal in cannabinoid therapeutics, positioned between evolving evidence, shifting regulations, and patient demand. Oncology and palliative care patients view nurses as trusted experts, yet many feel underprepared to address cannabis discussions confidently (McIntosh et al., 2024; Paiva et al., 2024). Empirical work from Australia, Portugal, Canada, and the United States shows that nurses overwhelmingly acknowledge the therapeutic potential of medical cannabis but report substantial deficits in understanding the endocannabinoid system, pharmacology, dosing, indications, and legal frameworks, and strongly endorse the need for targeted education (Balneaves & Alraja, 2019; McIntosh et al., 2024; Paiva et al., 2024). Professional bodies increasingly frame nurses as key advocates for patient autonomy, responsible for initiating non-judgmental conversations, educating patients and families, monitoring for benefits and harms, and integrating cannabis use into holistic care plans(Clark, 2018; Damsky Dell, Msn, Aprn, Aocn, Lnc & P. Stein, Md, 2021) .The recognition of "cannabis nursing" as a specialty practice underscores nursing's transition toward a more formalized, evidence-based role in cannabinoid therapeutics(Cho et al., 2025).

IV. PHARMALOGICAL AND BIOLOGICAL FOUNDATIONS

1. Overview of Cannabinoids Relevant to Oncology (THC, CBD, CBG, Minor Cannabinoids)

Cannabinoids represent a diverse pharmacological class with significant relevance to oncology, comprising three primary categories: phytocannabinoids derived from Cannabis sativa, endocannabinoids synthesized endogenously, and synthetic cannabinoids produced pharmaceutically(Alves et al., 2020; Blebea et al., 2024; Duczmal et al., 2024; Mashabela & Kappo, 2024; Teixeira, 2025; Walsh et al., 2021). Over 120 phytocannabinoids have been identified in Cannabis sativa, all biosynthetically derived from cannabigerolic acid (CBGA) (Blebea et al., 2024; Mashabela & Kappo, 2024; Walsh et al., 2021; Zagzoog et al., 2020). The most extensively studied phytocannabinoids include Δ9-tetrahydrocannabinol (THC), a CB1 and CB2 receptor partial agonist responsible for psychoactive effects yet demonstrating analgesic, antiemetic, and anticancer properties in preclinical models(Blebea et al., 2024; Calapai et al., 2022; Śledziński et al., 2018; Zagzoog et al., 2020).

cannabidiol (CBD), a non-psychoactive compound exhibiting anti-inflammatory, neuroprotective, and anti-proliferative effects through CB1/CB2, TRPV channels, PPARs, and receptor-independent pathways(Blebea et al., 2024; Mashabela & Kappo, 2024; Melo et al., 2025; Voicu et al., 2023) ; and cannabigerol (CBG), a non-psychotomimetic partial agonist with antioxidant, anti-inflammatory, and anti-tumoral activity(Blebea et al., 2024; Calapai et al., 2022; Walsh et al., 2021). Minor cannabinoids (e.g., cannabichromene, cannabinol, cannabidivarin) similarly display receptor-dependent and receptor-independent antitumor actions in preclinical models(Calapai et al., 2022; Patel et al., 2024; Śledziński et al., 2018; Walsh et al., 2021; Zagzoog et al., 2020). At the molecular level, cannabinoids primarily signal through CB1 receptors abundant in the central nervous system yet also expressed in numerous tumors and CB2 receptors predominantly found on immune cells and frequently upregulated in malignancies, while additionally engaging GPR55, TRPV1/2/4, TRPM8, PPARs, and 5-HT receptors, thereby creating a complex signaling network in cancer biology (Blebea et al., 2024; Duczmal et al., 2024; Mangal et al., 2021; Patel et al., 2024; Salum et al., 2025; Walsh et al., 2021).

2. Endocannabinoid System and Cancer Biology

The endocannabinoid system emerges as a promising target in cancer biology, with preclinical evidence consistently demonstrating that cannabinoids suppress cancer cell proliferation, trigger programmed cell death, and disrupt cellular invasion, tumor angiogenesis, and metastatic dissemination though effects vary substantially depending on tumor histology, cannabinoid dosage, and receptor context (Blebea et al., 2024; Mangal et al., 2021; Milian et al., 2020; Salum et al., 2025; Śledziński et al., 2018). These findings underscore the biological plausibility of cannabinoid-based therapeutic approaches yet highlight the complexity of translating preclinical observations into clinical benefit.

3. CB1/CB2-Mediated Anti-Tumor Mechanisms

Activation of CB1 and CB2 receptors on malignant cells and within the tumor microenvironment initiates multiple anti-tumor mechanisms. CB1/CB2 signaling triggers ceramide synthesis, precipitating endoplasmic reticulum stress, and subsequent autophagy and apoptosis(Mangal et al., 2021; Mashabela & Kappo, 2024; Salum et al., 2025; Śledziński et al., 2018). Cannabinoid receptor activation downregulates pro-survival pathways including AKT/mTORC1 and EGFR signaling, resulting in cell-cycle arrest and diminished proliferation(Blebea et al., 2024; Mangal et al., 2021; O'Reilly et al., 2023; Śledziński et al., 2018),while reducing angiogenesis, invasion, and metastatic potential through modulation of matrix metalloproteinases and pro-angiogenic factors (ALSalamat et al., 2024; Blebea et al., 2024; Mangal et al., 2021; Milian et al., 2020; Śledziński et al., 2018). Selective CB2 agonists substantially reduce cancer cell proliferation and survival across diverse cell lines while conferring less psychoactive liability than CB1-biased agonists(Alghamdi et al., 2025; Śledziński et al., 2018; Turgut et al., 2022). In colorectal cancer models, CBD's anti-proliferative and pro-apoptotic effects predominantly depend on CB2 engagement, operating through G1 cell-cycle arrest, downregulation of cyclins and cyclin-dependent kinases, and ER-stress induction (Mashabela & Kappo, 2024). Synthetic CB1/CB2 agonists similarly suppress proliferation and clonogenicity while inducing intrinsic apoptosis in pancreatic and breast cancer cells(Turgut et al., 2022).

4. Receptor-Independent Pathways

Many cannabinoid-mediated anti-cancer effects, particularly of CBD and CBG, operate substantially independent of CB1/CB2 signaling. CBD demonstrates broad anti-cancer activity across glioma, melanoma, leukemia, colorectal, breast, lung, and prostate malignancies, predominantly via TRPV1/2 activation, reactive oxygen species generation, calcium influx, and mitochondrial dysfunction triggering apoptosis or apoptosis-autophagy pathways(Blebea et al., 2024; Mangal et al., 2021; Mashabela & Kappo, 2024; Melo et al., 2025; Salum et al., 2025; Śledziński et al., 2018). In prostate cancer, CBD inhibits proliferation and invasiveness while suppressing cyclin and CDK expression, reducing AKT phosphorylation, and increasing E-cadherin expression effects unblocked by CB1/CB2 or TRPV1 antagonists, indicating alternative molecular targets (O'Reilly et al., 2023). Minor cannabinoids including CBG, CBC, CBDV, and CBN similarly display anti-proliferative and pro-apoptotic activity in colorectal, breast, and prostate cancer models, operating through TRPM8 antagonism, COX-2 modulation, or other non-CB1/CB2-dependent mechanisms (Blebea et al., 2024; Calapai et al., 2022; Śledziński et al., 2018).

5. Cannabinoid Receptors as Prognostic Markers

Cannabinoid receptor expression emerges as a potentially informative prognostic marker in select malignancies, with elevated CB1/CB2 levels correlating with improved survival and cannabinoid agonists demonstrating capacity to reverse epithelial-to-mesenchymal transition (EMT). In non-small cell lung cancer, patients with high CB1/CB2 expression exhibit prolonged survival; mechanistically, THC and CBD reduce EGFR expression, suppress proliferation, restore epithelial markers evidenced by increased E-cadherin and decreased vimentin/CDH2 and diminish migratory capacity, collectively suppressing EMT and invasion(Milian et al., 2020). These findings suggest that cannabinoid receptor status may help stratify patient risk and that cannabinoid-based interventions might specifically benefit tumors with dysregulated EMT programs, though validation in clinical trials is required.

6. Caveats, Translational Gaps, and Biological Complexity

While preclinical evidence predominantly demonstrates anti-proliferative and pro-apoptotic cannabinoid effects, critical caveats temper clinical optimism. Certain experimental contexts reveal pro-tumorigenic or proliferation-stimulating cannabinoid actions, underscoring that outcomes depend critically on tumor histology, cannabinoid dosage, receptor expression profiles, and the tumor microenvironment (Blebea et al., 2024; Salum et al., 2025; Śledziński et al., 2018). More fundamentally, the vast majority of evidence derives from preclinical cell lines and animal models; robust clinical data demonstrating that mechanistic insights translate into tangible improvements in patient outcomes remain sparse(Blebea et al., 2024; Mangal et al., 2021; Milian et al., 2020; Salum et al., 2025; Śledziński et al., 2018).

Cannabinoids modulate cancer hallmarks (proliferation, survival, angiogenesis, invasion, metastasis) through CB1/CB2-dependent and receptor-independent pathways, positioning the endocannabinoid system as a biologically plausible yet unproven therapeutic target. Closing this translational gap requires rigorous clinical trials, attention to patient heterogeneity, and recognition that in vitro efficacy does not guarantee clinical benefit.

V. CLINICAL EVIDENCE FOR MEDICAL CANNABIS IN ONCOLOGY

1. Overview of the Evidence Base

The clinical evidence base for cannabinoids in cancer care remains modest and methodologically heterogeneous, constraining confidence in therapeutic recommendations. Recent systematic reviews reveal that most published trials are small, employ diverse cannabinoid formulations including THC, CBD, synthetic analogues, and combinations administered via multiple routes, substantially limiting robust conclusions and evidence-based guideline development (Braun et al., 2024; Creangă-Murariu et al., 2025; Doppen et al., 2022; Häuser et al., 2023; Troyer & Tanco, 2024a). The certainty of evidence is uniformly rated as low or very low for most clinical outcomes, and high-quality randomized controlled trials remain conspicuously sparse (Braun et al., 2024; Doppen et al., 2022; Troyer & Tanco, 2024a; Wang et al., 2021). Patient use of cannabis for cancer symptom management has risen substantially, frequently advancing ahead of the empirical evidence supporting such practices (Braun et al., 2024; Kleckner et al., 2019; Vinette et al., 2022). This evidence-practice gap underscores an urgent need for well-designed trials to inform safe and effective cannabinoid integration into oncology practice.

a. Cancer-Related Pain

Cancer-related pain represents one of the most common indications for medical cannabis, yet clinical evidence remains disappointing. Nabiximols and THC preparations showed modest pain reduction in advanced cancer patients, but a Cochrane systematic review of nabiximols for opioid-refractory cancer pain concluded with moderate-certainty evidence that these agents failed to meaningfully reduce pain intensity or improve symptoms compared with placebo, nor did they demonstrate opioid-sparing effects (Häuser et al., 2023). Broader meta-analyses of non-inhaled medical cannabis for chronic pain show only marginal improvements offset by increased adverse effects(Wang et al., 2021). Major guidelines including MASCC and ASCO recommend against cannabinoid use as adjuvant analgesics for cancer pain(Braun et al., 2024; De Feo et al., 2023), highlighting the critical gap between patient expectations and clinical reality.

b. Other Supportive Indications (Chemotherapy-Induced Nausea/Vomiting, Appetite, Sleep, Anxiety, and Mood)

Chemotherapy-Induced Nausea and Vomiting (CINV) has historically represented the strongest indication for cannabinoid use in oncology, yet contemporary evidence reveals important nuances. A recent systematic review of cannabinoids for CINV synthesized 32 studies encompassing 1,889 patients, identifying that trials comparing cannabinoids with older, now-obsolete antiemetic regimens frequently demonstrated cannabinoid superiority, and most placebo-controlled trials suggested benefit (Kemmner et al., 2025). This favorable signal substantially diminishes when examining the single study employing modern, guideline-concordant antiemetic therapy comprising 5-HT3 receptor antagonists, NK1 antagonists, and dexamethasone in which cannabinoids improved nausea and vomiting yet incurred greater cannabinoid-related adverse effects, leading investigators to judge the evidence insufficient to support routine clinical use (Kemmner et al., 2025). MASCC consensus concluded that while THC and nabilone demonstrate superiority over placebo for CINV, they do not outperform standard antiemetics, and evidence for refractory CINV remains limited and inconsistent (Alderman et al., 2023). ASCO guidelines cautiously note that cannabinoids may modestly improve refractory CINV when added to guideline-based antiemetic regimens but underscore the low certainty of evidence and absence of benefit for other supportive outcomes (Braun et al., 2024). This pattern underscores that cannabinoids may occupy a narrow therapeutic niche in CINV management, relevant primarily when conventional antiemetics prove inadequate.

Appetite and Cachexia: Despite widespread clinical use and patient perception of efficacy, cannabinoids demonstrate limited evidence for appetite stimulation and weight gain in cancer populations. A systematic review and meta-analysis in palliative medicine found no convincing benefit of cannabinoids over placebo for appetite, caloric intake, or weight gain in cancer patients, and a head-to-head randomized trial demonstrated that megestrol acetate substantially outperformed dronabinol for cancer-associated anorexia (Mücke et al., 2018). Recent oncology-focused systematic reviews reinforce these conclusions, reporting that evidence supporting cannabinoids for appetite and cachexia remains limited and inconsistent (Creangă-Murariu et al., 2025; Doppen et al., 2022; Troyer & Tanco, 2024b; Valente et al., 2024). Current clinical guidelines from MASCC and ASCO do not recommend cannabinoids as first-line therapeutic agents for cancer-associated anorexia and cachexia (Alderman et al., 2023; Braun et al., 2024; Mücke et al., 2018).

Sleep Disturbance, Anxiety, and Mood: Cannabinoids are frequently sought by cancer patients for management of anxiety, mood disturbances, and sleep problems, yet the clinical evidence remains unconvincing. Systematic reviews of cannabinoids in palliative care report low-quality evidence of improvement in secondary outcomes including sleep, fatigue, and mood, though these effects are inconsistent and often not designated as primary endpoints (Doppen et al., 2022; Troyer & Tanco, 2024b). MASCC guidelines concluded that while some randomized trials suggested potential benefits for sleep or mood, no high-quality evidence supports cannabis as treatment for anxiety, depression, or insomnia in cancer populations (De Feo et al., 2023). A double-blind randomized controlled trial of CBD oil for advanced cancer symptom burden demonstrated no difference from placebo in total symptom scores (Good et al., 2019), while a subsequent trial of 1:1 THC:CBD oil similarly showed no reduction in overall symptom burden compared with palliative care alone, with only a small, statistically significant yet clinically modest pain benefit offset by increased psychotomimetic adverse effects (Hardy et al., 2025). Well-delivered palliative care itself produces substantial symptom improvement, and cannabinoids confer little additive benefit in unselected cancer populations.

c. Global Symptom Burden and Quality of Life

A recent large systematic review and meta-analysis synthesizing 98 interventional and observational studies across diverse cancer types found that cannabinoids reduced pain and anxiety compared with baseline measures, with mean pain and anxiety scores decreasing approximately 1.2–1.3 points on standardized assessment scales (Creangă-Murariu et al., 2025). Trends toward improvement emerged for appetite, CINV, and insomnia, though confidence intervals were wide and overlapped no effect, limiting interpretability(Creangă-Murariu et al., 2025). Critically, this comprehensive review documented a substantial increase in psychiatric, neurologic, and gastrointestinal adverse events associated with THC-predominant formulations, underscoring the importance of careful patient selection and cautious dose titration(Creangă-Murariu et al., 2025). Parallel scoping investigations mapping cannabis use patterns in oncology populations reveal that patients frequently report perceived benefits for pain, nausea, appetite, sleep, and emotional distress, and routinely integrate cannabis into personal symptom management strategies regardless of equivocal randomized controlled trial evidence(Kleckner et al., 2019; Valente et al., 2024; Vinette et al., 2022). This gap between patient-reported benefit and trial data reinforces the importance of shared decision-making and transparent communication of evidence limitations.

d. Safety Profile and Risk–Benefit Balance

The safety profile of cannabinoids in cancer and palliative populations reveals a pattern of frequent, though typically transient, adverse effects. Common side effects include dizziness, somnolence, cognitive impairment, dry mouth, nausea, and psychiatric manifestations such as anxiety or dysphoria, with THC-dominant formulations carrying particular risk(AminiLari et al., 2022; Creangă-Murariu et al., 2025; Mücke et al., 2018; To et al., 2023; Wang et al., 2021). Systematic reviews document significantly elevated rates of central nervous system and gastrointestinal adverse effects compared with placebo, with dizziness occurring in approximately 9% of patients in shorter trials and escalating to nearly 30% in longer-term studies(AminiLari et al., 2022; Mücke et al., 2018; Wang et al., 2021). While serious adverse events are not uniformly increased, the cumulative tolerability burden proves particularly problematic in frail patients with advanced cancer (AminiLari et al., 2022; Mücke et al., 2018; To et al., 2023; Wang et al., 2021). Additional concerns persist regarding potential pharmacokinetic and pharmacodynamic interactions with systemic cancer therapies and immunotherapies, though high-quality clinical data remain sparse(Braun et al., 2024; To et al., 2023; Troyer & Tanco, 2024a).

Balancing modest and uncertain therapeutic benefits against non-trivial toxicity risks, major guideline bodies including ASCO advocate for cautious, highly individualized cannabinoid use in oncology. These organizations recommend against cannabinoids as cancer-directed treatments, advise against routine use for cancer pain or psychological symptoms, and reserve cannabinoids primarily as adjunctive agents for refractory CINV in carefully selected patients, ideally within clinical trials or under close specialist supervision(Alderman et al., 2023; Braun et al., 2024; To et al., 2023). This conservative stance reflects the growing recognition that potential harms, combined with limited proven efficacy, necessitate a risk aware and evidence-based approach to cannabinoid integration in oncology practice.

VI. MEDICAL CANNABIS AND CANCER TREATEMENT INTERACTIONS

1. Pharmacokinetic Interactions

Cannabinoids present a clinically significant pharmacokinetic risk profile through their capacity to inhibit or induce major drug-metabolizing enzymes and membrane transporters critical to cancer drug disposition (**Tab.1**) . Both THC and CBD modulate key cytochrome P450 enzymes particularly CYP3A4 and CYP2C9 as well as uridine diphosphoglucuronosyl transferases and efflux transporters including P-glycoprotein, breast cancer resistance protein, and multidrug resistance proteins(Alves et al., 2020; Campos et al., 2024; Hanganu et al., 2022; Patel et al., 2024; Woerdenbag et al., 2023).

Table 1. Pharmacokinetic drug-drug interactions between cannabinoids and oncology medications: CYP450 enzyme and transporter mechanisms

Enzyme / Transporter	Interaction with THC / CBD	Oncology-Related Medications
CYP3A4	• Inducers may decrease THC/CBD levels	Rifampin
CYP3A4	• Inhibitors may increase THC/CBD levels	Azole antifungals (fluconazole), macrolides (clarithromycin, erythromycin), HIV protease inhibitors
CYP3A4	• CBD may increase levels of CYP3A4 substrates	Tacrolimus, cyclosporine, sirolimus, buprenorphine
CYP2C9	• Inhibitors may increase THC levels	Fluconazole
CYP2C9	• Inducers may decrease THC levels	Rifampin
CYP2C9	• THC/CBD may increase substrate drug levels	Warfarin, phenytoin
CYP2C19	• Inducers may decrease THC/CBD levels	Rifampin
CYP2C19	• Inhibitors may increase THC/CBD levels	Omeprazole, esomeprazole, fluconazole
CYP2C19	• CBD may increase substrate drug levels	Clopidogrel, diazepam, sertraline, escitalopram, pantoprazole
CYP1A1 / CYP1A2	• Smoking cannabis may increase metabolism of substrates	Amitriptyline, duloxetine, clozapine, olanzapine, mirtazapine
P-glycoprotein	• CBD may inhibit transport and increase toxicity risk	Digoxin, dabigatran

Source. Data adapted from MacCallum et al. (2021). THC = Δ9-tetrahydrocannabinol; CBD = Cannabidiol; CYP = Cytochrome P450. Original table presented comprehensive interactions across all therapeutic domains; current table focuses on oncology-related medications and clinical scenarios relevant to cancer treatment.

Since numerous cytotoxic and targeted anticancer agents including taxanes, tyrosine kinase inhibitors, tamoxifen, and bosutinib depend critically on these metabolic pathways for clearance, concurrent cannabinoid administration poses substantial risk of altered drug exposure that may increase toxicity through elevated plasma concentrations or conversely reduce efficacy through diminished bioavailability (Alves et al., 2020; Campos et al., 2024; Hanganu et al., 2022; Patel et al., 2024; Woerdenbag et al., 2023). For example, THC and CBD both inhibit CYP3A4, potentially increasing plasma concentrations of taxane-based chemotherapy (docetaxel, paclitaxel) and oral tyrosine kinase inhibitors (ibrutinib, sunitinib) by 20–40%, thereby raising toxicity risk(MacCallum et al., 2021). Narrative and systematic reviews underscore a fundamental evidentiary limitation: the overwhelming majority of interaction data derive from in vitro or animal model studies, and clinically validated dose-adjustment strategies for patients receiving concurrent cannabinoids and narrow-therapeutic-index anticancer agents remain absent from the literature(Woerdenbag et al., 2023; Alsherbiny & Li, 2018; Campos et al., 2024; Hanganu et al., 2022; Patel et al., 2024). Consequently, close therapeutic drug monitoring and vigilant clinical surveillance are strongly recommended.

2. Chemotherapy and Targeted Therapies

Preclinical studies show additive or synergistic tumor cell killing when cannabinoids are combined with several chemotherapeutics and targeted agents, and suggest that cannabinoids might also attenuate chemotherapy-induced toxicities such as neuropathy, nephrotoxicity, cardiotoxicity, and mucositis(Abrams, 2022; Buchtova et al., 2023a; Ramer & Hinz, 2025). However, most work is limited to cytotoxicity assays and animal models; robust human data demonstrating improved response rates or survival with cannabis–chemotherapy combinations are not available(Abrams, 2022; Ramer & Hinz, 2025; Woerdenbag et al., 2023). ASCO guidelines therefore recommend against using cannabis or cannabinoids as cancer-directed treatment outside clinical trials(Braun et al., 2024).

3. Immunotherapy

Cannabinoids present a distinct immunological concern when used with immune checkpoint inhibitors, a cornerstone of modern cancer treatment. Cannabinoids exert immunosuppressive effects primarily via CB2 receptor signaling, potentially undermining the antitumor immune activation that checkpoint inhibitors require(Ramer & Hinz, 2025; Vigano et al., 2025; Woerdenbag et al., 2023; Abrams, 2022). Observational studies in patients receiving checkpoint inhibitors report lower response rates with concurrent cannabis use, though overall survival outcomes remain inconsistently affected (Buchtova et al., 2023b; Patel et al., 2024; Ramer & Hinz, 2025; Vigano et al., 2025). Current expert consensus views cannabinoid-checkpoint inhibitor combinations skeptically, recommending caution or avoidance pending stronger clinical evidence(Abrams, 2022; Braun et al., 2024; Hinz & Ramer, 2022; Vigano et al., 2025; Woerdenbag et al., 2023). Given the high stakes of compromising a potentially curative immunotherapy, clinicians should explicitly discuss the potential risks of concurrent cannabis use with patients receiving checkpoint inhibitors.

4. Clinical Practice Implications

While cannabis products are generally well tolerated and may help with refractory chemotherapy-induced nausea and pain, oncologists should adopt a systematic approach. Clinicians must routinely inquire about all cannabis use including CBD-only products documenting route, dose, and frequency. They should assess potential cytochrome P450 and transporter-mediated interactions with each patient's cancer regimen, and exercise particular caution with patients receiving immune checkpoint inhibitors or narrow-therapeutic-index oral targeted therapies(Abrams, 2022; Braun et al., 2024; Campos et al., 2024; Hanganu et al., 2022; Patel et al., 2024; Woerdenbag et al., 2023), When cannabis use is pursued, standardized, non-smoked formulations should be preferred over herbal cannabis to ensure dose reliability and minimize unpredictable pharmacokinetic effects.

VII. THE EVOLVING ROLE OF ONCOLOGY NURSES IN CANNABIOIDS THERAPEUTICS

1. Clarifying Indications and Goals of Care

Before initiating cannabis, clinicians must establish clear therapeutic indication and realistic expectations grounded in available evidence. Practitioners should confirm that cannabis is being considered for evidence-supported indications including refractory chemotherapy-induced nausea and vomiting, adjunctive pain management, appetite stimulation, sleep disturbance, and anxiety while transparently acknowledging that evidence strength varies substantially across symptoms(Damsky Dell, Msn, Aprn, Aocn, Lnc & P. Stein, Md, 2021; Vinette et al., 2022; Woerdenbag et al., 2023). Explicit goal-setting conversations are essential, particularly in advanced and palliative care settings, to establish concrete therapeutic objectives and align patient expectations with realistic outcomes(Cyr et al., 2018, 2022). Oncology nurses play a critical role by eliciting patients' symptom priorities, proactively addressing misconceptions such as cannabis as a cancer "cure," and formally documenting mutually agreed treatment goals(Baral et al., 2025; Cyr et al., 2018).

2. Product Selection and Routes of Administration

Effective cannabinoid integration into oncology requires thoughtful product selection and route optimization. Clinical guidance recommends initiating, when feasible, with standardized pharmaceutical cannabinoid preparations rather than non-standardized herbal products, a strategy that substantially improves dose predictability and safety (Cyr et al., 2018, 2022). For baseline symptom control, oral or oromucosal administration is generally preferred due to superior dose precision, while inhaled formulations may be reserved for breakthrough or episodic symptoms in carefully selected clinical contexts(Cyr et al., 2022; Woerdenbag et al., 2023). The therapeutic landscape encompasses diverse formulations oils, capsules, edibles, oromucosal sprays, vaporized products, topicals, suppositories, and specialized routes including intramuscular and gastrostomy administration each presenting distinct onset times, duration of action, and safety profiles (Cyr et al., 2018, 2022; Vinette et al., 2022). Oncology nurses occupy a pivotal role in patient education, explaining that orally administered Δ9-THC undergoes first-pass hepatic metabolism to the substantially more potent 11-OH-THC metabolite, necessitating conservative starting doses and cautious titration to prevent adverse effects(Cyr et al., 2022). Nurses also ensure correct device operation, assess administration feasibility in frail or cognitively impaired patients, and provide ongoing support enabling safe and effective cannabinoid therapy (Cyr et al., 2022).

3. Dosing and Titration Principles

Systematic dosing and titration represent cornerstones of safe cannabinoid therapy in oncology and palliative care, and expert consensus affirms that clinicians with basic pharmacologic knowledge can safely authorize and monitor cannabinoid-based medicines within a structured framework(MacCallum & Russo, 2018). THC and CBD exhibit distinct indications, contraindications, and titration approaches, and available products span THC-dominant, CBD-dominant, and balanced formulations, necessitating individualized selection(Cyr et al., 2022).

Core dosing principles emphasize starting conservatively: cannabis-naïve and frail patients may experience adverse effects at oral THC doses as low as 5–10 mg, demanding careful titration over days to weeks to minimize neuropsychiatric and cardiovascular toxicity and reduce tolerance development(Cyr et al., 2018, 2022; MacCallum & Russo, 2018). Expert guidance generally recommends capping total daily THC at approximately 30 mg or less, ideally combined with CBD to attenuate THC-associated anxiety, tachycardia, and dysphoria(Cyr et al., 2018, 2022; MacCallum & Russo, 2018).

Titration must remain highly individualized, varying substantially based on patient-specific factors including comorbidities, concomitant medications, symptom burden, and susceptibility to adverse effects, with schedules flexibly adjusted according to symptom response and tolerability (Cyr et al., 2018, 2022; MacCallum & Russo, 2018).

Oncology nurses prove instrumental in supporting safe titration through frequent symptom and toxicity assessments, reinforcing adherence to individualized titration protocols, and educating patients and families about the risks of rapid dose escalation or unsupervised changes (Clark, 2018; Cyr et al., 2018, 2022). Nurses further empower patients by teaching recognition of early over-dosing signs including excessive sedation, anxiety, or confusion and establishing clear communication pathways for contacting the care team when concerns arise.

4. Safety Monitoring and Drug Interaction Management

Safe cannabinoid use in cancer care demands vigilant safety monitoring and proactive management of potential drug interactions, as cannabis products can substantially alter the pharmacokinetics and efficacy of anticancer agents and supportive medications through effects on efflux transporters and hepatic drug-metabolizing enzymes(Patel et al., 2024; Woerdenbag et al., 2023). Additional concerns emerge regarding cannabinoid combinations with immunotherapies, given potential immunosuppressive effects that could undermine checkpoint inhibitor activity (Tehranchi et al., 2025; Woerdenbag et al., 2023).

Safe cannabinoid initiation necessitates comprehensive baseline assessment including detailed review of comorbidities such as cardiovascular disease, psychiatric history, and hepatic function alongside careful cataloging of concomitant medications, with particular attention to agents with narrow therapeutic windows(Cyr et al., 2022). Clinicians should also systematically assess individual risk for cannabis use disorder, especially in patients with extended life expectancy, and establish explicit safety precautions regarding driving, machinery operation, and fall prevention, particularly in older adults(Cyr et al., 2018, 2022; MacCallum & Russo, 2018).

Oncology nurses occupy a critical frontline position in this safety framework, serving as primary monitors for adverse effects, potential drug interactions, and treatment adherence while frequently identifying unreported cannabis self-medication(Baral et al., 2025; Hughes & Casarett, 2021; Woerdenbag et al., 2023). Nursing assessments should incorporate standardized symptom scales, mental status evaluation, and periodic reassessment of quality of life and functional outcomes as cannabinoid doses are adjusted, ensuring that therapy remains proportionate to benefit and tolerable to the individual patient(Cyr et al., 2022; Damsky Dell, Msn, Aprn, Aocn, Lnc & P. Stein, Md, 2021; Vinette et al., 2022).

5. Shared Decision-Making and Communication

Effective cannabis integration into oncology requires transparent, non-judgmental shared decision-making grounded in realistic communication about evidence, benefits, and risks. Oncology practice data reveal that patients frequently initiate cannabis discussions and commonly self-medicate, yet many providers report insufficient knowledge to counsel confidently on dosing, efficacy, or safety profiles(Baral et al., 2025; Hughes & Casarett, 2021; Patel et al., 2024; Razmovski-Naumovski et al., 2022, 2025). National and expert guidelines accordingly emphasize open dialogue centered on treatment goals, potential adverse effects, evidence quality stratified by indication, and transparent acknowledgment of evidence limitations(Abrams, 2022; Razmovski-Naumovski et al., 2022; Tehranchi et al., 2025).

Oncology nurses bear an ethical obligation to champion patient autonomy and informed choice by providing balanced, evidence-based education regarding potential palliative benefits alongside genuine scientific uncertainties surrounding cannabis(-Clark, 2018; Damsky Dell, Msn, Aprn, Aocn, Lnc & P. Stein, Md, 2021) . Nursing responsibilities encompass creating psychologically safe environments with patient centered approach, where patients and families disclose cannabis use without fear of judgment, thereby dismantling stigma-related barriers to open communication(Baral et al., 2025; Clark, 2018; Khaldouni et al., 2025; Patel et al., 2024).

Nurses further translate complex pharmacologic and regulatory information into accessible language, clarifying distinctions between THC and CBD, product quality standards, contamination hazards, and legal constraints(Clark, 2018; Damsky Dell, Msn, Aprn, Aocn, Lnc & P. Stein, Md, 2021), while actively coordinating communication among oncology teams, primary care providers, and cannabis-authorizing clinicians to ensure comprehensive awareness of dosing, indications, and monitoring protocols a coordinated approach essential for managing interaction risks and providing coherent, consistent guidance(Hughes & Casarett, 2021, 2021; Tehranchi et al., 2025).

VIII. Medical Cannabis in Palliative Cancer Care

The integration of medical cannabis into cancer palliative and end-of-life care raises fundamental ethical questions that extend beyond clinical efficacy. Issues of patient autonomy, safety in vulnerable populations, equitable access, and the lasting impact of cannabis criminalization on stigma and disclosure all merit explicit consideration.

1. Ethical Considerations

Medical cannabis in cancer palliative care engages multiple ethical principles requiring explicit navigation. Autonomy versus evidence creates tension between honoring patient preferences and evidence-based practice, as many perceive cannabis as beneficial despite inconsistent efficacy data(Braun et al., 2024; Doppen et al., 2022; Nugent et al., 2020; To et al., 2023; Troyer & Tanco, 2024b). Beneficence and non-maleficence require balancing reported symptom relief against neuropsychiatric effects, drug interactions, and incompletely understood long-term harms, demanding vigilant monitoring (Bar-Lev Schleider et al., 2018; Doppen et al., 2022; Nimalan et al., 2022; To et al., 2023; Troyer & Tanco, 2024b; Woerdenbag et al., 2023). Justice concerns are pressing: high costs, limited insurance coverage, and uneven availability risk making cannabis a privilege of wealthier patients, amplifying health inequities (Bar-Lev Schleider et al., 2018; Croker et al., 2022; Gibson et al., 2024; Sura et al., 2022; Woerdenbag et al., 2023). Oncology nurses play a critical role in addressing these tensions by facilitating informed decision-making, transparently acknowledging evidence limitations, and advocating for equitable access to cannabis information and products.

2. Legal and Regulatory Challenges

Legal and regulatory fragmentation creates substantial barriers to safe cannabis integration in oncology. Laws vary dramatically across jurisdictions, and many clinicians remain uncertain about legality and regulatory requirements even in permissive jurisdictions, creating confusion and inconsistent practice(Filetti et al., 2021; Herbert & Hardy, 2021; Skórzewska & Gęca, 2024; Trapani et al., 2025; Woerdenbag et al., 2023). Schedule I or equivalent drug classifications in many regions substantially constrain clinical trials, product standardization, and pharmacovigilance systems, thereby impeding generation of robust, high-quality evidence(Braun et al., 2024; Castle et al., 2025; Doppen et al., 2022; Razmovski-Naumovski et al., 2025; Woerdenbag et al., 2023). Current clinical guidelines from major organizations including ASCO and MASCC advise against cannabis as a cancer-directed therapy and recommend against routine use for cancer pain, instead emphasizing thorough risk-benefit discussions with careful documentation to support informed shared decision-making(Braun et al., 2024; To et al., 2023; Troyer & Tanco, 2024b). These regulatory constraints and guideline recommendations underscore the critical need for policy reform that would facilitate rigorous research while maintaining patient safety.

3. Cultural and Stigma-Related Dimensions

Cannabis discussions in oncology are shaped profoundly by cultural beliefs, historical trauma, and persistent stigma that extend beyond pharmacology. Stigma and legal concerns create a significant clinician-practice gap: many providers intellectually support medical cannabis yet hesitate to prescribe due to moral discomfort, fear of legal consequences, or institutional barriers(Filetti et al., 2021; Luba et al., 2018; Nugent et al., 2020; Trapani et al., 2025). Racialized disparities compound these challenges, as the legacy of discriminatory drug policing, clinician bias regarding addiction potential, and stereotype threat collectively discourage patients of color from openly discussing cannabis or accessing it through legitimate medical channels, often forcing reliance on unregulated illicit sources (Bar-Lev Schleider et al., 2018; Gibson et al., 2024; Nugent et al., 2020; Woerdenbag et al., 2023). Generational and cultural norms further shape cannabis acceptability: older adults and certain cultural communities view cannabis as morally questionable, a perception that influences younger patients' willingness to use it or disclose use to family and clinicians(Gibson et al., 2024; Nugent et al., 2020). Equitable cancer care requires oncology teams to recognize bias and cultural factors in cannabis discussions, build trust with patients, and combat stigma.

IX. Synthesis and Future Directions - Key Takeaways for Oncology Nurses

Medical cannabis in cancer care presents a fundamental paradox: 25-33% of patients use cannabis despite weak evidence for most symptoms (Amin et al., 2024; Azizoddin et al., 2023; Donovan et al., 2023). This final section synthesizes key findings and highlights the critical role of oncology nurses in bridging the evidence-practice gap.

1. The Oncology Nurse as Clinical Leader

Four clinical priorities define safe cannabis integration, and oncology nurses lead in all four domains **(Cyr et al., 2022; Hughes & Casarett, 2021)**:

a. **Indication Clarification** Nurses establish clear therapeutic goals and realistic symptom improvement thresholds before initiation. Nurses proactively correct misconceptions (cannabis as "cancer cure") and document agreed treatment goals **(Baral et al., 2025; Cyr et al., 2022).**

b. **Safety Baseline Assessment** Nurses conduct comprehensive baseline assessments: comorbidities, medications (especially narrow-therapeutic-index agents and immunotherapies), cardiovascular history, psychiatric history, and cannabis use disorder risk (Cyr et al., 2022). Nurses identify unreported self-medication and perform medication reconciliation (Baral et al., 2025; Hughes & Casarett, 2021).
c. **Structured Monitoring** Nurses conduct standardized assessments at baseline and regular intervals, monitoring symptom relief, adverse effects, drug interactions, mental/functional status, and safety risks (driving, falls) (Cyr et al., 2022; Vinette et al., 2022).
d. **Shared Decision-Making & Communication** Nurses create non-judgmental environments for cannabis disclosure, translate complex pharmacology (THC vs. CBD, metabolism) into accessible language, and coordinate communication among oncology, primary care, and cannabis-authorizing clinicians to ensure consistent guidance.(Clark, 2018; Hughes & Casarett, 2021; Tehranchi et al., 2025).

2. Advancing Practice Through Policy and Research

Current regulatory restrictions paradoxically impede research needed to establish safe cannabinoid use (Braun et al., 2024; Castle et al., 2025). Oncology nurses should advocate for rescheduling cannabinoids from Schedule I to facilitate rigorous trials, standardizing product quality and dosing requirements, and establishing pharmacovigilance systems (Razmovski-Naumovski et al., 2022; Woerdenbag et al., 2023). Research priorities include investigation of equity and racial disparities in cannabis access and outcomes (Bar-Lev Schleider et al., 2018; Gibson et al., 2024).

Until stronger evidence emerges, cannabinoids should be reserved for carefully selected patients with refractory symptoms, used within close monitoring frameworks, and integrated into shared decision-making conversations (Braun et al., 2024; To et al., 2023).

CONCLUSION

Medical cannabis in cancer care requires investment in nursing education, clinician-patient communication, and rigorous research. Oncology nurses are essential clinical leaders who transparently educate patients about evidence limitations, conduct safety monitoring, implement shared decision-making, coordinate interdisciplinary communication, and advocate for equitable access. As evidence strengthens and regulatory barriers diminish, oncology nurses will remain at the intersection of patient autonomy, clinical safety, and evidence-informed care ensuring cautious, individualized, evidence-based practice grounded in transparent shared decision-making.

REFERNCES

Abrams, D. I. (2022). Cannabis, Cannabinoids and Cannabis-Based Medicines in Cancer Care. *Integrative Cancer Therapies*, *21*, 15347354221081772. DOI: 10.1177/15347354221081772 PMID: 35225051

Abu-Amna, M., Salti, T., Khoury, M., Cohen, I., & Bar-Sela, G. (2021). Medical Cannabis in Oncology: A Valuable Unappreciated Remedy or an Undesirable Risk? *Current Treatment Options in Oncology*, *22*(2), 16. DOI: 10.1007/s11864-020-00811-2 PMID: 33439370

Abuhasira, R., Shbiro, L., & Landschaft, Y. (2018). Medical use of cannabis and cannabinoids containing products – Regulations in Europe and North America. *European Journal of Internal Medicine*, *49*, 2–6. DOI: 10.1016/j.ejim.2018.01.001 PMID: 29329891

Aguilar, S., Gutiérrez, V., Sánchez, L., & Nougier, M. (2018). *Medicinal cannabis policies and practices around the world.*

Alderman, B., Hui, D., Mukhopadhyay, S., Bouleuc, C., Case, A. A., Amano, K., Crawford, G. B., De Feo, G., Sbrana, A., Tanco, K., To, J., Garsed, J., & Davis, M. (2023). Multinational Association of Supportive Care in Cancer (MASCC) expert opinion/consensus guidance on the use of cannabinoids for gastrointestinal symptoms in patients with cancer. *Supportive Care in Cancer*, *31*(1), 39. DOI: 10.1007/s00520-022-07480-x PMID: 36525085

Alghamdi, S. S., Albahlal, H. N., Aloumi, D. E., Bin Saqyah, S., Alsubait, A., Alamre, J., Alrashed, M., Alsuhabeny, N., & Mohammed, A. E. (2025). Revealing the therapeutic potential of synthetic cannabinoids : A systematic review of cannabinoid receptor binding dynamics and their implications for cancer therapy. *Journal of Cannabis Research*, *7*(1), 33. DOI: 10.1186/s42238-025-00289-5 PMID: 40483537

ALSalamat, H. A., Abuarab, S. F., Salamah, H. M., Ishqair, A. H., Dwikat, M. F., Nourelden, A. Z., Qandil, A. N., Barakat, Y., & Barakat, M.ALSalamat. (2024). Cannabis and cancer : Unveiling the potential of a green ally in breast, colorectal, and prostate cancer. *Journal of Cannabis Research*, *6*(1), 24. DOI: 10.1186/s42238-024-00233-z PMID: 38755733

Alsherbiny, M. A., & Li, C. G. (2018). Medicinal Cannabis—Potential Drug Interactions. *Medicines (Basel, Switzerland)*, *6*(1), 3. DOI: 10.3390/medicines6010003 PMID: 30583596

Alves, P., Amaral, C., Teixeira, N., & Correia-da-Silva, G. (2020). Cannabis sativa : Much more beyond Δ9-tetrahydrocannabinol. *Pharmacological Research, 157*, 104822. DOI: 10.1016/j.phrs.2020.104822 PMID: 32335286

Amin, S., Chae, S. W., Kawamoto, C. T., Phillips, K. T., & Pokhrel, P. (2024). Cannabis use among cancer patients and survivors in the United States : A systematic review. *JNCI Cancer Spectrum, 8*(1), pkae004. Advance online publication. DOI: 10.1093/jncics/pkae004 PMID: 38291891

AminiLari, M., Wang, L., Neumark, S., Adli, T., Couban, R. J., Giangregorio, A., Carney, C. E., & Busse, J. W.AminiLari. (2022). Medical cannabis and cannabinoids for impaired sleep : A systematic review and meta-analysis of randomized clinical trials. *Sleep (Basel), 45*(2), zsab234. Advance online publication. DOI: 10.1093/sleep/zsab234 PMID: 34546363

Azizoddin, D. R., Cohn, A. M., Ulahannan, S. V., Henson, C. E., Alexander, A. C., Moore, K. N., Holman, L. L., Boozary, L. K., Sifat, M. S., & Kendzor, D. E. (2023). Cannabis use among adults undergoing cancer treatment. *Cancer, 129*(21), 3498–3508. DOI: 10.1002/cncr.34922 PMID: 37354093

Balneaves, L. G., & Alraja, A. A. (2019). "Guarding their practice" : A descriptive study of Canadian nursing policies and education related to medical cannabis. *BMC Nursing, 18*(1), 66. DOI: 10.1186/s12912-019-0390-7 PMID: 31827392

Bar-Lev Schleider, L., Mechoulam, R., Lederman, V., Hilou, M., Lencovsky, O., Betzalel, O., Shbiro, L., & Novack, V. (2018). Prospective analysis of safety and efficacy of medical cannabis in large unselected population of patients with cancer. *European Journal of Internal Medicine, 49*, 37–43. DOI: 10.1016/j.ejim.2018.01.023 PMID: 29482741

Baral, A., Diggs, B.-N. A., Greengold, J., Foronda, C., Anglade, D., Camacho-Rivera, M., Islam, J. Y., & Vidot, D. C. (2025). State of the Science : Health Care Provider Communication of Cannabis Use Among Adults Living with Cancer. *Journal of Cancer Education, 40*(3), 329–347. DOI: 10.1007/s13187-024-02484-z PMID: 39160419

Baratta, F., Pignata, I., Ravetto Enri, L., & Brusa, P. (2022). Cannabis for Medical Use : Analysis of Recent Clinical Trials in View of Current Legislation. *Frontiers in Pharmacology, 13*, 888903. DOI: 10.3389/fphar.2022.888903 PMID: 35694246

Blebea, N. M., Pricopie, A. I., Vlad, R. A., & Hancu, G. (2024). Phytocannabinoids : Exploring Pharmacological Profiles and Their Impact on Therapeutical Use. *International Journal of Molecular Sciences, 25*(8), 4204. DOI: 10.3390/ijms25084204 PMID: 38673788

Braun, I. M., Abrams, D. I., Blansky, S. E., & Pergam, S. A. (2021). Cannabis and the Cancer Patient. *Journal of the National Cancer Institute. Monographs, 2021*(58), 68–77. DOI: 10.1093/jncimonographs/lgab012 PMID: 34850899

Braun, I. M., Bohlke, K., Abrams, D. I., Anderson, H., Balneaves, L. G., Bar-Sela, G., Bowles, D. W., Chai, P. R., Damani, A., Gupta, A., Hallmeyer, S., Subbiah, I. M., Twelves, C., Wallace, M. S., & Roeland, E. J. (2024). Cannabis and Cannabinoids in Adults With Cancer : ASCO Guideline. *Journal of Clinical Oncology, 42*(13), 1575–1593. DOI: 10.1200/JCO.23.02596 PMID: 38478773

Buchtova, T., Lukac, D., Skrott, Z., Chroma, K., Bartek, J., & Mistrik, M. (2023a). Drug–Drug Interactions of Cannabidiol with Standard-of-Care Chemotherapeutics. *International Journal of Molecular Sciences, 24*(3), 2885. DOI: 10.3390/ijms24032885 PMID: 36769206

Buchtova, T., Lukac, D., Skrott, Z., Chroma, K., Bartek, J., & Mistrik, M. (2023b). Drug–Drug Interactions of Cannabidiol with Standard-of-Care Chemotherapeutics. *International Journal of Molecular Sciences, 24*(3), 2885. DOI: 10.3390/ijms24032885 PMID: 36769206

Calapai, F., Cardia, L., Esposito, E., Ammendolia, I., Mondello, C., Lo Giudice, R., Gangemi, S., Calapai, G., & Mannucci, C. (2022). Pharmacological Aspects and Biological Effects of Cannabigerol and Its Synthetic Derivatives. *Evidence-Based Complementary and Alternative Medicine : eCAM, 2022*, 1–14. DOI: 10.1155/2022/3336516 PMID: 36397993

Campos, M. G., China, M., Cláudio, M., Capinha, M., Torres, R., Oliveira, S., & Fortuna, A. (2024). Drug–Cannabinoid Interactions in Selected Therapeutics for Symptoms Associated with Epilepsy, Autism Spectrum Disorder, Cancer, Multiple Sclerosis, and Pain. *Pharmaceuticals (Basel, Switzerland), 17*(5), 613. DOI: 10.3390/ph17050613 PMID: 38794183

Castle, R. D., Marzolf, J., Morris, M., & Bushell, W. C. (2025). Meta-analysis of medical cannabis outcomes and associations with cancer. *Frontiers in Oncology, 15*, 1490621. DOI: 10.3389/fonc.2025.1490621 PMID: 40303989

Cho, H., Kalina, E., Wu, J., Cook, R., Salloum, R., Liu, Y., Bian, J., Guo, J., & Starkweather, A. (2025). A Scoping Review of Observational Research on Cannabis Use for Symptom Management in HIV and Cancer : Implications for Cannabis Nursing. *Journal of Clinical Nursing, 34*(2), 422–429. DOI: 10.1111/jocn.17565 PMID: 39603980

Clark, C. (2018). Medical Cannabis : The Oncology Nurse's Role in Patient Education About the Effects of Marijuana on Cancer Palliation. *Clinical Journal of Oncology Nursing*, *22*(1), E1–E6. DOI: 10.1188/18.CJON.E1-E6 PMID: 29350699

Cohen, T., Ezra, M. B., Yanai, S., Oren-Azulay, T., Wein, S., & Hamama-Raz, Y. (2023). Use of Medical Cannabis by Patients With Cancer : Attitudes, Knowledge, and Practice. *Journal of Pain and Symptom Management*, *66*(3), 203–211.e1. DOI: 10.1016/j.jpainsymman.2023.05.010 PMID: 37244526

Cousins, M. M., Mayo, C., Devasia, T., Dykstra, M., Regan, S., Miller, S., Allen, S. G., Bryant, A. K., Morales-Rivera, K., Herr, D. J., Edwards, D. M., Takayesu, J., Birer, S., Egerer, N., Evans, J., Elliott, D., Henderson, C., Laucis, A. M., McFarlane, M., & Jagsi, R. (2023). Cannabis Use in Patients Seen in an Academic Radiation Oncology Department. *Practical Radiation Oncology*, *13*(2), 112–121. DOI: 10.1016/j.prro.2022.11.002 PMID: 36460181

Creangă-Murariu, I., Rezu , I.-I., Karami, R., Rancz, A., Zolcsák, Á., Engh, M. A., Obeidat, M., Tamba, B.-I., Hegyi, P., & Bunduc, S. (2025). Indications of Cannabinoids for the Palliation of Cancer-Associated Symptoms : A Systematic Review and Meta-Analysis. *Current Oncology Reports*, *27*(9), 1080–1096. DOI: 10.1007/s11912-025-01695-x PMID: 40748522

Croker, J. A., Bobitt, J., Arora, K., & Kaskie, B. (2022). Medical Cannabis and Utilization of Nonhospice Palliative Care Services : Complements and Alternatives at End of Life. *Innovation in Aging*, *6*(1), igab048. Advance online publication. DOI: 10.1093/geroni/igab048 PMID: 35047709

Cyr, C., Arboleda, M. F., Aggarwal, S. K., Balneaves, L. G., Daeninck, P., Néron, A., Prosk, E., & Vigano, A. (2018). Cannabis in palliative care : Current challenges and practical recommendations. *Annals of Palliative Medicine*, *7*(4), 463–477. DOI: 10.21037/apm.2018.06.04 PMID: 30180728

Cyr, C., Davis, M. P., Schecter, D., & Daeninck, P. (2022). *Cannabis and Cannabinoid-Based Medicines in Cancer Care : A Comprehensive Guide to Medical Management*. Springer International Publishing., DOI: 10.1007/978-3-030-89918-9

De Feo, G., Case, A. A., Crawford, G. B., Hui, D., To, J., Sbrana, A., Alderman, B., Mukhopadhyay, S., Bouleuc, C., Amano, K., Tanco, K., Garsed, J., & Davis, M. (2023). Multinational Association of Supportive Care in Cancer (MASCC) guidelines : Cannabis for psychological symptoms including insomnia, anxiety, and depression. *Supportive Care in Cancer*, *31*(3), 176. DOI: 10.1007/s00520-023-07628-3 PMID: 36809575

De Souza, M. R., Henriques, A. T., & Limberger, R. P. (2022a). Medical cannabis regulation : An overview of models around the world with emphasis on the Brazilian scenario. *Journal of Cannabis Research, 4*(1), 33. DOI: 10.1186/s42238-022-00142-z PMID: 35710586

De Souza, M. R., Henriques, A. T., & Limberger, R. P. (2022b). Medical cannabis regulation : An overview of models around the world with emphasis on the Brazilian scenario. *Journal of Cannabis Research, 4*(1), 33. DOI: 10.1186/s42238-022-00142-z PMID: 35710586

Dell, Damsky, Msn, Aprn, & Aocn, Lnc, D., & P. Stein, Md, D. (. (2021). Exploring the Use of Medical Marijuana for Supportive Care of Oncology Patients. *Journal of the Advanced Practitioner in Oncology, 12*(2). Advance online publication. DOI: 10.6004/jadpro.2021.12.2.6 PMID: 34109050

Donovan, K. A., Dolan, A., Lubrano Di Ciccone, B. B., Babilonia, M. B., Skinner, A., Reed, D. R., & Portman, D. G. (2023). Cannabis consumption in young adults with cancer : Descriptive study. *BMJ Supportive & Palliative Care, 13*(e3), e1133–e1140. DOI: 10.1136/bmjspcare-2021-003353 PMID: 35788467

Doppen, M., Kung, S., Maijers, I., John, M., Dunphy, H., Townsley, H., Eathorne, A., Semprini, A., & Braithwaite, I. (2022). Cannabis in Palliative Care : A Systematic Review of Current Evidence. *Journal of Pain and Symptom Management, 64*(5), e260–e284. DOI: 10.1016/j.jpainsymman.2022.06.002 PMID: 35705116

Duczmal, D., Bazan-Wozniak, A., Niedzielska, K., & Pietrzak, R. (2024). Cannabinoids—Multifunctional Compounds, Applications and Challenges—Mini Review. *Molecules (Basel, Switzerland), 29*(20), 4923. DOI: 10.3390/molecules29204923 PMID: 39459291

Eldering, L., Kiew, I., Lee, W., Seah, D., & Chye, R. (2025). Perceptions and interests of cannabis use among patients with cancer : A cross-sectional survey. *Palliative Medicine, 39*(8), 910–914. DOI: 10.1177/02692163251351550 PMID: 40637222

Ellison, G. L., Helzlsouer, K. J., Rosenfield, S. M., Kim, Y., Ashare, R. L., Blaes, A. H., Cullen, J., Doran, N., Ebbert, J. O., Egan, K. M., Heffner, J. L., Lee, R. T., McClure, E. A., McDaniels-Davidson, C., Meghani, S. H., Newcomb, P. A., Nugent, S., Hernandez-Ortega, N., Salz, T., & Zylla, D. M. (2024). Perceptions, prevalence, and patterns of cannabis use among cancer patients treated at 12 NCI-Designated Cancer Centers. *Journal of the National Cancer Institute. Monographs, 2024*(66), 202–217. DOI: 10.1093/jncimonographs/lgae029 PMID: 39108244

Filetti, M., Trapani, D., Cortellini, A., Cofini, V., Necozione, S., Pinato, D. J., Porzio, G., Marchetti, P., & Giusti, R. (2021). Knowledge and attitudes of Italian medical oncologists and palliative care physicians toward medical use of cannabis in cancer care : A national survey. *Supportive Care in Cancer*, *29*(12), 7845–7854. DOI: 10.1007/s00520-021-06383-7 PMID: 34176017

Gibson, L. P., Ferrer, R. A., Meghani, S. H., & Acevedo, A. M. (2024). Potential role of cannabis in ameliorating observed racialized disparities in cancer pain management. *Journal of the National Cancer Institute*, *116*(7), 1019–1025. DOI: 10.1093/jnci/djae058 PMID: 38471103

Gonzalez, B. D., Li, X., Martinez, Y. C., Jim, H. S. L., Oswald, L. B., Islam, J. Y., Turner, K., & Egan, K. M. (2024). Cannabis use and patient-reported outcomes among patients at a comprehensive cancer center. *Journal of the National Cancer Institute. Monographs*, *2024*(66), 259–266. DOI: 10.1093/jncimonographs/lgae012 PMID: 39108234

Good, P., Haywood, A., Gogna, G., Martin, J., Yates, P., Greer, R., & Hardy, J. (2019). Oral medicinal cannabinoids to relieve symptom burden in the palliative care of patients with advanced cancer : A double-blind, placebo controlled, randomised clinical trial of efficacy and safety of cannabidiol (CBD). *BMC Palliative Care*, *18*(1), 110. DOI: 10.1186/s12904-019-0494-6 PMID: 31810437

Hanganu, B., Lazar, D. E., Manoilescu, I. S., Mocanu, V., Butcovan, D., Buhas, C. L., Szalontay, A. S., & Ioan, B. G. (2022). Controversial Link between Cannabis and Anticancer Treatments—Where Are We and Where Are We Going? A Systematic Review of the Literature. *Cancers (Basel)*, *14*(16), 4057. DOI: 10.3390/cancers14164057 PMID: 36011049

Hardy, J. R., Greer, R. M., Pelecanos, A. M., Huggett, G. E., Kearney, A. M., Gurgenci, T. H., & Good, P. D. (2025). Medicinal cannabis for symptom control in advanced cancer : A double-blind, placebo-controlled, randomised clinical trial of 1:1 tetrahydrocannabinol and cannabidiol. *Supportive Care in Cancer*, *33*(8), 715. DOI: 10.1007/s00520-025-09763-5 PMID: 40705150

Häuser, W., Welsch, P., Radbruch, L., Fisher, E., Bell, R. F., & Moore, R. A. (2023). Cannabis-based medicines and medical cannabis for adults with cancer pain. *Cochrane Database of Systematic Reviews*, *2023*(6). DOI: 10.1002/14651858.CD014915.pub2

Helzlsouer, K. J., Rosenfield, S. M., Freedman, A. N., & Ellison, G. L. (2024). Overview of cancer patient perspectives on cannabis use during treatment. *Journal of the National Cancer Institute. Monographs*, *2024*(66), 199–201. DOI: 10.1093/jncimonographs/lgae025 PMID: 39108236

Herbert, A., & Hardy, J. (2021). Medicinal cannabis use in palliative care. *Australian Journal of General Practice, 50*(6), 363–368. DOI: 10.31128/AJGP-02-21-5831 PMID: 34059839

Hinz, B., & Ramer, R. (2022). Cannabinoids as anticancer drugs : Current status of preclinical research. *British Journal of Cancer, 127*(1), 1–13. DOI: 10.1038/s41416-022-01727-4 PMID: 35277658

Hossain, M. K., & Chae, H. J. (2024). Medical cannabis : From research breakthroughs to shifting public perceptions and ensuring safe use. *Integrative Medicine Research, 13*(4), 101094. DOI: 10.1016/j.imr.2024.101094 PMID: 39640076

Hughes, K. T., & Casarett, D. J. (2021). Education and communication are critical to effectively incorporating cannabis into cancer treatment. *Cancer, 127*(1), 27–30. DOI: 10.1002/cncr.33204 PMID: 32986251

Jardim, C., & Delgado-Charro, M. B. (2025). The Regulatory Environment Surrounding Cannabis Medicines in the EU, the USA, and Australia. *Pharmaceutics, 17*(5), 635. DOI: 10.3390/pharmaceutics17050635 PMID: 40430926

Kemmner, S. F., Dörfler, J., & Huebner, J. (2025). Cannabinoids for the prevention of chemotherapy-induced nausea and vomiting in oncological therapy : A systematic review. *Journal of Cancer Survivorship: Research and Practice*. Advance online publication. DOI: 10.1007/s11764-025-01876-4 PMID: 40797063

Khademi, S., Hallinan, C. M., Conway, M., & Bonomo, Y. (2023). Using Social Media Data to Investigate Public Perceptions of Cannabis as a Medicine : Narrative Review. *Journal of Medical Internet Research, 25*, e36667. DOI: 10.2196/36667 PMID: 36848191

Khaldouni, S., Amane, M., Lamtali, S., Boussaa, S., El Rhanbouri, M., Oussous, A., & Laghouasli, F. (2025). Implementation of Advanced Nursing Practices Through the Adoption of a Patient-Centered Approach. In Amane, M., & Boussaa, S. (Eds.), *Advanced Nursing Practices for Clinical Excellence* (pp. 305–348). IGI Global., DOI: 10.4018/979-8-3693-6730-8.ch014

Kleckner, A. S., Kleckner, I. R., Kamen, C. S., Tejani, M. A., Janelsins, M. C., Morrow, G. R., & Peppone, L. J. (2019). Opportunities for cannabis in supportive care in cancer. *Therapeutic Advances in Medical Oncology, 11*, 1758835919866362. DOI: 10.1177/1758835919866362 PMID: 31413731

Luba, R., Earleywine, M., Farmer, S., & Slavin, M. (2018). Cannabis in End-of-Life Care : Examining Attitudes and Practices of Palliative Care Providers. *Journal of Psychoactive Drugs*, *50*(4), 348–354. DOI: 10.1080/02791072.2018.1462543 PMID: 29714640

MacCallum, C. A., Lo, L. A., & Boivin, M. (2021). "Is medical cannabis safe for my patients?" A practical review of cannabis safety considerations. *European Journal of Internal Medicine*, *89*, 10–18. DOI: 10.1016/j.ejim.2021.05.002 PMID: 34083092

MacCallum, C. A., & Russo, E. B. (2018). Practical considerations in medical cannabis administration and dosing. *European Journal of Internal Medicine*, *49*, 12–19. DOI: 10.1016/j.ejim.2018.01.004 PMID: 29307505

Malabadi, R. B., Mammadova, S. S., Kolkar, K. P., Mr, S., Chalannavar, R. K., & Karen, V. C. C. (2024). Cannabis sativa : A therapeutic medicinal plant-global marketing updates. *World Journal of Biology Pharmacy and Health Sciences*, *17*(2), 170–183. DOI: 10.30574/wjbphs.2024.17.2.0044

Mangal, N., Erridge, S., Habib, N., Sadanandam, A., Reebye, V., & Sodergren, M. H. (2021). Cannabinoids in the landscape of cancer. *Journal of Cancer Research and Clinical Oncology*, *147*(9), 2507–2534. DOI: 10.1007/s00432-021-03710-7 PMID: 34259916

Mashabela, M. D., & Kappo, A. P. (2024). Anti-Cancer and Anti-Proliferative Potential of Cannabidiol : A Cellular and Molecular Perspective. *International Journal of Molecular Sciences*, *25*(11), 5659. DOI: 10.3390/ijms25115659 PMID: 38891847

McClure, E. A., Walters, K. J., Tomko, R. L., Dahne, J., Hill, E. G., & McRae-Clark, A. L. (2023). Cannabis use prevalence, patterns, and reasons for use among patients with cancer and survivors in a state without legal cannabis access. *Supportive Care in Cancer*, *31*(7), 429. DOI: 10.1007/s00520-023-07881-6 PMID: 37382737

McIntosh, N., Wilson, N. J., Povalej, P., Hunt, L., & Lewis, P. (2024). An Exploration of Registered Nurses' Experiences Caring for Patients Taking Medicinal Cannabis. *Nursing Open*, *11*(10), e70063. DOI: 10.1002/nop2.70063 PMID: 39455290

Melo, E. S. A., Asevedo, E. A., Duarte-Almeida, J. M., Nurkolis, F., Syahputra, R. A., Park, M. N., Kim, B., Couto, R. O. D., & Ribeiro, R. I. M. D. A. (2025). Mechanisms of Cell Death Induced by Cannabidiol Against Tumor Cells : A Review of Preclinical Studies. *Plants*, *14*(4), 585. DOI: 10.3390/plants14040585 PMID: 40006844

Milian, L., Mata, M., Alcacer, J., Oliver, M., Sancho-Tello, M., Martín De Llano, J. J., Camps, C., Galbis, J., Carretero, J., & Carda, C. (2020). Cannabinoid receptor expression in non-small cell lung cancer. Effectiveness of tetrahydrocannabinol and cannabidiol inhibiting cell proliferation and epithelial-mesenchymal transition in vitro. *PLoS One*, *15*(2), e0228909. DOI: 10.1371/journal.pone.0228909 PMID: 32049991

Mücke, M., Weier, M., Carter, C., Copeland, J., Degenhardt, L., Cuhls, H., Radbruch, L., Häuser, W., & Conrad, R. (2018). Systematic review and meta-analysis of cannabinoids in palliative medicine. *Journal of Cachexia, Sarcopenia and Muscle*, *9*(2), 220–234. DOI: 10.1002/jcsm.12273 PMID: 29400010

Nayak, M. M., Revette, A., Chai, P. R., Lansang, K., Sannes, T., Tung, S., & Braun, I. M. (2023). Medical cannabis-related stigma : Cancer survivors' perspectives. *Journal of Cancer Survivorship: Research and Practice*, *17*(4), 951–956. DOI: 10.1007/s11764-022-01297-7 PMID: 36435953

Nielsen, S. W., Ruhlmann, C. H., Eckhoff, L., Brønnum, D., Herrstedt, J., & Dalton, S. O. (2022). Cannabis use among Danish patients with cancer : A cross-sectional survey of sociodemographic traits, quality of life, and patient experiences. *Supportive Care in Cancer*, *30*(2), 1181–1190. DOI: 10.1007/s00520-021-06515-z PMID: 34453567

Nimalan, D., Kawka, M., Erridge, S., Ergisi, M., Harris, M., Salazar, O., Ali, R., Loupasaki, K., Holvey, C., Coomber, R., Platt, M., Rucker, J. J., Khan, S., & Sodergren, M. H. (2022). UK Medical Cannabis Registry palliative care patients cohort : Initial experience and outcomes. *Journal of Cannabis Research*, *4*(1), 3. DOI: 10.1186/s42238-021-00114-9 PMID: 34980282

Nugent, S. M., Meghani, S. H., Rogal, S. S., & Merlin, J. S. (2020). Medical cannabis use among individuals with cancer : An unresolved and timely issue. *Cancer*, *126*(9), 1832–1836. DOI: 10.1002/cncr.32732 PMID: 32012232

O'Reilly, E., Khalifa, K., Cosgrave, J., Azam, H., Prencipe, M., Simpson, J. C., Gallagher, W. M., & Perry, A. S. (2023). Cannabidiol Inhibits the Proliferation and Invasiveness of Prostate Cancer Cells. *Journal of Natural Products*, *86*(9), 2151–2161. DOI: 10.1021/acs.jnatprod.3c00363 PMID: 37703852

Paiva, C., Santos, T., Cunha-Oliveira, A., Rosendo, I., & Pita, J.-R. (2024). Knowledge, opinions and experiences of nurses and nursing students in Portugal regarding the use of medical Cannabis. *BMC Nursing*, *23*(1), 788. DOI: 10.1186/s12912-024-02443-5 PMID: 39468501

Patel, R., Patel, M., Patel, Z., Kavani, H., Patel, D., & Shaikh, S. (2024). Analyzing the medical use of cannabis for cancer patients : A critical perspective. *International Journal of Community Medicine and Public Health, 11*(3), 1349–1354. DOI: 10.18203/2394-6040.ijcmph20240644

Pergam, S. A., Woodfield, M. C., Lee, C. M., Cheng, G., Baker, K. K., Marquis, S. R., & Fann, J. R. (2017). Cannabis use among patients at a comprehensive cancer center in a state with legalized medicinal and recreational use. *Cancer, 123*(22), 4488–4497. DOI: 10.1002/cncr.30879 PMID: 28944449

Ramer, R., & Hinz, B. (2025). Effect of cannabinoids on the efficacy and side effects of anticancer therapeutic strategies – Current status of preclinical and clinical research. *Pharmacology & Therapeutics, 270*, 108851. DOI: 10.1016/j.pharmthera.2025.108851 PMID: 40221102

Rashid, Z., Lee, G. R., Khalil, M., Altaf, A., Zindani, S., Sarfraz, A., & Pawlik, T. M. (2025). Patterns of Cannabis Use Among Cancer Survivors : Insights From the Behavioral Risk Factor Surveillance System. *JCO Oncology Practice*, •••, OP-25–OP-00121. DOI: 10.1200/OP-25-00121 PMID: 40632994

Razmovski-Naumovski, V., Martin, J. H., Chye, R., Phillips, J. L., Lintzeris, N., Solowij, N., Lee, J., Lovell, M., Noble, B., Galettis, P., Brown, L., Fazekas, B., Clark, K., Luckett, T., McCaffrey, N., Currow, D. C., & Agar, M. R. (2025). Design Considerations for Medicinal Cannabis Clinical Trials in People Receiving Palliative Care. *Journal of Pain and Symptom Management, 69*(5), e395–e408. DOI: 10.1016/j.jpainsymman.2025.02.009 PMID: 39988015

Razmovski-Naumovski, V., West, P. A., Bellemore, F., Byfieldt, N., Bellamy, D., Chye, R., Clark, K., Martin, J. H., Fazekas, B., Phillips, J. L., & Agar, M. R. (2022). Defining the trials nurses' role in operationalising a medicinal cannabis clinical trial. *Collegian (Royal College of Nursing, Australia), 29*(3), 370–378. DOI: 10.1016/j.colegn.2021.10.003

Ruheel, M. A., Gomes, Z., Usman, S., Homayouni, P., & Ng, J. Y. (2021). Facilitators and barriers to the regulation of medical cannabis : A scoping review of the peer-reviewed literature. *Harm Reduction Journal, 18*(1), 106. DOI: 10.1186/s12954-021-00547-8 PMID: 34649577

Salum, K. C. R., Miranda, G. B. A., Dias, A. L., Carneiro, J. R. I., Bozza, P. T., Da Fonseca, A. C. P., & Silva, T. (2025). The endocannabinoid system in cancer biology : A mini-review of mechanisms and therapeutic potential. *Oncology Reviews, 19*, 1573797. DOI: 10.3389/or.2025.1573797 PMID: 40370489

Salz, T., Meza, A. M., Chino, F., Mao, J. J., Raghunathan, N. J., Jinna, S., Brens, J., Furberg, H., & Korenstein, D. (2023). Cannabis use among recently treated cancer patients : Perceptions and experiences. *Supportive Care in Cancer, 31*(9), 545. DOI: 10.1007/s00520-023-07994-y PMID: 37650961

Schubel, L. C., McCready, D. M., LoParco, C. R., Arem, H., & Berg, C. J. (2025). Cannabis Use Among Adolescents and Young Adults with Cancer : A Scoping Review. *Journal of Cancer Education*. Advance online publication. DOI: 10.1007/s13187-025-02693-0 PMID: 40764891

Shalata, W., Abu Saleh, O., Tourkey, L., Shalata, S., Neime, A. E., Abu Juma'a, A., Soklakova, A., Tourkey, L., Jama, A. A., & Yakobson, A. (2024). The Efficacy of Cannabis in Oncology Patient Care and Its Anti-Tumor Effects. *Cancers (Basel), 16*(16), 2909. DOI: 10.3390/cancers16162909 PMID: 39199679

Skórzewska, M., & Gęca, K. (2024). The Role of Cannabinoids in Advancing Cancer Treatment : Insights from Evidence-Based Medicine. *Current Oncology Reports, 26*(11), 1334–1348. DOI: 10.1007/s11912-024-01589-4 PMID: 39110350

Śledziński, P., Zeyland, J., Słomski, R., & Nowak, A. (2018). The current state and future perspectives of cannabinoids in cancer biology. *Cancer Medicine, 7*(3), 765–775. DOI: 10.1002/cam4.1312 PMID: 29473338

Sura, K. T., Kohman, L., Huang, D., & Pasniciuc, S. V. (2022). Experience With Medical Marijuana for Cancer Patients in the Palliative Setting. *Cureus*. Advance online publication. DOI: 10.7759/cureus.26406 PMID: 35915672

Taylor, J. S., Fradgley, E. A., Britton, B. B., Martin, J. H., Lucas, C., Carlson, M. A., Bridge, P., Morris, S., Watts, G., & Lynam, J. (2025). Patients' Perceptions of the Efficacy, Safety, and Quality of the Evidence of Medicinal Cannabis : A Survey of Australian Cancer Patients. *Asia Pacific Journal of Clinical Oncology, 21*(5), 545–551. DOI: 10.1111/ajco.14149 PMID: 39829052

Tehranchi, K., Patell, R., Bindal, P., Dodge, L., Freed, J., Buss, M., Schonberg, M. A., Braun, I., & Rangachari, D. (2025). Patterns and factors among oncology fellows recommending medical cannabis to adults with cancer. *Journal of Cannabis Research, 7*(1), 45. DOI: 10.1186/s42238-025-00293-9 PMID: 40660376

Teixeira, H. M. (2025). Phytocanabinoids and synthetic cannabinoids : From recreational consumption to potential therapeutic use – a review. *Frontiers in Toxicology, 6*, 1495547. DOI: 10.3389/ftox.2024.1495547 PMID: 39936019

To, J., Davis, M., Sbrana, A., Alderman, B., Hui, D., Mukhopadhyay, S., Bouleuc, C., Case, A. A., Amano, K., Crawford, G. B., De Feo, G., Tanco, K., & Garsed, J. (2023). MASCC guideline : Cannabis for cancer-related pain and risk of harms and adverse events. *Supportive Care in Cancer*, *31*(4), 202. DOI: 10.1007/s00520-023-07662-1 PMID: 36872397

Trapani, D., Nidhamalddin, S. J., Gandini, S., Filetti, M., Altuna, S. C., Carnevale Schianca, A., Petrillo, A., Murthy, S. M., Girardi, F., Bezuidenhout, J. B., El Bairi, K., Lombardi, P., Khan, S. Z., Lengyel, C. G., Seeber, A., Hussain, S., Seid, F. U., Elfaham, E., Odhiambo, A. O., & Giusti, R. (2025). An international survey on the knowledge, attitudes and clinical patterns of use of medical cannabis for cancer care : The TASMAN study. *European Journal of Cancer*, *215*, 115158. DOI: 10.1016/j.ejca.2024.115158 PMID: 39647216

Troyer, J., & Tanco, K. (2024a). Review of the Use of Medicinal Cannabis Products in Palliative Care. *Cancers (Basel)*, *16*(7), 1412. DOI: 10.3390/cancers16071412 PMID: 38611090

Troyer, J., & Tanco, K. (2024b). Review of the Use of Medicinal Cannabis Products in Palliative Care. *Cancers (Basel)*, *16*(7), 1412. DOI: 10.3390/cancers16071412 PMID: 38611090

Turgeman, I., & Bar-Sela, G. (2019). Cannabis for cancer – illusion or the tip of an iceberg : A review of the evidence for the use of Cannabis and synthetic cannabinoids in oncology. *Expert Opinion on Investigational Drugs*, *28*(3), 285–296. DOI: 10.1080/13543784.2019.1561859 PMID: 30572744

Turgut, N. H., Armagan, G., Kasapligil, G., & Erdogan, M. A. (2022). Anti-cancer effects of selective cannabinoid agonists in pancreatic and breast cancer cells. *Bratislava Medical Journal*, *123*(11), 813–821. DOI: 10.4149/BLL_2022_130 PMID: 36254639

Valente, A. C., Lopes, L. P. N., & Matheus, M. E. (2024). Medical cannabis use in oncology and associated outcomes : A scoping review. *Journal of Oncology Pharmacy Practice*, *30*(4), 737–751. DOI: 10.1177/10781552241239006 PMID: 38477532

Vigano, M., Wang, L., As'sadiq, A., Samarani, S., Ahmad, A., & Costiniuk, C. T. (2025). Impact of cannabinoids on cancer outcomes in patients receiving immune checkpoint inhibitor immunotherapy. *Frontiers in Immunology*, *16*, 1497829. DOI: 10.3389/fimmu.2025.1497829 PMID: 40109334

Vinette, B., Côté, J., El-Akhras, A., Mrad, H., Chicoine, G., & Bilodeau, K. (2022). Routes of administration, reasons for use, and approved indications of medical cannabis in oncology : A scoping review. *BMC Cancer*, *22*(1), 319. DOI: 10.1186/s12885-022-09378-7 PMID: 35331185

Voicu, V., Brehar, F.-M., Toader, C., Covache-Busuioc, R.-A., Corlatescu, A. D., Bordeianu, A., Costin, H. P., Bratu, B.-G., Glavan, L.-A., & Ciurea, A. V. (2023). Cannabinoids in Medicine : A Multifaceted Exploration of Types, Therapeutic Applications, and Emerging Opportunities in Neurodegenerative Diseases and Cancer Therapy. *Biomolecules*, *13*(9), 1388. DOI: 10.3390/biom13091388 PMID: 37759788

Walsh, K. B., McKinney, A. E., & Holmes, A. E. (2021). Minor Cannabinoids : Biosynthesis, Molecular Pharmacology and Potential Therapeutic Uses. *Frontiers in Pharmacology*, *12*, 777804. DOI: 10.3389/fphar.2021.777804 PMID: 34916950

Wang, L., Hong, P. J., May, C., Rehman, Y., Oparin, Y., Hong, C. J., Hong, B. Y., AminiLari, M., Gallo, L., Kaushal, A., Craigie, S., Couban, R. J., Kum, E., Shanthanna, H., Price, I., Upadhye, S., Ware, M. A., Campbell, F., Buchbinder, R., & Busse, J. W. (2021). Medical cannabis or cannabinoids for chronic non-cancer and cancer related pain : A systematic review and meta-analysis of randomised clinical trials. *BMJ (Clinical Research Ed.)*, (1034), n1034. Advance online publication. DOI: 10.1136/bmj.n1034 PMID: 34497047

Weisman, J. M., & Rodríguez, M. (2021). A systematic review of medical students' and professionals' attitudes and knowledge regarding medical cannabis. *Journal of Cannabis Research*, *3*(1), 47. DOI: 10.1186/s42238-021-00100-1 PMID: 34641976

Woerdenbag, H. J., Olinga, P., Kok, E. A., Brugman, D. A. P., Van Ark, U. F., Ramcharan, A. S., Lebbink, P. W., Hoogwater, F. J. H., Knapen, D. G., De Groot, D. J. A., & Nijkamp, M. W. (2023). Potential, Limitations and Risks of Cannabis-Derived Products in Cancer Treatment. *Cancers (Basel)*, *15*(7), 2119. DOI: 10.3390/cancers15072119 PMID: 37046779

Worster, B., Hajjar, E. R., & Handley, N. (2022). Cannabis Use in Patients With Cancer : A Clinical Review. *JCO Oncology Practice*, *18*(11), 743–749. DOI: 10.1200/OP.22.00080 PMID: 35749680

Zagzoog, A., Mohamed, K. A., Kim, H. J. J., Kim, E. D., Frank, C. S., Black, T., Jadhav, P. D., Holbrook, L. A., & Laprairie, R. B. (2020). In vitro and in vivo pharmacological activity of minor cannabinoids isolated from Cannabis sativa. *Scientific Reports*, *10*(1), 20405. DOI: 10.1038/s41598-020-77175-y PMID: 33230154

Zhou, E. S., Nayak, M. M., Chai, P. R., & Braun, I. M. (2022). Cancer patient's attitudes of using medicinal cannabis for sleep. *Journal of Psychosocial Oncology*, *40*(3), 397–403. DOI: 10.1080/07347332.2021.1910396 PMID: 33847549

Chapter 14
Cannabis Nursing:
Emergence of a New Nursing Specialty and Its Integration Into Contemporary Clinical Practice

Abdelati Oussous
http://orcid.org/0009-0002-9555-346X
Cadi Ayyad University, Morocco

Mounia Amane
http://orcid.org/0000-0002-9273-4284
Higher Institute of Nursing Professions and Health Techniques, Marrakech, Morocco

Mohammed El Rhanbouri
http://orcid.org/0009-0006-9643-5181
Cadi Ayyad University, Morocco

Mouna Khouchani
Faculty of Medicine and Pharmacy, Marrakech, Morocco

Fatiha Laghouasli
http://orcid.org/0009-0008-6716-812X
Cadi Ayyad University, Morocco

ABSTRACT

This chapter explores cannabis nursing as an emerging specialty shaped by the rapid uptake of medical cannabis in healthcare. Although access and demand have grown, clinical governance, professional training, and standardized practice have not kept pace, creating safety, ethical, and organizational risks. Drawing on international experience and recent professional frameworks, the chapter positions

DOI: 10.4018/979-8-2600-2035-7.ch014

cannabis nursing within advanced practice, emphasizing structured assessment, evidence-informed decision-making, therapeutic education, and interprofessional coordination. It reviews historical drivers, regulatory heterogeneity, training gaps, and stigma, and highlights nurses' roles in risk management, documentation, and continuity of care. By defining conceptual models, core competencies, educational needs, and institutional integration strategies, the chapter argues that cannabis nursing is essential for safe, equitable, person-centered implementation of medical cannabis.

INTRODUCTION

Throughout the history of nursing, some specialties emerge not because a new drug appears or a new technology is introduced, but rather from the need to fill a clinical gap that has become too visible to ignore. Medical cannabis falls into this category. Its rapid integration within contemporary care pathways has occurred in a paradoxical context: while legal access and patient demand have expanded considerably, clinical oversight, professional training, and standardization of practices long remained fragmented (Brooks et al., 2017). This disconnect between therapeutic accessibility and clinical governance now represents one of the primary challenges to integrating medical cannabis into health systems (Committee on the Public Health Consequences of Changes in the Cannabis Policy Landscape et al., 2024).

The therapeutic benefits of cannabis are real but modest, varying by indication and mode of administration (Montero-Oleas et al., 2020; Whiting et al., 2015; Committee on the Health Effects of Marijuana: An Evidence Review and Research Agenda et al., 2017). Levels of evidence remain uneven, with more robust data for certain neuropathic pain conditions, spasticity related to multiple sclerosis, or chemotherapy-induced nausea, and weak or insufficient evidence for many other indications frequently cited by patients (Busse et al., 2021; Stockings et al., 2018). At the same time, the risks associated with unsupervised use are well documented: drug interactions, cardiovascular and neuropsychiatric effects, and an increased risk of accidents, particularly when clinical monitoring is insufficient (Brown & Winterstein, 2019; Di Forti et al., 2019; Page et al., 2020). Recent population-level analyses confirm that the absence of structured clinical supervision can turn a potential benefit into an individual and systemic risk, particularly among vulnerable populations (Stall et al., 2024).

Faced with this clinical uncertainty and growing demand, the need for specific nursing expertise has become clear. The emergence of cannabis nursing is not the result of a sudden institutional recognition. Rather, it reflects a gradual process shaped by the increasing medicalization of cannabis, the growing complexity of care pathways, and the identification of a striking deficit in clinical expertise at the bedside. International experiences—particularly in Canada, the United States, the Netherlands, and Israel—show that nurses have progressively been called upon to play a pivotal liaison role among patients, physicians, pharmacists, and regulatory authorities. In often heterogeneous regulatory contexts, they provide therapeutic education, monitor adverse effects, and coordinate care (Clarke & Fitzcharles, 2023; Shim et al., 2023; Zarhin et al., 2018).

A major milestone was reached with the official recognition of cannabis nursing as a specialty by the American Nurses Association (ANA) in 2023, followed by the publication of the first *Cannabis Nursing: Scope and Standards of Practice* in collaboration with the American Cannabis Nurses Association (ACNA) (Moore, 2024) . This formalization of the specialty builds upon the National Nursing Guidelines for Medical Marijuana from the National Council of State Boards of Nursing which, as early as 2018, laid the foundations for safe nursing practice by emphasizing clinical assessment, harm reduction, rigorous documentation, and interprofessional collaboration (NCSBN, 2018). Together, these standardizing frameworks mark the shift from an informal practice to a structured specialty that can be taught, assessed, and institutionally integrated. Yet this professional recognition, while essential, has not resolved a deeper structural tension

However, this professional structuring continues to face a persistent problem: the readiness of health systems and nursing professionals remains largely insufficient relative to patient demand. A critical training deficit—extensively documented internationally—contributes to marked heterogeneity in clinical practices and undermines care safety. In this context, the absence of a clearly identified designated clinical expert limits therapeutic optimization.

Yet nurses occupy a strategic position to address these challenges. Their clinical proximity, continuous presence across care pathways, and bridging role within teams give them a unique capacity to gather reliable information. They can thus document actual cannabis use, therapeutic expectations, adverse effects, as well as medical or psychosocial vulnerabilities (NCSBN, 2018). The literature emphasizes that the quality of the therapeutic alliance and the adoption of non-judgmental communication are essential determinants of patient disclosure of cannabis use and the safety of clinical decisions (Troup et al., 2022; W. R. Miller & Rollnick, 2013). Moreover, in a field characterized by polarized social representations, coordination and interprofessional collaboration appear to be major drivers for coherence, continuity, and quality of care (Reeves et al., 2017; WHO, 2010).

From this perspective, cannabis nursing fully aligns with the paradigm of advanced practice nursing. It requires specialized clinical expertise, the capacity for structured risk assessment, rigorous evidence-based practice, leadership in interprofessional coordination, and an ethical responsibility in the face of scientific uncertainty and patient vulnerabilities (Tracy & O'Grady, 2019). Far from being a marginal or transient practice, it represents a professional response to a major contemporary issue: how can a therapy whose use often precedes clinical oversight be integrated into a safe, equitable, and person-centered manner?

This chapter engages with this question and proposes to examine cannabis nursing as an emerging nursing specialty at the intersection of therapeutic innovation and care safety. By integrating historical, conceptual, clinical, educational, and organizational dimensions, it aims to show that the development of cannabis nursing constitutes a logical and necessary evolution of contemporary nursing practice, responding to growing demands for quality, rigor, and equity in the integration of medical cannabis.

1. HISTORICAL BACKGROUND OF CANNABIS NURSING: THE GENESIS OF A SPECIALTY

The emergence of cannabis nursing as a specialty is part of a historical and geopolitical dynamic marked by the progressive medicalization of cannabis in certain pioneer countries—Canada, the United States, and Israel—. In these pioneering settings, regulatory, clinical, and cultural transformations created the conditions for increasing involvement of nursing professionals in care related to medical cannabis. This section traces the key stages of this genesis.

1.1 Roots and Pioneer Settings

In the United States, the movement began in the 1990s, primarily driven by advocacy from patients living with HIV/AIDS and cancer, calling for compassionate access to cannabis. The legalization of medical cannabis, starting with California in 1996, occurred in a context of regulatory fragmentation, with each state developing its own access and prescribing frameworks. This heterogeneity led to uneven involvement of health professionals and limited integration of cannabis into conventional care structures. Nevertheless, the growth of legal markets and the increasing number of patients using cannabis progressively necessitated clinical, educational, and harm-reduction competencies within the nursing domain, particularly in symptom assessment, therapeutic education, and monitoring of adverse effects (Committee on the Public Health Consequences of Changes in the Cannabis Policy Landscape et al., 2024).

Canada adopted a pioneering and structured approach as early as 2001. The Marihuana Medical Access Regulations (MMAR) established a federal framework for access to medical cannabis under supervision. This evolution continued through successive reforms: the Marijuana for Medical Purposes Regulations (MMPR)

(Health Canada, 2014), which introduced a commercialized system via licensed producers; the Access to Cannabis for Medical Purposes Regulations (ACMPR) (Garcia, 2019), which reintroduced personal cultivation under strict conditions; and the 2018 Cannabis Act, which promoted a gradual normalization of cannabis within the health system. However, this integration occurred largely outside traditional pharmaceutical channels, with clinical oversight sometimes limited. Nurses thus came to play a pivotal role among patients, physicians, and producers, particularly in supporting patients, assisting with patient-directed dosing, and providing education for safer use (Clarke & Fitzcharles, 2023; Shim et al., 2023).

The Netherlands represents another pioneering setting, characterized by strong state intervention in regulating medical cannabis. The creation in 2000 of the Office of Medicinal Cannabis (OMC) enabled centralized production, distribution, and clinical research on cannabis in accordance with the requirements of the Single Convention on Narcotic Drugs. This approach explicitly aimed to support rigorous clinical trials and ensure standardized pharmaceutical-grade product quality. In this context, cannabis is regarded as a therapeutic agent subject to scientific evaluation rather than as a tolerated exception, which facilitated the progressive integration of nursing competencies in clinical research, patient monitoring, and the prevention of diversion (Scholten, 2001).

Finally, Israel occupies a distinct place in the history of medical cannabis, combining an early national program (dating to the 1990s) with major investment in biomedical research. The Israeli model is based on a strict institutional distinction between medical cannabis and recreational use, reflected in a licensing system, specialized prescriber training, and centralized monitoring. Successive reforms expanded access while strengthening clinical and organizational requirements, creating an environment in which nurses have progressively assumed responsibilities in patient assessment, longitudinal follow-up, and care coordination (Aviram, 2025; Zarhin et al., 2018).

These divergent trajectories—state-level fragmentation (United States), federal centralization (Canada), scientific regulation (Netherlands), biomedical research (Israel)—reveal a consistent pattern: in all contexts, the absence of structured medical supervision compelled nurses to fill an unmet clinical need. While these historical settings enabled the grassroots emergence of nursing role, other contemporary factors accelerated their professional structuring: training gap, the opioid crisis, and the evolution of clinical evidence.

1.2. Catalyzing Factors

1.2.1. Training and Knowledge Gaps Among Clinicians

From the earliest phases of legalization, a lack of professional preparedness—both clinical and regulatory—was noted (Brooks et al., 2017). Recent syntheses confirm this gap: a majority of nurses and students have received no formal education on medical cannabis, undermining the safety of advice provided (Paiva et al., 2024; Weisman & Rodríguez, 2021; Zolotov et al., 2021). This deficit acts as a paradoxical catalyst: it increases patient demand directed toward nurses while limiting their capacity to respond safely—thereby deepening the clinical void that cannabis nursing seeks to fill.

1.2.2. Opioid Crisis

The opioid crisis positioned cannabis as a potential alternative in pain management. Although the opioid-sparing effect of cannabinoids remains debated, an updated meta-analysis indicates a modest but significant reduction in opioid consumption among patients treated with cannabis for chronic pain (Nielsen et al., 2022). However, Le Foll et al. (2021) emphasize the need to interpret these findings cautiously due to methodological limitations in observational studies.

Thus, while the opioid crisis is an important catalyst, it does not by itself justify generalized integration of medical cannabis without a structured clinical and professional framework.

Beyond societal and educational determinants, the evolution of clinical evidence and patient demand also shape the emerging landscape of this specialty.

1.2.3. Clinical Evidence, Recommendations, and Patient Demand

Concurrently, certain professional guidelines have helped legitimize and frame the use of medical cannabis for specific indications. ASCO guidelines illustrate this evolution by offering a pragmatic oncology framework based on a balanced analysis of benefits and risks (Braun et al., 2024). The evidence mapping by Montero-Oleas et al. (2020) nevertheless confirms that, despite a substantial volume of publications, the quality of evidence remains uneven across indications. Notably, the majority of included reviews relied on short-term trials with heterogeneous populations and outcome measures, limiting direct comparability across indications and reinforcing the need for clinician-led individualized benefit–risk appraisal. In this context of uncertainty, patient demand plays a driving role, placing nurses on the front line for therapeutic education, expectation management, and identification of at-risk situations (Clark et al., 2022).

In a nutshell, the development of cannabis nursing reflects a convergence of historical, clinical, professional, and societal factors. However, this empirical and fragmented emergence quickly revealed its limitations, demanding the shift from an informal practice to a formally recognized specialty. This professional structuring is discussed below.

1.3. Professional Structuring of Cannabis Nursing

Faced with practice variability and scientific uncertainty, professional structuring has emerged as an essential response. In 2023, the American Nurses Association (ANA) recognized cannabis nursing as a distinct specialty. In 2024, the ANA collaborated with the American Cannabis Nurses Association (ACNA) to publish the book *"Cannabis Nursing: Scope and Standards of Practice."* This professional reference provides a first framework for nursing practice in medical cannabis, guiding nurses in the delivery of safe, high-quality, competency-based care. It defines key concepts of cannabis nursing and addresses the endocannabinoid system, therapeutic applications of cannabis, ethical principles, cannabis use disorders, regulatory considerations, and social justice issues (Moore, 2024). This foundational document was preceded by the National Nursing Guidelines for Medical Marijuana from the National Council of State Boards of Nursing (NCSBN, 2018), which established principles for practice safety, nursing responsibilities, and competency requirements, thereby contributing to standardization and safer care.

Training plays a central role in this structuring process. Targeted educational programs have demonstrated improved knowledge and practitioner confidence, particularly among advanced practice nurses (Klein & Bindler, 2022). Moreover, the work of Kurtzman et al. (2022) highlights the importance of nursing leadership in the organizational integration of medical cannabis when approached through the lens of quality and patient safety.

1.4. Parallels With Advanced Practice Nursing Roles

The evolution of medical cannabis shows similarities with other clinical domains that have progressively matured into advanced nursing specialties, notably emergency nursing and oncology. As with these areas, legitimacy was built through the articulation of clinical evidence, recognition of unmet needs, and regulatory structuring.

The (NCSBN, 2018) recognizes that advanced practice nurses may be involved in certifying eligible medical conditions, depending on jurisdictional frameworks. In addition, the development of consensus-based competency frameworks—such as the one proposed by Zolotov et al. (2025)— marks disciplinary maturation. These frameworks provide a shared foundation for education, practice, and potential certification, positioning medical cannabis within the logic of an emerging clinical specialty rather than a marginal practice.

These historical parallels justify the conceptual anchoring of cannabis nursing in advanced practice models—a framework developed in the following section.

2. CONCEPTUAL FRAMEWORK: ADVANCED PRACTICE APPLIED TO CANNABIS NURSING

This section proposes a conceptual framework to define, structure, and operationalize cannabis nursing as an emerging specialty within advanced nursing practice. The objective is not to "reinvent" a discipline, but to ground this clinical field in robust models in order to: (a) clarify the scope of practice, (b) explicitly define expected and assessable competencies, and (c) facilitate organizational and medico-legal integration within heterogeneous regulatory contexts.

2.1. Role, Scope, and Competencies: Why a Theoretical Model is Necessary?

Advanced nursing practice corresponds to a level of practice characterized by heightened clinical autonomy, complex reasoning, and the ability to intervene in situations marked by uncertainty, risk, and multidimensionality—clinical, ethical, organizational. The International Council of Nurses defines the Advanced Practice Nurse as a nurse who has acquired an expert knowledge, complex clinical decision-making skills, and clinical competencies for expanded practice, the scope of which varies according to context and national regulation (International Council of Nurses, 2020). In this approach, the conceptual model is not a theoretical appendage; it is a practical tool to delineate and legitimize the role, directly linked to patient safety and professional accountability.

This perspective is particularly relevant for cannabis nursing because the domain encompasses multiple sources of variability and risk: (1) heterogeneity of indications and evidence levels across symptoms (pain, nausea, spasticity, sleep disorders, etc.); (2) product variability (formulations, THC/CBD ratios, routes of administration, titration); (3) drug interactions and patient vulnerabilities (psychiatric conditions, substance use disorders, pregnancy, driving safety, frailty); (4) stigma and frequent conflation of medical and recreational use; and (5) regulatory instability across jurisdictions. From an educational standpoint, the literature consistently documents a deficit in professional preparedness: the scoping review by Zolotov et al. (2021)

highlights training that is often limited or non-standardized and a perceived inadequacy in counselling patients safely.

In this context, a theoretical framework fulfills four operational functions:

- Delineate the clinical scope: structured assessment, therapeutic education, medication safety monitoring, outcome follow-up, documentation, and traceability.
- Standardize competencies: define expected knowledge, skills and attitudes; specify observable behaviours; and clarify boundaries of practice requiring referral.
- Facilitate institutional integration: align the role with existing procedures (pharmacy protocols, quality assurance, risk management, storage/administration policies, adverse event reporting pathways).
- Enable practice evaluation: establish indicators, impact metrics, continuous quality improvement mechanisms, and compliance monitoring.

For the concrete deployment of advanced roles, a second type of model proves valuable: a development and evaluation framework. The PEPPA model (Participatory, Evidence-based, Patient-focused Process for Advanced Practice Nursing) describes a structured process for designing, implementing, and evaluating advanced practice roles based on patient needs and health system characteristics (Bryant-Lukosius & DiCenso, 2004). In cannabis nursing, PEPPA can support a sequential approach: needs assessment (symptoms, patient requests, risks); clarification of objectives (safety, health literacy, care coordination); role design (competencies, activities, interprofessional interfaces); implementation (protocols, training); and evaluation (clinical outcomes, quality indicators, patient satisfaction, adverse events).

Finally, coherence among competencies, education, recognition, and authorization to practice is a critical determinant of safety. The U.S. consensus model for APRN regulation formalizes an alignment logic known as "LACE" (Licensure, Accreditation, Certification, Education), designed to reduce ambiguities between training, certification, and authorized scope (APRN Consensus Work Group & the National Council of State Boards of Nursing APRN Advisory Committee, 2008). Although regulatory architectures vary internationally, the principle remains transferable: without explicit alignment among competencies, training, and governance, cannabis nursing risks remaining an "implicit" practice—difficult to evaluate and vulnerable to medico-legal exposure.

This need for clear reference points is further amplified by evolving legal frameworks. In the United States, for example, the discrepancy between state-level legalization and federal prohibition illustrates regulatory complexity: cannabis remains classified as Schedule I at the federal level, while an administrative rescheduling process to Schedule III, initiated by a Department of Justice proposal, was explicitly accelerated by an executive order published in December 2025 (Congressional Research Service, 2025). Such contexts reinforce the value of an advanced practice framework that incorporates regulatory literacy, meticulous documentation, and proactive risk management.

2.2. Hamric Model of Advanced Practice Nursing Applied to Cannabis Nursing

To structure cannabis nursing, Hamric & Hanson's integrative model of advanced nursing practice (6th edition) is selected as the central framework. It proposes an architecture of seven core competencies that transcend specific clinical domains, making it particularly suitable for emerging specialties such as cannabis nursing (Tracy & O'Grady, 2019). The seven core competencies and their application areas in cannabis nursing are summarized in **Table 1**; their operationalization is detailed in Section 3.

Table 1. Application of the Hamric & Hanson model to cannabis nursing

Core Competency	Application Domain in Cannabis Nursing
1. Direct Clinical Practice	Expert delivery of direct care, including comprehensive assessment, clinical diagnosis, intervention, and longitudinal follow-up: evaluating indications, risk profiles, therapeutic efficacy, and adverse drug events (Kurtzman et al., 2022).
2. Guidance and Coaching	Supporting and educating patients and families to promote self-management and health-seeking behaviours: patient education; coaching for safe titration ("start low, go slow"); and strategies for stigma reduction (W. R. Miller & Rollnick, 2013; Zolotov et al., 2021).
3. Consultation	Providing specialized expertise to healthcare professionals or systems regarding complex cases: oncology, psychiatry; managing organizational interfaces with pharmacy services (risk mitigation, pathway design, and clinical protocols) (Tracy & O'Grady, 2019).
4. Evidence-Based Practice (EBP)	Systematic integration of high-quality evidence, clinical expertise, and patient preferences: reflective practice; critical appraisal of literature (e.g., Whiting et al., 2015); and the synthesis of evidence into care plans and clinical reasoning (Albarqouni et al., 2018; Committee on the Health Effects of Marijuana: An Evidence Review and Research Agenda et al., 2017).
5. Leadership	Influencing, inspiring, and leading systemic change to improve care quality: standardizing clinical practices; advocating for robust institutional policies; and spearheading quality and safety initiatives (NCSBN, 2018c; NHS England, 2025).

continued on following page

Table 1. Continued

Core Competency	Application Domain in Cannabis Nursing
6. Collaboration	Interprofessional partnership to achieve shared therapeutic goals: coordinating care with physicians, pharmacists, social workers, and other multidisciplinary stakeholders (Reeves et al., 2017; WHO, 2010).
7. Ethical Decision-Making	Resolving ethical dilemmas through the principles of autonomy, beneficence, non-maleficence, and justice: balancing patient self-determination with risk prevention (e.g., psychiatric vulnerability); ensuring equitable access; and managing stigma-related conflicts (Tracy & O'Grady, 2019).

2.3. Regulatory Integration and Practice Safeguards

The conceptual framework must also integrate the regulatory dimension— characterized by instability and heterogeneity—that defines medical cannabis practice. This complexity reinforces the value of an advanced practice framework incorporating regulatory literacy, rigorous documentation, and proactive management of medico-legal risks. The ability to navigate evolving regulatory landscapes and adapt practice accordingly constitutes an essential cross-cutting competency for the cannabis nurse.

3. CLINICAL IMPLEMENTATION—EBP COMPETENCIES AND TOOLS OF THE CANNABIS NURSE

The core competencies of the cannabis nurse, grounded in evidence-based practice (EBP), form an integrated framework. This section outlines their practical implementation, drawing on the current evidence base and emerging standards, building on the advanced practice framework presented in Section 2.

3.1 Applied Pharmacological and Assessment Competencies

Pharmacological competency forms the foundation of safe practice. It requires a solid understanding of the endocannabinoid system, pharmacokinetics across routes of administration, and the clinical implications of varying THC/CBD ratios (NCSBN, 2018). This knowledge enables clinically reasoned counselling, for example, prioritizing sublingual oils for stable chronic pain management and vaporized formulations for acute chemotherapy-induced nausea (Huestis, 2007). It also requires critical appraisal of evidence to calibrate patient expectations, such as referencing the meta-analysis by Whiting et al. (2015), which reports "moderate" evidence for neuropathic pain relief but "limited" evidence for anxiety reduction. It should be noted that this review included trials of variable quality and duration, with most using synthetic cannabinoids rather than whole-plant preparations—a distinction clinically relevant to current practice, where product heterogeneity remains considerable Accordingly, this competency demands ongoing vigilance in response to the rapid growth of unregulated commercial products.

Pre-treatment assessment, in turn, extends beyond standard history-taking to identify cannabis-specific risks. The NCSBN Guidelines (NCSBN, 2018) delineate essential components, including evaluation of comorbidities (cardiovascular, respiratory, psychiatric), potential drug interactions, and individual vulnerability factors such as history of psychosis or age under 25 years — populations in which THC exposure is associated with an elevated risk of psychotic disorders (Di Forti et al., 2019; Volkow et al., 2014). The nurse must systematically analyze clinically significant interactions, such as increased clobazam levels with concomitant CBD use in patients with epilepsy (Morrison et al., 2019) or the need for warfarin dose adjustment when CBD is co-administered (Brown & Winterstein, 2019). This dual competency positions the nurse as a critical safety checkpoint in the therapeutic pathway.

3.2 Decision-Making Competency: Developing Evidence-Based Care Plans

In jurisdictions permitting collaborative prescribing, the nurse practitioner contributes to developing a structured therapeutic plan built around three EBP principles: realistic goals, cautious titration, and predefined discontinuation criteria (NCSBN, 2018c). Practical recommendations, such as the simplified Canadian guidelines (Allan et al., 2018), support shared decision-making.

- Evidence-aligned goals: objectives must be specific (e.g., "30% reduction in neuropathic pain intensity on the VAS within 4 weeks") and calibrated to indication-specific evidence quality—robust for neuropathic pain and sclerosis–related spasticity, but moderate or insufficient for many others (Busse et al., 2021; Committee on the Health Effects of Marijuana: An Evidence Review and Research Agenda et al., 2017; Stockings et al., 2018).
- Cautious titration ("start low, go slow"): This principle is supported by consensus recommendations favouring gradual dosing. For inhaled cannabis, guidelines recommend starting with a single inhalation and waiting 15 minutes before considering additional doses to achieve symptom control while minimizing adverse effects (MacCallum & Russo, 2018).

This competency places the nurse as a guarantor of scientific rigor in medical cannabis practice, preventing expansion of use beyond evidence-supported indications.

3.3 Safe Monitoring and Risk Prevention

Monitoring is a dynamic competency that goes far beyond routine side-effect surveillance to encompass multiple safety dimensions:

- Road and occupational safety: Explicit counselling on abstaining from driving (at least 6 hours post-inhalation), supported by data demonstrating increased collision risk (Rogeberg & Elvik, 2016; Sevigny, 2021).
- Screening for cannabis use disorder: Use of validated instrument such as the ASSIST (Alcohol, Smoking and Substance Involvement Screening Test) to identify problematic use patterns (Hasin et al., 2015).
- Psychiatric vigilance: Active monitoring for emergence of psychotic or anxiety symptoms, particularly among adolescents, young adults or individuals with personal or family psychiatric histories (Volkow et al., 2014; Di Forti et al., 2019).
- Cardiovascular assessment: Monitoring for tachycardia, orthostatic hypotension, and other cardiovascular effects (Page et al., 2020).

Through these activities, the nurse serves as the linchpin of longitudinal safety, especially critical for vulnerable populations.

3.4 Contextual Competency: Adaptation to Specific Clinical Settings

Excellence in cannabis nursing requires nuanced adaptation based on patient populations and levels of evidence available for each indication.

- Oncology/palliative care: Application of evidence supporting THC or nabiximols for refractory chemotherapy-induced nausea and vomiting, with careful management of interactions with conventional antiemetics (Smith et al., 2015).
- Pediatric neurology: Integration of trial data on purified CBD (Epidiolex®) for or treatment-resistant epileptic encephalopathies, including coordination of dose adjustments for concomitant anticonvulsants (Devinsky et al., 2017; Thiele et al., 2018).
- Noncancer chronic pain: Implementation of recommendations, such as those of Busse et al.(2021), which position cannabis as an option only after failure of first-line therapies, accompanied by transparent informed consent regarding the modest magnitude of expected benefits.

This contextual competency prevents rigid, one-size-fits-all protocols ill-suited to clinical realities.

3.5 Mastery of Tools and Commitment to Continuing Education

The cannabis nurse must master an arsenal of validated tools to anchor practice in EBP: risk assessment grids (NCSBN, 2018), dosing algorithms (Allan et al., 2018), informed-consent templates, and shared decision-making aids (Busse et al., 2021). These instruments are essential for structuring practice and reducing variability.

This competency also entails an active commitment to continuing professional development—an imperative given internationally documented training deficits (Paiva et al., 2024; Weisman & Rodríguez, 2021). The consensus competency framework (Zolotov et al., 2025), detailed in Section 4, provides a valuable structure for self-assessment and ongoing learning. This metacognitive competency—the ability to recognize the limits of one's knowledge and actively seek updates—constitutes both the ethical foundation and a critical safety safeguard of the specialty.

Collectively, the core competencies of the cannabis nurse form an integrated framework in which pharmacology, assessment, clinical decision-making, monitoring, contextual adaptation, and tool mastery converge to deliver safe, evidence-based care. In a rapidly evolving therapeutic landscape, these competencies are inherently dynamic, requiring ongoing reflection grounded in critical appraisal of emerging evidence and intellectual humility regarding current knowledge limitations. Integrating medical cannabis into nursing care cannot be conceived without an evidence-based approach attentive to risks, uncertainties, and patient values. This section underscores the need to structure education and clinical tools to support the emergence of a robust nursing specialty capable of addressing contemporary challenges in medical cannabis care.

4. EDUCATION, CURRICULUM, AND PROFESSIONAL DEVELOPMENT IN CANNABIS NURSING

The development of cannabis nursing as a specialty requires redesigning nursing education pathways to address knowledge and competency gaps specific to the therapeutic use of cannabis. This section examines current training deficits, approaches to continuing professional development, existing competency frameworks, and proposes a structured model curriculum, which constitutes a foundational lever for the legitimation and institutional recognition of this specialized practice.

4.1 Foundational Deficits and Continuing Professional Development Strategies

The emergence of cannabis nursing as a structured specialty is hindered by a systemic training deficit documented internationally. Prelicensure nursing education programs rarely include substantive content on therapeutic cannabis or the endocannabinoid system —the pathophysiological cornerstone of cannabinoid therapeutic (Zolotov et al., 2021). This gap manifests consistently across settings: in Canada, 76.3% of nurse practitioners report a noticeable need for training on dosing and individualized therapeutic planning, while in Portugal, 71.7% of nurses and 79.5% of students report never having encountered the concept of the endocannabinoid system (Balneaves et al., 2018; Paiva et al., 2024).

These knowledge deficits generate a troubling disconnect between theoretical acceptance and clinical competence. In U.S. long-term care facilities, 94.2% of professionals consider medical cannabis a viable therapeutic option, but only 37.2% believe they have received adequate training; lack of education and clinical guidance thus represents the primary barrier to its recommendation, despite a significant association between knowledge and professional confidence ($p = 0.002$) (Attonito et al., 2024). This gap between acceptance and competence compromises patient safety and impedes the integration of cannabis into care plans (McIntosh et al., 2024).

In response to this foundational deficit, several continuing education strategies demonstrate effectiveness in closing the competence gap. E-learning enhances accessibility: a systematic meta-review indicates that digital modules significantly improve nursing knowledge while generating high learner satisfaction (Rouleau et al., 2019). A brief digital training program produced significant gain in nurse practitioners' understanding of pharmacokinetics and drug–drug interactions, while also increasing their willingness to inquire about cannabis use and provide patient counselling (Klein & Bindler, 2022). Clinical simulation, guided by INACSL standards, is particularly relevant for practicing management of complex scenarios (overdosing, opioid interactions) and strengthening interprofessional collaboration(Inacsl Standards Committee et al., 2025). Finally, adopting educational strategies that target implicit bias appears essential in a field marked by persistent stigma, to support clinical practice grounded in evidence rather than social stereotypes (Kruse et al., 2022).

This multimodal combination—digital, experiential, and reflective—extends beyond factual knowledge acquisition: it builds the clinical confidence required for safe practice, progressively transforming theoretical understanding into demonstrable, transferable expertise.

4.2 Cannabis Nursing Competency Frameworks

Several organizations have structured cannabis nursing through professional standards. The NCSBN (2018b) guidelines and the ANA/ACNA Cannabis Nursing: Scope and Standards of Practice (Moore, 2024)—both presented in detail in Section 1.3—provide the foundational regulatory and professional framework for the specialty.

An international consensus statement published by Zolotov et al.(2025) complements these frameworks by identifying six core competencies for medical education: (1) understanding the fundamentals of the endocannabinoid system; (2) describing the main components of the cannabis plant and their biological effects; (3) examining the legal and regulatory framework for cannabis; (4) describing the evidence base for conditions commonly managed with cannabis; (5) recognizing potential risks associated with medical cannabis use; and (6) applying basic principles of clinical care using medical cannabis. These frameworks provide an essential foundation for program accreditation and practice evaluation.

4.3 Proposed Model Curriculum

A model curriculum for cannabis nursing should build on the competency framework of Zolotov et al. (2025), the NCSBN guidelines (2018), and the ANA/ACNA standards (2024) (American Cannabis Nurses Association, 2023; American Nurses Association, 2021; NCSBN, 2018). Accordingly, essential content domain should include: (a) pharmacological fundamentals of cannabinoids and the endocannabinoid system; (b) legislation, regulation, and professional ethics across jurisdictions; (c) assessment of target symptoms; (d) risk management (cannabis use disorder, drug interactions); and (e) therapeutic communication and stigma reduction. Learning objectives should adhere to the SMART criteria and align with Miller's pyramid of clinical competence (G. E. Miller, 1990): progressing from "knows" (factual knowledge) to "knows how" (comprehension), "shows how" (demonstration in simulation), and ultimately "does" (application in supervised clinical practice. Competency assessment should combine validated knowledge questionnaires (assessing the "knows" level) with high-fidelity simulations using structured observation grids aligned with INACSL standards (McMahon et al., 2021).

4.4 Curriculum as the Foundation for Specialty Recognition

Formalizing a standardized curriculum extends beyond addressing to an educational need; it constitutes the decisive step toward official recognition of cannabis nursing as a specialty. By codifying a core set of assessable competencies, it defines a distinct domain of expertise—a prerequisite for recognition by professional regulatory bodies. The robust evaluation embedded within it renders mastery measurable, thereby establishing the credibility needed for specialty certification pathways (NCSBN, 2018). Finally, integration into accredited academic programs and shared governance anchors the specialty institutionally. Thus, the curriculum does more than train; it demonstrates, standardizes, and certifies expertise. It serves as the indispensable catalyst in the transition from an emerging practice to an established nursing specialty.

5. INTERPROFESSIONAL COLLABORATION AND CLINICAL COMMUNICATION

Within cannabis nursing as an emerging specialty, the nurse's role extends beyond implementing prescribed treatments. Rather, the nurse functions as a pivotal integrator within an interprofessional care network, ensuring safety, coherence, and continuity across the care continuum. This section examines the collaboration and communication models that underpin this advanced practice.

5.1 Why IPE and Coordination are Central?

In the emerging field of medical cannabis—characterized by heterogeneous knowledge across disciplines and persistent social stigma— interprofessional education (IPE) and structured coordination are not an organizational luxury but a prerequisite for clinical safety. A meta-analysis including 15 studies found that seven reported overall positive effects of IPE on team collaboration, quality of care, and reductions in clinical errors across diverse settings, while four reported mixed results (Reeves et al., 2018). Three imperatives justify this centrality in medical cannabis: (1) patient safety, threatened by undocumented drug–drug interactions or inappropriate dosing; (2) consistency of patient education, critical when patients receive contradictory advice regarding titration or administration routes; and (3) continuity across fragmented care pathways spanning specialized, primary, and community settings (Reeves et al., 2018). The World Health Organization emphasizes that IPE promotes effective collaboration and improves health outcomes (WHO, 2010), while National Council of State Boards of Nursing guidelines explicitly position the nurses as responsible for interprofessional communication to prevent treatment conflicts (NCSBN, 2018)—a pre-eminent risk in a field where perceptions remain polarized (Zolotov et al., 2018).

5.2 Operational Models to Structure Collaboration

Translating collaborative intent into practice requires explicit operational frameworks. Clarifying professional roles using tools such as the RACI matrix (Responsible, Accountable, Consulted, Informed) formalizes responsibilities at each care stage: prescribing (physician), symptom assessment and ongoing nursing surveillance, dosing guidance (pharmacist), and psychosocial support (social worker) (Brower et al., 2021). This role clarification prevents ambiguity that can lead to therapeutic delays or critical omissions. Effective collaborative practice relies on structured governance models, shared protocols, joint decision-making processes, and standardized communication strategies—supported by enabling leadership, appropriate institutional policies, and a work environment conductive to interprofessional coordination (WHO, 2010). Additionally, communication tools such as SBAR (Situation–Background–Assessment–Recommendation) serve as practical frameworks for interprofessional exchanges. When integrated into multimodal organizational interventions, SBAR has been shown to improve team communication and safety culture (Lo et al., 2021). A systematic review confirms that SBAR implementation yields moderate improvement in patient safety outcomes (Müller et al., 2018)—a critical advantage when patients navigate complex care transitions across hospital, home, and multiple provider settings.

5.3 Nonjudgmental Communication and Stigma-Informed Care

Non-judgmental communication is an essential competency for mitigating stigma surrounding medical cannabis—a core ethical challenge developed in Section 8.1. A "stigma-informed" attitude requires nurses to adopt a non-directive communication style grounded in motivational interviewing principles (W. R. Miller & Rollnick, 2013). This evidence–based method —validated in substance use contexts (Smedslund et al., 2011)— enables clinicians to explore patients' expectations, prior experiences, and concerns without judgement while strengthening autonomous decision-making. Within the interprofessional team, nurses serve as mediators who challenge implicit biases (e.g., equating therapeutic cannabis with a "recreational drug use") through contextualized evidence sharing. This dual competency—patient-centered communication and interprofessional mediation— fosters psychological safety within teams, a prerequisite for authentic collaboration and high-reliability care.

5.4 Clinical Illustrations: When Theory Meets Practice

To anchor these principles in clinical reality, three vignettes illustrate how structured interprofessional collaboration and non-judgmental communication transform potentially conflictual situations into coherent and safe therapeutic pathways.

Vignette 1: Chronic pain and opioid reduction. Ms. L., 58, lives with chronic low back pain treated with oxycodone (60 mg/day) but experiences debilitating side effects. During a multidisciplinary team meeting (physician, specialized nurse, pharmacist), the team proposes a trial of low-THC cannabis (<5% THC) alongside gradual opioid tapering, consistent with recommendations from Busse et al.(2021). The nurse, trained in motivational interviewing, explores the patient's fears about cannabis without judgment, documents effects using a shared symptom diary, and ensures weekly information relay with the pharmacist to support coordinated dose adjustments.

Vignette 2: Oncology and chemotherapy-induced nausea. Mr. K., receiving chemotherapy for pancreatic adenocarcinoma, experiences nausea refractory to standard antiemetics. The specialized nurse initiates an urgent consultation with the oncologist and hospital pharmacist. Drawing on evidence from Smith et al. (2015), the team adds a THC/CBD oromucosal spray to his regimen. The nurse structures handoffs between hospital and home care using a standardized SBAR protocol, preventing communication breakdowns during care transitions.

Vignette 3: Psychiatric vulnerability and safety. A young adult with an anxiety disorder reports self-medicating with recreational cannabis. Alerted by data from Di Forti et al. (2019) regarding increased psychosis risk in vulnerable individuals, the nurse facilitates a non-stigmatizing referral for joint evaluation by a psychiatrist and the prescribing clinician. At the same time, the nurse provides factual education about risks documented by Volkow et al. (2014), illustrating how clinical vigilance and respect for patient autonomy can coexist.

6. INSTITUTIONAL INTEGRATION AND REGULATORY NAVIGATION

The institutional integration of cannabis for therapeutic purposes presents a particular organizational challenge because it combines: (1) a therapeutic agent whose legal and pharmaceutical status varies widely across jurisdictions; (2) supply chains that may fall under conventional medicinal regulation (marketing authorization) or specialized medical cannabis frameworks; (3) traceability requirements comparable to those for controlled substances; and (4) medication-related risks (dosing errors, drug interactions, neurocognitive effects) that require robust quality-

and-safety systems (WHO, 2017). In this context, the value of cannabis nursing extends beyond individual clinical competence: it is fully realized when institutions formalize a defined scope of practice, standardized documentation, and system-wide clinical governance—rather than relying on fragmented, case-by-case management (Committee on the Public Health Consequences of Changes in the Cannabis Policy Landscape et al., 2024).

6.1. Regulatory Heterogeneity and the Need for Institutional Policies

Legal frameworks directly determine access (who can initiate/authorize, where and how the product is obtained), scope of practice (administration vs self-administration, storage protocols, inventory management), and documentation requirements (prescription, "medical authorization," written order, consent forms, registries, incident reporting). This heterogeneity operates across multiple dimensions:

Product status: medicine vs medical-cannabis regime.

In some jurisdictions, access occurs through cannabinoid-based medicines with full pharmaceutical status (e.g., approved products), whereas elsewhere it occurs under specialized medical cannabis regulations where products lack formal medicinal classification. Within the European Union, cannabis-derived products may follow multiple regulatory pathways (medicine, preparation, herbal substance, etc.), requiring institutions to clarify "what comes in" and under what status, before defining who administers and how to document (EMCDDA, 2023).

Federal vs regional level: intra-country variability.

In the United States, discrepancies between state policies and federal law have long generated institutional uncertainty. Although federal administrative actions under consideration (including a proposal to reschedule cannabis) may affect research access and certain supply channels, they do not automatically standardize clinical practice within healthcare facilities (U.S. Department of Justice, 2024).

Facility-level supply models: patient-supplied versus pharmacy-integrated.

Health systems must choose between (a) a "patient-supplied" model (patients bring the product; the hospital oversees storage and administration) and (b) a "pharmacy-integrated" model (products enter through institutional supply chains). This choice determines traceability (lot numbers, THC/CBD concentrations, dosage forms), quality assessment (reliable labeling), and error-risk management. Safety alerts have highlighted the frequency of labeling problems (missing information, inaccurate concentrations) on certain medical cannabis products, reinforcing the need for structured verification prior to administration and precise documentation of strength and dose (ISMP, 2020).

Implications for clinical documentation.

When products are authorized through mechanisms other than conventional prescriptions (e.g., "recommendation or certification"), nursing and medical documentation must compensate by explicitly recording: clinical indication; therapeutic goals (pain, spasticity, nausea…); benefit–risk assessment; dosing regimen (THC/CBD ratio, frequency, route); monitoring, and stopping criteria. Professional nursing recommendations emphasize the responsibility to verify local legal requirements and integrate structured, auditable documentation into the plan of care (National Safety Council, 2019).

Finally, heterogeneity is not only legal—it is also programmatic. Some countries have relied on access/experimentation programs with transitional arrangements. In France, the national authority communicated continuity of care provision for patients enrolled in the experimentation, with a specified deadline, illustrating the need for "bridge" protocols and close administrative follow-up (ANSM, 2024).

Despite jurisdictional diversity—federal versus state frameworks in the United States, a dedicated regime in Canada, multi-pathways in Europe—one consistent imperative emerges: the need for an explicit institutional policy covering secure storage, rigorous traceability, standardized documentation, and incident management. Guidelines for preventing diversion of controlled substances within hospital pharmacies offer transferable principle for the secure handling of THC-containing products (Clark et al., 2022). Exemplar hospital policies demonstrate the value of codifying rules regarding patient-supplied cannabis, restrictions on recreational cannabis within facilities, and mandatory documentation in the clinical record—to reduce reliance on informal practices (Canadian Society of Hospital Pharmacists, 2021). Without this organizational foundation, nurses encounter ambiguities that may lead to therapeutic delays, critical omissions, or defensive practice patterns.

A detailed comparative synthesis of regulatory frameworks and their operational implications across jurisdictions (United States, Canada, Europe, Israel) is presented in Appendix A.

6.2. Quality and Safety: Committees, Audits, Indicators, and Protocol Updates

The safety of cannabis/cannabinoid therapeutics should be approached as a conventional medication safety issue, requiring standardization, error prevention, and organizational learning (WHO, 2017). Two structural components are central:

1) Cross-cutting quality-and-safety governance (a committee or subgroup within medication governance) overseeing authorized product lists, required competencies, periodic audits, and feedback integration. Contemporary incident-response frameworks advocate for a proportionate, systems-oriented approach that prioritize

analysis of contributing factors and process improvement over individual attribution of blame (NHS England, 2025).

2) Pragmatic performance indicators spanning processes (documentation completeness, reconciliation rates, storage compliance), outcomes (adverse event rates, safety signals), and competencies (staff training rates, reassessment frequency)—a comprehensive selection of validated Key Performance Indicators (KPIs) is provided in Appendix G.

Protocol updates should be triggered by regulatory changes, introduction of new products, safety signals (e.g., inaccurate labeling), or internal incidents. Safety advisories underscore that strength and labeling errors can lead to inappropriate intake and clinical consequences, justifying heightened vigilance regarding product information quality (ISMP, 2020)

6.3. Organizational Rationale: Toward a Dedicated Clinical "Stream"

Three arguments support establishing a dedicated, structured pathway for medical cannabis:

- Reducing variability and ensuring equitable access: when frameworks are heterogeneous, access and safety may depend on the clinical service, individual prescriber preference, or staff familiarity. Public policy analyses emphasize that inconsistent protections and fragmented governance increase risk of inequities and lack of coherence in public health safeguards (Committee on the Public Health Consequences of Changes in the Cannabis Policy Landscape et al., 2024). A unified institutional framework standardizes assessment, documentation, and education across all care setting.
- Medication safety and risk control: a dedicated pathway facilitates targeted training, standardized tools (order sets, checklists, patient handouts), regular audits, and structured interface with pharmacy to reduce errors and diversion risk (Clark et al., 2022; WHO, 2017).
- Natural clinical integration: the most coherent hospital applications are embedded within already-structured pathways (chronic/complex pain, oncology, supportive care, palliative care, neurology…), where regular reassessment, benefit–risk balancing, and interdisciplinary coordination are already standardized. The dedicated pathway then functions as a clinical–regulatory interface that secures the circuit, standardizes documentation, and ensures admission-to-discharge continuity (Health Canada, 2018; Règlement sur le cannabis, 2018).

In summary, institutional integration is not merely a "legal" concern: it is a system challenge. Cannabis nursing delivers its full value when it is translated into concrete mechanisms—governance, internal policies, standardized documentation—that transform a therapy with modest evidence into a safe, equitable, and patient-centered intervention. This organizational foundation constitutes the indispensable prerequisite to the effective realization of patient-centered added value—symptom benefits, enhanced safety, and improved care experience— these components are analysed in the next section.

7. ADDED VALUE AND PATIENT-CENTERED OUTCOMES OF MEDICAL CANNABIS: IMPLICATIONS FOR CANNABIS NURSING

Integrating medical cannabis into care pathways requires rigorous assessment of its therapeutic value across three complementary dimensions: patient-reported outcomes, health system impact, and the robustness of the underlying evidence base. This triangulated approach clarifies the distinctive nursing contribution to optimizing these therapies in a safe, person-centered manner.

7.1 Clinical Outcomes and Patient Experience

Evidence from recent literature indicates modest but clinically meaningful benefits of medical cannabis for quality of life and symptom control (Stockings et al., 2018). A systematic meta-analysis reports statistically significant improvements in health-related quality-of-life scores (Tait et al., 2026). However, the authors acknowledge substantial heterogeneity across included studies in terms of cannabinoid formulations, dosing regimens, and follow-up durations, which tempers the generalizability of these findings to specific patient populations. These findings are corroborated by clinical registries documenting reductions in pain-related burden and improvements in sleep quality (Datta et al., 2025).

Nevertheless, a critical gap persists between patient needs and the clinical support they receive. An oncology survey reveals that a majority of patients withhold disclosure of cannabis use due to fear of judgment or perceived provider incompetence (Camp et al., 2025). This non-disclosure compromises safety and limits therapeutic optimization. Although benefits are genuine, they remain variable and necessitate individualized titration—an area where cannabis nurses provide decisive added value through longitudinal follow-up and therapeutic education (NCSBN, 2018).

7.2 Impact on the health system

The systemic impact of medical cannabis presents a dual profile. Some observational data suggest a potential to alleviate pressure on acute care services, such as reductions in hospitalizations for chronic pain and a temporal decline in opioid-related overdose deaths (Shover et al., 2019).

Conversely, legalization has been accompanied by marked increases in emergency department utilization and hospitalizations among vulnerable populations: among older adults (≥ 65 years) in Ontario, visits for cannabis-related intoxication rose sharply between 2015 and 2022 (Stall et al., 2024); an increase in emergency visits for anxiety disorders involving cannabis has also been documented (McCarthy et al., 2024); Canadian data report rising hospitalizations for acute psychiatric disorders or drug interactions (Governement of Canada, 2023); and in the United Kingdom, an upsurge in accidental paediatric ingestions of edible products has been observed (Myran et al., 2022). These trends underscore that, in the absence of clinical supervision, a potential benefit may become a systemic risk. In this context, cannabis nurses serve as essential safeguards—preventing adverse events and reducing inappropriate emergency care utilization (NCSBN, 2018).

7.3 Evidence limitations and the Distinctive role of cannabis nursing

Interpretation of benefits must be tempered by the limited certainty of current evidence, due to products and dosing heterogeneity and the predominance of observational study design (Committee on the Health Effects of Marijuana: An Evidence Review and Research Agenda et al., 2017; Vinette et al., 2022). Additionally, although rare, cardiovascular risks warrant particular vigilance (Page et al., 2020).

Amid this complexity, cannabis nursing positions itself as the pivotal specialty to maximize therapeutic value while minimizing risks. The specialized nurse ensures: (1) evidence- informed therapeutic education to address documented knowledge deficits; (2) individualized titration guided by patient-reported outcomes measures (PROMs); and (3) proactive monitoring for adverse effects. By embedding these functions into care pathways, cannabis nurses transform a therapy supported by modest evidence into a safe, patient-centered intervention that demonstrates value for the health system.

Although therapeutic benefits are real yet moderate in magnitude, their equitable and safe deployment raises substantial ethical challenges—stigma, access disparities, and clinical governance—addressed in the following section.

8. ETHICAL CHALLENGES, STIGMA, AND EQUITY

8.1. Stigma and Professional Resistance

Stigma associated with cannabis remains a major barrier to its clinical integration, even in contexts of supervised therapeutic use. It operates across multiple levels: negative social representations, persistent conflation of therapeutic and recreational use, fear judgment among patients, and professional reticence among providers. Clinically, this stigma carries tangible costs when it compromises transparency essential for safe follow-up—concealing adverse effects, dose adjustments, concomitant substance use, or drug–drug interactions—and undermines shared decision-making.

Certain patient populations appear particularly vulnerable. Among cancer survivors, stigma related to medical cannabis is frequently reported within clinical settings, fostering secrecy and impairing care coordination (Nayak et al., 2023). Among older adults, fear of judgment and social caution may limit disclosure, despite heightened vulnerability due to frailty, polypharmacy, and fall risk—factors that make clinical monitoring especially critical (Dahlke et al., 2024). More broadly, patients describe cannabis as a "stigmatized medicine", shaping their interactions with healthcare professionals and influencing their disclosure strategies (Bottorff et al., 2013). Non-disclosure or partial disclosure compromises medication history accuracy and safety, particularly when cannabis is used alongside analgesics, sedatives, or other treatments (King et al., 2024).

On the provider side, resistance often stems from (1) uncertainty regarding benefit–risk profiles (product variability, THC/CBD ratios, administration routes, titration protocols); (2) lack of formal training; and (3) concerns about regulatory compliance (responsibilities, pathways, documentation). These factors perpetuate heterogeneous practices and hoc integration rather than standardized, auditable care pathways.

Strategies for destigmatization. Three priority approaches include:

- Normalize cannabis assessment within routine clinical evaluation and medication reconciliation using non-judgmental language and standardized inquiries (therapeutic goals, formulation/route/dose, perceived benefits, adverse effects, modalities of access/use), thereby improving information quality and follow-up safety (King et al., 2024).
- Train interprofessional teams in shared decision-making, implicit bias recognition, and patient-centered communication that distinguishes clinical assessment from moral judgment about substance use (Bottorff et al., 2013; Nayak et al., 2023).

- o Strengthen institutional frameworks (policies, care pathways, documentation standards) to reduce organizational ambiguity that fuels secondary stigma and fear of "doing something wrong" (Balneaves & Alraja, 2019; NCSBN, 2018).

8.2. Clinical Governance and Research Needs: Toward Evidence-Based Integration

Safe integration of medical cannabis requires explicit clinical governance capable of addressing both regulatory heterogeneity and limitations in the current evidence base. These dimensions—organizational and epistemic—are intrinsically linked: without structured institutional frameworks, scientific uncertainties translate into fragmented practices; without implementation-oriented research, institutional policies lack empirical foundations for standardizing care pathways.

A minimal institutional framework in the face of regulatory instability

Tensions surrounding scope of practice and clinical governance complicate the integration of therapeutic cannabis. Heterogeneous legal frameworks generate ambiguities within healthcare facilities regarding storage, administration, traceability, and documentation, hindering interprofessional standardization. In the United States, the historical mismatch between federal regulation (Schedule I classification) and state policies has long contributed to organizational uncertainty (Haffajee et al., 2018). Although recent federal administrative actions (including a proposal for rescheduling) are reshaping this landscape (U.S. Department of Justice, 2024), persistent instability reinforces the need for robust local governance centered on safety, traceability, and role clarification.

In jurisdictions where authorization or prescribing is primarily the responsibility of physicians (or, less commonly, advanced practice nurses depending on regulatory context), nursing contributions is mainly focussed in clinical integration: structured assessment, therapeutic education, screening for interactions, monitoring of therapeutic and adverse effects, and care coordination. However, systemic barriers—knowledge deficits, practice uncertainties, product access challenges—promote informal governance in which decisions vary by team or setting, to the detriment of equity and safety (Hachem et al., 2022).

In response, a minimal governance framework should explicitly define four components: accountability structure, secure handling protocols, documentation guidelines, and a quality and safety system—each developed in Section 6 (NCSBN, 2018). Without these elements, organizations foster defensive practice patterns, interprofessional ambiguity, and uneven integration—precisely undermining the safety and equity objectives that cannabis nursing aims to achieve (Hachem et al., 2022; NCSBN, 2018).

"Integration"-oriented research: bridging evidence and practice

Heterogeneity in scientific evidence constitutes a second governance challenge. Evidence quality varies according to indications, products, and study designs, limiting translatability of results to real-world clinical pathways. Moreover, many studies remain disconnected from organizational questions critical to safety and equity: who provides monitoring, how follow-up is structured, which outcomes matter most to patients, and what minimum documentation is required (Busse et al., 2021; Committee on the Health Effects of Marijuana: An Evidence Review and Research Agenda et al., 2017).

To support cannabis nursing maturation, three research priorities are directly useful to clinical governance:

- Pragmatic comparative effectiveness trials: comparing formulations, cannabinoid ratios, administration routes, and titration strategies using standardized outcomes (target symptoms, functional status, quality of life) with rigorous adverse events monitoring (Busse et al., 2021; Committee on the Health Effects of Marijuana: An Evidence Review and Research Agenda et al., 2017).
- Safety in vulnerable populations: investigating drug interactions and treatment- related harms (sedation, falls, cognitive impairment) among poly-medicated, frail patients or those with psychiatric comorbidities to develop tailored monitoring plans (Dahlke et al., 2024; Renard et al., 2024).
- Implementation science: comparing organizational models (dedicated consultation vs integration into pain/oncology/palliative/primary care) on clinical and organizational outcomes (documentation quality, access delays, care continuity, unscheduled healthcare use) (Hachem et al., 2022; NCSBN, 2018).

The objective is to produce "integration"-oriented evidence: what works, for whom, in which organizational context, and at what cost to the system? Such data are crucial for guiding protocols, reducing practice variability, and clarifying the distinctive contribution of nursing in securing care pathways (Committee on the Health Effects of Marijuana: An Evidence Review and Research Agenda et al., 2017; Renard et al., 2024).

In summary, clinical governance and research are not separate challenges but complementary requirements for transforming a therapy with moderate evidence and an unstable regulation into a safe, equitable, patient-centered intervention. Cannabis nursing emerges precisely as the professional specialty positioned to bridge this gap—provided institutions formalize explicit policies and research directs those policies toward empirically validated integration models.

8.3. Future Directions: Competencies, Integrated Pathways, Public Health, and Telemonitoring

Immediate priorities focus on competency development. As detailed in Section 4, training deficits are internationally documented—with nurses and students consistently reporting limited exposure to dedicated curricula and inadequate confidence for safe practice(Paiva et al., 2024; Zolotov et al., 2025). Within the structured competency framework of (Zolotov et al., 2025), cannabis nursing functions as an integrative specialty bridging an expanding therapeutic domain and established quality–safety imperatives: patient education, risk stratification, structured follow-up, meticulous documentation, and interprofessional coordination (NCSBN, 2018b).

Concurrently, institutional policies must be harmonized. A Canadian study highlights variability in nursing policies and education and underscores the need to clarify administration protocols within care settings to support coherent, non-judgmental practice (Balneaves & Alraja, 2019). Medium-term integration within established clinical pathways (chronic pain, oncology, palliative care) via dedicated tracks can standardize cautious titration, strengthen adverse-effect monitoring, and improve care continuity. This requires: (1) standardized documentation procedures; (2) therapeutic education and shared decision-making tools; and (3) continuous quality improvement system (audit, indicators, feedback) (NCSBN, 2018c; Renard et al., 2024).

Finally, remote monitoring and digital tools are a logical extension, provided they align with privacy, security, and safety requirements. Structured patient self-monitoring (symptoms, sleep, pain, anxiety), adverse events reporting, adherence tracking, and gradual dose adjustments under supervision. This approach is particularly relevant for patients using cannabis over prolonged periods, for whom therapeutic alliance and follow-up quality condition safety and perceived effectiveness (King et al., 2024; Paiva et al., 2024).

In summary, challenges related to stigma, governance, and evidence are not merely obstacles: they define the maturation agenda for cannabis nursing. Competency consolidation, institutional harmonization, and generation of "integration"-oriented evidence appear to be crucial conditions for safe, coherent, patient-centered deployment (Balneaves & Alraja, 2019; Zolotov et al., 2025).

9. OPERATIONAL TOOLKIT: CLINICAL PRACTICE, TRAINING, AND GOVERNANCE

This section brings together operational tools intended to reduce variability in practice, enhance care safety, and facilitate institutional integration. Interpretive principles and decision criteria are integrated into the text, while "ready-to-use" resources (checklists, algorithm, RACI matrix, audit grids, and indicators) are to be found in appendices and simply referenced throughout.

9.1. Tools for the Clinician: Assessment, Shared Decision-Making, Documentation

Safety primarily depends on the quality of the clinical process: explicit indication, measurable objectives, risk screening, cautious titration, structured reassessment, and standardized documentation (NCSBN, 2018c; Busse et al., 2021). To support interprofessional continuity and auditability, **Table 2** presents a shared minimal dataset for assessment and documentation.

Table 2. Initial assessment checklist and minimal documentation (clinical dataset)

Domain	Minimum Fields (to be documented in the EHR*)
1. Indications & Objectives	Target symptom(s); therapeutic goals; continuation and discontinuation criteria.
2. Risks / Major Contraindications	History of psychosis or mania; pregnancy and breastfeeding; cardiovascular risk; fall risk; Substance Use Disorder (SUD).
3. Medications & Interactions	Concurrent use of sedatives, opioids, anticoagulants, or AEDs**; interaction mitigation plan.
4. Product & Route	Route of administration; THC:CBD ratio; concentration; source and quality; batch traceability.
5. Titration Protocol	Starting dose; titration increments (steps); dosing schedule; management of Adverse Events (AE).
6. Safety Education	Driving and machinery warnings; alcohol interactions; secure storage; non-diversion (non-sharing); red flags/warning signs.
7. Follow-up & Outcomes	Outcome measures (PROMs***); reassessment schedule; clinically meaningful benefit threshold.
8. Documentation & Incidents	Prescription/protocol adherence; Adverse Events (AE); discrepancies or diversion; corrective actions taken.

* Electronic Health Record. ** Anti-Epileptic Drugs. ***Patient-Reported Outcome Measures

Note. A detailed version (screening items, scale examples, suggested DPI fields) is provided in Appendix B.

9.1.1. Titration and Follow-Up: Standardize Decisions, not Doses

Product heterogeneity limits the utility of fixed milligram-based regimens. More valuable standardization concern clinical decision points: when to initiate, when to adjust dosing, when to stop, and how to objectively evaluate benefit-risk balance. Recommendations converge toward gradual titration ("start low, go slow"), close reassessment at initiation, and a priori definition of clinically meaningful benefit threshold (Bhaskar et al., 2021; MacCallum & Russo, 2018). Accordingly, a stepwise workflow for initiation, titration, documentation, and escalation safety actions is summarized in **Table 3**. For chronic pain, (Busse et al., 2021) recommendation favours non-inhaled formulations and emphasizes transparent benefit–risk discussion. An adaptable clinical algorithm is proposed in Appendix C.

Table 3. Synthetic clinical algorithm for initiation, titration, and escalation safety actions

Step	Action
1	Verify indication, objectives, contraindications, and interactions; document baseline status
2	Choose an initial formulation with a low-risk profile; counsel on onset latency
3	Start at a low dose; adjust only one parameter at a time; space dose steps
4	Reassess benefit and tolerability at planned intervals; document outcomes and adverse effects
5	In the event of severe adverse effects (confusion, hallucinations, syncope, chest pain), stop treatment and refer according to severity

9.1.2. Patient Education and Teach-Back: Mitigating Avoidable Risk

Adverse effects (drowsiness, dizziness, attentional disturbances) increase fall and accident risk, especially during initiation and dose changes (NCSBN, 2018c; Busse et al., 2021). The teach-back method (having the patient restate key messages) improves medication education quality and provided documented evidence of understanding (Prochnow et al., 2019). To standardize counseling and support documentation, essential patient safety messages are consolidated in **Table 4**. An education handout is provided in Appendix D, with a mini teach-back to document.

Table 4. Essential patient safety messages for medical cannabis therapy

Theme	Patient safety message
Dose adherence	Respect the prescribed dose and avoid rapid adjustments
Driving and machinery	Do not drive or operate machinery if drowsy or dizzy, especially soon after a dose
Alcohol and interactions	Avoid alcohol and report all medications taken (risk of interactions and sedation)
Storage and sharing	Store the product securely, out of children's reach; do not share
Red flags	Seek care in case of confusion, hallucinations, syncope, chest pain, or worsening psychiatric symptoms

9.2. Tools for the Educator: Curriculum, Simulation, Competency Assessment

Studies among nurses/nursing students often show a knowledge gap and heterogeneity in educational practices, supporting the need for structured curricula and standardized competency assessments (Balneaves & Alraja, 2019; Paiva et al., 2024). A competency-based curriculum should be grounded in: professional standards for the specialty published by the American Nurses Association and the American Cannabis Nurses Association (American Cannabis Nurses Association, 2023; American Nurses Association, 2021), consensus competencies for health professionals (Zolotov et al., 2025).

9.2.1. Interprofessional Scenarios and Simulation

Care typically involves multiple stakeholders: prescribing physicians, pharmacy services, nursing staff, quality and risk management, security, and IT/DPI. Simulation scenarios benefit from explicit role clarification and coordination protocols, aligned with interprofessional education competencies (Interprofessional Education Collaborative, 2023). Standards from the International Nursing Association for Clinical Simulation and Learning support aligning objectives–briefing–debriefing to transform experience into transferable learning (Charnetski & Jarvill, 2021).

9.2.2. Assess "Know," "Show," and "Do"

A multimodal assessment approach yields greater validity: structured MCQs (knowledge), mini-OSCE/simulation (clinical and communication skills), and chart audits (real-world performance). Miller's pyramid (1990) provides a pragmatic progression (know → know-how → show → do). At the institutional level, training evaluation can incorporate the Kirkpatrick model (reaction, learning, behaviours, results) to link educational training to clinical and organizational outcomes (Kirkpatrick & Francisco, 1996).

9.3. Tools for the Administrator/Decision-Maker: Policies, Accountability, Quality and Safety

9.3.1. Minimal Institutional Policy. "Non-Negotiable" Clauses

An institutional policy must, at minimum, clarify:

- o Supply pathway(s) (institutional product versus patient's personal product; conditions for acceptance and traceability).
- o Administration/documentation modalities (who administers; where to document in the EHR; double-check rules if applicable).
- o Storage and access (security, chain of responsibility, inventory if required by the framework).
- o Management of EI and incidents (reporting, analysis, corrective actions).
- o Updating (regulatory monitoring + feedback/lessons learned, at least annually).

9.3.2. Preventing Diversion and Securing Processes

Regardless of legal status, governance must incorporate a "high-alert medication" approach: restricted access, traceability, standardized discrepancy management, a reporting culture, and regular audits. The American Society of Health-System Pharmacists' hospital guidelines on preventing diversion of controlled substances provide transferable principles (Clark et al., 2022). Behavioral research further identifies diversion risk factors and underscores the importance of explicit patient education regarding secure storage and non-sharing (Sznitman et al., 2020).

9.3.3. Clarify Roles: RACI Matrix and Validation Pathways

The RACI matrix is a simple tool to clarify responsibilities, reduce ambiguity, and accelerate decision-making during traceability incidents (Brower et al., 2021). An adaptable example is proposed in Appendix E (roles adjustable to the organizational chart). A practical rule: each critical task should have exactly one "A" (accountable) and at least one "R" (responsible).

9.3.4. Manage Through Indicators: Structure, Process, Outcomes

Performance management benefits from framing within the structure–process–outcomes triad of Donabedian, (2005). Appendices E and F provide an audit grid (structure/process) and a selection of indicators. The goal is to identify actionable gaps (e.g., absence of teach-back, incomplete documentation, noncompliant storage) and close continuous quality improvement cycle.

9.3.5. Regulatory Monitoring and Updating: Treating Instability as a Safety Variable

Regulatory frameworks evolve rapidly and must be formally integrated into quality management systems. For example, in the United States, a federal rescheduling dynamic was relaunched in late 2025 in the context of an ongoing regulatory process, which requires formal mechanisms for updating procedures and internal communication. Similar developments in other jurisdictions (e.g., amendments in Canada, extension of the therapeutic experimentation in France through March 31, 2026) illustrate the value of establishing scheduled review triggers (at least annually, and after any major change).

CONCLUSION

In closing, medical cannabis is now incorporated into multiple care pathways, yet its clinical integration remains characterized by heterogeneity in products, levels of evidence, and legal frameworks. This situation creates a gap between (sometimes facilitated) access and teams' capacity to deliver standardized, safe, and person-centered care. The challenges extend beyond pharmacology to include documentation, traceability, benefit–risk evaluation, and the consistency of messages delivered to patients. In this context, cannabis nursing can be understood as a professional response to a need for structuring: clarifying the scope of practice, securing care delivery, reducing avoidable variability, and supporting interprofessional continuity.

The conceptual frameworks examined in this chapter converge on an operational premise: advanced nursing practice provides a robust architecture for defining the role, boundaries, and competencies of an emerging specialty. At the level of direct care, cannabis nursing translates into structured clinical assessment, documented shared decision-making, education grounded in teach-back, and outcomes monitoring with explicit continuation or discontinuation criteria. At the team level, this role helps harmonize clinical language, streamline referrals to prescribers, and strengthen risk management—particularly when patients are in situations of vulnerability.

From an educational standpoint, the central need is to transform fragmented knowledge into actionable, assessable competencies. The effectiveness of a training program rests on explicit clinical objectives, representative case scenarios, appropriate assessment methods, and a shared interprofessional language. In practice, this requires integrating pharmacology, indication-specific evidence, and safety with essential relational competencies: nonjudgmental communication, motivational interviewing, exploration of expectations and values, and management of social representations (stigma, confusion between medical and recreational use). Useful training must also prepare professionals for documentation and traceability, because clinical writing materializes the decision, protects the patient, and supports organizational learning.

Institutional dimensions constitute a major lever of maturity. Even when access is legal, the absence of procedures (storage, traceability, administration, documentation, adverse event reporting, discrepancy management, and diversion prevention) transforms a clinical risk into an organizational and medico-legal risk. Conversely, coherent internal policies that are regularly updated make it possible to integrate medical cannabis like any intervention with uncertain benefit and non-zero risk. The tools presented in this chapter share a common purpose: making practice explicit, measurable, and improvable. A minimal dataset supports continuity of care; a titration algorithm enables cautious, reproducible escalation; an education handout strengthens safety; a RACI matrix clarifies responsibilities; and an audit grid and indicators translate observations into corrective actions.

Several directions emerge to consolidate the field. First, the evidence base and recommendations remain evolving; systematic surveillance and risk-based reasoning are essential to adjust practice and protocols. Second, outcomes assessment must go beyond symptom intensity alone and incorporate functionality, quality of life, safety, treatment adherence, and, when relevant, the risk of substance use disorders. Third, equity of access and health literacy must be considered from the design phase of care pathways, to avoid a “niche specialty” reserved for patients who are already informed. Finally, the development of cannabis nursing would benefit from integration into existing quality-and-safety programs and priority clinical pathways (pain, oncology, neurology, palliative care), with implementation evaluations and shared indicators.

Overall, viewing cannabis nursing as an emerging specialty means recognizing that integrating medical cannabis is not a simple therapeutic add-on, but a transformation that is simultaneously clinical, educational, and organizational. Owing to their proximity to patients and their coordinating role, nurses are particularly well positioned to support this integration, provided that expertise is recognized, trained, assessed, and anchored in coherent institutional policies. This approach offers a pragmatic trajectory: strengthen safety, improve the patient experience, and make decisions more transparent, regardless of future regulatory developments.

REFERENCES

Albarqouni, L., Hoffmann, T., Straus, S., Olsen, N. R., Young, T., Ilic, D., Shaneyfelt, T., Haynes, R. B., Guyatt, G., & Glasziou, P. (2018). Core Competencies in Evidence-Based Practice for Health Professionals : Consensus Statement Based on a Systematic Review and Delphi Survey. *JAMA Network Open*, *1*(2), e180281. DOI: 10.1001/jamanetworkopen.2018.0281 PMID: 30646073

Allan, G. M., Ramji, J., Perry, D., & Ton, J. (2018). Simplified guideline for prescribing medical cannabinoids in primary care. *Journal of Nursing Regulation*, *9*(2), S5. DOI: 10.1016/S2155-8256(18)30082-6 PMID: 29449241

American Cannabis Nurses Association. (2023). Cannabis Nursing : Scope and Standards of Practice (4th éd.).

American Nurses Association. (2021). Herapeutic Use of Marijuana and Related Cannabinoids (p. 03).

ANSM. (2024). Mise en place de l'expérimentation du cannabis médical. https://ansm.sante.fr/dossiers-thematiques/cannabis-a-usage-medical/mise-en-place-de-lexperimentation-du-cannabis-medical

APRN Consensus Work Group & the National Council of State Boards of Nursing APRN Advisory Committee. (2008). *Regulation : Licensure*. Accreditation, Certification & Education.

Attonito, J., Freeman, K., Bone, M. K., Howard, H., Blum, C., & Luck, G. (2024). Knowledge, Attitudes, and Beliefs Regarding Medical Cannabis Among Patients and Providers in Florida's Long-Term Care Facilities. *Cureus*. Advance online publication. DOI: 10.7759/cureus.66115 PMID: 39229412

Aviram, J. (2025). Medical cannabis in Israel : A comprehensive review of trends and regulations, 2011–2025. *Journal of Cannabis Research*, *7*(1), 90. DOI: 10.1186/s42238-025-00344-1 PMID: 41233935

Balneaves, L. G., Alraja, A., Ziemianski, D., McCuaig, F., & Ware, M. (2018). A National Needs Assessment of Canadian Nurse Practitioners Regarding Cannabis for Therapeutic Purposes. *Cannabis and Cannabinoid Research*, *3*(1), 66–73. DOI: 10.1089/can.2018.0002 PMID: 29588917

Balneaves, L. G., & Alraja, A. A. (2019). "Guarding their practice" : A descriptive study of Canadian nursing policies and education related to medical cannabis. *BMC Nursing*, *18*(1), 66. DOI: 10.1186/s12912-019-0390-7 PMID: 31827392

Bhaskar, A., Bell, A., Boivin, M., Briques, W., Brown, M., Clarke, H., Cyr, C., Eisenberg, E., De Oliveira Silva, R. F., Frohlich, E., Georgius, P., Hogg, M., Horsted, T. I., MacCallum, C. A., Müller-Vahl, K. R., O'Connell, C., Sealey, R., Seibolt, M., Sihota, A., & Moulin, D. E. (2021). Consensus recommendations on dosing and administration of medical cannabis to treat chronic pain : Results of a modified Delphi process. *Journal of Cannabis Research*, *3*(1), 22. DOI: 10.1186/s42238-021-00073-1 PMID: 34215346

Bottorff, J. L., Bissell, L. J., Balneaves, L. G., Oliffe, J. L., Capler, N. R., & Buxton, J. (2013). Perceptions of cannabis as a stigmatized medicine : A qualitative descriptive study. *Harm Reduction Journal*, *10*(1), 2. DOI: 10.1186/1477-7517-10-2 PMID: 23414118

Braun, I. M., Bohlke, K., Abrams, D. I., Anderson, H., Balneaves, L. G., Bar-Sela, G., Bowles, D. W., Chai, P. R., Damani, A., Gupta, A., Hallmeyer, S., Subbiah, I. M., Twelves, C., Wallace, M. S., & Roeland, E. J. (2024). Cannabis and Cannabinoids in Adults With Cancer : ASCO Guideline. *Journal of Clinical Oncology*, *42*(13), 1575–1593. DOI: 10.1200/JCO.23.02596 PMID: 38478773

Brooks, E., Gundersen, D. C., Flynn, E., Brooks-Russell, A., & Bull, S. (2017). The clinical implications of legalizing marijuana : Are physician and non-physician providers prepared? *Addictive Behaviors*, *72*, 1–7. DOI: 10.1016/j.addbeh.2017.03.007 PMID: 28319813

Brower, H. H., Nicklas, B. J., Nader, M. A., Trost, L. M., & Miller, D. P. (2021). Creating effective academic research teams : Two tools borrowed from business practice. *Journal of Clinical and Translational Science*, *5*(1), e74. DOI: 10.1017/cts.2020.553 PMID: 33948292

Brown, J., & Winterstein, A. (2019). Potential Adverse Drug Events and Drug–Drug Interactions with Medical and Consumer Cannabidiol (CBD) Use. *Journal of Clinical Medicine*, *8*(7), 989. DOI: 10.3390/jcm8070989 PMID: 31288397

Bryant-Lukosius, D., & DiCenso, A. (2004). A framework for the introduction and evaluation of advanced practice nursing roles. *Journal of Advanced Nursing*, *48*(5), 530–540. DOI: 10.1111/j.1365-2648.2004.03235.x PMID: 15533091

Busse, J. W., Vankrunkelsven, P., Zeng, L., Heen, A. F., Merglen, A., Campbell, F., Granan, L.-P., Aertgeerts, B., Buchbinder, R., Coen, M., Juurlink, D., Samer, C., Siemieniuk, R. A. C., Kumar, N., Cooper, L., Brown, J., Lytvyn, L., Zeraatkar, D., Wang, L., & Agoritsas, T. (2021). Medical cannabis or cannabinoids for chronic pain : A clinical practice guideline. *BMJ (Clinical Research Ed.)*, (2040), n2040. Advance online publication. DOI: 10.1136/bmj.n2040 PMID: 34497062

Camp, L., Babicheva, V., Conahan, C., Hayes, S., & Sherburne Hawkins, S. (2025). Cannabis Use and Disclosure in the Oncology Setting : A Cross-Sectional Survey Exploring Information Needs Among Cancer Survivors. *Clinical Journal of Oncology Nursing*, *29*(2), 157–164. DOI: 10.1188/25.CJON.157-164 PMID: 40096564

Canadian Society of Hospital Pharmacists. (2021). Cannabis for the Hospitalized Patient : Position Statement. www.cshp.ca

Charnetski, M., & Jarvill, M. (2021). Healthcare Simulation Standards of Best PracticeTM Operations. *Clinical Simulation in Nursing*, *58*, 33–39. DOI: 10.1016/j.ecns.2021.08.012

Clark, J., Fera, T., Fortier, C., Gullickson, K., Hays, A., Murdaugh, L., Ogden, R.Jr, O'Neal, B., Rush, J., & Vest, T. (2022). ASHP Guidelines on Preventing Diversion of Controlled Substances. *American Journal of Health-System Pharmacy*, *79*(24), 2279–2306. DOI: 10.1093/ajhp/zxac246 PMID: 36208462

Clarke, H., & Fitzcharles, M. (2023). The evolving culture of medical cannabis in Canada for the management of chronic pain. *Frontiers in Pharmacology*, *14*, 1153584. DOI: 10.3389/fphar.2023.1153584 PMID: 37089954

Committee on the Health Effects of Marijuana. An Evidence Review and Research Agenda, Board on Population Health and Public Health Practice, Health and Medicine Division, & National Academies of Sciences, Engineering, and Medicine. (2017). The Health Effects of Cannabis and Cannabinoids : The Current State of Evidence and Recommendations for Research (p. 24625). National Academies Press. DOI: 10.17226/24625

Committee on the Public Health Consequences of Changes in the Cannabis Policy Landscape. Board on Population Health and Public Health Practice, Health and Medicine Division, & National Academies of Sciences, Engineering, and Medicine. (2024). Cannabis Policy Impacts Public Health and Health Equity (S. Teutsch, Y. Hurd, & E. Boyle, Éds.; p. 27766). National Academies Press. DOI: 10.17226/27766

Congressional Research Service. (2025). Rescheduling Marijuana : Implications for Criminal and Collateral Consequences. https://www.congress.gov/crs-product/IF12715

Dahlke, S., Butler, J. I., Hunter, K. F., Toubiana, M., Kalogirou, M. R., Shrestha, S., Devkota, R., Law, J., & Scheuerman, M. (2024). The Effects of Stigma : Older Persons and Medicinal Cannabis. *Qualitative Health Research*, *34*(8-9), 717–731. DOI: 10.1177/10497323241227419 PMID: 38305270

Datta, I., Erridge, S., Holvey, C., Coomber, R., Guru, R., Holden, W., Darweish Medniuk, A., Sajad, M., Searle, R., Usmani, A., Varma, S., Rucker, J. J., Platt, M., & Sodergren, M. H. (2025). UK medical cannabis registry : A clinical outcome analysis of medical cannabis therapy in chronic pain patients with and without co-morbid sleep impairment. *Pain Practice*, *25*(1), e13438. DOI: 10.1111/papr.13438 PMID: 39545361

Devinsky, O., Cross, J. H., Laux, L., Marsh, E., Miller, I., Nabbout, R., Scheffer, I. E., Thiele, E. A., & Wright, S. (2017). Trial of Cannabidiol for Drug-Resistant Seizures in the Dravet Syndrome. *The New England Journal of Medicine*, *376*(21), 2011–2020. DOI: 10.1056/NEJMoa1611618 PMID: 28538134

Di Forti, M., Quattrone, D., Freeman, T. P., Tripoli, G., Gayer-Anderson, C., Quigley, H., Rodriguez, V., Jongsma, H. E., Ferraro, L., La Cascia, C., La Barbera, D., Tarricone, I., Berardi, D., Szöke, A., Arango, C., Tortelli, A., Velthorst, E., Bernardo, M., Del-Ben, C. M., & Van Der Ven, E. (2019). The contribution of cannabis use to variation in the incidence of psychotic disorder across Europe (EU-GEI) : A multicentre case-control study. *The Lancet. Psychiatry*, *6*(5), 427–436. DOI: 10.1016/S2215-0366(19)30048-3 PMID: 30902669

Donabedian, A. (2005). Evaluating the Quality of Medical Care.

EMCDDA. (2023). Cannabis laws in Europe. https://www.emcdda.europa.eu/publications/cannabis-laws-in-europe_en

Garcia, A. (2019). COUNCIL ON SCIENCE AND. *Public Health*.

Governement of Canada. (2023). Data on cannabis adverse reactions : 2023 annual report—Canada.ca.

Groce, E. (2018). The Health Effects of Cannabis and Cannabinoids : The Current State of Evidence and Recommendations for Research. *Journal of Medical Regulation*, *104*(4), 32–32. DOI: 10.30770/2572-1852-104.4.32

Hachem, Y., Abdallah, S. J., Rueda, S., Wiese, J. L., Mehra, K., Rup, J., Cowan, J., Vigano, A., & Costiniuk, C. T. (2022). Healthcare practitioner perceptions on barriers impacting cannabis prescribing practices. *BMC Complementary Medicine and Therapies*, *22*(1), 237. DOI: 10.1186/s12906-022-03716-9 PMID: 36076191

Haffajee, R. L., MacCoun, R. J., & Mello, M. M. (2018). Behind Schedule—Reconciling Federal and State Marijuana Policy. *The New England Journal of Medicine*, *379*(6), 501–504. DOI: 10.1056/NEJMp1804408 PMID: 29996065

Hasin, D. S., Saha, T. D., Kerridge, B. T., Goldstein, R. B., Chou, S. P., Zhang, H., Jung, J., Pickering, R. P., Ruan, W. J., Smith, S. M., Huang, B., & Grant, B. F. (2015). Prevalence of Marijuana Use Disorders in the United States Between 2001-2002 and 2012-2013. *JAMA Psychiatry*, *72*(12), 1235. DOI: 10.1001/jamapsychiatry.2015.1858 PMID: 26502112

Health Canada. (2014). MARIHUANA FOR MEDICAL PURPOSES REGULATIONS: The Canadian Journal of Addiction, 5(4), 20. DOI: 10.1097/02024458-201412000-00010

Health Canada. (2018). Information for Health Care Professionals : Cannabis (marihuana, marijuana) and the cannabinoids. Government of Canada = Gouvernement du Canada. https://www.canada.ca/content/dam/hc-sc/documents/services/drugs-medication/cannabis/information-medical-practitioners/information-health-care-professionals-cannabis-cannabinoids-eng.pdf

Huestis, M. A. (2007). Human Cannabinoid Pharmacokinetics. *Chemistry & Biodiversity*, *4*(8), 1770–1804. DOI: 10.1002/cbdv.200790152 PMID: 17712819

International Council of Nurses. (2020). *Guidelines on Advanced Practice Nursing*.

Interprofessional Education Collaborative. (2023). IPEC Core Competencies for Interprofessional Collaborative Practice : Version 3.

ISMP. (2020). SMP Warns that Medical Marijuana Product Labeling Problems Have Led to Errors. www.ismp.org

King, D. D., Gill, C. J., Cadieux, C. S., & Singh, N. (2024). The role of stigma in cannabis use disclosure : An exploratory study. *Harm Reduction Journal*, *21*(1), 21. DOI: 10.1186/s12954-024-00929-8 PMID: 38273362

Kirkpatrick, D. L., & Francisco, S. (1996). Evaluating Training Programs : The Four Levels,.

Klein, T. A., & Bindler, R. (2022). Ask Your Provider About Cannabis : Increasing Nurse Practitioner Knowledge and Confidence. *Cannabis and Cannabinoid Research*, *7*(5), 700–705. DOI: 10.1089/can.2021.0061 PMID: 34432530

Kruse, J. A., Collins, J. L., & Vugrin, M. (2022). Educational strategies used to improve the knowledge, skills, and attitudes of health care students and providers regarding implicit bias : An integrative review of the literature. *International Journal of Nursing Studies Advances*, *4*, 100073. DOI: 10.1016/j.ijnsa.2022.100073 PMID: 38745633

Kurtzman, E. T., Greene, J., Begley, R., & Drenkard, K. N. (2022). "We want what's best for patients." nurse leaders' attitudes about medical cannabis : A qualitative study. *International Journal of Nursing Studies Advances*, *4*, 100065. DOI: 10.1016/j.ijnsa.2022.100065 PMID: 38745605

Le Foll, B. (2021). Opioid-sparing effects of cannabinoids : Myth or reality? *Progress in Neuro-Psychopharmacology & Biological Psychiatry*, *106*, 110065. DOI: 10.1016/j.pnpbp.2020.110065 PMID: 32828853

Lo, L., Rotteau, L., & Shojania, K. (2021). Can SBAR be implemented with high fidelity and does it improve communication between healthcare workers? A systematic review. *BMJ Open*, *11*(12), e055247. DOI: 10.1136/bmjopen-2021-055247 PMID: 34921087

MacCallum, C. A., & Russo, E. B. (2018). Practical considerations in medical cannabis administration and dosing. *European Journal of Internal Medicine*, *49*, 12–19. DOI: 10.1016/j.ejim.2018.01.004 PMID: 29307505

McCarthy, S. D. S., Xiao, J., Pugliese, M., Perrault-Sequeira, L., & Myran, D. T. (2024). Changes in cannabis involvement in emergency department visits for anxiety disorders after cannabis legalization : A repeated cross-sectional study. *Lancet Regional Health. Americas*, *36*, 100815. DOI: 10.1016/j.lana.2024.100815 PMID: 38974381

McIntosh, N., Wilson, N. J., Povalej, P., Hunt, L., & Lewis, P. (2024). An Exploration of Registered Nurses' Experiences Caring for Patients Taking Medicinal Cannabis. *Nursing Open*, *11*(10), e70063. DOI: 10.1002/nop2.70063 PMID: 39455290

McMahon, E., Jimenez, F. A., Lawrence, K., & Victor, J. (2021). Healthcare Simulation Standards of Best PracticeTM Evaluation of Learning and Performance. *Clinical Simulation in Nursing*, *58*, 54–56. DOI: 10.1016/j.ecns.2021.08.016

Miller, G. E. (1990). The Assessment of Clinical Skills/Competence/Performance. *Journal of Medical Education*. PMID: 2400509

Miller, W. R., & Rollnick, S. (2013). Motivational interviewing : Helping people change.

Montero-Oleas, N., Arevalo-Rodriguez, I., Nuñez-González, S., Viteri-García, A., & Simancas-Racines, D. (2020). Therapeutic use of cannabis and cannabinoids : An evidence mapping and appraisal of systematic reviews. *BMC Complementary Medicine and Therapies*, *20*(1), 12. DOI: 10.1186/s12906-019-2803-2 PMID: 32020875

Moore, E. (2024). Connecting the dots with cannabis care. *American Nurse Journal*, *19*(7), 30–32. Advance online publication. DOI: 10.51256/ANJ072430

Morrison, G., Crockett, J., Blakey, G., & Sommerville, K. (2019). A Phase 1, Open-Label, Pharmacokinetic Trial to Investigate Possible Drug-Drug Interactions Between Clobazam, Stiripentol, or Valproate and Cannabidiol in Healthy Subjects. *Clinical Pharmacology in Drug Development*, *8*(8), 1009–1031. DOI: 10.1002/cpdd.665 PMID: 30791225

Müller, M., Jürgens, J., Redaèlli, M., Klingberg, K., Hautz, W. E., & Stock, S. (2018). Impact of the communication and patient hand-off tool SBAR on patient safety : A systematic review. *BMJ Open*, *8*(8), e022202. DOI: 10.1136/bmjopen-2018-022202 PMID: 30139905

Myran, D. T., Tanuseputro, P., Auger, N., Konikoff, L., Talarico, R., & Finkelstein, Y. (2022). Edible Cannabis Legalization and Unintentional Poisonings in Children. *The New England Journal of Medicine*, *387*(8), 757–759. DOI: 10.1056/NEJMc2207661 PMID: 36001718

National Safety Council. (2019). Appropriate Labeling of Cannabis- and Marijuana-Derived Products. ttps://www.nsc.org/getattachment/74b9f446-ef96-412b-91f3-a0c4983d7112/hc-appropriate-labeling-cannabis-marijuana-derived-products-156

Nayak, M. M., Revette, A., Chai, P. R., Lansang, K., Sannes, T., Tung, S., & Braun, I. M. (2023). Medical cannabis-related stigma : Cancer survivors' perspectives. *Journal of Cancer Survivorship: Research and Practice*, *17*(4), 951–956. DOI: 10.1007/s11764-022-01297-7 PMID: 36435953

NCSBN. (2018a). *APRNs Certifying a Medical Marijuana Qualifying Condition.*, DOI: 10.1016/S2155-8256(18)30097-8

NCSBN. (2018b). *Medical Marijuana Education in Pre-Licensure Nursing Programs.*, DOI: 10.1016/S2155-8256(18)30095-4

NCSBN. (2018c). The NCSBN National Nursing Guidelines for Medical Marijuana. *Journal of Nursing Regulation*, *9*(2), S5. DOI: 10.1016/S2155-8256(18)30082-6

NHS England. (2025). Guide to responding proportionately to patient safety incidents.

Nielsen, S., Picco, L., Murnion, B., Winters, B., Matheson, J., Graham, M., Campbell, G., Parvaresh, L., Khor, K.-E., Betz-Stablein, B., Farrell, M., Lintzeris, N., & Le Foll, B. (2022). Opioid-sparing effect of cannabinoids for analgesia : An updated systematic review and meta-analysis of preclinical and clinical studies. *Neuropsychopharmacology : Official Publication of the American College of Neuropsychopharmacology*, *47*(7), 1315–1330. DOI: 10.1038/s41386-022-01322-4 PMID: 35459926

Page, R. L.II, Allen, L. A., Kloner, R. A., Carriker, C. R., Martel, C., Morris, A. A., Piano, M. R., Rana, J. S., & Saucedo, J. F.American Heart Association Clinical Pharmacology Committee and Heart Failure and Transplantation Committee of the Council on Clinical Cardiology. (2020). Medical Marijuana, Recreational Cannabis, and Cardiovascular Health : A Scientific Statement From the American Heart Association. *Circulation*, *142*(10). Advance online publication. DOI: 10.1161/CIR.0000000000000883 PMID: 32752884

Paiva, C., Santos, T., Cunha-Oliveira, A., Rosendo, I., & Pita, J.-R. (2024). Knowledge, opinions and experiences of nurses and nursing students in Portugal regarding the use of medical Cannabis. *BMC Nursing*, *23*(1), 788. DOI: 10.1186/s12912-024-02443-5 PMID: 39468501

Persico, L., Wilson-Keates, B., DiGregorio, H., Decker, S., & Xavier, N.Inacsl Standards Committee. (2025). Preamble : Grounded in Excellence: The Cornerstone Healthcare Simulation Standards of Best Practice®. *Clinical Simulation in Nursing*, *105*, 101774. DOI: 10.1016/j.ecns.2025.101774

Prochnow, J. A., Meiers, S. J., & Scheckel, M. M. (2019). Improving Patient and Caregiver New Medication Education Using an Innovative Teach-back Toolkit. *Journal of Nursing Care Quality*, *34*(2), 101–106. DOI: 10.1097/NCQ.0000000000000342 PMID: 30198943

Reeves, S., Pelone, F., Harrison, R., Goldman, J., & Zwarenstein, M. (2017). Interprofessional collaboration to improve professional practice and healthcare outcomes. *Cochrane Database of Systematic Reviews*, *2018*(8). Advance online publication. DOI: 10.1002/14651858.CD000072.pub3 PMID: 28639262

Règlement sur le cannabis, DORS/2018-144 Lois du Canada (2018). http://laws-lois.justice.gc.ca

Renard, J., Sanger, N., & Gabrys, R. (2024). Clearing the Smoke on Cannabis.

Rogeberg, O., & Elvik, R. (2016). The effects of cannabis intoxication on motor vehicle collision revisited and revised. *Addiction (Abingdon, England)*, *111*(8), 1348–1359. DOI: 10.1111/add.13347 PMID: 26878835

Rouleau, G., Gagnon, M.-P., Côté, J., Payne-Gagnon, J., Hudson, E., Dubois, C.-A., & Bouix-Picasso, J. (2019). Effects of E-Learning in a Continuing Education Context on Nursing Care : Systematic Review of Systematic Qualitative, Quantitative, and Mixed-Studies Reviews. *Journal of Medical Internet Research*, *21*(10), e15118. DOI: 10.2196/15118 PMID: 31579016

Scholten, W. K. (2001). Dutch Measures to Control Medical Grade Marijuana : Facilitating Clinical Trials. *Drug Information Journal*, *35*(2), 481–484. DOI: 10.1177/009286150103500217

Sevigny, E. L. (2021). Cannabis and driving ability. *Current Opinion in Psychology*, *38*, 75–79. DOI: 10.1016/j.copsyc.2021.03.003 PMID: 33839427

Shim, M., Nguyen, H., & Grootendorst, P. (2023). Lessons from 20 years of medical cannabis use in Canada. *PLoS One*, *18*(3), e0271079. DOI: 10.1371/journal.pone.0271079 PMID: 36952564

Shover, C. L., Davis, C. S., Gordon, S. C., & Humphreys, K. (2019). Association between medical cannabis laws and opioid overdose mortality has reversed over time. *Proceedings of the National Academy of Sciences of the United States of America*, *116*(26), 12624–12626. DOI: 10.1073/pnas.1903434116 PMID: 31182592

Smedslund, G., Berg, R. C., Hammerstrøm, K. T., Steiro, A., Leiknes, K. A., Dahl, H. M., & Karlsen, K. (2011). Motivational interviewing for substance abuse. Cochrane Database of Systematic Reviews, 2011(11). DOI: 10.1002/14651858.CD008063.pub2

Smith, L. A., Azariah, F., Lavender, V. T., Stoner, N. S., & Bettiol, S. (2015). Cannabinoids for nausea and vomiting in adults with cancer receiving chemotherapy. *Cochrane Database of Systematic Reviews*, *2021*(11). Advance online publication. DOI: 10.1002/14651858.CD009464.pub2 PMID: 26561338

Stall, N. M., Shi, S., Malikov, K., Wang, S., Rochon, P. A., Hillmer, M. P., & Zipursky, J. S. (2024). Edible Cannabis Legalization and Cannabis Poisonings in Older Adults. *JAMA Internal Medicine*, *184*(7), 840. DOI: 10.1001/jamainternmed.2024.1331 PMID: 38767898

Stockings, E., Campbell, G., Hall, W. D., Nielsen, S., Zagic, D., Rahman, R., Murnion, B., Farrell, M., Weier, M., & Degenhardt, L. (2018). Cannabis and cannabinoids for the treatment of people with chronic noncancer pain conditions : A systematic review and meta-analysis of controlled and observational studies. *Pain*, *159*(10), 1932–1954. DOI: 10.1097/j.pain.0000000000001293 PMID: 29847469

Sznitman, S. R., Goldberg, V., Sheinman-Yuffe, H., Zolotov, Y., Flechter, E., & Bar-Sela, G. (2020). Long-term medical cannabis use and risk factors for diversion : Report on physician's guidance and patients' behaviour. *Palliative & Supportive Care*, *18*(1), 18–23. DOI: 10.1017/S1478951519000348 PMID: 31190678

Tait, M.-A., Acret, L., Costa, D. S. J., Campbell, R., White, K., & Rutherford, C. (2026). Health-related quality of life in patients receiving medicinal cannabis : Systematic review and meta-analysis of primary research findings 2015–2025. *Quality of Life Research: An International Journal of Quality of Life Aspects of Treatment, Care and Rehabilitation*, *35*(3), 56. DOI: 10.1007/s11136-026-04170-7 PMID: 41621036

Thiele, E. A., Marsh, E. D., French, J. A., Mazurkiewicz-Beldzinska, M., Benbadis, S. R., Joshi, C., Lyons, P. D., Taylor, A., Roberts, C., Sommerville, K., Gunning, B., Gawlowicz, J., Lisewski, P., Mazurkiewicz Beldzinska, M., Mitosek Szewczyk, K., Steinborn, B., Zolnowska, M., Hughes, E., McLellan, A., & Wilfong, A. (2018). Cannabidiol in patients with seizures associated with Lennox-Gastaut syndrome (GWPCARE4) : A randomised, double-blind, placebo-controlled phase 3 trial. *Lancet*, *391*(10125), 1085–1096. DOI: 10.1016/S0140-6736(18)30136-3 PMID: 29395273

Tracy, M. F., & O'Grady, E. T. (2019). Hamric and Hanson's Advanced Practice Nursing (6th éd.).

Troup, L. J., Erridge, S., Ciesluk, B., & Sodergren, M. H. (2022). Perceived Stigma of Patients Undergoing Treatment with Cannabis-Based Medicinal Products. *International Journal of Environmental Research and Public Health*, *19*(12), 7499. DOI: 10.3390/ijerph19127499 PMID: 35742748

U.S. Department of Justice. (2024). Schedules of Controlled Substances : Rescheduling of Marijuana.

Vinette, B., Côté, J., El-Akhras, A., Mrad, H., Chicoine, G., & Bilodeau, K. (2022). Routes of administration, reasons for use, and approved indications of medical cannabis in oncology : A scoping review. *BMC Cancer*, *22*(1), 319. DOI: 10.1186/s12885-022-09378-7 PMID: 35331185

Volkow, N. D., Baler, R. D., Compton, W. M., & Weiss, S. R. B. (2014). Adverse Health Effects of Marijuana Use. *The New England Journal of Medicine*, *370*(23), 2219–2227. DOI: 10.1056/NEJMra1402309 PMID: 24897085

Weisman, J. M., & Rodríguez, M. (2021). A systematic review of medical students' and professionals' attitudes and knowledge regarding medical cannabis. *Journal of Cannabis Research*, *3*(1), 47. DOI: 10.1186/s42238-021-00100-1 PMID: 34641976

Whiting, P. F., Wolff, R. F., Deshpande, S., Di Nisio, M., Duffy, S., Hernandez, A. V., Keurentjes, J. C., Lang, S., Misso, K., Ryder, S., Schmidlkofer, S., Westwood, M., & Kleijnen, J. (2015). Cannabinoids for Medical Use : A Systematic Review and Meta-analysis. *Journal of the American Medical Association*, *313*(24), 2456. DOI: 10.1001/jama.2015.6358 PMID: 26103030

WHO. (2010). Framework for Action on Interprofessional Education & Collaborative Practice. World Health Organization. https://www.who.int/publications/i/item/framework-for-action-on-interprofessional-education-collaborative-practice

WHO. (2017). Medication Without Harm—Global Patient Safety Challenge on Medication Safet.

Zarhin, D., Negev, M., Vulfsons, S., & Sznitman, S. R. (2018). Rhetorical and regulatory boundary-work : The case of medical cannabis policy-making in Israel. *Social Science & Medicine*, *217*, 1–9. DOI: 10.1016/j.socscimed.2018.09.047 PMID: 30278412

Zolotov, Y., Mendoza Temple, L., Isralowitz, R., Gorelick, D. A., Abraham, R., Abrams, D. I., Barich, K., Boehnke, K. F., Dahmer, S., Friedman, J., Frye, P., Haramati, A., Isaac, J., Mathre, M. L., McNabb, M. E., Ring, M., Russo, E. B., Slawek, D. E., Temple, B. R., & Kogan, M. (2025). Developing Medical Cannabis Competencies : A Consensus Statement. *JAMA Network Open*, *8*(10), e2535049. DOI: 10.1001/jamanetworkopen.2025.35049 PMID: 41055914

Zolotov, Y., Metri, S., Calabria, E., & Kogan, M. (2021). Medical cannabis education among healthcare trainees : A scoping review. *Complementary Therapies in Medicine*, *58*, 102675. DOI: 10.1016/j.ctim.2021.102675 PMID: 33539943

Zolotov, Y., Vulfsons, S., Zarhin, D., & Sznitman, S. (2018). Medical cannabis : An oxymoron? Physicians' perceptions of medical cannabis. *The International Journal on Drug Policy*, *57*, 4–10. DOI: 10.1016/j.drugpo.2018.03.025 PMID: 29653439

KEY TERMS AND DEFINITIONS

Clinical Governance: An organizational framework ensuring safe, evidence-based integration of medical cannabis through explicit policies on storage, traceability, documentation, role clarification, adverse event reporting, and continuous quality improvement—transforming informal practices into auditable, standardized care. It encompasses accountability chains, secure pathways, documentation rules, and quality-safety systems that transform a therapy with moderate evidence into a safe, equitable intervention.

Endocannabinoid System: A complex physiological network of receptors (CB1, CB2), endogenous ligands (anandamide, 2-AG), and metabolic enzymes that modulates pain, mood, appetite, and immune function. Understanding this system is foundational for rational cannabis therapeutics and patient education; it serves as the pathophysiological cornerstone of cannabinoid action and a foundational knowledge domain for cannabis nursing practice.

Evidence-Based Practice (EBP): The systematic integration of best available research evidence, clinical expertise, and patient values to guide cannabis-related decisions—calibrating expectations to variable evidence levels (e.g., robust for neuropathic pain/spasticity; weak for anxiety) while acknowledging scientific uncertainty. It requires critical appraisal of literature, reflective practice, and synthesis of evidence into structured care plans and clinical reasoning.

Hamric and Hanson Model: An integrative conceptual framework for advanced nursing practice outlining seven core competencies: direct clinical practice, guidance and coaching, consultation, evidence-based practice, leadership, collaboration, and ethical decision-making. This model provides the conceptual foundation for structuring cannabis nursing as a recognized specialty.

Interprofessional Education (IPE): An educational approach in which members of different health professions learn with, from, and about each other to improve collaboration and patient outcomes.

National Council of State Boards of Nursing (NCSBN): A U.S. regulatory body that published National Nursing Guidelines for Medical Marijuana (2018), establishing foundational safety principles for nursing practice: structured assessment, harm reduction, rigorous documentation, and interprofessional communication regarding medical cannabis. These guidelines define mandatory frameworks for risk assessment, drug interaction screening, and clinical responsibilities.

Patient Safety: The prevention of harm through systematic risk mitigation: screening for contraindications (psychosis history, cardiovascular risk), managing drug interactions (e.g., CBD with clobazam/warfarin), counseling on driving restrictions, preventing diversion, and monitoring for adverse events (falls, confusion, psychiatric symptoms). It encompasses structured risk assessment, explicit safety counseling, and systematic documentation to support organizational learning.

Regulatory Frameworks: The legal and policy structures governing access to, authorization of, and clinical use of medical cannabis across jurisdictions. These frameworks determine product status (medicine versus medical-cannabis regime), scope of practice, documentation requirements, and institutional pathways, requiring nurses to develop regulatory literacy as a core competency.

Stigma: Negative social representations and judgments associated with cannabis that persist even in therapeutic contexts, creating barriers to patient disclosure, clinical transparency, and equitable access. Stigma-informed care requires nonjudgmental communication, motivational interviewing, and explicit institutional policies to reduce organizational ambiguity and secondary stigma.

Therapeutic Education: Structured patient teaching on product selection, dosing, onset/offset kinetics by route, realistic expectations aligned with evidence, safety precautions, and self-monitoring—often reinforced through teach-back methodology to verify comprehension and reduce avoidable risks.

APPENDIX

Appendix A

Table 5. Comparative Synthesis of Regulatory Frameworks and Operational Implications for Medical Cannabis

Jurisdiction	Access / Status (Macro Level)	Hospital Pathway (Meso Level)	Documentation & Traceability (Micro Level)	Implications for Nursing Practice
United States	Evolving federal framework; rescheduling proposal under discussion (DEA, 2024).	High variability by State; local institutional policies required (AMA, 2019; NCSBN, 2018).	Often hybrid documentation (recommendation vs. order; facility-specific rules).	Clarify administration vs. self-administration; secure storage requirements; escalation/incident criteria.
Canada	Federal regime under the *Cannabis Act*; regulates hospital administration/ distribution via dedicated provisions (Gov. of Canada, 2018).	Hospitals may receive products from licensed holders and administer via "medical document" or written order; specific labeling/ packaging constraints.	Mandatory labeling (practitioner, patient, daily quantity, date); quantity limits; standardized documentation.	High traceability requirements; nursing procedures for verification (dose/ potency/route), storage, and EHR documentation.
Europe (EU examples)	Multi-pathway regulation (medicines, preparations); EMA clarification pending national implementation (EMA, 2023).	Often structured via hospital pharmacy; transitional programs available (e.g., ANSM, France).	Variable requirements; need for institutional standardization (internal forms: batch, concentration, consent).	Focus on local harmonization, "bridge" protocols, and risk management (interactions, neurocognition, falls).
Israel	Dedicated national regime for medical cannabis with specific authorizations/ dispensing (MoH Israel).	Pathway depends on authorized suppliers; institutional policy is essential.	Documentation focused on authorization, indication, and dose; traceability must be formalized.	Need for a clear institutional framework and interprofessional coordination (MD-Pharmacy-Nurse).

Appendix B

Table 6. Extended Checklist: Initial Assessment and Minimum Documentation

Domain	Items to Document (Detailed)	Notes / Examples
Indication & Objectives	Target symptom(s); SMART goals; previously attempted alternatives; clinical justification.	Ex: neuropathic pain, refractory nausea; Goals: -2 points on NRS within 2–4 weeks.
History & Vulnerabilities	Psychiatric history; cognitive impairment; fall risk; pregnancy/breastfeeding; advanced age; professional driving.	*Screening for psychosis/mania risk factors; caution if family history is present.*
Medications & Interactions	Current medication list; psychoactive substances; potential CYP interactions; mitigation plan.	*Specific attention to sedatives, opioids, benzodiazepines, anticoagulants, AEDs, and alcohol.*
Product & Quality	Formulation; THC:CBD ratio; concentration; batch/traceability; source of supply.	*Prioritize standardized products; record label details (mg/mL).*
Route & Schedule	Route (sublingual/oral/inhaled); timing; administration rules; meal adjustments.	*Note: Inhalation provides rapid onset; oral administration has a longer latency.*
Titration Plan	Starting dose; increments (steps); frequency of increase; maximum comfort dose; management of adverse events.	*"Start low, go slow" principle; reduce/delay increments if AEs occur.*
Outcome Evaluation	Baseline measures; selected scales; reassessment date; clinically meaningful benefit threshold.	Pain: NRS; Sleep: ISI; Anxiety: GAD-7 (according to protocol).
Safety & Counseling	Driving/machinery; alcohol; secure storage; non-diversion; red flags; informed consent.	*Red flags: severe confusion, hallucinations, syncope, chest pain.*
Documentation & Incidents	Prescription/protocol adherence; discrepancies; adverse events; reporting; corrective actions.	*Document counseling and understanding (teach-back); report suspected diversion.*

This tool is a detailed version of the clinical dataset, intended for adaptation into local Electronic Health Records (EHR).

Appendix C

Figure 1. Clinical decision algorithm for medical cannabis titration

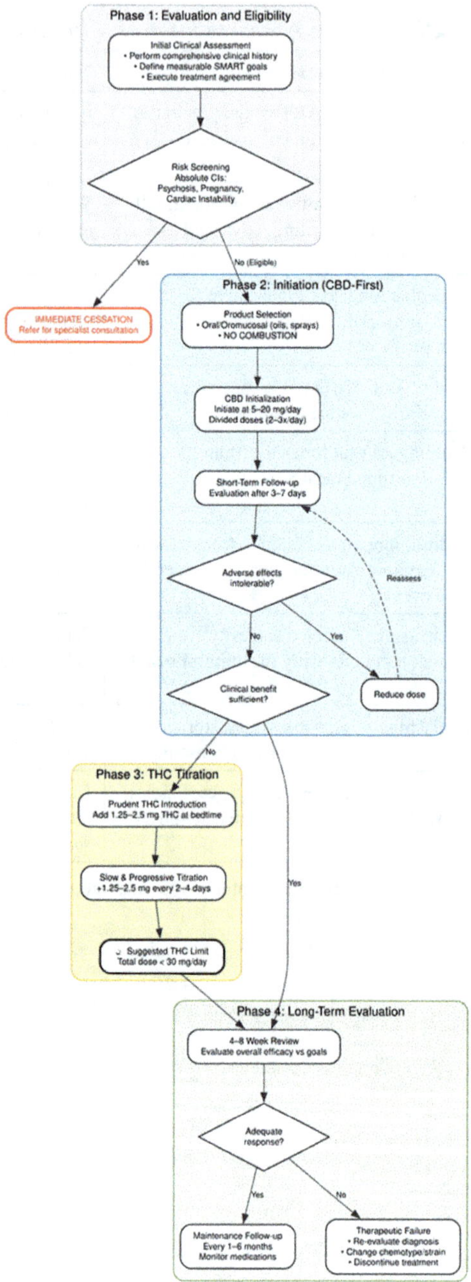

Appendix C: Clinical Decision Algorithm for Medical Cannabis Titration

Adapted primarily from MacCallum and Russo's practical evidence-informed framework for medical cannabis dosing, emphasizing "start low, go slow, and stay low" principles, with integration of advanced nursing clinical governance, patient safety screening, and longitudinal therapeutic monitoring (MacCallum & Russo, 2018). Supplemental dosing and safety considerations are further informed by contemporary consensus recommendations and broader evidence reviews in cannabinoid therapeutics (Bhaskar et al., 2021; Busse et al., 2021; Groce, 2018).

Psychosis, pregnancy, and cardiac instability categories reflect precautionary screening domains derived from safety-first clinical frameworks and should be individualized according to patient-specific risk–benefit assessment, jurisdictional regulations, and specialist consultation where clinically indicated. This algorithm is intended as an educational clinical decision-support tool and does not replace individualized medical judgment or multidisciplinary evaluation.

Appendix D — Patient Education Fact Sheet: Medical Cannabis and Safety

1. Why has this treatment been prescribed?
   - Objective: To improve specific symptoms (e.g., pain, sleep, nausea) while maintaining safety.
   - Ongoing Evaluation: Clinical benefits are reassessed regularly; treatment may be discontinued if efficacy is insufficient or if adverse effects become significant.
2. How to use your treatment
   - Adherence: Strictly follow the prescription regarding dose, frequency, and route of administration.
   - Onset of Action: Wait for the full effect before taking a subsequent dose, as oral forms have a longer onset latency.
   - Consistency: Do not modify multiple parameters (such as dose and frequency) simultaneously.
3. Safety Precautions and Restrictions
   - Substance Interactions: Avoid alcohol and other sedative substances unless specifically cleared by your medical team.
   - High-Risk Activities: Do not drive, work at heights, or operate dangerous machinery if you experience drowsiness or dizziness, or immediately following a dose.
   - Non-Diversion: Do not share your medication with anyone else.

4. Possible Side Effects
   - Common side effects include drowsiness, dizziness, dry mouth, anxiety, palpitations, and attention disturbances.
   - The risk of side effects increases with THC content, higher doses, the use of multiple medications (polypharmacy), or certain underlying health conditions.
5. Warning Signs: Seek Medical Attention Immediately
   Consult a healthcare professional or emergency services if you experience:
   - Significant confusion, hallucinations, or unusual agitation.
   - Syncope (fainting), chest pain, or shortness of breath.
   - Repeated falls, uncontrollable vomiting, or suicidal ideation.
6. Storage and Traceability
   - Storage: Keep the product in its original packaging, out of reach of children, and away from heat.
   - Records: If requested by your care team, record the product name, batch number, and the exact dose taken.
7. Clinical Follow-up
   - Ensure you attend scheduled reassessment appointments to evaluate the treatment's effectiveness and tolerability.
   - Always provide an updated list of all medications and report any changes, including new prescriptions or over-the-counter self-medication

Appendix E

Table 7. RACI Matrix: Governance and Responsibilities

Key Activities	MD	PH	NS	RN	QRM	IT	PT
1. Eligibility & Continuation Decision	A/R	C	I	C	I	I	I
2. Compliance & Labeling Verification	A	R	I	C	I	I	C
3. Definition of Authorized Forms	A	C	C	I	I	I	I
4. EMR/MAR Order Configuration	A	C	C	I	I	R	I
5. Secure Storage & Sealing (ADC/Safe)	I	A/R	C	C	I	I	I
6. Initial Inventory & Perpetual Log	I	A/R	I	R	I	I	C
7. Administration & MAR Documentation	C	C	A	R	I	C	I
8. Supervision of Self-administration	A	C	A	R	I	I	R
9. Adverse Event Monitoring & Notes	C	I	I	A/R	I	I	I

continued on following page

Table 7. Continued

Key Activities	MD	PH	NS	RN	QRM	IT	PT
10. Discrepancy/Diversion Escalation	I	A/R	C	C	C	I	I
11. Pharmacovigilance Reporting	C	C	C	R	A/R	I	I
12. Anti-diversion Program Management	I	A/R	C	I	R	I	I
13. Training & Competency Validation	I	C	A	C	C	I	I
14. Patient Education & Teach-back	C	C	I	A/R	I	I	C
15. Discharge Reconciliation & Restitution	A	R	C	R	I	I	C
16. Quarterly KPI Review (PDSA)	I	C	C	I	A/R	C	I

(R = Responsible; A = Accountable; C = Consulted; I = Informed) (**MD**: Physician; **PH**: Pharmacist; **NS**: Nursing Supervisor/Manager; **RN**: Staff Nurse; **QRM**: Quality/Risk Management; **IT**: Information Technology; **PT**: Patient).

Appendix F: Audit Grids (Structure and Process)

Table 8. Structure Audit (Institutional Readiness)

Item	Expected Evidence	Score (0-2)	Gaps & Actions
S1. Formal Policy	Validated policy on usage/exclusions.		
S2. Role Definition	Signed/distributed RACI matrix.		
S3. EMR/MAR Readiness	"Continuation of therapy" screenshots.		
S4. Secure Storage	ADC/Safe procedure + physical audit.		
S5. Traceability Tools	Inventory logs and waiver templates.		
S6. Anti-diversion Strategy	Committee minutes and annual plan.		

Table 8. Process Audit (Clinical Execution)

Item	Expected Evidence	Score (0-2)	Gaps & Actions
P1. Eligibility Verification	EHR note + registry check.		
P2. Clinical Decision Logic	Documented rationale for continuation.		
P3. Storage Compliance	Observation of secure handling.		
P4. Inventory Documentation	Signed perpetual log.		
P5. MAR Accuracy	Consistency between MAR and dosc.		
P7. Standardized Education	Trace of education + teach-back.		

Appendix G

Table 9. Key Performance Indicators (KPIs)

Indicator	Definition / Calculation	Type	Source	Frequency
Documentation Completion Rate	% of files with a complete minimal clinical dataset.	Process	EHR	Monthly
Reassessment Lead Time	Median days between initiation and 1st reassessment.	Process	EHR	Monthly
Reported Adverse Event Rate	Number of cannabis-related AEs / total patients.	Outcome	Vigilance	Quarterly
Intolerance Cessation Rate	Number of stops due to AE / total initiations.	Outcome	EHR	Quarterly
Clinical Benefit Achievement	% of patients reaching defined benefit threshold.	Outcome	PROMs	Quarterly
Safety Signals (Falls/MVA)	Number of events (falls/accidents) / total patients.	Outcome	Vigilance	Quarterly
Diversion Incidents	Number of suspected or confirmed diversion cases.	Outcome	Vigilance	Quarterly

About the Contributors

Kathleen Pinto Araya is a Psychiatric Nurse Practitioner and brings over thirty years of experience in nursing, leadership, and higher education. She has spent her nursing career working in both New Jersey and Florida primarily in community health, neurology, and pediatrics, and continues to actively practice nursing. Dr. Pinto Araya has served in academia as a faculty member, and in leadership roles including Dean of Nursing, Program Chair, and Subject Matter Expert for undergraduate and graduate nursing students. Additionally, she held roles including Doctoral Advisor/ Chair, and facilitator for Executive Leadership, Nursing Education, and Population Health. During her career, she has contributed to the nursing profession through her active research in debriefing following high fidelity simulation. In addition to her current research, Dr. Pinto Araya has presented on community health issues to several public and private organizations in the U.S. and internationally including the Global Council on Nursing and Health Education as a Scientific Committee Member and Keynote Speaker. She has been politically involved in the State Nurses Association as a forum committee member. She has also volunteered as a practicum mentor for nursing students at several local and national universities and has been recognized for excellence in practice and education by organizations including the National Society for Leadership and Success, Sigma Theta Tau, and Delta Mu Delta. Her research interests include Business, Research, Nursing, Administration, Education, Simulation, and Population/Community Health. Dr. Pinto Araya earned her PhD, Doctor of Philosophy in Nursing, Master of Science in Nursing, and Bachelor of Science in Nursing from the University of Phoenix. She earned her Psychiatric Nurse Practitioner Degree from Chamberlain University, Master of Business Administration, and Master of Healthcare Management from Capella University. Her undergraduate degree in Social Science was earned from Ocean County College and Diploma in Nursing from Ann May School of Nursing.

Rana Zeine, MD, PhD, MBA is Adjunct Faculty at Kean University Department of Biological Sciences (1/2020-present), and Union College of Union County STEM-Biology (9/2023-present) Union, New Jersey, USA, and also Visiting Professor III at Chamberlain University College of Nursing (10/2021-11/2025), North Brunswick, NJ, USA. Dr. Zeine is presently serving as associate editor with Springer-Nature, London, UK, for the Journal of Cannabis Research, and as Clinical Thematic Book Collection Editor with IGI Global Publishing, PA, USA. She currently teaches Neuroscience, Immunology, Microbiology, Anatomy & Physiology, Biological Aspects of Aging, Genetics, Biology of Cancer, Independent Research, and formerly taught Pathology at the Saint James School of Medicine. She also serves as a judge at the annual Terra North Jersey STEM Fair (TNJSF). Dr. Zeine received her B.S. in Biology '83, Teaching Diploma '83, and M.D. '87 degrees from the American University of Beirut (AUB) in Lebanon and her PhD from McGill University, Canada, and her MBA from the Keller Graduate School of Management from DeVry College of New York.

***

Lesley Affeldt, BSN, RN, CHPN, is a Palliative and Hospice Nurse Educator based in Southern California with clinical expertise in Oncology, Palliative Care, Hospice, and Medical Cannabis. She holds a national certification in Hospice and Palliative Nursing and a Medical Cannabis Certificate from both Pacific Colleges of Health and Sciences as well as Dr. Ethan Russo's Advanced Cannabis Pharmacology and Therapeutics course. Lesley integrates evidence-based cannabis therapeutics into her educational and clinical practice, founding Integrative Holistics, DBA CannaMedRN. She serves on the board of the Ventura County Chapter of the American Association of Critical-Care Nurses and was a recent candidate for the Board of Directors of the American Cannabis Nurses Association. Lesley is a passionate advocate for patient autonomy, clinician education, and community empowerment through compassionate care.

Samia Boussaa is currently Professor in ISPITS (Institut Supérieur des Professions Infirmières et des Techniques de Santé) of Rabat (Morocco). She obtained her PhD, in Ecology and Epidemiology, at Cadi Ayyad University (Morocco) and at Strasbourg University (France) in 2008. Her research is focused on Medical Entomology, Vector Borne Disease and especially on Epidemiology of leishmaniasis in Morocco.

M'lissa Duncan is a board-certified holistic baccalaureate nurse, wellness educator, and integrative health advocate specializing in cannabis and plant-based medicine. She holds a Master's degree in Cannabinoid Therapeutics, with graduate training focused on the endocannabinoid system, cannabis pharmacology, clinical application, and ethical integration within healthcare. Grounded in holistic nursing principles, her work emphasizes whole-person care that honors the interconnectedness of body, mind, spirit, and environment. Her approach integrates evidence-informed nursing practice, patient education, trauma-informed care, and respect for autonomy, with particular attention to individuals navigating chronic conditions, stress-related illness, and gaps within conventional healthcare systems. M'lissa serves on the Board of Directors of the American Cannabis Nurses Association (ACNA) and is an active member of the organization, contributing to professional standards and education in cannabis-informed nursing practice. As a writer, she brings a balanced, evidence-informed voice to discussions on cannabis, holistic nursing, and integrative care, advancing cannabis literacy.

Arun Kumar Garov, working as Assistant Professor, RIMT University, Mandi Gobindgarh, Punjab, India. His research areas are time series analysis and forecasting analysis, Reliability.

Mike Harvey, MS (Medical Cannabis Science and Therapeutics), BSN, Mike Harvey is a Cannabis Nurse Educator and retired Army Nurse Corps officer with over 40 years of distinguished military service, including 23 years of active federal service. A dedicated nurse leader and educator, Mike Harvey earned an Associate Degree in Nursing in 1993 from Clark Community College, Vancouver, Washington, followed by a Bachelor of Science in Nursing in 2004 from North Carolina Central University, Durham, NC. In 2023, Mike Harvey completed a Master of Science in Medical Cannabis Science and Therapeutics from the University of Maryland School of Pharmacy—the first graduate program in the United States dedicated to the study of medical cannabis. Throughout a career spanning both military and civilian healthcare systems, Mike Harvey has demonstrated a deep commitment to advancing evidence-based, patient-centered care. As a Veterans Affairs (VA) nurse for a decade, including seven years in the Cardiac Intensive Care Unit at the Durham VA Medical Center, Mike Harvey developed a strong foundation in critical care and Veteran health. This experience informs Mike Harvey's current work in cannabis nursing, where they focus on educating healthcare professionals and the public about the science of cannabis and its therapeutic potential—particularly for Veterans. A sought-after speaker and advocate, Mike Harvey has presented at the American Cannabis Nurses Association (ACNA) annual conference and has been invited to speak at the South Carolina Nurses Association's annual nursing conference on three occasions. These educational sessions emphasize the pharmacological principles of cannabis and the importance of individualized cannabis pharmacotherapy for veterans and other patient populations. Mike Harvey continues to champion the integration of cannabinoid therapeutics into nursing practice, aiming to empower nurses with the knowledge and tools necessary to support safe, effective, and compassionate care in this rapidly evolving field.

Said Khaldouni is a nurse researcher with a Master's degree in Advanced Nursing Practice in Oncology and Palliative Care. He is currently pursuing a PhD at Cadi Ayyad University in Morocco.

Zaoui Khalifa, Advanced Practice Nurse specialized in Oncology and Palliative Care and PhD candidate at Cadi Ayyad University (Marrekch, Morocco). Holder of a Master's degree in Advanced Practice Nursing and a DUT in Computer Engineering. Research interests include advanced nursing practice, oncology and palliative care, health systems, and the implementation of advanced practice roles in Morocco and comparable contexts.

Daniel King is an internationally recognized nurse anesthesiologist, educator, and researcher advancing interdisciplinary care and evidence-based policy. He earned his BSN from the University of Southern Indiana (2010) where he was awarded the David L. Rice Alumni Achievement Award, a Master of Nurse Anesthesia from Mayo Clinic College of Medicine and Science (2016), where he was awarded the Virginia B. Hartridge Achievement Award, and a DNP from The University of Alabama (2020), where he was named a Centennial Scholar. Dr. King is an Associate Professor in the DNP Nurse Anesthesia Program at Rosalind Franklin University of Medicine and Science and the owner of DreamLion Anesthesia & Wellness. In elected leadership roles, he has helped shape national practice guidance and professional development initiatives. A prolific scholar and speaker, his cannabis-focused research on assessment and stigma reduction—including development of the Cannabis Use and Behaviors Assessment Tool (CUBAT)—has informed perioperative risk assessment and health equity conversations. He also mentors doctoral learners and supports interprofessional scholarship.

Mary Lynn (ML) Mathre, RN, MSN, has more than 50 years of experience as a nurse and has specialized in addictions nursing since 1987 and cannabis education since 1990. ML is a Veteran of the Navy Nurse Corps (1973-1979) and from 1985-1987 she was a Med-Surg instructor at the UVA SON before accepting the role of charge nurse on the Addictions Treatment Unit at the now closed Blue Ridge Hospital. Mary Lynn was the first nurse to achieve Clinician V status at UVA and when Blue Ridge Hospital closed, she served as the Addictions Consult Nurse for the UVA Health System until 2002. Ms. Mathre is a co-founder and President of Patients Out of Time (incorporated in 1995) as a non-profit organization devoted to educating health care professionals and the public about the therapeutic uses of cannabis. ML is the editor of Cannabis in Medical Practice: A Legal, Historical and Pharmacological Overview of the Therapeutic Use of Marijuana (1997) and co-editor of Women and Cannabis: Medicine, Science and Sociology (2002). Ms. Mathre has authored several chapters on the topic of medical cannabis, numerous peer-reviewed articles on the topic, and written resolutions for several professional organizations in support of patient access to medical marijuana, including those of the Virginia Nurses Society on Addictions, the Virginia Nurses Association, the National Nurses Society on Addictions, and the American Public Health Association. She has served on the planning committee for Patients Out of Time's accredited National Clinical Conference on Cannabis Therapeutics conference series since it began in 2000 (now an annual event beginning in 2015). Ms. Mathre is also a founding member and Past President of the American Cannabis Nurses Association.

Christobal Mozingo Goodwin D.Div, MSN, RN, CDE has earned a Doctorate of Divinity through United Life Church and is a Board-Certified Holistic Nurse and Certified Diabetes Educator. Due to his long name, Christobal goes by "Dr. MoGo". He is internationally recognized as a promoter of mind-body-spirit health. He is a celebrated & award-winning educator who serves on the faculty at The Oregon School of Massage. As a Master's-Prepared Registered Nurse with over 30 years of combined experience in healthcare, wellness, and workplace safety, Dr. MoGo is regarded by his peers and students as a rare gem in the challenging landscape of our current healthcare crisis. His areas of holistic healthcare expertise include Haptic Healing techniques such as therapeutic bodywork and intentional touch.

Ramya Raghavan Assistant Professor, Sri Sathya Sai University for Human Excellence, India. Her recent editorial work on a book dedicated to advancing cancer treatment through spatial omics approaches underscores her commitment to innovation. Her expertise extends to the critical intersection of the exposome and Social Determinants of Health (SDOH). Dr. Raghavan's work underscores how a holistic understanding of environmental exposures, from the molecular level to population-wide influences, is crucial for addressing health disparities and advancing a more equitable approach to disease prevention. With a robust background in biology and a dedication to science communication, Dr. Raghavan ensures the clarity, accuracy, and accessibility of cutting-edge medical advancements, particularly in the evolving fields of omics, exposomics, and their implications for public health.

Alexandria Scoggins, DNP, RN-BC, is the Chief Nursing Officer of Cannability Consulting, LLC and the Corporate Director of Quality Improvement for Westminster Canterbury on Chesapeake Bay. She also serves as a Healthcare

Quality Consultant for Chiles Healthcare Consulting. Dr. Scoggins earned her Doctor of Nursing Practice and Master of Nursing Administration and Leadership degrees from Virginia Commonwealth University, where her DNP project on Fostering Cannabis Safety and Literacy for Older Adults and Healthcare Providers won VCU's Ann B. Hamric Award for sustainable practice improvement. Actively engaged in professional leadership, she serves on the Education and Research Committees for the American Cannabis Nurses Association. Her work focuses on integrating cannabis therapeutics into healthcare, particularly within post-acute and long-term care settings, where she champions evidence-based practice and healthcare quality.

Index

A

B

C

D

E

F

G

O

P

S

T

U

W

www.ingramcontent.com/pod-product-compliance
Lightning Source LLC
LaVergne TN
LVHW081330021026
849161LV00008BA/1810